Handbuch der experimentellen Pharmakologie
Handbook of Experimental Pharmacology

Heffter-Heubner   New Series

XXX

Modern Inhalation Anesthetics

Contributors

P. Bass · J. W. Bellville · D. R. Bennett · J. Bimar · A. Bracken
H. W. Brewer · J. P. Bunker · T. H. S. Burns · H. W. Calderwood
M. B. Chenoweth · E. N. Cohen · R. M. Featherstone · B. R. Fink
A. Galindo · R. W. Gardier · N. M. Greene · E. R. Larsen · W. W. Mapleson
R. I. Mazze · L. E. Morris · E. S. Munson · R. Naquet · S. H. Ngai
N. T. Smith · Penelope C. Smith · L. R. Soma · C. Trey · L. D. Vandam
R. A. Van Dyke · A. Van Poznak

Editor

Maynard B. Chenoweth

With 90 Figures

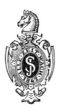

Springer-Verlag Berlin · Heidelberg · New York 1972

Maynard B. Chenoweth, Biochemical Research Laboratory
The Dow Chemical Company, Midland, MI 48640, USA

ISBN 3-540-05135-X Springer-Verlag Berlin · Heidelberg · New York
ISBN 0-387-05135-X Springer-Verlag New York · Heidelberg · Berlin

Druck: Carl Ritter und Co., Wiesbaden

Table of Contents

Section 1.0

Section 2.0

Section 3.0. Clinical Monographs

Section 4.0. Comparative Action on Vital Systems of Man

List of Contributors

Bass, Paul, School of Pharmacy, 425 N, Charter Street, University of Wisconsin, Madison, WI 53706/USA

Bellville, J. Weldon, Department of Anesthesia, Stanford University, Stanford, CA 94305/USA

Bennett, Donald R., Biomedical Research Laboratory, Dow Corning Corporation Midland, MI 48640/USA

Bimar, J., Département d'Anesthésie, C.H.U. Nord, 13-Marseille/France

Bracken, A., Chief Chemist-Medical, The British Oxygen Company, Deer Park Road, London, S.W. 19/Great Britain

Brewer, H. Winslow, Department of Anesthesia, Stanford University School of Medicine, Stanford Medical Center, Stanford, CA 94305/USA

Bunker, John P., Department of Anesthesia, Stanford University Medical Center, Stanford, CA 94305/USA

Burns, T. H. S., Department of Anesthetics, St. Thomas' Hospital, London, S.E. 1/Great Britain

Calderwood, Hugh W., Department of Anesthesiology, College of Medicine, University of Florida, Gainsville, FL 32601/USA

Chenoweth, Maynard B., Biochemical Research Laboratory, The Dow Chemical Company, Midland, MI 48640/USA

Cohen, Ellis N., Department of Anesthesia, Stanford University School of Medicine, Stanford Medical Center, Stanford, CA 94305/USA

Featherstone, Robert M., Department of Pharmacology, University of California School of Medicine, San Francisco, CA 94122/USA

Fink, B. Raymond, Department of Anesthesiology, University of Washington, School of Medicine, Seattle, WA 98105/USA

Galindo, Anibal, University of Washington, Department of Anesthesiology, Research Laboratories, Seattle, WA 98105/USA

Gardier, Robert W., The Ohio State University, College of Medicine, Departments of Anesthesiology and Pharmacology, Columbus, OH 43210/USA

Greene, Nicholas M., Department of Anesthesiology, Yale University School of Medicine, Yale-New Haven Hospital, New Haven, CT 06504/USA

Larsen, Eric R., Halogens Research Laboratory, 768 Building, The Dow Chemical Company, Midland, MI 48640/USA

Mapleson, William W., Reader in the Physics of Anaesthesia, Department of Anaesthetics, Welsh National School of Medicine, Heath Park, Cardiff, CF4 4XN/Great Britain

Mazze, Richard I., Department of Anesthesia, Stanford University Medical School, Stanford, CA 94305/USA

Morris, Lucien E., Department of Anesthesia, Medical College of Ohio at Toledo, Toledo, OH 43614/USA

Munson, Edwin S., Department of Anesthesiology, University of California, School of Medicine, Davis, CA 95616/USA

Naquet, R., Institut de Neurophysiologie et de Psychophysiologie, C.N.R.S., I.N.P. 3, 31, Chemin Joseph-Aiguier, Marseille/France

Ngai, S. H., Department of Anesthesiology, Columbia University, College of Physicians and Surgeons, 630 West 168th Street, New York, NY 10032/USA

Smith, N. Ty, Department of Anesthesia, Stanford University School of Medicine, Stanford, CA 94305/USA

Smith, Penelope Cave, Departments of Anesthesia and Pediatrics, Stanford University School of Medicine, Stanford, CA 94305/USA

Soma, Lawrence R., Associate Professor of Anesthesia, Department of Clinical Studies, School of Veterinary Medicine, University of Pennsylvania, Philadelphia, PA 19104/USA

Trey, Charles, Associate Professor, Tufts Medical School, Lecturer, Harvard Medical School, Head, Gastroenterology, St. Elisabeth's Hospital and New England Deaconess Hospital, Boston, MA 02215/USA

Vandam, Leroy D., Department of Anesthesia, Harvard Medical School, Boston, MA 02115/USA

Van Dyke, Russell A., Section of Anesthesia Research, Mayo Clinic and Mayo Foundation, Rochester, MN 55901/USA

Van Poznak, Alan, Department of Anesthesiology, New York Hospital, Cornell University Medical Center, 525 East 68th Street, New York, NY 10021/USA

Foreword and Commentary

M. B. Chenoweth

This seems a particularly good point in the century to produce this work, for enough time has elapsed since their introduction to assure a meaningful body of knowledge about these drugs. Furthermore, the outburst of chemical discovery which permitted their synthesis seems to have slackened and only occasionally do new variations on the multihalogenated compounds appear. Unless a new drug of this class has unexpectedly great advantages over those now available, it is unlikely that the many hurdles will ever be cleared to put the drug in the hands of such anesthesiologists as might want it. Thus, this volume, hopefully, will be both a documentation of the past and a take-off point for a different future.

The decision as to what was to be a „Modern Inhalation Anesthetic" was made quite simply. Any drug in use when the Editor graduated from Medical School well over a quarter century ago was, *ipso facto*, not modern. Immediately, no one else was totally satisfied. A recent newspaper account of the death of an ancient Indian "nurse" in Florida at the age of 132 even raised the possibility that the entire history of anesthesia could have been encompassed in a single human lifetime. But some way needed to be found to exclude such antiquities as ethylene. A non-medical aspect of the volatile and gaseous anesthetics has thus become the criterion for inclusion. Lack of fire hazard is the essence of modernity and no one would attempt to turn back the clock by introduction of a flammable compound. While we see in Chapter 2 that definition of flammability still leaves something to be desired, it can be well-assessed in a practical and relative way.

No pharmacologist or anesthetist can teach about an anesthetic without reference to "classical" drugs and such references appear throughout the work and in the Index, even though they escaped from the Table of Contents.

It is difficult for an individual to grasp much more than his immediate environment and there may well be places where ether is still the main volatile anesthetic in use. By looking at the other end of the sequence — the actual amounts of these materials being made or purchased — a broader view of a changing picture can be had.

Table 1 was obtained for me in mid 1968 by Dr. Jack M. Tadman of our organization. It clearly shows a rapid decline in ether purchases while the purchase of halothane greatly increased about 1960. There is a slight recovery of ether purchases, but 1964, '65, '66 show a real decline in cyclopropane. Probably to no-one's surprise, nitrous oxide gained steadily throughout that period. A newcomer, methoxyflurane, had a fast start and then seems to have plateaued, although Table 2 shows it to have a considerable share of Federal Government (U.S.A.) purchases. Table 3 shows 1965 sales for a wider variety of drugs. Thanks to the courtesy of Dr. Sanford Cobb of Abbott Laboratories, Hospital Products Division, the following Table 4 presents his knowledgeable estimate of the number of anesthesias performed using methoxyflurane in the United States. Perhaps the most that can be gleaned from these tables is a sense of awe at the quantities consumed in the United States alone.

Table 1. *Estimated U.S.A. annual purchases of selected inhalant anesthetics*

	1957	1958	1959	1960	1961
	$ 000				
Total inhalant anes. market	2,207.2	2,624.0	3,048.2	4,370.4	6,940.7
Nitrous oxide	116.0	259.8	158.0	165.4	355.2
Cyclopropane	143.6	256.8	190.6	92.9	202.0
Ether	1,084.3	1,142,8	1,083.0	932.9	818.8
Halothane	—	284.9	971.0	2,589.2	4,933.0
Methoxyflurane	—	—	—	—	—

	1962	1963	1964	1965	1966
	$ 000				
Total inhalant anes. market	8,934.1	9,907.7	21,789.8	22,949.1	24,789
Nitrous oxide	380.7	159.6	3,187.3	3,372.0	3,977
Cyclopropane	215.9	139.9	2,398.2	1,878.0	1,471
Ether	754.0	751.2	847.2	818.0	982
Halothane	6,353.2	7,257.5	12,832.6	13,990.0	15,518
Methoxyflurane	587.0	805.4	1,842.5	2,000.0	2,333

	1967				1968			
	$ 000	67/66 Var. %	Share %	Units 000	$ 000	68/67 Var. %	Share %	Units 000
Total inhalant anes. market	26,404	+ 6.5	100	—	13,459	+ 0.2	100	—
Nitrous oxide	3,926	− 1.3	15	—	1,848	+12	14	—
Cyclopropane	1,088	−26.1	3	—	438	− 4	3	—
Ether	880	−10.4	3	390 lb	365	−29	3	110 lb
Halothane	17,935	+15.6	68	107 l	9,016	+ 0.4	70	59.5 l
Methoxyflurane	2,214	− 5.1	8	12.5 l	1,379	+14	11	7.9 l

Table 2. *Estimated federal government [U.S.A.] purchases of selected general inhalation anesthetics* 1967

	Units	$ (000)	% of $
Halothane	79,000 l	1,086	62
Methoxyflurane	36,000 l	498	26
Ether	13,700 l	219	11

Certain comments on the format and style of the actual text may be worthwhile. A degree of consistency has been imposed on spelling and on drug names. As the work is edited in the midst of the Great Lakes area of the United States, the Editor has arbitrarily chosen *his* way of usage. The authors turned in polished manuscripts befitting their positions. The Editor would not dare, nor desire, to modify their style and only tried to catch the minor errors introduced by capricious typewriters. Thus, the reader gets the original teacher, undiluted by editorial ink.

Table 3. *General inhalation anesthetics — 1965*

Product	Estimated 1965 sales		Selling price $	Relative anesthesia cost[a]
	$ 000	000 units		
Chloroform	24	13 (pt.)	1.69/pt.	1
Cyclopropane	1,878	5,225 (gal. gas)	0.36/gal.	141
Ether	818	551 (lb.)	1.49/lb.	2
Fluoroxene	189	2,025 (ml)	9.45/100 ml	210
Halothane	13,990	80,000 (ml)	21.90/125 ml	18—67
Methoxyflurane	2,000	11,250 (ml)	22.20/125 ml	25—51
Nitrous Oxide	3,372	224,800 (gal. gas)	0.015/gal.	19
Vinyl Ether	219	4,977 (ml)	0.44/10 ml	31

$$^a\text{ Relative anesthesia cost} = \frac{S/L \text{ (gas or vapor)} \times \text{anesthesia concentration}}{S/L \text{ vapor of chloroform} \times 1.5}$$

Table 4. *Estimated anesthesias with methoxyflurane in the United States*

Year	Millions of anesthesias
1962	0.378
1963	0.672
1964	0.966
1965	1.372
1966	1.708
1967	1.806
1968	2.289
1969	2.592

It is said that the Navajo Indians deliberately weave an imperfection into each blanket. Thus, they can not possibly offend the Gods by the creation of perfection. No such insurance is needed in this work for despite all vigilance, there are undoubtedly errors enough to protect us all from the offense of perfection.

Section 2.0

The Chemistry of Modern Inhalation Anesthetics

Eric R. Larsen

With 3 Figures

I. Introduction

During the past 10 years, several new anesthetic agents have come into wide-spread use. Three of these agents, halothane, methoxyflurane, and fluroxene, are commercial drugs and are dealt with in considerable depth in the following section. Several others, roflurane and teflurane, are still in clinical evaluation and are covered in a less extensive fashion.

The physical chemistry of these compounds as it applies to the field of anesthesiology has been reviewed a number of times and will not be dealt with in this section.

The chemistry of these compounds that is applicable to their synthesis, purification, stability, and chemical reactivity is less well known. The bulk of this information is scattered through-out the patent literature of several countries, and it is the author's object to try to bring this information together into a meaningful compilation. In this maze of patents can be found at least a dozen processes for the synthesis of halothane, four for the synthesis of teflurane, and two each for methoxyflurane, roflurane, and fluroxene. There are, in addition, at least three processes for the removal of olefinic impurities that occur in halothane when it is manufactured by the thermal bromination of 2-chloro-1,1,1-trifluoroethane.

It will be obvious to the reader that the amount of work that has been done to delineate the chemistry of these compounds is meager. This is principly due to the fact that as drugs, the compounds are not readily accessible to the average chemist, and the chemists who do have access to the drugs are normally more concerned with obtaining data required for the development of its end use than in exploring its other chemistry.

II. Halothane

Halothane, 2-bromo-2-chloro-1,1,1-trifluoroethane, is a clear, heavy, colorless liquid having a sweet non-irritating odor resembling that of chloroform. The compound was first prepared, and its anesthetic properties discovered, at Imperial Chemical Industries, Ltd. (ICI) in the United Kingdom by Suckling and Raventos (1957). In a little over a decade halothane has established itself as the leading anesthetic agent by capturing over 50% of the anesthetic market.

Halothane is a relatively inert compound and participates in few chemical reactions. This chemical inertness is in general due to the strong inductive effects of the fluorine atoms in the trifluoromethyl group which effectively strengthen the carbon-chlorine and carbon-bromine bonds adjacent to it.

Table 1. *Physical properties of the newer anesthetic agents*

Formula	Halothane[a] CF$_3$CHBrCl	Methoxyflurane[b] CH$_3$OCF$_2$CHCl$_2$	Fluroxene[c] CF$_3$CH$_2$OCH=CH$_2$	Teflurane[d] CF$_3$CHBrF	Roflurane[b] CH$_3$OCF$_2$CHBrF
Molecular weight	198	165	126	181	193
Boiling point (760 mmHg)	50.2	104.65	43.1	8.66	88
Vapor pressure (20 °C, mmHg)	241.5	23	295	1240	55
Refractive index (n^t_D)	1.3700[20]	1.3849[25]	1.3198[20]	1.3171[0]	1.3649[25]
Specific gravity (d^t_4)	1.86[20]	1.4223[25]	1.135[20]	1.862[0]	1.7146[25]
Freezing point (°C)		−35.00			
Solubility in H$_2$O (g/100 g α 37 °C)	0.345	0.195		0.04	~0.2
Lower explosion limit (oxygen) vol.-%	~17[e]	5.4	4.0	~19	10
Lower explosion limit (nitrous oxide) vol-%	5	2.7	—	4	—

[a] ANON, 1963   [b] LARSEN, 1961; ANON, 1968   [c] CONWAY, 1965, SHUKYS, 1958   [d] LARSEN, 1959   [e] BROWN and MORRIS, 1966

A. Synthesis

The bulk of the halothane produced today is manufactured by the original process developed by Suckling and Raventos (1957), that is, the thermal bromination of 2-chloro-1,1,1-trifluoroethane. The remainder is made by a process developed by Scherer et al. (1960) at Farbwerke Hoechst in Germany. The Hoechst process is based upon the aluminum bromide catalyzed rearrangement of 1-bromo-2-chloro-1,1,2-trifluoroethane ($CF_2BrCHClF$). A number of other processes have been disclosed in the patent literature and will be discussed below. None of these other processes have as yet been commercially exploited by their inventors.

1. ICI Process

The ICI process for the manufacture of halothane is based upon the thermal bromination of 2-chloro-1,1,1-trifluoroethane according to the equation (Suckling and Raventos, 1957; Chapman et al., 1966):

$$CF_3CH_2Cl + Br_2 \xrightarrow{425-475°} CF_3CHBrCl + HBr .$$

The bromination is carried out by passing a mixture of the haloethane and bromine vapor through a heated silica tube at a temperature between 425 and 475 °C and with a contact time of between 1 and 2 sec. Because the product, $CF_3CHBrCl$, will also react with bromine under these conditions, i.e.

$$CF_3CHBrCl + Br_2 \longrightarrow CF_3CBr_2Cl + HBr$$

the molar ratio of 2-chloro-1,1,1-trifluoroethane to bromine fed to the reactor is maintained in the range of 1.5 : 1 to 2 : 1 (Suckling and Raventos, 1957). The use of this large excess of the ethane reduces the amount of over bromination but does not eliminate it. Gains in yield made by minimizing over-bromination are off-set to a large extent by increases in the amount of 2-chloro-1,1,1-trifluoroethane that must be recovered and recycled.

In any high temperature free radical process numerous side reactions are possible and that used in the manufacture of halothane is no exception. Two studies have been published in recent years in which the by-products resulting from these extraneous side reactions have been elucidated [Chapman et al., 1967; Scipioni et al., 1967 (1, 2)]. The by-products which have been reported by these studies are listed in Table 2.

In the original ICI process, the effluent gases from the reactor were introduced to a continuous still operated so that the hydrogen bromide passed away at the head of the still, while unreacted bromine, 2-chloro-1,1,1-trifluoroethane and the organic reaction products collected in the boiler. The boiler contents overflowed continuously to a second still in which the 2-chloro-1,1,1-trifluoroethane was removed and recycled to the reactor. The crude brominated products were withdrawn from the boiler of the second still and passed to continuous washing and separating devices where they were washed with aqueous 10% sodium hydroxide and then with water. The crude product was then collected, dried and distilled. The fraction boiling at 50.2 °C at 760 mm was collected as the final product. The yield for the process, based upon the 2-chloro-1,1,1-trifluoroethane consumed, was reported to be about 73% (Suckling and Raventos, 1957).

The over-brominated product, CF_3CBr_2Cl, which amounts to 5—10% of the organic product may be recycled to the reactor along with 2-chloro-1,1,1-trifluoroethane. Disproportion occurs according to the equation

$$CF_3CBr_2Cl + CF_3CH_2Cl \longrightarrow 2\,CF_3CHBrCl .$$

This reaction, like the bromination, is not clean and results in the formation of the same by-products as reported in Table 2 (SUCKLING and RAVENTOS, 1960).

The discovery by COHEN et al. (1963) of certain higher boiling olefinic impurities in halothane, mainly $CF_3CCl=CClCF_3$, has led to the development of several methods for their removal.

The simplest, and the one most likely employed, is the oxidation of the olefins with aqueous potassium permanganate (VINEY, 1967). The process consists of vigorously agitating the halothane with dilute alkaline permanganate at ambient

Table 2. *By-products found in crude halothane prepared by the thermal bromination of 2-chloro-1,1,1-trifluoroethane*

Compound	Boiling point °C	Reference
CF_3CH_2Cl[a]	6.2	1,2
CF_3CHCl_2[a]	27	1
CF_3CH_2Br[a]	26.5	1
$CF_3CH=CClF_3$ (trans)[a]	35.2	1,2
$CF_3CH=CClCF_3$ (cis)[a]	—	1,2
$CF_2=CBrCl$[a]	43	1,2
CF_3CCl_3	46	2
CF_2ClCH_2Cl[a]	46.8	1
$CBrCl_2F$[a]	51—52	1
$CF_3CBr=CHCF_3$ (trans)[a]	55	1,2
$CHCl_3$[a]	61.2	1
$CF_3CCl=CCl\ CF_3$ (trans)[a]	65.3	1,2
$CF_3CCl=CClCF_3$ (cis)[a]	69.2	1,2
CF_3CBrCl_2[a]	69.2	1,2
CF_3CHBr_2[a]	73	1,2
$CF_2=CBr_2$	73	1,2
$CF_3CBr=CClCF_3$ (trans)	80.5	1,2
$CF_3CBr=CClCF_3$ (cis)	86.2	1,2
CF_3CBr_2Cl[a]	92.5	1,2
$CF_3CBr=CBrCF_3$ (trans)	106.4	1,2
$CF_3CBr=CBrCF_3$ (cis)	108.2	1,2

1. CHAPMAN et al., 1967
2. SCIPIONI et al., 1967 (2)
[a] Compounds detected in flucthane (ICI) (CHAPMAN et al., 1967)

temperatures for several hours. HENNE and TROTT (1947) showed that $CF_3CCl=CClCF_3$ is oxidized to trifluoroacetic acid under these conditions. The trifluoroacetic acid formed is removed, as a salt, in the water phase. When the oxidation is complete the halothane is separated and dried. The purification step may be carried out either before or after the final distillation step in the original process discussed above. The olefinic impurities are reduced by this treatment to less than 10 ppm.

CROPP and GILMAN (1967) reported the removal of olefinic impurities of the type $CF_3CX=CYCF_3$, wherein X stands for hydrogen, bromine, and chlorine and Y stands for bromine or chlorine, by refluxing the impure halothane with aluminum bromide. This process is based on the fact that the fluorine atoms in $CF_3CX=CYCF_3$ are allylic in nature and undergo an exchange reaction with aluminum bromide to give aluminum fluoride and highly brominated organic compounds, i.e.

$$CF_3CX=CYCF_3 + AlBr_3 \longrightarrow CBr_2=CXCY=CBr_2 \,.$$

Since the boiling points of organic fluorine compounds are markedly increased by the substitution of fluorine by bromine, the higher brominated compounds are readily removed by distillation. The amount of fluorine-containing olefinic impurities in the halothane are reported to be decreased to less than 10 ppm by this process.

A third purification process has been developed by SCHERER and KUHN (1967). This process involves treating the impure halothane with alcoholic caustic at ambient temperatures, washing away the excess alcohol, drying, and distilling. The process is based on the reaction of $CF_3CCl=CClCF_3$ with alcoholic caustic reported by HENNE and LATIF (1953). The fluorobutene undergoes both allylic and vinylic replacement of the halogens to give high boiling ethers which are readily removed by distillation.

$$CH_3OH + CF_3CCl=CClCF_3 \xrightarrow{excess\ KOH} CF_3CHClC(OCH_3)_2CF_3 + $$
$$CF_3CCl=C(OCH_3)CF(OCH_3)_2$$

2. Hoechst Process

The Hoechst process for the manufacture of halothane is a two step process based on the reactions:

a) $CF_2=CFCl + HBr \xrightarrow[\text{or peroxide}]{\text{light}} CF_2BrCHClF$

b) $CF_2BrCHClF \xrightarrow[50\ ^\circ C]{AlBr_3} CF_3CHBrCl$

The first step in the processes was developed by SHERER et al. (1964) and is carried out by passing equimolar amounts of chlorotrifluoroethylene and hydrogen bromide into a stirred reactor containing 1-bromo-2-chloro-1,1,2-trifluoroethane (the reaction product). Both light and peroxides are reported to be active catalysts for the reaction. Light is probably the catalyst of choice since the use of peroxides leave bromine-containing residues which must be removed. The reaction is carried out at temperatures of about 40—50 °C with the rate of reaction being determined by the solubility of the olefin and hydrogen bromide in the product, by the light intensity, or peroxide concentration, and by the ability of the equipment to remove the heat of reaction.

The reaction may be carried out in a continuous manner by removing the product from the reactor as it is formed. The crude product is washed free of hydrogen bromide and rectified; the fraction boiling at 52—53 °C is collected as the product. The higher boiling impurities formed in the reaction, $CF_2BrCFBrCl$ and coupled products, are removed by the distillation. Conversions for this step are reported to be about 86% and yields are about 90%.

The second step of the process, developed by SHERER and KUHN [1962, 1962 (1)], is carried out by passing 1-bromo-2-chloro-1,1,2-trifluoroethane into a reactor containing halothane along with a small amount of either aluminum chloride or aluminum bromide. The halothane isomer ($CF_2BrCHClF$) undergoes an exothermic intramolecular rearrangement to halothane; the reaction temperature is maintained at 50 °C by evaporative cooling.

While it is possible to carry out this reaction in a continuous manner, it is probable that in the actual manufacture of halothane a batch reaction is used. This is postulated since in a continuous process small amounts of unconverted halothane isomer, which is extremely difficult to remove by distillation, would almost certainly be present in the product.

The only impurity reported to be present, to date, is the compound 1,2-dichloroperfluorocyclobutane (bp 60.4 °C). This cyclobutane arises from the dimerization of chlorotrifluoroethylene, and is probably present in the raw material used.

The yields obtained in reaction b are reported to be about 90%. Consequently the overall yield of halothane, based on chlorotrifluoroethylene, is about 75—80%.

3. Miscellaneous Processes

In addition to the above two commercial process for the manufacture of halothane a number of other more or less elegant processes have been reported.

McGINTY (1963) has shown that the compound CF_3CBr_2Cl may be converted to halothane by reduction with "nascent" hydrogen produced by the reaction of hydrochloric acid on mild steel, that is:

$$CF_3CBr_2Cl + HCl + Fe \xrightarrow[H_2O]{reflux} CF_3CHClBr \ (45\%) + CF_3CCl{=}CClCF_3 \ (20\%) \, .$$

This reaction is of little more than cursory interest, however, because of the large amounts of the highly toxic 2,3-dichlorohexafluorobutene-2 formed as a by-product.

An improved process for the reduction of 2,2-dibromo-2-chloro-1,1,1-trifluoro-ethane has been reported by MADAI (1963). This reduction can be illustrated by the following equation:

$$CF_3CBr_2Cl + Na_2SO_3 + NaOH \xrightarrow[reflux]{H_2O} CF_3CHBrCl + Na_2SO_4 + NaBr \, .$$

The reduction is carried out in an aqueous medium at reflux and essentially pure halothane distills away from the reaction mixture as it is formed. Yields are reported to be about 90%.

The starting material for the above reductions may be prepared by the addition of bromine to chlorotrifluoroethylene followed by an aluminum bromide catalyzed rearrangement (MADAI, 1963), i.e.

$$CF_2{=}CFCl + Br_2 \longrightarrow CF_2BrCFBrCl \xrightarrow{AlBr_3} CF_3CBr_2Cl \, .$$

This same dibromide is the principle by-product of the ICI halothane process.

CHAPMAN and McGINTY (1960, 1964) have reported the synthesis of halothane by the Swartz reaction, or antimony catalyzed fluorination of 1,2-dibromo-1,1,2-trichloroethane, i.e.

$$CCl_2BrCHClBr + HF \xrightarrow[SbCl_5]{SbCl_3} CF_3CHClBr + CF_2ClCHClBr \, .$$

The reaction, carried out at about 130 °C under an autogeneous pressure of 200 psig., gives generally low, about 20%, conversions to halothane. The principle product, 2-bromo-1,2-dichloro-1,1-difluoroethane, may be treated further with hydrogen fluoride and antimony chlorides to yield additional halothane. The Swartz process is not particularly suited to the fluorination of bromine-containing compounds since the antimony fluorobromides formed in the reaction do not react with hydrogen fluoride to reform the active fluorination catalysts (RUH and DAVIS, 1957).

CROWTHER and ROBERTS (1962) have reported the synthesis of halothane from bromochloroacetic acid and sulfur tetrafluoride.

$$CHClBrCO_2H + SF_4 \xrightarrow[\substack{autogeneous \\ pressure}]{100—120°} CF_3CHClBr + SOF_2 \, .$$

This reaction is of particular interest since Edamura and Larsen (1968) have employed a modification of it in order to prepare the optical isomers of halothane.

4. Synthesis of Optically Active Halothane

Halothane has an asymmetric carbon atom and therefore has two optically active forms. To date no direct means of resolving the compound into its enantiomorphs has been reported.

Edamura and Larsen (1968) have, however, reported the synthesis of both the d- and l-enantiomorphs by the procedure outlined below. (B represents an alkaloid base; brucine or cinchonidine):

$$\text{I. } CHBrClCO_2H \xrightarrow{\text{B}} CHBrClCO_2H \cdot B$$

$$\text{II. } CHBrClCO_2H \cdot B \longrightarrow *CHBrClCO_2H \cdot B$$

$$\text{III. } *CHBrClCO_2H \cdot B + H_3PO_4 \longrightarrow *CHBrClCO_2H$$

$$\text{IV. } *CHBrClCO_2H + SF_4 \xrightarrow[\substack{7 \text{ days} \\ \text{HF catalyst}}]{70\,°C} CF_3*CHBrCl$$

Racemic bromochloroacetic acid was converted to the salt of an alkaloid base in methanol (Step I). Depending on the alkaloid used either the salt of d- or l-bromochloroacetic acid crystallized out (Step II), leaving the other isomer in solution. The alkaloid salt was then decomposed with syrupy phosphoric acid (Step III) to release the optically active bromochloroacetic acid ($[\alpha]_D^{25}\ 15 \pm 2°$). The optically active bromochloroacetic acid was then fluorinated at 70 °C for a period of at least 7 days under autogeneous pressure. A series of runs were made which indicate that racemization does not take place under these conditions but that the use of the higher temperatures employed by Crowther and Roberts (1966) can cause racemization.

The optical purity of the d-halothane obtained ($[\alpha]_D^{25} + 1.5$, $[\alpha]_{365}^{25} + 2.4$) was approximately 60%, while the l-isomer ($[\alpha]_D^{25} - 0.64°$, $[\alpha]_{365}^{25} - 1.9$) obtained had an optical purity of approximately 50%. Extrapolation of these values indicate that the pure enantiomorphs of halothane should show specific rotations $[\alpha]_\lambda^T$ of $1.5° \pm 0.2°$ for the sodium D line, and $4.2° \pm 0.5°$ for light having a wavelength of 365 millimicrons at 25 °C.

5. Synthesis of Isotopically Labeled Halothane

Halothane has been prepared in which various of the atoms have been replaced by the corresponding isotopes, i.e. deuterium, carbon-14 and chlorine-36.

Hine et al. [1961 (1)] prepared deuterio-halothane ($CF_3CDClBr$) by shaking halothane with a solution of NaOD in D_2O for 24 h. Isotopic purity was determined by the disappearance of the 8.875 μ infrared absorption band of the protium compound, and the appearance of the 11.025 μ absorption band of the deuterium-containing analog. The isotopic purity of the deuterio-halothane was reported to be 97%.

Halothane-1-C^{14} was synthesized (Vandyke et al.) from chloroacetic-1-C^{14} acid. This acid, reacted with a 3.5 fold excess of sulfur tetrafluoride at 198 °C (2100 psig) for 62 h, gave a 70% yield of trifluoroethyl chloride-1-C^{14}. The trifluoroethyl chloride was converted to halothane-1-C^{14} by thermal bromination, using a 1:1 molar ratio of the haloethane to bromine, at 540°. The crude halothane-1-C^{14}

(30% yield) was purified by gas phase chromatography to give a 15% yield of halothane-1-C^{14} having a purity of greater than 99.9%, and free of 1,1,1,4,4,4-hexafluoro-2,3-dichlorobutene-2.

B. Chemical Reactions of Halothane

1. Thermal Decomposition

SCIPIONI et al. [1967 (2)] studied the thermal decomposition of halothane at 500 °C and found that the principle products, besides hydrogen bromide and bromine, were $CF_3CCl=CClCF_3$, $CF_3CBr=CClCF_3$, $CF_2=CBrCl$, CF_3CH_2Cl, CF_3CBr_2Cl, CF_3CHBr_2, $CF_3CCl=CHCF_3$, and $CF_3Br=CHCF_3$. Miscellaneous other minor products are also reported. Decomposition is relatively rapid at this temperature, being 24% complete within 2 sec, and 38% within 4 sec.

The reaction mechanism probably involves the initial homolytic cleavage of the carbon-bromine bond to yield the free radical $CF_3CHCl \cdot$, i.e.

$$CF_3CHBrCl \longrightarrow CF_3CHCl \cdot + Br \cdot$$

This radical is the same one formed by the abstraction of hydrogen in the thermal bromination of 2-chloro-1,1,1-trifluoroethane. Unlike the bromination reaction, little free bromine is present during the thermal decomposition and radical coupling becomes the primary reactions, i.e.,

$$2CF_3CHCl \cdot \longrightarrow CF_3CHClCHClCF_3$$
$$CF_3CHClCHClCF_3 \longrightarrow CF_3CH=CClCF_3 + HCl$$

or

$$CF_3CHClBr + CF_3CHCl \cdot \longrightarrow CF_3CH_2Cl + CF_3CClBr \cdot$$
$$CF_3CHCl \cdot + CF_3CBrCl \cdot \longrightarrow CF_3CHClCBrClCF_3$$
$$CF_3CHClCBrClCF_3 \longrightarrow CF_3CCl=CClCF_3 + HBr.$$

In practice a large number of abstraction, coupling, dehydrohalogenation, and dehalogenation reactions are possible under these conditions and nearly any product that can be written can probably be found.

The threshold temperature required to bring about homolytic cleavage of the carbon-bromine bond is normally about 400 °C. Considerable reduction in this temperature may take place in the presence of catalysts such as the iron and copper halides. The author has found that coupling products may be formed from halothane during gas chromatography when the inlet temperature is in the range of 150—200 °C and iron salts are present in the inlet tube.

2. Reactions with Metals

Halothane does not react readily with most metals, such as iron, copper, nickel, etc. It does, however, react readily with such active metals as zinc. Unlike most vincinyl halides which are dehalogenated by zinc to give the corresponding olefins, halothane is reduced to 2-chloro-1,1,1-trifluoroethane (CHAPMAN and McGINTY, 1960).

$$2CF_3CHBrCl + Zn \xrightarrow[\text{reflux}]{\text{ethanol}} 2CF_3CH_2Cl + ZnBr_2.$$

COHEN et al. (1965) have reported that halothane reacts at elevated temperatures (> 150 °C) with copper and oxygen to yield small amounts of coupled products, principally $CF_3CCl=CClCF_3$. As mentioned above, the author found small amounts of coupled products believed to be due to thermal cracking in the presence of metal salts in a similar temperature range.

In an attempt to determine whether halothane does in fact react with copper the author stored halothane in the presence of air over a very finely divided copper dust of the type used to catalyze the Ullmann reaction for a period of 3 months. If coupling reactions do occur in the presence of copper under ambient conditions, copper bromide should be found on the surface of the copper particles. Examination of the copper surface by x-ray fluorescence failed to show any significant formation of copper bromide. It can be concluded, therefore, that while halothane may react with copper near the temperature required for thermal decomposition, it does not react under conditions likely to be found in anesthetic equipment such as the Copper Kettle (Larsen, 1964).

Albin et al. (1964) found that there was no significant enrichment of either 2,3-dichloro-hexafluorobutene-2, or 2-bromo-1,1,1,4,4,4-hexafluorobutene-2 in halothane in samples taken from the Copper Kettle vaporizers after long-term use.

3. Reaction with Base

Halothane does not react with either soda lime or barium hydroxide at an appreciable rate in either dry or aqueous systems and consequently is stable enough to be used in the presence of carbon dioxide absorbers.

Hine et al. [1961 (1)] have shown that the hydrogen atom in halothane undergoes a relatively rapid base catalyzed exchange reaction with deuterium oxide to give deuterohalothane ($CF_3CDClBr$). The reaction mechanism was shown to be

$$CF_3CHClBr + B^- \longrightarrow CF_3CClBr^- + HB$$

$$CF_3CClBr^- + DB \longrightarrow CF_3CDClBr + B^-$$

The presence of a base (B) was found to be necessary to the exchange and no appreciable exchange took place with the solvent alone under the conditions used. The kinetics of the reaction were found to be second order with rate constants of about 21.8×10^{-3} l · mole^{-1} sec^{-1} in deuterium oxide, 11.1×10^{-3} in water, and 1.66×10^{-3} in methanol. All reactions were carried out at 0 °C.

It was further shown by Hine et al. [1961 (2)] that halothane is dehydrohalogenated by caustic.

$$CF_3CHClBr \xrightarrow{OH^-} [CF_3CClBr^-] \longrightarrow CF_2{=}CBrCl + F^- + H_2O .$$

The rate constant (k = 2.9×10^{-6} l · mole^{-1} sec^{-1} at 55 °C) for this reaction is, however, too small for this reaction to represent a source of hazard during anesthesia.

In methanol solution the olefin reacts rapidly with the solvent to yield $CH_3OCF_2CHClBr$. The stability of halothane to base is attributed to the stabilizing effect of the fluorines upon the intermediate carbanion. This effect is such that in the presence of a proton donating solvent such as water and methanol the return of the carbanion to the saturated compound is several thousand times more likely to occur than is the loss of the β-fluorine.

Seyferth et al. (1969) have shown that halothane reacts with potassium t-butoxide and phenylmercuric chloride to give phenyl(1-bromo-1-chloro-2,2,2-trifluoroethyl)-mercury in 86% yield.

$$PhHgCl + Me_3COK + CF_3CHBrCl \xrightarrow[-10\ to\ 0°]{THF} PhHgCBrClCF_3 + Me_3COH + KCl .$$

Presumably the phenylmercuric chloride acts as a trap for the CF_3CBrCl^- anion which is formed by the reaction of halothane with base. Thermolysis of $PhHgCBrClCF_3$ in a refluxing solution of cyclooctene in chlorobenzene results in the extrusion of the carbene CF_3CCl which is trapped by the cyclooctene to give 9-chloro-9-trifluoromethylbicyclo[6 · 1 · 0]nonane (64% yield). A small amount of the carbene CF_3CBr is simultaneously formed which gives the analogous 9-bromo compound (5%).

Displacement of the $CF_3CCl_2^-$ anion from the analogous phenyl(1,1-dichloro-2,2,2-trifluoromethyl)-mercury by sodium iodide results in the formation of 1,1-dichloro-2,2-difluoroethylene by β-elimination of fluoride, rather than in carbene formation which would result from α-elimination of chloride.

$$PhHgCCl_2CF_3 + Na^+I^- \xrightarrow{DME} PhHgI + Na^+CCl_2CF_3^- \longrightarrow NaF + CCl_2{=}CF_2 \, .$$

These results are in agreement with those reported by HINE et al. [1961 (2)]. Similar results would be expected with the organomercurial formed from halothane.

4. Photochemical Reactions

Halothane when exposed to light having a wavelength of less than 5400 Å undergoes homolytic cleavage of the carbon-bromine bond. The free radical formed, $CF_3CHCl \cdot$, in the presence of oxygen, forms peroxy radicals which in turn decompose to give volatile acids. To prevent this reaction halothane is normally stored in amber glass bottles and is inhibited with 0.01% of thymol which acts as an anti-oxidant.

5. Halothane Azeotrope

Halothane forms a maximum boiling point azeotrope (B.P. 51.5 °C) with diethyl ether that has been evaluated clinically as an anesthetic agent (BOIVIN et al., 1958). This mixture, patented by HUDON (1963) in Canada and by LOTT and YALE (1960) in the United States, consists of 68.3 vol-% halothane and 31.7 vol-% diethyl ether, has a specific gravity of 1.24 and has a vapor pressure of 213 mmHg at 20 °C.

III. Methoxyflurane

Methoxyflurane, 2,2-dichloro-1,1-difluoroethyl methyl ether, is a clear, colorless liquid having a characteristic fruity odor. A crude reaction product containing this compound was first prepared by GOWLAND (1940) who reported it to be unstable and to be oxidized by air. Later workers, including TARRANT and BROWN (1951), and PARK et al. (1951), concluded that the product was inherently unstable and decomposed by the loss of hydrogen fluoride. It should be noted that when the product is prepared in the manner described in the early literature the material is decidedly toxic and causes delayed death when administered as an anesthetic.

The discovery by LARSEN (1961, 1963) that the reputed instability was not inherent in the compound per se, but was in fact due to the presence of a small amount, less than 1%, of 2,2-dichloro-1-fluorovinyl methyl ether, lead to the development of a product suitable for use as an anesthetic agent.

While methoxyflurane is an ether, the strong inductive effect of the α-fluorines decrease the electron donor (basic) properties of the ether (C–O–C) linkage to such an extent that little, if any, ether character remains. In contrast to typical ethers, i.e. diethyl ether, which are readily protonated by concentrated sulfuric acid to form oxonium salts, methoxyflurane shows little tendency to be protonated by this acid. In fact less than one drop of sulfuric acid is soluble in 100 ml of methoxy-flurane at 100 °C. In spite of this very limited solubility methoxyflurane does react with concentrated sulfuric acid. This reaction will be discussed below.

The inductive effect of the α-fluorines tend to strengthen the adjacent carbon-chlorine bonds in much the same manner as the trifluoromethyl group in halothane tends to stabilize the adjacent carbon-halogen bonds.

A. Synthesis

Methoxyflurane is manufactured by The Dow Chemical Company in the United States by the process developed by LARSEN (1966). The process consists of two discrete steps. The first's the addition of methanol to 1,1-dichloro-2,2-difluoro-ethylene,

$$CH_3OH + CF_2{=}CCl_2 \xrightarrow{OH^-} CH_3OCF_2CHCl_2 \text{ (99\%)} + CH_3OCF{=}CCl_2 \text{ (}<1\%\text{)}$$

in a manner similar to that employed by TARRANT and BROWN (1951) and PARK et al. (1951). In this reaction small amounts of 2,2-dichloro-1-fluorovinyl methyl ether are formed which must be removed in order to obtain a stable product.

The second process step consists of the oxidation of the vinyl ether. While a number of oxidizing agents have been shown to be suitable, ozonization is preferred.

$$CH_3OCF{=}CCl_2 + O_3 \longrightarrow CH_3OCF{-}O{-}CCl_2 \longrightarrow CH_3OCOF + COCl_2$$
$$\underset{O\text{——}O}{\big|\qquad\big|}$$

+ other by products

In a preferred embodiment of the process the first step is carried out by adding the olefin, $CF_2{=}CCl_2$, to methanol and passing the mixture through a strong base ion exchange resin; the reaction is carried out at approximately 10—20 °C in order to minimize side reactions. When the addition is complete the crude product is washed free of excess methanol, dried over calcium chloride, and sent forward to the purification step.

In the purification process oxygen containing up to 4% ozone is passed into the crude methoxyflurane at a temperature of 10—15 °C until the solution turns a bright blue due to dissolved ozone. At this point the concentration of vinyl ether, and any other olefinic impurities, is less than ten parts per million. The crude ozonized product is heated to reflux to destroy the ozonide, and then distilled. The cut boiling at 104.6 °C at 760 mm of mercury is collected, washed with dilute caustic, washed with water and dried over calcium chloride.

Material that passes specifications at this point is inhibited with 0.01% butylated hydroxytoluene prior to packaging.

The original synthesis employed by GOWLAND (1940) consisted of slowly adding a methanolic solution of potassium hydroxide to 1,2,2-trichloro-1,1-difluoroethane contained in an ice cooled vessel. While the ether is apparently formed in accordance with the equation

$$CHCl_2CF_2Cl + KOH + CH_3OH \longrightarrow CHCl_2CF_2OCH_3 + KCl + H_2O$$

the reaction apparently consists of two steps. The haloethane is first dehydro-chlorinated to give 1,1-dichloro-2,2-difluoroethylene which then undergoes a base catalyzed addition of methanol to yield the product.

1. $CHCl_2CF_2Cl + KOH \longrightarrow CCl_2{=}CF_2 + KCl + H_2O$

2. $CF_2{=}CCl_2 + CH_3OH \xrightarrow{OH^-} CH_3OCF_2CHCl_2$

That this is probably the actual reaction sequence can be shown by employing the corresponding tribromodifluoroethane ($CF_2BrCHBr_2$) in the process. In this case, little or no ether is formed until all of the haloethane is converted to the olefin. The addition of a small amount of excess base leads to a highly exothermic reaction to form the ether.

The crude product prepared by this process contains small amounts (less than 3%) of the vinyl ether $CH_3OCF=CCl_2$ and other by products, which must be removed in order to obtain a material that is usable as an anesthetic agent.

B. Synthesis of Isotopically Labeled Methoxyflurane

A number of isotopically labeled forms of methoxyflurane have been prepared.

HINE et al. [1961 (1)] reported the synthesis of 2-deuterio-2,2-dichloro-1,1-difluoroethyl methyl ether having an isotopic purity of about 97% by the reaction of methoxyflurane with NaOD in D_2O. In the reaction product, the 11.35 μ band of the protium compound had decreased to less than 3% of its original value within 24 h. This absorption band was replaced by the 10.620 μ band of the deuterium compound.

LARSEN (1962, 1968) prepared the compounds $^{14}CH_3OCF_2CHCl_2$, and $CT_3OCF_2CHCl_2$ by the reaction of 1,1-dichloro-2,2-difluoroethylene with $^{14}CH_3OH$ and CT_3OH respectively. The reactions were carried out by slowly adding the olefin to a suspension of Dowex-21K anion exchange resin (OH^-form) in a methanol solution of isotopically labeled methanol.

LARSEN (1964) prepared methoxyflurane-^{36}Cl by slowly adding 1,2,2-trichloro-1,1-difluoroethane-^{36}Cl to methanolic KOH at 0 °C. The excess methanol was extracted with water, and the crude product separated and purified by gas liquid chromatography. The 1,2,2-trichloro-1,1-difluoroethane-^{36}Cl used was obtained by adding chlorine-36 to 1,1-difluoro-2-chloroethylene.

C. Chemical Reactions of Methoxyflurane

1. Thermal Decomposition

Methoxyflurane is decomposed slowly at elevated temperatures (> 200 °C) to methyl fluoride and dichloroacetyl fluoride in metal equipment according to the equation:

$$CHCl_2CF_2OCH_3 \longrightarrow CHCl_2COF + CH_3F .$$

At 105 °C LARSEN (1964) has shown that no decomposition takes place upon heating the compound in a nickel container for as long as 72 h. Prolonged heating in glass, however, resulted in the reaction of the methoxyflurane with the container to yield silicon tetrafluoride and methyl dichloroacetate. This reaction will be discussed further below (III, C, 4).

2. Reactions with Metals

Methoxyflurane is stable in the presence of such metals as mild steel, nickel, copper, and aluminum. Long term storage tests (10 years) with copper and aluminum have shown no evidence of either corrosion of the metal or degradation of the methoxyflurane.

The discoloration of methoxyflurane that occurs when methoxyflurane is stored in contact with copper, brass or bronze is due to the oxidation of the inhibitor, butylated hydroxytoluene, rather than to any reaction between the methoxyflurane and the metal surface. In one study methoxyflurane was stored for 3 months in the presence of extremely fine copper dust of the type used to catalyze the Ullmann reaction. Examination of the copper dust at the end of this period by x-ray fluorescence showed no significant increase in the chloride content of the surface of the copper particles. Since any reaction between methoxyflurane and copper would result in the formation of copper chloride it was concluded that neither reduction, nor coupling, takes place when methoxyflurane is used in the presence of copper.

Methoxyflurane, unlike many polyhalogenated compounds such as carbon tetrachloride, chloroform, trichloroethylene, etc., is stable in the presence of aluminum. In a recent patent (LARSEN et al., 1966) the use of methoxyflurane as an inhibitor for the reaction between polyalkyl halides and aluminum was taught.

3. Reaction with Bases

Methoxyflurane exhibits a high degree of stability toward bases such as soda lime and barium hydroxide, and presents no hazard when used in the presence of carbon dioxide absorbers. Samples of methoxyflurane stored over sodium hydroxide pellets for 2 weeks at 130 °F showed no evidence of decomposition.

HINE et al. [1961 (1, 2)] have shown that methoxyflurane reacts with sodium hydroxide and sodium methylate in the same manner as does halothane. The following reaction sequence takes place with sodium methylate in methanol:

$$CH_3OCF_2CHCl_2 \xrightarrow[k_1]{OH^-} CH_3OCF_2CCl_2^- \xrightarrow[k_2]{CH_3OH} CH_3OCF_2CHCl_2$$

$$\downarrow k_3$$

$$CH_3OCF=CCl_2 + F^-$$

Using deutero-methoxyflurane HINE et al. [1961 (1)], showed that the reaction proceeds by an initial abstraction of the β-hydrogen atom by the methoxide ion to yield the carbanion $CH_3OCF_2CCl_2^-$. This carbanion may either return to the

Table 3. *Kinetics of Dehydrofluorination of Halothane and Methoxyflurane by Methanolic Sodium Methoxide*

	10^6 k l mole^{-1} sec.$^{-1}$	
	55 °C	70 °C
$CF_3CHBrCl$	2.9	33
$CH_3OCF_2CHCl_2$	3.0	27

[HINE, et al., 1961 (2)]

saturated ether by abstraction of a proton from the solvent, or undergo β-elimination of a fluoride ion to yield the vinyl ether. The rate constant (k_1, 20 °C) reported for the abstraction of the proton was found to be about 7×10^{-5} l · mole^{-1} sec^{-1} or about one five hundredth as rapid as the abstraction of the proton in halothane under the same conditions. The rate constant for the abstraction reaction with halothane was found to be 2.2×10^{-3} l · mole^{-1} sec^{-1}. The tendency of the carbanion to undergo elimination once it is formed is, however, considerably greater in the case of methoxyflurane. In the overall reaction leading to dehydrofluorination the decreased tendency of methoxyflurane to form a carbanion with base is offset by the increased tendency of the carbanion to undergo β-elimination. The net result is that halothane and methoxyflurane show almost identical rates of dehydrofluorination. The rate constants determined by HINE et al. [1961 (2)] for the dehydrofluorination of these compounds are shown in Table 3.

4. Reaction with Acids

The hydrolysis of methoxyflurane by concentrated (96%) sulfuric acid has been reported by YOUNG and TARRANT (1949). The reaction results in the loss of the fluorine atoms and gives good yields of methyl dichloroacetate.

$$CH_3OCF_2CHCl_2 + H_2SO_4 \xrightarrow{10\,°C} CHCl_2CO_2CH_3 + HSO_3F$$

LARSEN (1963) later reported that methoxyflurane undergoes an acid catalyzed reaction with glass in the presence of strong mineral acids such as concentrated sulfuric acid. Phosphoric acid (85%) and 2,2,3,3,3-pentafluoropropionic acids were ineffective as catalysts. The reaction is autocatalytic when the ether is heated in sealed glass ampoules (LARSEN, 1961). The mechanism proposed for the autocatalytic reaction of methoxyflurane with glass is:

$$4HF + SiO_2 \longrightarrow SiF_4 + H_2O$$

The ether oxygen is protonated, which should significantly weaken or polarize the C–F bond. Nucleophilic displacement of the fluorine by water, or another base such as the sulfate ion, could then result in ester formation.

Since the ether linkage in methoxyflurane is an extremely poor electron donor, protonation to give the oxonium ion intermediate does not take place when significant amounts of water are present. In the autocatalytic reaction with glass the presence of enough water to result in the formation of a second phase essentially stops the reaction.

5. Photochemical Reactions

Methoxyflurane sold for drug use contains small amounts (0.01%) of butylated hydroxytoluene as an antioxidant and is packaged in opaque glass bottles. These safety measures were incorporated into the drug during its early development, though long term storage tests show them to be superfluous under normal storage conditions.

Samples of uninhibited methoxyflurane have been stored in clear glass bottles for periods as long as 9 years under normal laboratory lighting conditions with no evidence of photochemical decomposition. However, exposure to high intensity ultraviolet light will cause homolytic cleavage of the carbon-chlorine bond with the resulting decomposition of the molecule.

Although methoxyflurane does not normally react with light, the photochemically induced oxidation of the anti-oxidant does lead to the slow formation of a yellow to brown coloration. This change does not affect the quality of the anesthetic agent (ANON, 1968).

IV. Fluroxene

Fluroxene, trifluoroethyl vinyl ether, is a colorless, relatively low boiling liquid (bp. 42.7 °C) having a mild non-objectionable odor in anesthetic concentrations. Unlike halothane and methoxyflurane, fluroxene is both flammable and explosive at the concentrations normally used during anesthesia. The compound is, however, less flammable than diethyl ether, ethyl vinyl ether, divinyl ether, and cyclopropane (SHUKYS, 1958). The danger of explosion and fire during use of this compound is to a large extent minimized by the fact that the minimum spark energy required for ignition is much greater than that needed to ignite the non-halogenated ethers (LAWRENCE, 1959). Fluroxene, prepared by SHUKYS in 1951 at Air Reduction Company, was first employed as a clinical anesthetic by KRANTZ et al. (1953).

A. Synthesis

1. Air Reduction Process

Fluroxene is probably manufactured by a two step process from trifluoroethanol and acetylene:

1. $CF_3CH_2OH + HC \equiv CH \longrightarrow (CF_3CH_2O)_2CHCH_3$

2. $(CF_3CH_2O)_2CHCH_3 \xrightarrow[\text{catalyst}]{240-280°} CF_3CH_2OCH = CH_2 + CF_3CH_2OH$

The first step of the process is carried out by passing acetylene into trifluoroethanol containing a catalyst consisting of either mercuric oxide and boron trifluoride (TOWNSEND, 1959), or mercuric oxide and sulfuric acid (LAWLOR et al., 1964). The reaction temperature is controlled at a temperature of between 40 and 50 °C. When the absorption of acetylene slows, the reaction mixture is neutralized with aqueous sodium carbonate, dried, and rectified. The fraction boiling between 110—117 °C is collected; di-(2,2,2-trifluoroethyl) acetaldehyde acetal boils at 114 °C. The reported yield of acetal is 98% based upon the trifluoroethanol consumed (ANON, 1958).

The conversion of di-(2,2,2-trifluoroethyl) acetaldehyde acetal to trifluoroethyl vinyl ether is carried out by passing the acetal in the vapor phase through a fluidized catalyst bed consisting of an acid-activated clay of the montmorillonite type. The reaction temperature is maintained at about 240—280 °C.

The crude fluroxene is separated from unreacted acetal and trifluoroethanol, which are recycled, by distillation. The fluroxene fraction is washed with aqueous sodium hydroxide, dried, and then refluxed over alkali pellets. This treatment ensures the removal of residual trifluoroethanol, water and any aldehydes. The washed and dried product is then fractionally distilled, and the fluroxene fraction (B.P. 43° at 760 mm) is collected separately in pure form substantially free of toxic and other undesirable impurities. The final product is then stabilized by the addition of a small amount (0.01%) of N-phenyl-α-napthylamine prior to packaging (ANON, 1958; TOWNSEND, 1958).

2. Miscellaneous Processes

The original procedure employed by SHUKYS (1958) to prepare trifluoroethyl vinyl ether consisted of reacting acetylene with potassium trifluoroethylate in trifluoroethanol in a pressure vessel at 150 °C and 250 psig acetylene pressure.

The reaction, although it yields trifluoroethyl vinyl ether directly is relatively hazardous and would be difficult to employ on a commercial scale.

$$CF_3CH_2OH + HC \equiv CH \xrightarrow[\substack{150° \\ 250\ psig}]{CF_3CH_2OK} CF_3CH_2OCH=CH_2$$

BREY and TARRANT (1957) reported the preparation of trifluoroethyl vinyl ether by the following sequence of reactions.

a) $CF_3CH_2OH + \overset{\displaystyle O}{\overset{\displaystyle /\ \backslash}{CH_2-CH_2}} \xrightarrow[\substack{70° \\ autogeneous \\ pressure}]{KOH} CF_3CH_2OCH_2CH_2OH$

b) $CF_2CH_2OCH_2CH_2OH + PCl_5 \xrightarrow[CHCl_3]{reflux} CF_3CH_2OCH_2CH_2Cl$

c) $CF_3CH_2OCH_2CH_2Cl + KOH \xrightarrow[propanol]{} CF_3CH_2OCH=CH_2$

CROIX (1957) found that trifluoroethanol reacts with ethyl vinyl ether in the presence of p-toluenesulfonic acid to yield a mixed acetal:

$$CF_3CH_2OH + CH_2=CHOC_2H_5 \xrightarrow[\substack{35-40°}]{\substack{p\text{-toluene} \\ sulfonic\ acid}} CH_3\overset{\displaystyle OCH_2CF_3}{\underset{\displaystyle OCH_2CH_3}{\overset{\displaystyle /}{\underset{\displaystyle \backslash}{CH}}}}$$

This mixed acetal may be converted to trifluoroethyl vinyl ether either by further treatment with p-toluenesulfonic acid or by thermal cracking at 200 to 400 °C over pumice.

$$CH_3\overset{\displaystyle OCH_2CF_3}{\underset{\displaystyle OCH_2CH_3}{\overset{\displaystyle /}{\underset{\displaystyle \backslash}{CH}}}} \xrightarrow[heat]{acid\ or} CF_3CH_2OCH=CH_2 + CH_3CH_2OH$$

B. Chemical Reactions of Fluroxene

Little has been published concerning the chemical reactivity of trifluoroethyl vinyl ether, though on the basis of its structure it would be expected to undergo the same chemical reactions as non-fluorinated vinyl ethers.

KRANTZ et al. (1953) report that the compound neither hydrolyzed nor decomposed when incubated for 3 h at 38 °C in solutions buffered over a pH range of 2—11. Some acetaldehyde formation was found, however, when the compound was warmed with normal hydrochloric acid.

$$CF_3CH_2OCH=CH_2 + HCl \xrightarrow{H_2O} CF_3CH_2OH + CH_3CHO.$$

BELL and KRANTZ (1953) showed that trifluoroethyl vinyl ether is readily brominated in aqueous solution. LINDE (1956) took advantage of this ease of bromination to develop a method of analyzing the concentration of fluroxene in blood. In Linde's procedure the blood sample is steam distilled and the distillate is collected in a dilute solution of bromine in methanol. Potassium iodide is then added and titrated with sodium thiosulfate. As little as 1 mg of fluroxene is detectable by this method.

TARRANT and STUMP (1964) reported the light catalyzed addition of several bromine containing polyhalomethanes to trifluoroethyl vinyl ether, for example:

$$CCl_3Br + CF_3CH_2OCH=CH_2 \xrightarrow{\ h\nu\ } CF_3CH_2OCHBrCH_2CCl_3$$

$$CF_2Br_2 + CF_3CH_2OCH=CH_2 \xrightarrow{\ h\nu\ } CF_3CH_2OCHBrCH_2CF_2Br$$

Trifluoroethyl vinyl ether has been shown to undergo both homo- and copolymerization with relative ease. This phase of the chemistry has been investigated by a number of workers and is reported in a series of patents.

SCHILDKNECHT (1958) reported that trifluoroethyl vinyl ether readily forms a high molecular weight homopolymer when treated with a Friedel-Crafts catalyst such as boron trifluoride. The reaction occurs at temperatures as low as $-100\,°C$ and requires the presence of a small amount of a chlorinated solvent such as chloroform, or methylene chloride. Similar homopolymers have been reported by LUTTINGER et al. (1964) who found that polymerization could be catalyzed by gamma radiation, and by HECK (1965) who reported the use of aluminum isopropoxide as the catalyst.

Trifluoroethyl vinyl ether has been reported to undergo copolymerization with a wide variety of other monomers, such as chlorotrifluoroethylene (BARR, 1957), tetrafluoroethylene (SCHILDKNECHT, 1961), vinyl acetate and other vinyl esters (SCHILDKNECHT, 1958), and perfluorobutadiene (BOVEY et al., 1958). Catalysts employed in these polymerizations were generally peroxides and persulfates, however, both elemental oxygen and ozone were employed by BARR (1957).

Fluroxene Azeotropes

Fluroxene ((b.p. 42.7 °C) was found by CROIX (1962) to form minimum boiling azeotropic mixtures with 1,1,2-trichloro-1,2,2-trifluoroethane (Halon-113). These azeotropic mixtures are readily prepared by the isobaric distillation of simple mixtures of the two compounds. The lowest boiling fraction is the azeotropic mixture corresponding to a particular temperature and pressure. Some representative azeotropes of fluroxene-Halon-113 are:

B.P. °C °C	Vapor pressure mm of Hg	Fluroxene wt. %	Halon-113 wt. %
21.4	345	41.6	58.4
28.0	460	45	55
40.7	751	51.2	48.8

V. Teflurane

Teflurane, 2-bromo-1,1,1,2-tetrafluoroethane, is a colorless low boiling (8.66°C) liquid which is generally packaged in pressure containers and removed as a gas. The compound has been in clinical evaluation for several years, but due to the occurrence of cardiac arhythmias similar to those occurring with cyclopropane the agent has not been commercialized.

A. Synthesis

The process used to prepare teflurane for clinical evaluation has not been disclosed. However, a number of processes have appeared in the patent literature.

LARSEN (1961) reported the synthesis of teflurane in 70% yield via the high temperature (500—600 °C) bromination of 1,1,1,2-tetrafluoroethane in a manner similar to the ICI process for the synthesis of halothane.

$$CF_3CH_2F + Br_2 \xrightarrow[\text{1—5 sec}]{\text{500—600}°} CF_3CHBrF + HBr.$$

As with the ICI process over bromination, coupling reactions produce a number of undesirable by-products which are analogous to those obtained in the bromination of 2-chloro-1,1,1-trifluoroethane.

SUCKLING and RAVENTOS (1961) reported the synthesis of teflurane by the fluorination of either 2,2-dibromo-1,1,1-trifluoroethane or 1,2-dibromo-1,1,2-trifluoroethane, with pentavalent antimony chlorofluorides and hydrogen fluoride. The reaction was carried out at 110 °C and 250 psig. The product was distilled from the reaction as it was formed. The yield of teflurane, about 50%, was the same for both starting materials.

DAVIS and LARSEN (1967) reported the fluorination of a number of polybromofluoroethanes to teflurane with either chlorine trifluoride, or bromine trifluoride, in liquid bromine solvent, i.e.

$$CF_3CHBr_2 + ClF_3 \xrightarrow{Br_2} CF_3CHBrF \ (92\%)$$

$$CF_2BrCHBr_2 + BrF_3 \xrightarrow{Br_2} CF_3CHBrF \ (77\%)$$

$$CFBr_2CHBrF + BrF_3 \xrightarrow{Br_2} CF_3CHBrF \ (65\%)$$

RAUSCH et al. (1963) prepared teflurane by the addition of fluorine to 2-bromo-1,1-difluoroethylene using cobalt fluoride. In this process the bromodifluoroethylene is passed through a stirred bed of cobaltic fluoride (CoF_3) at about 35 °C. The reported yield of teflurane was 60%.

$$CF_2{=}CHBr + 2CoF_3 \longrightarrow CF_3CHBrF + 2CoF_2.$$

B. Chemical Properties

1. Reaction with Base

Teflurane is stable in the presence of solid sodium hydroxide pellets for prolonged periods at 75—80 °F. The formation of impurities was not observed (LARSEN, 1967). In view of HINE et al. [1961 (1, 2)] it is postulated that teflurane will react with base in a manner similar to that reported for halothane although at a somewhat slower rate.

2. Photochemical Stability

Studies carried out with teflurane in clear sealed glass ampoules indicate the compound is not degraded by prolonged exposure to ambient laboratory light, and consequently an antioxidant is not needed (LARSEN, 1960).

VI. Roflurane

Roflurane (2-bromo-1,1,2-trifluoroethyl methyl ether) is a clear, colorless, heavy, liquid having an odor similar to that of methoxyflurane. The compound was first reported by DEMIEL (1960) who prepared it by the base catalyzed addition of methanol to bromotrifluoroethylene in a manner similar to that described above for the manufacture of methoxyflurane.

The synthesis of the compound has also been reported by DAVIS and LARSEN (1965) via the fluorination of 2,2-dibromo-1,1-difluoroethyl methyl ether with bromine trifluoride in liquid bromine solvent.

$$CH_3OCF_2CHBr_2 + BrF_3 \xrightarrow{Br_2} CH_3OCF_2CHBrF.$$

The chemistry of this compound has not been studied extensively. In view of its structural similarity to methoxyflurane, it is not surprising that it is also similar to methoxyflurane in its chemical behavior.

Roflurane does not react with metals such as steel, nickel, copper, and aluminum (LARSEN, 1962), and inhibits the reaction of haloalkanes with aluminum [LARSEN et al., 1966 (2)]. The compound is stable in the presence of soda lime, or sodium hydroxide pellets, but does react slowly in a manner similar to that reported by HINE et al. [1961 (1, 2)] for halothane and methoxyflurane.

As with methoxyflurane, roflurane is defluorinated by concentrated sulfuric acid to give methyl bromofluoroacetate, and reacts with glass in the presence of strong mineral acids to yield the ester and silicon tetrafluoride [LARSEN, 1963 (2), 1964 (1)].

$$CHBrFCF_2OCH_3 \xrightarrow[H_2SO_4 \text{ catalyst}]{glass} CHBrFCO_2CH_3 + SiF_4.$$

VII. Flammability

One of the commonest chemical reactions in nature is that between oxygen and other compounds known as oxidation. Most reactions of this type take place with the liberation of heat and are therefore exothermic reactions. If this reaction takes place at a rapid enough rate, the mixture heats to high temperatures, combustion occurs and the heat liberated is referred to as the heat of combustion. When the combustion is associated with the emission of an appreciable amount of light or other radiation, the oxidation process is referred to as a flame. The rapid combustion of a quantity of premixed gaseous material and oxygen can lead to the sudden formation of large quantities of gaseous products which expand violently producing an explosion or detonation.

A principle incentive behind the development of the newer anesthetic agents has been the elimination of the fire and explosion hazard attendant with the older agents, i.e. diethyl ether, cyclopropane, etc. In order for a substance to offer a hazard of either fire or explosion, four factors must occur together. The elimination of any one of them effectively eliminates the hazard. First, it is necessary to have a fuel which can be either a gas, a liquid, or a solid. Second, it is necessary to have an oxidizing agent such as oxygen, nitrous oxide, etc.

Third, it is necessary that the fuel and oxidizing agent be in intimate contact so that the heat liberated in the combustion of one part of the mixture can raise the temperature of the adjacent layer of mixture above the autoignition temperature. Fourthly, it is necessary to have a source of ignition, or heat, sufficient to initiate the reaction. In standard anesthetic practice both the first and second factors are always present. The third may or may not be present, and depends on the concentration of the agent being employed. With the older agents the hazard of fire and explosions were minimized by attempting to eliminate the fourth factor, the source of ignition. The risk of fire and explosions with the older agents is significant in spite of extensive fire codes.

The risk could more effectively be eliminated by either developing agents that are not capable of being oxidized (elimination of the fuel), or by developing agents potent enough so that the necessary concentration of fuel needed for deflagration need not be employed. It is these two approaches that have been pursued in the development of the newer agents. Since the introduction of halogen into organic compounds is a relatively standard method of making compounds non-flammable in air it is natural that this technique should be extended to anesthetic agents, and this has worked well in those few cases where the compounds prepared were still useful as anesthetic agents.

Before discussing the effect of halogenation upon the relative flammability of organic compounds, it is necessary to define several items.

In any pair of gases consisting of a fuel and an oxidizing agent there is a range of concentrations within which the energy liberated by the combustion of any one layer is sufficient to ignite the adjacent layer of unburned gas and these mixtures are therefore capable of self propagation of flame. That mixture in which the minimum concentration of fuel is present (a lean mixture) corresponds to the lower limit of flammability, or the lower explosion limit, for that pair of fuel and oxidant. The mixture containing the maximum amount of fuel which will propagate a flame corresponds to the upper limit of flammability, or upper explosion limit. It must be recognized that the flammability limits of a compound define the minimum and maximum concentration of the compound which will propagate a flame and is by definition independent of all other factors.

The source of ignition can be any source of heat, i.e. flame, spark, hot wire, etc., of sufficient size and intensity so as to be capable of igniting a combustible, or more precisely a limit mixture. "As the test concerns the capability of the mixture to propagate flame, not the capacity of the source of energy to initiate flame, it is axiomatic that the limits are unaffected by variations in the nature and strength of the source of ignition" (COWARD and JONES, 1952).

Since the propagation of flame depends upon the transfer of energy from the burned to the unburned gas, and because in a limit mixture the energy available for transfer is only just enough to maintain flame propagation, anything which affects this transfer will have an effect upon the apparent value of the limits. In general, the direction of flame propagation, diameter of the vessel, pressure, temperature, turbulence, presence of an inert gas and the intensity of the ignition source will all have an effect upon the limit value obtained. When these factors can affect the value obtained then it is the limits of ignitability of a mixture that is being measured rather than the limits of flammability. For example, ... "when the limits vary according to the means of ignition, it is clear that the observers used either such strong sources of ignition that the caps of flame gave the appearance of general inflammation or such weak sources that flame was not started in mixtures which were in fact flammable. Under these conditions they were determining the limits of ignitibility by the particular sources of ignition they used, not the limits of flammability of the mixture itself" (COWARD and JONES, 1952).

Near each limit there is a range of mixtures that will propagate a mixture upward and not downward in a vertical test system. Mixtures within these ranges are properly "flammable mixtures" since placing the source in their lower confines will produce a self propagating flame. Similarly if the vessel diameter is too small the heat losses through the walls will tend to quench the flame and effectively narrow the limits. This phenomena is used to design "flame arresters".

Recently LARSEN (1969) has compiled the explosion limits for a wide variety of halogenated compounds. The atmospheres reported, air, oxygen, and nitrous oxide, are of special interest to the anesthesiologist. Fig. 1 shows a plot of the lower flammability limits of a number of these compounds in air, or oxygen, versus the total halogen content of the molecule, regardless of whether the halogen is fluorine, chlorine, or bromine. The curve shows the lower limit expected for any new compound. Compounds having more than two carbon atoms would be expected to fall below this line, although exceptions will probably be found. Those points which do fall significantly above the line were obtained using a spark generated by an automobile ignition (Ford) spark coil (< 5 J) and the values probably represent the limits of ignitability for this particular source rather than the true lower explosion limits (Larsen, 1969). Highly halogenated compounds appear to require a spark source in the range of 10—30 J in order to obtain values

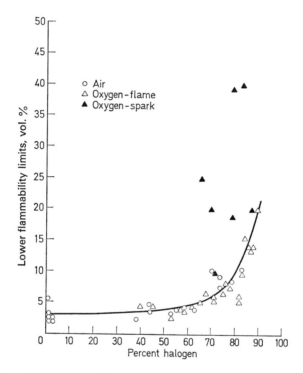

Fig. 1. Plot of lower limit of flammability versus the total halogen content of the molecule in oxygen and air atmospheres. No distinction is made among fluorine, chlorine, and bromine. The curve shows only the value that the author would explore for the lower flammability limit of a new compound when a flame or spark source having an energy of greater than 10 J is used for ignition. Compounds having more than two carbon atoms will normally fall below the line. Reprinted from Larsen (1969) with permission of Marcel Dekker, Inc.

approaching those obtained with a flame source. It is this enormous increase in energy required for ignition that renders the halogenated compounds non-flammable in clinical use, rather than any great increase in the lower flammability limits, since a static spark developing within the anesthetic apparatus will seldom if ever, exceed a few hundred millijoules.

Nitrous oxide, an endothermic compound, has an adverse effect upon the flammability of organic compounds, probably because an additional 19 kcal/mole of energy is imparted to the flame by the decomposition of the compound. With halothane the lower explosive limit decreases from about 14 vol-% in oxygen to about 2 vol-% in pure nitrous oxide, and the minimum ignition energy decreases from greater than 5 J to about 0.3 J (BROWN and MORRIS, 1966).

The flammability characteristics of halothane have been extensively studied. SEIFLOW (1957), using the methods developed by the United States Bureau of Mines (JONES, KENNEDY and MILLER, 1942; JONES, SCOTT and MILLER, 1942), found that any concentration of halothane and oxygen is non-explosive, and that mixtures of halothane in oxygen and nitrous oxide are non-flammable under conditions likely to be encountered in anesthetic practice.

BROWN and MORRIS (1966) re-examined the flammability of halothane and found that while halothane was non-flammable in oxygen at all concentrations up to saturation at room temperature using a cerium-magnesium (Ce-Mg) fusehead igniter in an open tube, a lower limit of 20—22.5 vol-% was obtained in a closed tube using the same ignition source. Using a heated platinum wire they obtained a lower limit of 17.5—20 vol-% at a wire temperature of 1000 °C, but no ignition at lower temperatures. In a closed steel bomb using a fusehead igniter the lower limit of inflammability was found to be 12.5—15 vol-%. PERLEE et al. (1965) using a glass sphere (2 l) combustion chamber and a guncotton igniter found no limits for halothane in air, but a range of 21 vol-% (LL) to 59 vol-% (UL) for halothane in oxygen, with the maximum pressure and rate of pressure rise occurring at a mixture containing 41 vol-% halothane and 59 vol-% oxygen.

It is obvious then that even though the halothane-oxygen mixture which is present in the saturated vapor space of an anesthetic vaporizer (~ 32 vol-% at 20 °C) is by definition a flammable mixture, this being a closed system for all practical purposes, it is ignitable only by the strongest sources, none of which could conceivably be present during normal use. The vapor concentration normally found in other parts of the anesthetic equipment (< 4 vol-%) are well below the lower flammable limit and no conceivable hazard is present. When more than two parts of nitrous oxide to one part of oxygen are present the lower limit in a closed tube decreases to 4—5 vol-%. A still lower value (1—2 vol-%) was found in pure nitrous oxide (BROWN and MORRIS). In view of the above information BROWN and MORRIS came to the following conclusions concerning the use of halothane. "So long as gas mixture being administered to the patient is known to be non-flammable to any ignition source in the theater, then there is no risk of explosion. These limiting concentrations of halothane in anesthetic practice are extremely remote from the normal usage of halothane. For example, the concentration of halothane in oxygen (20% V/V) which is required to produce an ignition is unlikely to be met with in anesthesia. When mixtures of at least one part of oxygen to three of nitrous oxide were tested, the results do not appear to limit the use of halothane in anesthesia."

Methoxyflurane was developed as an non-flammable anesthetic even though it's lower flammability limit in oxygen was known to be relatively low. In this case the low vapor pressure of the compound at normal operating room temperatures effectively prevents flammable concentrations from building up in the anesthetic apparatus. Fig. 2 shows the relationship between the vapor pressure-temperature curve for methoxyflurane, the normal anesthetic concentrations, and the lower flammability limits in various atmospheres (LARSEN, 1969).

In the case of Penthrane (a brand of methoxyflurane) the lower limit of flammability was determined in three different research laboratories (ANON, 1968). The values obtained are shown in Table 4. The values in column A were determined using flame propagation up a closed tube and a spark generated by a spark coil (> 10 J) as the ignition source [LARSEN, 1964 (2)]. The values in column B were reported by the laboratories of Physikalisch-Technische Bundesanstalt using flame propagation down a closed tube (NABERT, 1963). The strength of the igniting source was not cited but was probably as strong as the source employed by LARSEN. The third column values (C), obtained from WILTON-DAVIS and BRACKEN (1964), were determined in the laboratories of the British Oxygen Company. The

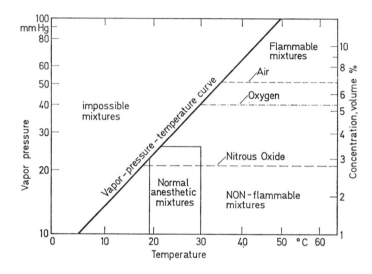

Fig. 2. Methoxyflurane — the relationships among vapor pressure-temperature curve, the normal anesthetic concentrations, and the lower flammability limits in various atmospheres. Reprinted from LARSEN (1969) with permission of Marcel Dekker, Inc.

Table 4. *Lower flammability limits of methoxyflurane*

Atmosphere	Aa	Bb	Cc
Air	8.7	6.0	6.97
Oxygen	5.4	5.5	6.15
50% O_2—50% N_2O	4.6		4.67
30% O_2—70% N_2O	4.0		
20% O_2—80% N_2O	3.7		
Nitrous oxide	2.7		2.46

[a] LARSEN (1946) — flame propagation upward in a closed tube, 10 to 20 J spark source.
[b] NABERT (1963) — flame propagation downward in a closed tube and temperature rise, spark source energy unknown.
[c] WILTON-DAVIS and BRACKEN (1964) — modified Pensky-Martin closed cup flash point apparatus, flame source.

method used employed a flame source and a modified Pensky-Marten closed cup flash point apparatus.

Fig. 3 shows the lower limits of flammability for methoxyflurane in various oxygen-nitrous oxide mixtures as a function of ignition source; spark (< 5 J) versus flame. The curve for the spark source is more properly the lower limit of ignitability with the rise in the curve probably being due to changes in the energy of the spark brought about by changes in the dielectric properties of the gas as the composition changes. The use of a more energetic spark brings the upper curve down until it is superimposable on the lower curve.

It is improbable that a hazard would exist even assuming that the concentration in the vaporizer exceeded the normal 3—4% because of the strength of the ignition source required to cause inflammation of the mixtures. It is difficult to conceive that sources of the required strength could be present during normal use.

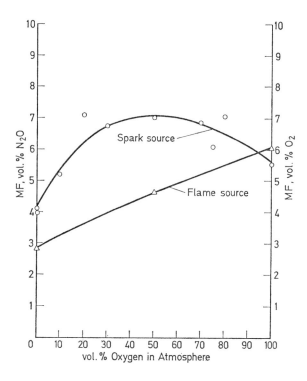

Fig. 3. Lower limits of flammability of methoxyflurane in oxygen-nitrous oxide atmospheres as a function of ignition source. The upper curve shows the lower limit of ignitability using an automobile ignition (Ford) spark coil (< 5 J). The lower curve shows the actual lower limit of flammability using a flame, or a high energy spark, source (> 10 J). Concentration of nitrous oxide in the atmosphere is 100 − vol.-% oxygen

The lower flammable limits for methoxyflurane were investigated at hyperbaric conditions by LARSEN [1946 (2)]. The results are shown in Table 5. It is interesting to note that the lower limit stays relatively constant at 6.1 vol-% up to three atmospheres of oxygen pressure. Since the volume percent of methoxyflurane present actually decreases as the oxygen pressure increases, it would appear that methoxyflurane is safe to use under hyperbaric conditions (3 vol-% at 20 °C at one atmosphere is equivalent to 1 vol-% at three atmospheres pressure). This evaluation must however be employed with caution since the laboratory conditions under which the tests are conducted differ more or less from conditions met with in practice, and the behavior of a vapor or gas on a laboratory scale is not always in full conformity with its performance under field conditions.

The lower flammability limit of fluroxene has been reported by Lawrence and Bastress (1959) to be 4.0 vol-% in dry oxygen. Later work by Miller and Dornette (1961) reported a lower limit of 7.5 vol-% which is probably the limit of ignitability for their system. Using a similar system Gramling and Volpitto (1963) found concentrations of 4.5 vol-% and above were flammable. Patterson et al. (1965) report that when a 20 ml plastic syringe was used as a test chamber the lowest concentration of fluroxene in mixtures of dry oxygen and nitrous oxide found to be flammable was 4.28 vol-%. In this later case it is probable that the value obtained is the limit of ignitability rather than the lower limit of flammability since a 20 ml syringe has a diameter much too small to avoid some quenching of the flame produced by a limit mixture. On the basis of chemical composition and structure it is probable that the lower limit for fluroxene is not greater than 4.0 vol-% and may be lower in rich nitrous oxide mixtures.

Table 5. *Lower flammability limits of methoxyflurane under hyperbaric condition in an oxygen atmosphere at 70 °C*

Oxygen pressure (atm)	Lower limit (vol-%)
1	6.1
2	6.0
3	6.2

Determinations carried out in a steel pressure vessel using spark ignition. Limits determined by rise in temperature and pressure.

Burns (Chapter 7.0, p. 409) raises a serious question of whether the exclusion of a compound from development because of flammability considerations alone is justifiable. In the author's opinion exclusion on this basis alone is not justified, provided of course that the developers can show that there is no increase in the overall danger, from a combined flammability and clinical viewpoint, to the patient. This approach was in fact the approach used in the development of methoxyflurane. The difficulty arises from the fact that because of a poor understanding of the role of halogenation in reducing the flammable hazard of organic compounds by many investigators some compounds are being classified as non-flammable agents when they burn freely in air. This is especially true with those compounds having halogen contents in the range of 40—60%. The hazard here is usually that the minimum ignition energies are not known and may well fall into the region where static sparks can ignite them. In addition spillage in an area where there are flames, or electrical switches which may spark, can lead to fires.

In the authors experience it is unlikely that any compound having more than two carbon atoms and less than 70% halogen content will be found which does not have finite flammability limits in air, although if the boiling point of the compound is sufficiently high it may not be possible to obtain the necessary vapor concentration at room temperature needed to create a hazard.

VIII. Foaming in Halogenated Anesthetics

Occasionally, during the use of out-of-circuit vaporizers (bubble-through type) methoxyflurane has been observed to foam, sometimes seriously (ARTUSIO, 1959; DORNETTE, 1967; SWEATMAN and YOUNG, 1968). How extensively the phenomenon exists is not known, but since it could conceivably represent a safety hazard, not only with methoxyflurane but with all halogenated anesthetics, the phenomenon warrants discussion in any treatise on the chemistry of these drugs.

Foams consist of a mass of gas bubbles dispersed in a liquid, the bubbles being separated by thin films of liquid and most of the volume being the gas phase. The formation of foam is a complex process involving changes in the surface tension of a liquid (pure liquids do not foam) brought about by the presence of a surface active agent. Whether or not a given surface active agent will cause foaming in a pure liquid depends upon the mechanics of the system, the temperature, the presence of impurities, the relative densities of the liquid and gas phases, and a number of other factors. The type of gas flow employed in bubble-through type vaporizers is highly conducive to foam formation.

An important cause of foaming with methoxyflurane is the inadvertent contamination of the agent by polydimethyl siloxane fluids, and greases, used to lubricate the moving parts of the vaporizers, or auxiliary equipment. Polydimethyl siloxane, which is the base silicone fluid used in many silicone greases as well as the base for some antifoaming agents, produces significant foaming in methoxyflurane at concentrations above 17 ppm. The foam height is related to both the gas flow and the silicone concentration; at low gas flow little foam is seen even at high silicone concentrations (> 100 ppm), while at high flow rates the foam height increases sharply at concentrations between about 20 and 50 ppm. Little additional foam is formed as the concentration of silicone exceeds 50 ppm. The foam produced is relatively unstable and collapses rapidly (< 30 sec) after the gas flow is stopped (LARSEN, 1959, 1968).

The interactions between the silicone and the anesthetic agent that result in foam formation are quite sensitive to changes in the structure of the silicone. Of the two commonly available types of silicones, the dimethyl and the methyl and phenyl fluids, only the polydimethyl siloxanes caused foaming with methoxyflurane; the methyl and phenyl polysiloxanes did not. Similarly with the newer, and still relatively uncommon, fluorosilicones those fluids having a relatively low fluorine content (< 40%) produced foam; those fluids having a high fluorine content (< 60%) did not. In screening tests the other halogenated anesthetic agents, e.g., trichloroethylene, halothane, roflurane, and anesthetic compound 347, could all be made to foam with one or another of the silicone fluids tested. No one silicone fluid would produce foam in all agents, and halothane appeared to be the most resistant to the problem (LARSEN, 1968). It is interesting to note that while foaming caused by silicones is relatively common when trichloroethylene is used as a solvent, the author has found no reference with respect to foaming when the compound is used as an anesthetic agent.

Because new silicone fluids, and greases made from them, are constantly being introduced to the marketplace, and because there is no way to assure that foaming cannot occur occasionally with any agent, it is recommended that silicones not be used as lubricants in anesthetic vaporizers, or in auxiliary equipment such as oxygen lines.

References

ALBIN, M. S., HORROCKS, L. A., KRETCHMER, H. E.: Halothane impurities and the Copper Kettle. Anesthesiology 25, 672—675 (1964).

ANON: Improvements in the compound di-(2,2,2-trifluoroethyl) acetal of acetaldehyde, process for producing the compound, and process for producing 2,2,2-trifluoroethyl vinyl ether. British Patent 790,824 (1958).

— Ayerst "Fluothane" (Halothane). Ayerst Laboratories brochure, issued April 1963.

— Penthrane, methoxyflurane, Abbott. Abbott Laboratories brochure 01-2068/R 11-200-Rev. June 1968.

ARTUSIO, J. F., JR.: Private communication (1959).

BARR, J. T.: Copolymers of 1-chloro-2,2-difluoroethylene and 2,2,2-trifluoroethyl vinyl ether. U.S. Patent 2,813,848 (1957).

BELL, F. K., KRANTZ, J. C., JR.: Anesthesia. XLIII. Estimation of anesthetic trifluoroethyl vinyl ether in aqueous solution. J. Am. Pharm. Assoc. 42, 633—634 (1953).

BOIVIN, P. A., HUDON, F., JACQUES, A.: Properties of the fluothane-ether anesthetic. Canad. Anaesth. Soc. J. 5, 409—413 (1958).

BOVEY, F., SMITH, S., ABERE, J. F.: Verfahren zur Herstellung kautschukartiger fluorhaltiger Mischpolymerisate. German Patent 1,040,248 (1958).

BREY, M. L., Tarrant, P.: Preparation and properties of some vinyl and glycidyl fluoro ethers. J. Am. Chem. Soc. 79, 6533—6536 (1957).

BROWN, T. A., MORRIS, G.: The ignition risk with mixtures of oxygen and nitrous oxide with halothane. Brit. J. Anaesthesia 38, 164—173 (1966).

CHAPMAN, J., HILL, R., MUIR. J., SUCKLING, C. W., VINEY, D. J.: Impurities in halothane: their identities, concentrations and determination. J. Pharm. and Pharmacol. 19, 213—239 (1967).

— McGINTY, R. L.: Process for the manufacture of 1-bromo-1-chloro-2,2,2-trifluoroethane. U.S. Patent 3,134,821 (1964).

— — Process for the preparation of bromochlorofluoro ethanes. U.S. Patent 2,921,099 (1960).

COHEN, E. N., BELLVILLE, J. W., BUDZIKIEWICZ, H., WILLIAMS, D. H.: Impurities in halothane. Science 141, 899 (1963).

— WINSLOW, H. W., BELLVILLE, J. W., SHER, R.: The chemistry and toxicology of di-chlorohexafluorobutene. Anesthesiology 26, 140—153 (1965).

CONWAY, C. M.: The anesthetic ethers. Brit. J. Anaesthesia 37, 644—654 (1965).

COWARD, H. F., JONES, G. W.: Limits of flammability of gases and vapors. Bur. Mines Bull. 1952, 503.

CROIX, L. S.: Trifluoroethyl alkyl acetals. U.S. Patent 2,809,218 (1957).

— Preparation of 2,2,2-trifluoroethyl vinyl ether. U.S. Patent 2,872,487 (1959).

— Anesthetic composition comprising halovinyl ether and halo hydrocarbon. U.S. Patent 3,027,299 (1962).

CROPP, D. T., GILMAN, D. J.: Process for purifying 2,2,2-trifluoro-1-chloro-1-bromoethane. U.S. Patent 3,349,137 (1967).

CROWTHER, A. F., ROBERTS, H. L.: Process for the preparation of 1,1,1-trifluoro-2-bromo-2-chloroethane. British Patent 908,290 (1962).

DAVIS, R. A., LARSEN, E. R.: Selective fluorination. Canadian Patent 704,494 (1965).

— — Chemistry of bromine trifluoride. The fluorination of bromofluoroethanes. J. Org. Chem. 32, 3478—3481 (1967).

DEMIEL, A.: Addition of alcohols to fluorinated ethylenes. J. Org. Chem. 25, 993—996 (1960).

DORNETTE, W. H. L.: Out-of-circuit methoxyflurane vaporizers and their application. No. 11 of a series of monographs on specific applications of methoxyflurane (Penthrane). Abbott Laboratories, North Chicago, Illinois, 6 (1967).

EDAMURA, F. Y., LARSEN, E. R.: Preparation of optically active halothane. Paper presented at the Meeting of the Midland Section, American Chemical Society, Midland, Michigan, October (1968).

GOWLAND, T. B.: Ethers containing fluorine. British Patent 523,449 (1940).

GRAMLING, Z. W., VOLPITTO, P. P.: Flammability of flucromar in the circle absorption system. Anesthesiology 24, 194—197 (1963).

HECK, R. F.: Crystalline poly (2,2,2-trifluoroethyl vinyl ether). Canadian Patent 655,609 (1963).

HENNE, A. L., LATIF, K. A.: Behavior of fluorinated olefins toward anionic reagents. J. Indian Chem. Soc. 30, 809—814 (1953).

— TROTT, P.: Preparation of trifluoroacetic acid. J. Am. Chem. Soc. 69, 1820 (1947).

HINE, J., WIESBOECK, R., GHIRARDELLI, R. G.: (1) The kinetics of the base-catalyzed deuterium exchange of 2,2-dihalo-1,1,1-trifluoroethanes. J. Am. Chem. Soc. 83, 1219—1221 (1961).

HINE, J., WIESBOECK, R., RAMSY, O. B.: (2) The carbanion mechanism for the dehydro-halogenation of 2,2-dihalo-1,1,1-trifluoroethane. J. Am. Chem. Soc. 83, 1222—1226 (1961).
HUDON, F.: Anesthetic compositions. Canadian Patent 658,678 (1963).
JONES, G. W., KENNEDY, R. E., MILLER, W. E.: (1) Limits of inflammability and ignition temperature of ethyl mercaptan in air. U.S. Bur. Mines; Rpt Invest. 1942, 3648.
— SCOTT, G. S., MILLER, W. E.: (2) Limits of inflammability and ignition temperature of styrene in air. U.S. Bur. Mines; Rpt Invest. 1942, 3630.
KRANTZ, J. C., JR., CARR, C. J., LU, G., Bell, F. K.: Anesthesia XL. The anesthetic action of trifluoroethyl vinyl ether. J. Pharmacol. Exptl Therap. 108, 488—495 (1953).
LARSEN, E. R.: Unpublished results (1959).
— The chemistry of methoxyflurane. Paper presented at the 140th Meeting of the American Chemical Society, Chicago, Illinois, September 3—8, (1961).
— 2-bromo-1,1,1,2-tetrafluoroethane. U.S. Patent 2,971,990 (1961).
— Unpublished results (1962).
— (1) Inhalation anesthetic: 2,2-dichloro-1,1-difluoroethyl methyl ether. U.S. Patent 3,104,202 (1963).
— (2) Hydrolysis of fluorinated ethers. J. Org. Chem. 28, 1133 (1963).
— (1) Decomposition of alpha-fluoroethers. Paper presented at the 148th Meeting of the American Chemical Society, Chicago, Illinois, September 1—3 (1964).
— (2) Unpublished results (1964).
— (1) Dichloro-difluoro ether. U.S. Patent 3,264,356 (1966).
— Unpublished results (1968).
— Fluorine compounds in anesthesiology. In: Fluorine chemistry reviews, Vol. III (Tarrant, P. Ed.). Marcel Dekker, Inc. Publisher 1969.
— DAVIS, R. A., LACOUME, J. R.: (2) Stabilization of haloalkanes with fluoroethers of the type R_1-O-CF_2R_2. U.S. Patent 3,278,615 (1966).
LAWLOR, F. E., BRAID, M., BARR, J. T.: The product prepared by reacting acetylene with trifluoroethanol. U.S. Patent 3,129,250 (1964).
LAWRENCE, J. S., BASTRESS, E. K.: Combustion characteristics of anesthetics. Anesthesiology 20, 192—197 (1959).
LINDE, H. W.: Estimation of trifluoroethyl vinyl ether in blood. Anesthesiology 17, 777—781 (1956).
LOTT, W. A., Yale, H. L.: Anesthetic. U.S. Patent 2,930,732 (1960).
LUTTINGER, M., SLIEMERS, F. A., JR., KIRCHER, J. F., LEININGER, R. E.: U.S. Atomic Energy Comm. Report BMI 1678 (1964); Chem. Abstr. 61, 14786 (1964).
MADAI, H.: Process for the production of 1,1,1-trifluoro-2-chloro-2-bromoethane. British Patent 939,920 (1963).
McGINTY, R. L.: Process for the manufacture of 2-bromo-2-chloro-1,1,1-trifluoroethane. U.S. Patent 3,082,263 (1963).
MILLER, G. L., DORNETTE, W. H. L.: Flammability studies of fluoromar-oxygen mixtures used in anesthesia. Anesthesia and Analgesia, Current Researches 40, 232—237 (1961).
NABERT, K.: Private communication (1963).
PARK, J. D., SNOW, C. M., LACHER, J. R.: Physical properties of some 1,1-difluoro-2,2-dichloroethyl alkyl ethers. J. Am. Chem. Soc. 73, 861—862 (1951).
PATTERSON, J. F., ADAMS, J. G., JR., JOHNSON, C. G.: Flammability of fluroxene. Anesthesiology 26, 825—826 (1965).
PERLEE, H. E., MARTINDILL, G. H., ZABETAKIS, M. G.: Flammability characteristics of selected halogenated hydrocarbons. U.S. Bur. Mines; Rept Invest. 1965, 6748.
RAUSCH, D. A., DAVIS, R. A., OSBORNF, D. W.: The addition of fluorine to halogenated olefins by means of metal fluorides. J. Org. Chem. 28, 494—497 (1963).
RUH, R. P., DAVIS, R. A.: Production of an antimony-containing fluorinating agent. U.S. Patent 2,786,738 (1957).
SCHERER, O., KAHN, H., KUHN, H.: Process for the manufacture of fluorobromo- or fluoro-bromohalo alkanes. Canadian Patent 692,039 (1964).
— KUHN, H.: (1) Process for preparing 1,1,1-trifluoro-2-chloro-2-bromoethane. Canadian Patent 650,600 (1962).
— — (2) Process for the manufacture of 2,2,2-trifluoro-1-chloro-1-bromoethane. Canadian Patent 652,239 (1962).
— — Process for eliminating fluorinated halogen butenes from 2,2,2-trifluoro-1-chloro-1-bromoethane. U.S. Patent 3,321,383 (1967).
SCHILDKNECHT, C. E.: Homopolymers from 2,2,2-trifluoroethyl vinyl ether. U.S. Patent 2,820,025 (1958).
— Copolymers of trifluoroethyl vinyl ether and halo-olefins and methods for preparing same. U.S. Patent 2,991,278 (1961).

Scipioni, A., Gambaretto, G., Troilo, G.: (1) Kinetics of the bromination of 1,1,1-trifluoro-2-chloroethane. Chim. e ind. (Milan) **49**, 583—586 (1967).

— — — Fraccaro, C.: (2) By-products of the high temperature bromination of 1,1,1-trifluoro-2-chloroethane. Chim. e ind. (Milan) **49**, 577—582 (1967).

Seiflow, G. H. F.: The non-inflammability of fluothane. Brit. J. Anaesthesia **29**, 438—439 (1957).

Seyferth, D., Mueller, D. C., Lambert, R. L., Jr.: New functional halomethylmercury compounds and halocarbenes. J. Am. Chem. Soc. **91**, 1562—1563 (1969).

Shukys, J. G.: Fluoroethers and methods of preparation. U.S. Patent 2,781,405 (1957).

— Trifluoroethyl vinyl ether compositions and methods for preparing and using same. U.S. Patent 2,830,007 (1958).

Suckling, C. W., Raventos, J.: A new halohydrocarbon and method of making the same. British Patent 767,779 (1957); see also U.S. Patent 2,849,502 (1958).

— — Process for the preparation of 1,1,1-trifluoro-2-bromo-2-chloroethane. U.S. Patent 2,921,098 (1960).

Sweatman, F., Young, J.: Private communication (1968).

Tarrant, P., Brown, H. J.: The addition of alcohols to some 1,1-difluoroethylenes. J. Am. Chem. Soc. **73**, 1781—1783 (1951).

— Stump, E. C., Jr.: Free-radical additions involving fluorine compounds. VII. The addition of perhaloalkanes to vinyl ether and vinyl 2,2,2-trifluoroethyl ether. J. Org. Chem. **29**, 1198—1202 (1964).

Townsend, P. W.: Method of preparing 2,2,2-trifluoroethyl vinyl ether. U.S. Patent 2,870,218 (1959).

van Dyke, R. A., Chenoweth, M. B., Larsen, E. R.: Synthesis and metabolism of halothane-1-[14]C. Nature **204**, 471—472 (1964).

Viney, D. J.: Purification of halothane. Canadian Patent 774,621 (1967).

Wilton-Davis, C. C., Bracken, A.: Private communications (1964).

Section 3.0

Clinical Monographs

3.1. Halothane

S. H. Ngai

Halothane as one of the modern inhalation anesthetics has a relatively short history. Its first clinical trial was conducted by Johnstone (1956) at the Manchester Royal Infirmary and the Crumpsall Hospital in England. Halothane soon gained wide acceptance because of its many pharmacological attributes and because of the need for a versatile, potent and nonflammable agent. The growth in popularity of halothane is phenomenal. Wherever modern anesthesia is being practiced halothane is the most frequently used general anesthetic.

Publications concerning the pharmacologic and clinical aspects of halothane continue at a fast pace from many sources. Monographs (Stephen and Little, 1961; Sadove and Wallace, 1962; Greene, 1968) and reviews [Johnstone, 1961 (1, 2); Black, 1965] cover the purview of this agent. Therefore, this section will discuss only some aspects of the pharmacology of halothane. Emphasis will be placed upon more recent advances. The medical library of The Ayerst Laboratories have rendered invaluable assistance in providing bibliography and pertinent reprints. Medlars service of The National Library of Medicine also searched the literature from January 1966 to November 1968. The author is grateful to both organizations.

I. Development of Halothane and Early Clinical Trials

Ferguson (1964) gave a lucid account of the discovery of halothane (Fluothane) on the occasion of the 25th Hurter Memorial Lecture. The Pharmaceuticals and General Chemicals Divisions of The Imperial Chemical Industries jointly considered the desirability of a new inhalation anesthetic in 1950. They laid down specifications for the anesthetic yet to be synthesized: a liquid with boiling point of about 60 °C so that it will have a suitable vapor pressure for easy administration, nonflammability, a reasonably high anesthetic action at low concentration and a good safety margin. The agent should also be inert and free from liability to cause damage to vital organs. Knowledge of fluorine chemistry already existant at that time directed the synthetic work to fluoro-alkanes. Fluoro-alkanes are generally more stable and have lower boiling points than their chlorine and bromine analogues. Halothane was one of 12 such compounds first prepared by Suckling in 1952 (Suckling, 1957, 1958). Subsequent pharmacologic studies by Raventós (1956) were exhaustive and indeed showed that halothane meets the original specifications. Further pharmacologic assessment was made by the Committee on Non-explosive Anaesthetic Agents of the British Medical Research Council (Burn et al., 1957).

Report of the first clinical trials of halothane by Johnstone appeared in 1956. The initial series of 500 cases was followed by another report on 2,500 cases (Brennen et al., 1957). These authors described the method of administration and clinical observations in some detail. With few exceptions these descriptions remain true 13 years later.

The use of halothane soon spread to other centers in England as well as in other countries. The immediate acceptance of this anesthetic in spite of its potency and the tendency to depress cardiovascular functions attests to its many advantages over other anesthetics available at that time. In the history of modern anesthetic practice the introduction of halothane and other fluorinated hydrocarbons and ethers may be considered "revolutionary," as were the cases of thiobarbiturates in the 1930s and succinylcholine in the early 1950s.

The state of art and science of anesthesia played an important role in the rapid advances of halothane. The development of precision vaporizers helped to make halothane a safe anesthetic. Accidental overdose became rare after a number of episodes occurred initially. The safety of halothane was further improved by studies on pharmacokinetics. Modern physical methods for measuring anesthetic concentration made this possible. The many faceted physiological studies confirmed earlier clinical observations for the most part. Progress in the knowledge about a single drug is indeed impressive.

II. Physical and Chemical Properties of Halothane

Larsen has discussed the chemistry of halothane in Section 2 of this monograph. Briefly, halothane is a heavy colorless liquid having a boiling point of 50.2 °C. The liquid specific gravity at 20 °C is 1.86 (Raventós, 1956). Its vapor pressure, in the range of 50°—55 °C has been determined by Bottomley and Seiflow (1963) by a static isoteniscope method; at 20 °C, the vapor pressure measures 243.5 mmHg. The vapor density is important in the design and calibration of precision vaporizers. At saturation vapor pressure the vapor density varies from 1.13 at 0 °C to 3.92 g/l at 30 °C. At a vapor pressure of 200 mmHg the vapor density approximates 2 g/l over a wide range of temperature (Bottomley and Seiflow, 1963).

Halothane is stable when stored in tinted glass containers or in clinical vaporizers. Exposure to light causes unstability evolving bromine with slow formation of volatile acids. Addition of thymol (0.01%, w/w) prevents this by mopping up free radicals produced by light, which would lead to bromine evolution by a chain reaction (Suckling, 1957). Halothane is compatible with all currently used anesthetic gases and vapors. Carbon dioxide absorbents such as soda lime and Baralyme do not cause decomposition (Raventós, 1956). Mixtures of halothane and oxygen (0.5—50%, v/v) are not flammable. Under hyperbaric conditions with halothane vapor pressures of 7.6—49 mmHg and oxygen pressure up to four atmospheres (absolute) the mixtures are not flammable or explosive (Gottlieb, 1966). However, direct contact with open flame or sparks causes halothane to break down, forming noxious products such as phosgene (for a more detailed discussion see Larsen). Also, exposure of halothane to gamma radiation forms dichlorohexafluorobutene (Pennington, 1968). The extent of this radiation induced transformation has not been measured quantitatively; its practical significance is uncertain at present.

Earlier commercial preparation contained a number of impurities in trace amounts, largely the intermediary products in the manufacturing process (Raven-

Tós and Lemon, 1965). One of these, dichlorohexafluorobutene ($CF_3CCl=CClCF_3$) in both trans- and cis-forms had an approximate concentration of 0.01 % (v/v), with ranges of 0.008—0.03 %. The presence of this contaminant was of concern in regard to hepatic toxicity (see Cohen, Section 9). Since 1965 the butenes and a number of other saturated impurities have been largely eliminated by changing the manufacturing process. Current commercial halothane marketed by the Imperial Chemical Industries, Ltd. and the Ayerst Laboratories contains less than 0.0075 % (w/w) or impurities. Any single unsaturated impurities are present in amounts less than 0.0005 % or five parts per million (Raventós and Lemon, 1965). Halothane manufactured by Hoechst is equally pure.

III. Methods of Assaying Halothane Concentration

In the original pharmacologic studies of Raventós (1956) vapor concentration delivered to the anesthetic chamber was calculated from the volume of liquid halothane added to the diluent gas (oxygen or air) according to standard gas laws. He measured tissue or blood halothane concentration with a method developed by Goodell (Appendix to Raventós, 1956). Extracts in petroleum ether were heated in sealed vials with sodium amoxide to release bromide, measured nephalometrically as silver bromide. Duncan (1959) and Burns and Snow (1961) modified the method, using lithium aluminum hydroxide and dispersed sodium respectively. These modifications improved the recovery rate as well as ease of analytical procedures.

However, studies on pharmacokinetics of halothane depend upon rapid and accurate measurement of vapor concentrations. Evaluation of various clinical vaporizers would be difficult and cumbersome without using some physical methods of measurement. Kalow (1957) first determined the ultraviolet and infrared spectra of halothane vapor using a spectrophotometer. At a wave length of 228 μ (in the ultraviolet range) the absorbance measures the vapor concentration without interference from other anesthetics such as nitrous oxide. An ultraviolet analyzer has been subsequently developed by Robinson and Denson (1962) using a mercury lamp (emission, 2537 Å). Only trichloroethylene among all commonly used anesthetics has absorptivity at this wave length. With a cell volume of 15 ml, a flow rate of 100 ml/min through the cell, the response time is about 20 sec. Evaluation of subsequent commercial models shows that this type of instrument is of adequate accuracy provided that it is calibrated with known vapor concentrations of halothane (Wolfson, 1968).

Infrared analyzers with smaller detector cells have a faster response time. Analyzers such as Beckman Model LB-1 use the whole infrared spectrum without dispersion. For halothane or other halogenated hydrocarbons the cell windows are constructed with crushed zinc sulfite (Irtran II). The detector cell is filled with the vapor to be analyzed at a low pressure (10—50 mmHg) or appropriate mixture of other gases. To eliminate the cross over effect of other gases, such as carbon dioxide or nitrous oxide, the analyzer case has to be filled with these gases. Again, frequent calibration with mixtures of known vapor concentrations is essential to insure accuracy.

Gas chromatography is an accurate and convenient method for measuring anesthetic concentrations in gas mixtures as well as in blood and tissues. Published methods vary in the use of instrument, column, adsorbent and other specifications. Both thermal conductivity and flame ionization detectors are applicable for halothane. For gas mixtures the method presents little problem except for careful

3*

calibration. Detection of halothane in blood and tissues requires reliable extraction of the anesthetic. Blood or tissue samples may be introduced directly into the carrier gas stream (BUTLER and FREEMAN, 1962; LOWE, 1964). Frequent cleaning of the injection port becomes necessary. Others used organic solvent extraction with heptane (RUTLEDGE et al., 1963) or carbon tetrachloride (WOLFSON et al., 1966) with a recovery of 96.5—100%. Equilibration of blood with known volume of gas has also been reported by several groups of investigators (YAMAMURA et al., 1966; SAIDMAN et al., 1967 (2); BUTLER et al., 1967; THEYE, 1968; and many others]. Knowing the blood/gas partition coefficient, anesthetic content in the liquid phase may be calculated. Complete extraction of anesthetic vapor from blood samples can be accomplished by refluxing. The vapor is condensed in a liquid nitrogen trap at —195 °C. The trapped vapor is then introduced into the gas chromatograph (RACKOW et al., 1966).

IV. Methods of Administration: Anesthetic Circuits and Vaporizers

Halothane may be used as the sole agent to produce the state of anesthesia. The onset of anesthesia is fast with appropriate vapor concentration. All depths of anesthesia may be achieved, although the skeletal muscles relax only at relatively deep levels. Deep anesthesia usually results in significant circulatory depression. For this reason the common practice is to administer halothane as the primary agent in conjunction with others as originally described by JOHNSTONE (1956). After preanesthetic medication with appropriate doses of belladonna, narcotic and/or hypnotics, anesthesia is induced with a fast-acting barbiturate. Succinylcholine provides muscular relaxation for endotracheal intubation when indicated. Halothane vapor is then added to the inspired mixture consisting of oxygen or nitrous oxide-oxygen. The relative merits of using halothane alone or with nitrous oxide are still under debate. Those favoring the use of halothane-oxygen claim that the high inspired oxygen concentration insures tissue oxygenation in spite of decreased cardiac output and hypotension (SHINOZAKI et al., 1968). MARTINEZ and NORLANDER (1967) also question the advisability of using nitrous oxide-oxygen mixture based upon their studies on elderly patients with cardiovascular and pulmonary diseases. During anesthesia maintained with halothane and nitrous oxide-oxygen mixtures, unexpected low arterial oxygen tensions were observed frequently. The arterial hypoxemia may be explained by many factors, among them the patient's age and pre-existing diseases; its clinical significance is not defined as no immediate sequelae occurred. However, the findings of MARTINEZ and NORLANDER point out the need for individual consideration in the choice of anesthetic mixture.

Administration of nitrous oxide with halothane considerably reduces the halothane concentration required to provide a given level of anesthesia (see below). Cardiovascular function is depressed to a lesser degree. The use of neuromuscular blocking agents when required makes it possible to keep the anesthesia at a light level. Early pharmacologic studies (RAVENTÓS, 1956) and clinical experience (JOHNSTONE, 1956) indicated that the concomitant administration of halothane and d-tubocurarine may result in profound arterial hypotension and cardiovascular collapse. Later experience of others disproved this impression. As expected, the degree of hypotension is related to the doses of halothane and d-tubocurarine (CHATAS et al., 1963). Therefore, depending on clinical circumstances and the anesthetist's preference, various muscle relaxants are being used with safety during halothane anesthesia.

A. Anesthetic Circuits

Halothane vapor mixture has been administered in all manners including the open drop method. With a non-rebreathing system the inspired anesthetic concentration equals that delivered. In practice when using this system a pressure equalizing valve is necessary to allow the escape of excess gas (STEEN and LEE, 1960). The most commonly used are the semi-open system such as the McGill circuit and the partial rebreathing circuit with carbon dioxide absorption. The McGill circuit is simple and easy to clean, a customary gas inflow rate being 7 l/min. Recently KAIN and NUNN (1968) re-evaluated this circuit and found that a fresh gas flow of 3.1—4.6 l/min (mean, 3.6) is adequate to prevent rebreathing in patients having a minute volume of respiration ranged from 3.4—8.8 l/min (mean, 5.3), the ratio of minimum adequate fresh gas flow to minute volume averaged 0.71 ± 0.17 (S.D.). However, the arrangement of McGill circuit offers no possibility of assisted or controlled ventilation.

In the circle system the extent of rebreathing depends upon the rate of fresh gas flow. As pulmonary uptake of halothane continues during the course of most clinical anesthesia (although at a decreasing rate) halothane concentration in the reservoir bag is expected to be lower than that delivered into the circuit. Rubber components of an anesthetic circuit also takes up halothane, the rubber/gas partition coefficient being 120 (EGER et al., 1962; TITEL and LOWE, 1968). The loss of halothane to rubber can delay the induction of anesthesia when the fresh gas flow is low. Higher gas flow minimizes this effect.

Several arrangements of circle system components have been tested for best economy to conserve fresh gas and to eliminate alveolar gas (EGER and ETHANS, 1968). The most economical arrangement has both inspiratory and expiratory valves close to the patient and the outflow valve immediately downstream from the expiratory valve.

The use of halothane-air mixture with portable equipment has been proposed for field use under unusual circumstances of disaster (PAPANTONY and LANDMESSER, 1960). However, hypoxemia can occur during anesthesia unless ventilation is assisted (MARKELLO and KING, 1964).

FOLKMAN and his associates (1968) administered halothane and other anesthetics to dogs by diffusion through silicone rubber coils. An arterial-venous shunt diverts blood through the coils immersed in the anesthetic liquid. For halothane the shunt measures $0.125 \times 0.250 \times 38$ in. (1 in. = 2.5 cm). The amount of halothane diffused into the blood can induce and maintain surgical anesthesia provided that pulmonary excretion is prevented by rebreathing. The possibility of administering halothane or other anesthetics clinically with this method is uncertain.

B. Vaporizers

JOHNSTONE (1956) used a trichloroethylene vaporizer and the Boyle's apparatus to administer halothane for his initial clinical trials. A mixture of nitrous oxide and oxygen (total flow, 10 l/min) was delivered to a semi-open circuit. Subsequently a partial rebreathing system was employed primarily for economy (BRENNEN et al., 1957). It soon became apparent that a more precise vaporizer is essential for the safe conduct of anesthesia. A number of vaporizers have been designed or adopted for halothane, for instance, HILL's vaporizer [1958 (1)], Rowbotham's bottle (BURTON, 1958), FNS vaporizer (FABIAN et al., 1958), Marett inhaler (WOODS and BROWN, 1959), and GOLDMAN's vaporizer (1962). These devices deliver variable vapor concentrations depending upon ambient temperature and total gas flow.

A draw-over precision vaporizer compensated for temperature and gas flow variations, the Fluotec vaporizer [MACKAY, 1957; HILL, 1958 (2)], stood the test of popular use over the years. The delivered vapor concentration is stable over a temperature range of 13—32 °C and a gas flow from 4—15 l/min. Another reliable vaporizer is the copper kettle designed by MORRIS (1952). The carrier gas is dispersed by a sintered disc into fine bubbles through liquid anesthetic to achieve full saturation. Knowing the gas flow through the vaporizer, liquid temperature and the vapor pressure, the volume of anesthetic vapor delivered can be calculated. Desired vapor concentration is obtained by appropriate dilution with oxygen or oxygen-gas mixtures. Both of these devices are used as an out-of-circuit vaporizer. The delivered vapor concentration is therefore not influenced by the minute volume of respiration. The original method of RAVENTÓS (1956) has also been used clinically. HART (1958) fed liquid halothane to the fresh gas input. HAMPTON and FLICKINGER (1961) added increments of liquid halothane to a closed circle system. However, this method is inherently dangerous, requiring close attention and frequent monitoring of vapor concentration.

With both Fluotec and copper kettle type of vaporizers, delivery of halothane is subject to error during intermittent positive pressure ventilation. Pressure fluctuations force additional gas in and out of the vaporizing chamber. Thus, with the Fluotec setting at 0.5%, as much as 3.2% halothane can be delivered (oxygen flow, 500 ml/min, circuit pressure, 30 cm water) (HILL and LOWE, 1962). Similarly, with a Vernitrol vaporizer, with intermittent positive pressure to the reservoir bag, 2% halothane has been measured in the delivery line even when no oxygen flows through the vaporizer (KEET et al., 1963). This source of error is great with low total gas flow (500 ml/min) but minimal with higher flows (4 l/min or more) (EGER and EPSTEIN, 1964). HILL and LOWE (1962) proposed to pressurize the Fluotec to eliminate the pressure effect. Others placed an unidirectional valve down stream from the vaporizer so that the circuit pressure is not transmitted back to the vaporizer (KEENEN, 1963; KEET et al., 1963).

Accidental overdose can occur even with precision vaporizers. The hazard of tipping Fluotec vaporizer and overfilling of kettle type vaporizer is well recognized. Defective valve seats in the flow-through gas meter can allow high oxygen flow to bubble liquid halothane into the delivery line (KOPRIVA and LOWENSTEIN, 1969). More subtle sources of error in vapor metering have been discussed by EGER and EPSTEIN (1964). As the kettle type of vaporizer is already 100% efficient (MORRIS and FELDMAN, 1958) attempts to further increase vapor delivery by devices such as a spraying tower or thermostatically controlled heating would seem unnecessary and potentially hazardous.

V. Uptake and Distribution of Halothane — Clinical Considerations

MAPLESON will discuss the principles of pharmacokinetics of gaseous anesthetics in section 5. Measurement in man or studies with mathematical model and electric analogues help to put the clinical administration of anesthetics on a more rational basis. These investigations also provided a sound approach to many works on pharmacodynamics. The monograph on uptake and distribution of anesthetic agents (PAPPER and KITZ, 1963) collectively surveyed the state of knowledge since KETY (1951) formulated his concept on this subject. Subsequent reviews by others (BUTLER, 1964; EGER, 1964; EPSTEIN and PAPPER, 1965; SAIDMAN, 1968) further defined factors which influence the uptake of anesthetics.

Halothane has a relatively low blood/gas partition coefficient (2.3) among anesthetic vapors (LARSON et al., 1962). This, together with other factors such as absence of airway irritation and the use of "overpressure" during induction, account for the rapid induction of anesthesia with halothane. SECHZER et al. (1963) studied in man the rate of anesthetic equilibration by administering subanesthetic concentration of halothane (0.2%) with a non-rebreathing system. As predicted, the rate was considerably slower than that of nitrous oxide or cyclopropane (gases less soluble in blood than halothane). At 5 min the alveolar halothane concentration approaches 50% of the inspired. Two hours elapse before the alveolar concentration reaches approximately 80% of the inspired. In contrast, with cyclopropane the alveolar gas tensions are 55 and 90% of the inspired at 1 and 5 min, respectively (SECHZER, 1963). On the other hand, the rate of equilibration with halothane is faster than that of more soluble anesthetics such as diethyl ether and methoxyflurane.

Studies using halothane in subanesthetic concentrations do not necessarily reflect the course of events under clinical conditions. Pharmacologic effects of trace amounts of halothane may be minimal. For the most part changes in ventilation and circulation, if any, are considered negligible. Experimental results indeed correspond closely with data derived from mathematical models or electric analogues constructed with known values of anesthetic solubility in blood and tissues, standard functions such as alveolar ventilation, cardiac output and its distribution to various body compartments (EGER, 1963; MAPLESON, 1963). However, these functions do change upon the induction of surgical anesthesia (see below). BUTLER (1963) has amply demonstrated wide fluctuations of the rate of halothane uptake under clinical circumstances as influenced by ventilatory and circulatory changes.

EGER and GUADAGNI (1963) used a different approach to study the uptake of halothane in man. They measured the volume of halothane vapor taken up by the body at a constant alveolar concentration. Thus, to maintain an alveolar concentration of 0.8%, 81 ml of halothane is absorbed during the first minute, 47 ml during the 5th min, and 28 ml during the 20th min. Pulmonary uptake continues to the 4th h at a rate of 5.6—10.8 ml/min, apparently because of the relatively high fat/blood partition coefficient (60). The inspired halothane concentrations calculated to maintain a constant alveolar concentration at 0.8% are high initially, about 4% with an alveolar ventilation of 4 l/min. At approximately 10 min, the inspired concentration required is reduced to 2%. At 3 h an inspired concentration of about 1% maintains the alveolar concentration at 0.8% because of the continued uptake.

The effect of hyperventilation on the rate of anesthetic equilibration has been calculated with a mathematical model (MUNSON and BOWERS, 1967). While hyperventilation considerably hastens the rate of rise of alveolar anesthetic concentration, reduction in cerebral blood flow as a result of hypocarbia would partially delay the cerebral equilibration with anesthetic in the arterial blood. In the case of halothane, time required to reach 95% equilibration between brain and arterial blood is 28 min with an alveolar ventilation of 4 l/min and an arterial carbon dioxide tension of 40 mmHg. Doubling the alveolar ventilation without a change in carbon dioxide tension shortens the 95% equilibration time to 13 min. But with a reduction in arterial carbon dioxide tension to 20 mmHg and cerebral blood flow from 44—25 ml/100 g/min, 20 min is required for 95% equilibration. Considering alterations in ventilation and cerebral blood flow together, the rate of rise in cerebral halothane concentration remains the same as under normal circumstances during the first 10 min of administration. If these computations can be applied to clinical conditions it would seem that hyperventilation alone would not necessarily hasten the induction of anesthesia. Furthermore, the rate of rise in alveolar and arterial anesthetic concentrations does accelerate with hyperventilation. This common clinical practice can be potentially hazardous in respect to cardiovascular depression when using overpressure.

MUNSON et al. [1968 (1)] further examined the influence of changes in cardiac output upon the rate of cerebral anesthetic equilibration. Using a similar mathematical model they predicted that with a reduced cardiac output (such as during shock) and a differential decrease in blood flow to tissues other than brain, the rate of rise of brain halothane concentration would be accelerated. This would explain in part the well known clinical observation that patients with reduced blood volume and low cardiac output are inordinately sensitive to anesthetic depression. With an increase in cardiac output such as during excitement, again with a change in cardiac output distribution preferentially to muscles and vessel-rich organs other than brain, "induction" can be expected to be slow. However, hyperventilation accompanying excitement would compensate for this change. The clinical implication of this computation as described cannot be well defined as excitement usually does not persist and the anesthetist is expected to take measures to terminate the excitement.

A few other factors affect the rate of equilibration with halothane. EPSTEIN et al. (1964) showed in dogs that when nitrous oxide in high concentration (70%) is administered together with halothane, the rate of equilibration of halothane is faster. This phenomena has been called the second gas effect, occurring because the uptake of nitrous oxide (second gas) increase the inspiratory flow. Ordinarily the second gas effect can be expected to take place only with nitrous oxide because of its solubility (blood/gas partition coefficient, 0.47) and the concentration administered. The second gas effect would be negligible with ethylene, as ethylene is less soluble (blood/gas partition coefficient, 0.17). Its uptake is much less than that of nitrous oxide, taking place in a shorter time (SALANITRE et al., 1965). Other anesthetics are not usually administered in concentrations high enough to produce the second gas effect.

Recently, STOELTING and EGER [1969 (1)] offered an additional explanation for the second gas effect. They showed in dogs *after* equilibration with halothane, the addition of 70% nitrous oxide to the inspired mixture causes an increase in the alveolar halothane concentration to about 8% higher than that inspired. This occurs because of a concentrating effect secondary to nitrous oxide uptake from the lung.

In infants and children equilibration of alveolar anesthetic concentration toward that inspired proceeds at a faster rate than in adults (SALANITRE et al., 1969). These authors suggested that the faster rate of anesthetic equilibration in children is related to physiologic differences. Children have a larger ventilatory volume, higher cardiac output and a proportionately lager percentage of vessel-rich tissues relative to body weight than adults. As discussed above, increased ventilation hastens equilibration. The higher cardiac output, although expected to delay the rate of rise of alveolar anesthetic concentration, has an overall effect to increase the total body uptake. Furthermore, the vessel-rich tissues, estimated to be 19% of body weight in children (7% in adults), receive a large share of cardiac output, and come to anesthetic equilibration with arterial blood sooner. Thus, the mixed venous blood anesthetic concentration increases at a faster rate.

Distribution of halothane in the body depends on two factors: perfusion and tissue/blood partition coefficients. The vessel-rich tissues have a relatively low tissue/blood partition coefficient (brain, 2.6; liver, 2.6; kidney, 1.6) (LARSON, 1962).

These tissues come to equilibrium after 10—15 min (EGER, 1964). The muscle comprises a large mass (40—50% of the body weight), but is perfused with only about 20% of the cardiac output. Therefore the muscle comes to equilibrium much later. The fat has a relatively high tissue/blood partition coefficient (60) and is poorly perfused. Although halothane may also enter the fat through intertissue diffusion (PERL et al., 1965) under usual clinical circumstances the fat does not come to anesthetic equilibrium with blood. Uptake of halothane by fat continues at a slow rate.

Metabolism of halothane plays a significant role in its disposition in the body. In man, as much as 11—12% of an administered dose has been recovered from the urine as bromide or trifluoro-acetic acid (REHDER et al., 1967). The rate at which halothane degradation proceeds is essentially unknown. Possible metabolic pathways are being discussed by VAN DYKE in section 5.2 of this monograph. Halothane may also diffuse through skin but the amount lost is very small ($0.0076 \, ml/min/m^2$) and of little consequence [STOELTING and EGER, 1969 (2)]. Comparing anesthetics of different fat solubilities, the rate of percutaneous loss appears to vary inversely with fat solubility, suggesting that with halothane the subcutaneous adipose tissue may act as a sink to drain the skin of its halothane content.

VI. Anesthetic Requirement of Halothane

EGER and his co-workers [1965 (1, 2)] developed the concept of minimum anesthetic concentration (MAC). As defined, MAC is the alveolar concentration of an anesthetic that will prevent muscular movement upon painful stimulation in 50% of test subjects, assuming that the anesthetic tension in the brain closely approximates that in the lung. The stimulus consists of tail clamping or electric shock in experimental animals and skin incision in man. Others have used spinal reflexes to study anesthetic potency and depth [DE JONG et al., 1967, 1968 (1); FREUD et al., 1969]. The measurement of MAC allows some degree of precision in studies of anesthetic potency and factors influencing anesthetic requirement. The concept is also useful in comparing physiological effects of different anesthetics at equipotent concentrations. However, the anesthetic depth at MAC represents but one point (movement in response to pain) along a stratum of different physiologic effects with increasing anesthetic concentrations. Clinically, the anesthetic depth at MAC probably provides amnesia and analgesia but higher anesthetic concentration is usually required for skeletal muscle relaxation (DE JONG et al., 1967).

MAC of halothane in man is 0.77% [SAIDMAN et al., 1967 (1)]. The addition of 70% nitrous oxide reduces the MAC to about 0.3% (SAIDMAN and EGER, 1964; FREUND et al., 1969). The corresponding arterial concentrations are approximately 15 and 6 mg% respectively. Premedication with 8—15 mg of morphine reduces the MAC of halothane slightly from 0.74—0.69%.

A number of other factors influence the required concentration of halothane for anesthesia. Age of patient seems to have an inverse relationship with anesthetic requirements (GREGORY et al., 1969). MAC for infants younger than 6 months is 1.08%; for teenagers 0.92%, for young adults 0.84% and for elderly patients (70 years and older) 0.64%. It would seem that Guedel's original observation now finds support with quantitative data. REGAN and EGER (1967) showed in dogs that with moderate hypothermia to 27—29 °C MAC changes rectilineally with body temperature. For a 10 °C decrease in temperature MAC of halothane reduces by 0.44%. Extreme changes in metabolic activity also affect the anesthetic requirement. Dogs with hypothyroidism and lowered basal metabolic rate are found to require 0.84% halothane for anesthesia. Euthyroid dogs require 0.90% and those with hyperthyroidism, 1.03% (BABAD and EGER, 1968).

Pretreatment with certain drugs which alter the central nervous system norepinephrine stores has been found to change MAC of halothane. In dogs chronic treatment with drugs which deplete CNS norepinephrine stores such as alpha methyl dopa and reserpine decreased the anesthetic requirement of halothane by as much as 30% (MILLER et al., 1968). These findings suggest that changes in central norepinephrine concentrations may influence anesthetic requirement. The relationship between central norepinephrine and serotonin stores, release and state of consciousness have been implicated (see JOUVET, 1969).

Earlier studies indicate that carbon dioxide in small concentrations (5—10%) may add to the narcotic action of anesthetics (KLEINDORFER, 1931; McALEAVY et al., 1961). With halothane the additive effect of carbon dioxide is not evident until the arterial carbon dioxide tension rises to above 95 mmHg (EISELE et al., 1967). Conversely, hypocarbia (Pa_{CO_2} 15—20 mmHg) does not change the MAC of halothane (BRIDGES and EGER, 1966; EISELE et al., 1967).

Chronic alcoholics appear to require greater than usual amount of anesthetics. MAC of halothane has been determined in these subjects and compared to that of normal adults (HAN, 1969). Alcoholics require an alveolar halothane concentration of 0.94—1.68% (mean 1.31) to prevent movement upon skin incision, MAC for normal adults being 0.78%. This difference has been attributed to a change in CNS excitability and a higher Ostwald solubility coefficient of halothane in the cerebral white matter of alcoholic subjects.

VII. Effects on Physiological Systems

Section 4 of this monograph will discuss the action of halothane on vital systems in comparison with other modern anesthetics. The review of pharmacologic effects here includes certain relevant observations in experimental animals and in man and where possible, their clinical implications.

A. Nervous System

Halothane, like other general anesthetics, depresses neuronal activity and interferes with synaptic transmission. In the visceral ganglion of *Aplysia* and nerve cells of *Helix* halothane reduces excitability as it hyperpolarizes the synaptic membrane. The excitatory postsynaptic potential (EPSP) upon threshold stimulation is abolished. The amplitude of EPSP with supraliminal stimulus decreases and its rate of decay increases. In autorhythmic neurons halothane reduces the firing frequency and spike amplitude (CHALAZONITIS, 1967). GISSEN et al. (1966) studied the action of halothane on the neuromuscular junction with single fiber preparations of the frog sartorius. Halothane (0.1% V/V in Ringer's solution) does not change the resting potential of postsynaptic membrane. Response to indirect stimulation decreases. Of interest is the fact that halothane, like diethyl ether, reduces the amplitude of miniature potentials. GISSEN et al. interpreted these effects of halothane as a result of desensitization (or stabilization) of the postsynaptic membrane, probably through changes in ionic permeability. In dogs, halothane (2%, inspired) inhibits transmission through sympathetic ganglion (GARFIELD et al., 1968). Although these studies used simple models of synapse, the results probably reflect the depressant action of the anesthetic in the central nervous system.

The action of halothane on evoked potential, along afferent pathways and in the cerebral cortex has been studied. In encephale isolé preparation of cats 1—3% halothane (inspired) depresses the evoked potentials in the auditory cortex earlier than that in the inferior colliculus (SASA et al., 1967). The evoked potentials and the spontaneous multiple unit activity in the midbrain reticular formation of cats show progressive depression with increasing depth of halothane anesthesia (MORI et al., 1968). In man, however, the evoked potentials over the visual cortex do not change significantly during light halothane anesthesia except for a longer latency (DOMINO et al., 1963). More subtle changes in cerebral cortical activity have been shown in the cat (KITAHATA, 1968). Using paired click stimuli spaced at various intervals, halothane in concentrations of 0.9—2% (inspired) causes a dose related depression of the neuronal revovery cycle as recorded from the primary auditory cortex. The shortest inter-click interval to evoke the second response (absolute refractory period) is prolonged from 5—7 to 12—18 msec with 2% halothane. The maximum ratio of the second evoked response to the first (when the interclick interval is longer than 100 msec) decreased from 0.9—1 during wakefulness to about 0.6 during anesthesia. These changes could result from cortical depression, or, more likely, from depression of subcortical structures as shown earlier by KING et al. (1957) with barbiturates.

In cats and in man halothane produces essentially similar changes in electro-encephalographic patterns. With increasing anesthetic concentrations EEG shows progressive slowing with increasing amplitude (GAIN and PALETZ, 1957; BACKMAN et al., 1964; KITAHATA, 1968). Periods of suppression occur during deep anesthesia. Arterial hypotension may contribute to these changes not usually observed under clinical circumstances when the depth of anesthesia is not excessive.

Early clinical impressions indicated that halothane has relatively poor analgesic action as compared with other anesthetics such as nitrous oxide and trichloro-ethylene. DUNDEE and MOORE (1960) confirmed this in volunteers. Pain threshold as measured with sustained pressure on/the tibia is not significantly altered with 0.5% halothane but elevated with 50% nitrous oxide or 0.35—0.5% trichloro-ethylene. ROBSON et al. (1965) have made similar studies. Pain was elicited by cutaneous heating or tibial pressure. Although 0.5% halothane significantly elevates the pain threshold to both stimuli, the analgesic action appears to be less than that of 25—30% nitrous oxide.

Skeletal muscle relaxation is usually not adequate for intra-abdominal operations during light surgical anesthesia with halothane. Although a neuromuscular blocking action has been demonstrated in vitro (see above), halothane in anesthetic concentrations does not affect muscle response to indirect stimulation in vivo [NGAI et al., 1965 (1); KATZ and GISSEN, 1967]. Therefore, muscle relaxation must result from central depression. In the cat somatic reflexes are readily abolished during inhalation of halothane in inspired concentrations varying from 0.4—1.0% [NGAI et al., 1965 (1)]. Multisynaptic reflexes appear more liable to anesthetic depression than the monosynaptic reflex [NGAI, unpublished data; DE JONG et al., 1968 (2)]. In man the monosynaptic H-reflex is reduced to about 30% of control with 0.8% halothane (alveolar) and to 9% when 70% nitrous oxide is administered in addition (FREUND et al., 1969). As judged clinically abdominal muscle relaxation is only "fair" when the H-reflex is depressed to about 25% and "good" when the reflex is less than 25% of control (DE JONG et al., 1967). These measurements thus confirm earlier clinical observations that adequate muscle relaxation requires moderate or deep level of anesthesia with halothane.

Current clinical practice usually provides muscle relaxation with neuromuscular blocking agents. Although halothane has no demonstrable effect on indirectly

evoked muscle response in vivo, it considerably potentiates the action of d-tubocurarine (KATZ and GISSEN, 1967). d-Tubocurarine (0.1 mg/kg) reduced the ulnar
nerve stimulation 60—100% (mean 76%) during halothane anesthesia but only
30—70% (mean 53%) during anesthesia with nitrous oxide-meperidine. Halothane
also prolongs the duration of action of d-tubocurare: 19—48 min (mean 36 min)
as compared with 10—12 min (mean 16.5 min) with nitrous oxide. It should be
noted that this effect is not unique with halothane but common with other potent
anesthetics such as diethyl ether (KATZ, 1966) and methoxyflurane (HEISTERKAMP
et al., 1969). The subtle action of anesthetics on neuromuscular transmission
becomes evident only in the presence of d-tubocurarine.

B. Cerebral Circulation and Metabolism

Halothane appears to have a direct action on the cerebral vessels. Autoregulation of cerebral circulation in terms of tissue oxygen requirement appears abolished.
This action of halothane is in contrast with that of thiopental which reduces
cerebral blood flow (CBF) and cerebral metabolism (CMR_{O_2}) and increases cerebral
vascular resistance (CVR) (PIERCE et al., 1962).

Except for the earlier work of McDOWALL et al. (1963) subsequent studies in
dogs are in general agreement showing that halothane dilates cerebral vessels.
Changes in cerebral hemodynamics are related to the dose (concentration) of
halothane. According to THEYE and MICHENFELDER (1968) who measured the
sagittal sinus blood flow directly, CBF increases from a control value of 59.2 to
70.0 and 84.5 ml/100 g/min during light and deep halothane anesthesia respectively. The partial pressures of halothane in sagittal sinus blood range 2.8 to
5.7 mmHg during light anesthesia and 6.6—9.4 mmHg during deep anesthesia.
Correspondingly, CVR decreases from a control of 2.19—1.44 (light anesthesia)
and 0.80 (deep anesthesia) mmHg/ml/100 g/min, or 66% and 37% of control
respectively. The A–V oxygen difference decreases (from 9,89—7.31 and 6.15 ml/
100 ml) with an increased venous oxygen tension (from 27.8—33.3 and 37.5 mmHg).
Except for a decrease in perfusion pressure the arterial oxygen and carbon dioxide
tension as well as the body temperature were maintained constant. McDOWALL
(1967) reported similar results in dogs. Two % halothane increases the blood flow
through the cerebral cortex. With 4% halothane marked arterial hypotension
results but the cerebral blood flow is maintained near that of control due to vasodilation.

In man cerebral vasodilation has been demonstrated by WOLLMAN at al. (1964)
and CHRISTENSEN et al. (1967). With the arterial carbon dioxide and body temperature maintained constant at 41 mmHg and 37 °C respectively, CBF increases
27% and CVR decreases 26% (CHRISTENSEN et al., 1967). Reactivity of cerebral
vessels to changes in arterial carbon dioxide tension (Pa_{CO_2}) is maintained. With
an end-tidal halothane concentration of about 1%, hypocarbia (Pa_{CO_2}, 23 mmHg)
reduces CBF from 51—23 ml/100 g/min and increases CVR from 1.1—2.6 mmHg/
ml/100 g/min (WOLLMAN et al., 1964). Hypercarbia further increases CBF
(CHRISTENSEN et al., 1967). The same authors also found that hypotension potentiates the cerebral vasodilating action of halothane even in elderly patients with
cerebrovascular disease.

In dogs and in man halothane decreases CMR_{O_2} ranging from 15—33%. The
minimal reduction of 15% observed by COHEN et al. (1964) in man has been
attributed to a lowered body temperature. But later work by McHENRY et al.
(1965) and CHRISTENSEN et al. (1967) showed a 26% reduction in CMR_{O_2} during
halothane anesthesia without a significant fall in body temperature. The degree of

CMR_{O_2} depression seems to be related to the depth of anesthesia. In the dog, 0.5% halothane reduces the cerebral cortex oxygen uptake by 14% and 2% halothane produces a decrease of 33% (McDowall, 1967). As there are no significant shifts in cerebral pathways of carbohydrate utilization or a reduction in oxygen supply, the decrease in CMR_{O_2} is most likely a direct result of cerebral depression (Theye and Michenfelder, 1968).

The increased CBF together with a lowered oxygen utilization have been considered useful in clinical management of patients with compromized cerebral perfusion, for instance, carotid artery stenosis (Christensen et al., 1967). On the other hand, intracranial pressure increases significantly during halothane anesthesia. Marx et al. (1962) correlated the elevated cerebro-spinal fluid pressure with increases in systemic venous pressure and the halothane concentration administered. More recent observations of Jennett et al. (1969) showed that the intracranial pressure increases without a significant change in central venous pressure and that methoxyflurane and trichloroethylene share similar effects. These authors further found that the anesthetic induced increases in intracranial pressure are not always related to the arterial carbon dioxide tension, although in certain instances attentuated by hyperventilation and hypocarbia. In patients with normal cerebrospinal fluid pathways the increase in intracranial pressure (mean 68 mm water) is probably not of significance clinically. But in patients with space occupying lesions the increase can be considerable (means 180 and 278 mm water with 0.5 and 1% halothane, respectively). With the concomitant decrease in the arterial pressure the effective cerebral perfusion pressure falls strikingly (Jennett et al., 1969).

C. Respiratory System

Halothane, like other potent anesthetics, depresses respiration. Earlier clinical observations and more recent quantitative studies in animals and in man amply demonstrated this effect. While respiratory homeostasis may be maintained during light surgical anesthesia, moderate to deep anesthesia progressively decreases respiratory amplitude and increases respiratory rate, accompanied by an elevated arterial carbon dioxide tension (Burnap et al., 1958; Devine et al., 1958; Deutsch et al., 1962; Munson et al., 1966).

Respiratory depression during anesthesia with halothane or any other anesthetics may be attributed to reduced general cerebral activity and/or specific depression of the respiratory control mechanisms. Fink and his associates (1961, 1962) showed in man that while the state of wakefulness support rhythmic breathing in the absence of chemical drive, apnea can be produced readily by moderate decrease in Pa_{CO_2} with hyperventilation. During spontaneous breathing with 1—1.5% halothane (inspired) Pa_{CO_2} averages 47 mmHg. Lowering Pa_{CO_2} to 41 mmHg results in apnea — the respiratory threshold. With 2—2.5% halothane, the resting Pa_{CO_2} is 54 mmHg and the threshold Pa_{CO_2}, 47 mmHg. Fink et al. (1962) proposed that the depressed cerebral activity during anesthesia leaves the respiratory control almost entirely to chemical drive. Progressive respiratory neuronal depression explains the elevated respiratory threshold during deep halothane anesthesia.

Further evidence for the decreased responsiveness of the respiratory control system has been obtained in dogs and in man. In dogs, the resting Pa_{CO_2} rises from 45.6—115 mmHg with increasing alveolar halothane concentration from 0.55—1.8% (Merkel and Eger, 1963). Spontaneous breathing ceases when the alveolar concentration is about 2.2 times the minimal anesthetic requirement — MAC (Brandstater et al., 1965). Munson et al. (1966) provided detailed data on breathing and respiratory response to inhaled carbon dioxide in man. Respiratory rate increases from 16—36 min with an alveolar halothane concentration of 1.88% (2.5 MAC). The tidal volume as calculated from their results decreases progressively from an average of 425 ml (awake) to 93 ml during anesthesia with halothane (2.5 MAC). Pa_{CO_2} increases from 35.5—74.3 mmHg. The respiratory responsiveness to carbon dioxide as measured by the slope of the stimulus-response curve also decreases to only 6% of the control response.

The decreased respiratory amplitude may be readily explained on the basis of neuronal depression and failure of recruitment at the brain stem and/or the spinal cord level. The increase in respiratory rate is not easily explained. CESSI et al. (1963) and COLERIDGE et al. (1968), based upon their findings in animals, suggested that halothane causes tachypnea through its sensitizing action on the pulmonary stretch receptors. However, tachypnea can still develop during deep halothane anesthesia after bilateral vagotomy [NGAI et al., 1965 (2)]. Further attempts to elucidate the basis for tachypnea gave inconclusive results because of accompanying circulatory depression. In all likelihood, sensitization of pulmonary receptors and activation of Hering-Breuer reflex cannot account for the observed tachypnea. PASKIN et al. (1968) showed that this reflex appears not operative in man. Lung inflation does not result in inspiratory inhibition as expected.

More relevant is the fact that during anesthesia with halothane, as with other potent anesthetics, compensatory mechanisms against disturbances in carbon dioxide homeostasis, hypoxia and mechanics of breathing may fail. The elevated Pa_{CO_2} and decreased ventilatory response to inhaled carbon dioxide (see above) illustrate that anesthesia impairs the primary function of the regulatory system. The work of PASKIN et al. (1968) also showed that response to increased airway resistance is absent during anesthesia. Awake man attempts to overcome increased airway resistance by augmented inspiratory effort and a larger tidal volume. An anesthetized subject is not able to do so. Therefore, the anesthetic circuit must have the lowest possible resistance to airflow. Except for the light planes of anesthesia, breathing will have to be assisted or controlled to provide adequate gas exchange. As mentioned above, during halothane anesthesia the carbon dioxide threshold for rhythmic breathing falls near the normal level of P_{CO_2} (FINK et al., 1962). Apnea or feeble inspiratory effort would ensue if Pa_{CO_2} is kept around normal range. One often finds that assisted respiration leads to apnea and controlled respiration.

The clinical practice of controlled respiration commonly results in hypocarbia. The possible harm of hypocarbia has been a subject of extensive discussion. As the cerebral vessels retain their reactivity to changes in Pa_{CO_2} rather marked cerebral vasoconstriction occurs. CBF decreases to half of that during normocarbia. The jugular venous P_{O_2} falls from 54—31 mmHg (COHEN et al., 1964). However, biochemical indication of cerebral hypoxia during hyperventilation has not been found. Extensive clinical experience also gives no evidence of cerebral damage.

At the end of anesthesia conducted with controlled respiration, the resumption of adequate rhythmic breathing depends on several factors: the depth of anesthesia determining the respiratory threshold of Pa_{CO_2}; the level of Pa_{CO_2} as related to the degree of preceding ventilation; the rate of rise of Pa_{CO_2} during apnea as controlled respiration is discontinued and lastly, afferent stimulation. Surgical manipulation usually ceases at this time. The rate of rise of Pa_{CO_2} during apnea averages 6 mmHg/sec (ALLEN et al., 1967). Therefore, efforts should be made to eliminate halothane from the body (to lower the respiratory carbon dioxide threshold) before attempts to initiate rhythmic breathing are undertaken. If nitrous oxide is being administered with halothane controlled respiration should be continued with oxygen for a few minutes to first eliminate nitrous oxide so that hypoxemia will not occur during the necessary period of apnea.

Halothane does not irritate the upper respiratory tract. Halothane also suppresses the cough reflex. Cough induced by a transient airway irritation lasts considerably shorter during nitrous oxide, oxygen and halothane anesthesia than during equal levels of anesthesia with diethyl ether, cyclopropane or thiopental-nitrous oxide (HARRISON, 1962). CALVERT et al (1966) found that halothane suppresses cough reflex at a blood concentration ranging from 6—13 mg%; less when nitrous oxide is administered with halothane, 5—8 mg%. Cough suppression is certainly a desirable property during anesthesia with an endotracheal airway.

Relaxation of tracheo-bronchial smooth muscle by halothane has been demonstrated in vitro with guinea pig tracheal chain (FLETCHER et al., 1968). Studies in dogs also showed that halothane reduces lung resistance to airflow and increases bronchial distensibility and lung compliance (COLGAN, 1965; KLIDE and AVIADO, 1967). The bronchoconstriction induced by intravenously administered histamine or vagal stimulation is effectively abolished by halothane (COLGAN, 1965; HICKEY et al., 1969). Clinicians recognize this property of halothane and utilize it to alleviate bronchial spasm during anesthesia. SNIDER and PAPPER (1961) analyzed their experience. In 27 patients who had wheezing prior to induction of anethesia or developed bronchial spasm during anesthesia, halothane cleared the wheezing in 24.

However, a number of other reports appear to indicate that in man halothane has no appreciable effect on the airway resistance. Values for respiratory resistance on passive exhalation in subjects anesthetized with halothane are not remarkably different from those in conscious individuals (BERGMAN, 1969). During cardio-pulmonary bypass when the lungs are functionally isolated from the systemic circulation, halothane administered to the airway or the systemic circulation does not change the pulmonary mechanics such as dynamic compliance, airway resistance and work of breathing significantly (PATTERSON et al., 1968).

Halothane appears to decrease the surface activity of the lung. Lung extracts from rabbits anesthetized with halothane have higher surface tension values than those from control animals (MOTOYAMA et al., 1969). In excised dogs' lungs with constant volume ventilation, the lung volume during deflation decreases progressively with halothane (WOO et al., 1969). These authors suggested that halothane may depress the synthesis of surfactant or its transport. The clinical significance of these findings is not yet defined.

Although not unique with halothane, the effect of anesthesia on some other pulmonary mechanics deserves mention. In normal adults the anatomical dead space does not change appreciably but the ratio of dead space ventilation (V_D) to tidal volume amounts to 33% during spontaneous breathing (NUNN, 1964; MARSHALL, 1966) and increases during controlled respiration (ASKROG et al., 1964). Calculated right to left shunting averages 11—14% of the cardiac output but values over 30% have been obtained at lower levels of Pa_{O_2}, presumably the result of uneven ventilation perfusion ratios (maldistribution) (NUNN, 1964). With high inspired oxygen concentration the alveolar-arterial oxygen tension gradient has a mean value of 184 mmHg. Based upon these findings NUNN (1964) suggested that an inspired oxygen concentration of 35% is required to provide a $P_{A_{O_2}}$ at about 200 mmHg, if arterial hypoxemia is to be avoided in most patients. In patients with cardiopulmonary diseases even 35% oxygen in the inspired mixture may not be adequate. Arterial oxygen tension as low as 60 mmHg has been recorded (MARTINEZ and NORLANDER, 1967).

Increased physiological shunting as reported by NUNN (1964) raises the possibility of progressive atelectasis with spontaneous shallow breathing. MARSHALL (1966) and COLGAN and WHANG (1968) reexamined this problem in surgical patients. Most of these subjects were free from cardiopulmonary diseases except four in MARSHALL's series. During halothane anesthesia the mean tidal volume decreases from 579—250 ml. Alveolar ventilation also decreases in spite of a faster respiratory rate, resulting in moderate hypercarbia (mean Pa_{CO_2}, 48—51 mmHg). However, compared with values obtained immediately before the induction of anesthesia, there are no significant changes in alveolar-arterial oxygen tension difference (range, 142—196 mmHg) or in shunting (approximately 10% of cardiac output). In addition, COLGAN and WHANG (1968) found no change in the functional residual capacity and lung compliance. These authors concluded that progressive atelectasis is not a predictable consequence of unassisted ventilation. To explain the apparent increase in shunting reported by others, MARSHALL (1966) suggested that a significant fall in cardiac output during halothane anesthesia would increase the arterial-mixed venous (a–v) oxygen content difference. This in turn would result in a greater alveolar-arterial oxygen tension gradient with the true shunt remaining constant. Therefore, if shunting is calculated assuming a given a–v oxygen difference, the shunt would appear to have increased.

D. Circulatory System

Cardiovascular effects of halothane have been studied extensively. Experimental and clinical observations agree on the overall depressant action related to the dose (concentration) of halothane. But a great deal of controversies and confusion still exist on the site of action, understandably because of the varieties of experimental design and methodology, interfering factors such as surgical trauma, concomitant use of other drugs, and above all, interpretation of experimental data. GOLDBERG (1968) gave an excellent review recently. Section 4.2 of this monograph discusses comparative action of anesthetics on the cardiovascular system.

Central Action. It would seem reasonable to assume that the hypotensive action of halothane is attributable to a large extent to the depression of the vasomotor regulatory mechanism. Indeed this has been shown in experimental animals. PRICE et al. (1963) administered halothane (1—2%) to the vascularly isolated head of the dog and produced systemic hypotension, bradycardia and decreased myocardial contractility. Subsequently, the same group of investigators demonstrated in dogs that microinjection of 5 µl of saline equilibrated with 5% halothane into the medullary vasomotor areas depresses arterial pressure responses (both pressor and depressor) to direct stimulation of these centers (PRICE et al., 1965). To avoid the use of basal anethesia NGAI and BOLME (1966) studied the action of halothane on hypothalamic vasomotor mechanisms in dogs with chronically implanted stimulating electrodes, carotid tunnels and aortic catheters. In this preparation halothane also depresses the pressor responses to central and reflex stimulation. However, it should be noted that the entire organism is being exposed to halothane which could act on both the central mechanisms and circulatory apparatus in the periphery.

There are evidences, to the contrary, that halothane probably has little or no action on the vasomotor regulatory mechanisms. MILLAR and BISCOE (1965, 1966) found in rabbits that halothane increases both the preganglionic and postganglionic sympathetic activity. In cross-circulation experiments (dogs) when the gracilis muscle is being perfused with blood from a donor, administration of halothane to the donor does not change the vascular resistance in the muscle [CHRISTOFORO and BRODY, 1968 (1)]. This finding appears to indicate that halothane may not affect the resting sympathetic activity. The work of EPSTEIN et al. (1968) and WANG et al. (1968) using major vessel occlusion and cross circulation preparations in dogs offers good evidence to indicate that halothane has minimal effect on the central vasomotor activity or its responsiveness to direct or reflex stimulation. After ligating all anastomotic vessels across the diaphragm, simultaneous occlusions of the descending aorta and inferior vena cava effectively isolate the cephalic and caudal halves of the body in respect to circulation. Caudal arterial and venous pressures reflect vasomotor tone in these beds without the influence of cardiac action but do reflect activity of the vasomotor control mechanisms. When halothane is administered in high concentration (6%) after major vessel occlusion, it reduces the cephalic arterial pressure but not the caudal arterial or venous pressures. As halothane distribution is limited to the cephalic circulation, these findings presumably indicate that halothane has little effect on the vasomotor center (EPSTEIN et al., 1968). In the cross circulation preparation the recipient's head is perfused with donor's blood through the carotid arteries, draining through jugular venous anastomosis. When halothane (1—2%, inspired) is administered to the body of the recipient, hypotension results as expected. However, when halothane is administered to the donor, thus only to the head of the recipient, the resting arterial pressure of the recipient does not change significantly. Pressor response to direct stimulation of the medullary vasomotor center is not affected either. These findings would indicate that halothane depresses cardiovascular function without an appreciable effect on the central control mechanisms (WANG et al., 1968).

It is difficult to resolve the divergent observations and disparate points of view. The effect of basal anesthetics on experimental results is largely unknown. The prevalent sympathetic activity before administration of halothane does appear to influence its central action. Data of WANG et al. (1968) showed that in one series of experiments where the cross-circulation involved thoracotomy of the recipient, administration of halothane to the head circulation results in moderate hypotension. The pressor response to direct central stimulation remains the same. Presumably the added surgical trauma and blood loss from thoracotomy increase the resting vasomotor activity. Halothane may attenuate this activity. The responsiveness of medullary vasomotor mechanisms however is not affected. The depressant effect of intramedullary microinjection of saline equilibrated with halothane vapor (PRICE et al., 1965) is difficult to interpret. The vapor concentration of 5% is rather high and not usually used in other studies.

The sensitizing action of halothane on the baroreceptors (BISCOE and MILLAR, 1964) may or may not have a bearing on the circulatory control system. An increased baroceptor activity would induce arterial hypotension reflexly. Indeed, BISCOE and MILLAR (1966) showed in rabbits that while halothane inhibits the depressor responses to afferent aortic nerve stimulation, such response can usually still be evoked. Perhaps the findings of MILLAR and BISCOE (1965, 1966) that halothane increases sympathetic discharge can be explained on the basis of barostatic reflexes. In their studies the arterial pressure decreased to 40—70% of control levels. Such hypotension could result in increased firing of excitatory vasomotor neurons. However, species difference may be an important consideration. Further work in this area would seem desirable. In any case, the failure of barostatic reflex during halothane anesthesia apparently results not from central depression but presumably through interference with ganglionic transmission and peripheral receptor response to humoral transmitters (see below).

Peripheral Actions. There are ample evidences for the depressant action of halothane in the periphery. Halothane interferes with sympathetic ganglionic transmission (see above), decreases heart rate and myocardial contractility, and relaxes vascular smooth muscles.

Ganglionic Transmission. Sympathetic ganglionic transmission, as indicated by the change in heart rate upon preganglionic (stellate) stimulation in spinal dogs, appears unaffected with lower concentrations of halothane (0.25—1%, inspired). In fact some potentiation has been observed. Two % halothane depresses the response. Atropine (1 mg/kg) exaggerates the ganglionic blocking action of halothane (GARFIELD et al., 1968). PRICE and PRICE (1967) obtained similar results. In dogs pretreated with atropine (0.4 mg/kg) 0.5% halothane (inspired) has negligible effect on ganglionic transmission; 1% halothane, 50% inhibition while 2% halothane blocks ganglionic transmission completely. In all likelihood, ganglionic blockade is not complete under most clinical circumstances. It probably contributes in part to the cardiovascular depressant action of halothane.

Heart. Depressant action of halothane on the heart has been shown with myocardial preparations in vitro, heart-lung preparations, as well as in intact animals and in man (see GOLDBERG, 1968).

In isolated rat ventricular trabeculae carneae muscle preparations stimulated with currents of threshold intensity, halothane depresses the force velocity relationship in direct relation to the concentration. The maximum initial velocity of isotonic shortening (V_{max}) and the tension developed isometrically (P_0) are lowered. Halothane also reduces the peak-developed isometric tension as well as the work and power (GOLDBERG and ULLRICK, 1967; GOLDBERG and PHEAR, 1968). At maximum load the degree of extension of the series elastic component increases by 12—13%. These finding led GOLDBERG and his coworkers to conclude that halothane decreases the active state intensity. The increased extensibility of series elastic element is thought to contribute to the reduced peak-developed tension due to diminished effectiveness of the contractile element. GOLDBERG (1968) further suggested that the depressant action of halothane on the myocardium is indirect, possibly through decreased ATPase activity of myofibrils and diminished availability of intracellular calcium at sites critical for actin and myosin binding. Many others have also demonstrated direct myocardial depression by halothane with a variety of isolated heart preparations.

All evidence obtained with the heart in situ corroborates the results of studies in vitro. In dog heart-lung preparations a direct depressant effect of halothane has been shown (FLACKE and ALPER, 1962). Both the heart rate and contractility decrease in proportion to the concentration of halothane. With 1% halothane, the systemic output decreases and the right atrial pressure rises. The heart is no longer able to compensate for an increase in venous inflow. Norepinephrine infusion cannot completely reverse the action of halothane in concentrations higher than 2% (inspired), supporting the view that reflex compensation for hypotension would be ineffective.

Direct measurement of myocardial contractility with Walton-Brodie strain gauge in intact dogs (MORROW et al., 1961; PRICE and PRICE, 1966) and in man (MORROW and MORROW, 1961; BLOODWELL et al., 1961) also demonstrated the depressant action of halothane in clinically used concentrations (0.5—3%). Prior sympathectomy (MORROW et al., 1961) or pretreatment with reserpine (REIN et al., 1963; MORROW and MORROW, 1963) does not exaggerate the action of halothane. Again, this would indicate that sympathetic nervous activity may have little influence on performance of the heart during halothane anesthesia.

Cardiac output decreases during halothane anesthesia (SEVERINGHAUS and CULLEN, 1958; WALTHER et al., 1964; SMITH et al., 1968; EGER et al., 1968; and many others). The magnitude of decrease is related to the alveolar halothane concentration, varying from 0.8—2.4%. An interesting observation is that as halothane anesthesia is continued at the same alveolar concentration, cardiac output and stroke volume tend to return toward control (EGER et al., 1968). This phenomenon has not been satisfactorily explained, as the total peripheral resistance remains decreased and the administration of hexamethonium produces no significant change in cardiovascular function at a given alveolar halothane concentration.

The addition of nitrous oxide to halothane appears to reverse partially the cardiovascular effects of halothane. In dogs with a given arterial halothane concentration (up to 24 mg%) nitrous oxide increases the rate of rise of right ventricular pressure. The cardiac output changes little but arterial pressure and total peripheral resistance increase considerably toward control values (SMITH and CORBASCIO, 1966). Subsequently, SMITH et al. (1968) and MARTIN et al. (1969) observed similar changes in man. These authors suggested that nitrous oxide may have a sympathetic "stimulating" effect. While this explanation remains speculative, the fact that nitrous oxide spares anesthetic requirement of halothane (see above, section on Anesthetic Requirements) and partially antagonizes the cardiovascular action of halothane would lend support to the common clinical practice of administering nitrous oxide with halothane.

On the other hand, SHINOZAKI et al. (1968) obtained data in man to conclude that the decreased cardiac output with halothane is a consequence of homeostatic adjustment to reduced oxygen demand. They hypothesized that the heart remains functionally intact as demonstrated by its ability to respond to differing needs. Earlier, PAYNE et al. (1959) also found variable changes in cardiac output under halothane anesthesia during surgical procedures. 7 of 12 patients had an increase, and the rest, 5, a decrease in cardiac output, presumably the resultant of many factors, including depth of anesthesia and surgical stimulation. It seems that although halothane depresses cardiovascular function, under usual clinical circumstances no overt effect is evident.

Since hypercarbia may develop during halothane anesthesia, its modifying effects on cardiovascular function are interest. MARTIN et al. (1969) found in man that a stepwise increase in Pa_{CO_2} from 20—60 mmHg improves myocardial performance at various levels of anesthesia with halothane (0.8 and 1.5%, alveolar) or halothane-nitrous oxide mixtures (70% nitrous oxide, 0.3 and 0.8% halothane). Mean arterial pressure, cardiac output, stroke volume and the rate of rise of arterial pressure all increase. However, the slope of response to increasing Pa_{CO_2} decreases with higher concentrations of halothane (see also PRICE et al., 1960).

As mentioned above, halothane decreases the heart rate. The negative chronotropic effect may be attributable to a direct action and possible vagal action. Early clinical observation and more recent data show that atropine increases the heart rate, considerably reverses the hypotensive effect of halothane. Direct action of halothane on the rabbit sinoatrial node has been studied in vitro (HAUSWIRTH and SCHAER, 1967). Intracellular recordings of the pacemaker tissue showed that 1—2% halothane reduces the slope of pacemaker potential, an effect expected to slow the rate of discharge. Halothane also decreases the maximum diastolic potential, approaching the threshold potential which is not significantly changed. Taking this action alone, the heart rate would be expected to increase. The combined effect, nevertheless, is a net decrease in discharge rate of the node.

Earlier clinical experience indicated that various arrhythmias may occur during halothane anesthesia. These arrhythmias are usually transient in nature and often associated with surgical manipulation during light anesthesia or hypercarbia. In adults, ventricular arrhythmias occur at a mean Pa_{CO_2} of 86 mmHg and a pHa of 7.10 (FUKUSHIMA et al., 1968). In children anesthetized with halothane a Pa_{CO_2} of 104—150 mmHg is the threshold for the development of ventricular arrhythmia (BLACK, 1967). With modern practice of anesthesia where close attention to ventilation is the accepted doctrine, one usually would not expect this degree of hypercarbia to occur.

The administration of a catecholamine during halothane anesthesia poses a different problem. The original pharmacologic study of RAVENTÓS (1956) and earlier clinical experience suggested that halothane may sensitize the heart to the action of catecholamines leading to serious ventricular arrhythmias. Indeed, episodes of asystole and ventricular fibrillation still occur after injection of epinephrine for hemostatic purposes. KATZ et al. (1962) questioned the absolute contraindication between epinephrine and halothane. They believe that the occurrence of ventricular arrhythmia is related to the dose of epinephrine administered. In a series of 100 surgical patients under halothane anesthesia subcutaneous infiltration of epinephrine (100 μg, 6 ml of 1:60,000 solution) does not increase the incidence of ventricular arrhythmia as compared with a control group of patients. KATZ et al. (1962) recommended that if local hemostasis is desired epinephrine should be used in dilute solutions (1:100,000) and not more than 10 ml (100 μg of epinephrine) should be given in any 10 min and not more than 30 ml (300 μg) in any hour. Strict attention to adequate ventilation is also recommended.

However, the proposed guide has not always been possible to follow. The safety of other vasopressors has been explored. Octapressin (2-phenylalanine-8-lysine vasopressin, PLV-2) has a local vasoconstrictor effect suitable for hemostatic purposes or even superior to that of epinephrine (KLINGERSTRÖM and WESTERMARK, 1963). It does not produce ventricular arrhythmia in anesthetized man when up to ten units is injected intravenously (SHANKS, 1963; KATZ, 1965). Octapressin is being used in Europe but is not yet available in the United States.

Beta-adrenergic receptor blockade with pronethalol or propranolol effectively terminates ventricular arrhythmia (JOHNSTONE, 1964; PAYNE and SENFIELD, 1964; FUKUSHIMA et al., 1968). This therapy may be indicated on rare occasions of persistent and serious arrhythmias such as multifocal ventricular extrasystoles and ventricular tachycardia. But as discussed above, the usual arrhythmias encountered during anesthesia are transient with little consequence on hemodynamics. Although beta receptor blockade has minimal cardiovascular effects on the heart rate and myocardial contractility (CRAYTHORNE and HUFFINGTON, 1966) these consequences should be seriously considered before propanolol or other similar drugs are administered, particularly in patients with frank or incipient congestive heart failure (KATZ and EPSTEIN, 1968). ELLIOTT et al (1968) also suggested that propanolol should be used with caution during halothane anesthesia. In asthmatic patients, propanolol increases airway resistance and decreases forced expiratory volume considerably (MACDONALD and MCNEILL, 1968). Beta receptor blocking drugs would seem unsuitable in these subjects.

Lidocaine in doses of 1—2 mg/kg intravenously is an effective antiarrhythmic agent. Its action lasts about 10—20 min, a duration considered sufficient to correct underlying causes for the arrhythmias (see KATZ and EPSTEIN, 1968).

Peripheral Circulation. Halothane reduces total peripheral resistance (TPR) in dogs (STIRLING et al., 1960; SMITH and CORBASCIO, 1966; THEYE, 1967) and in man (MORROW and MORROW, 1961; DEUTSCH et al., 1962; EGER et al., 1968).

DEUTSCH et al. (1962) observed a decrease of 17—19% in TPR during inhalation of about 2% halothane (inspired). With an alveolar halothane concentration varying from 0.8—2%, TPR decreases, ranging from 10—35% (EGER et al., 1968). However, halothane does not dilate all vascular beds. In certain organs halothane appears to cause vasoconstriction.

The increase in cerebral blood flow and decrease in cerebral vascular resistance has been discussed earlier in this section (see above). In dogs changes in coronary blood flow are variable [PRICE et al., 1968; NGAI et al., 1969 (1)], presumably the sum of anesthetic action on the coronary vessels per se and influences of other variables which determine coronary vascular resistance and blood flow. These may include the perfusion pressure, heart rate, myocardial tension, work of the heart and oxygen demand.

Halothane (1.2—1.6%, inspired) does not change the splanchnic vascular resistance in man (EPSTEIN et al., 1966). The splanchnic blood flow decreases from a mean of 1,880—1,320 ml/min, apparently related to the reduced perfusion pressure. However, a decrease in the intravascular distending force (pressure) and a probable increase in viscosity of blood secondary to decrease in blood flow should result in an apparent increase in resistance. The fact that the measured resistance does not change would imply that halothane may in fact cause vasodilation in this vascular bed. As the splanchnic circulation usually participates actively in hemodynamic adjustments, the absence of splanchnic vasoconstriction in the face of hypotension indicates that halothane interferes with reflex compensatory mechanisms or vascular response to sympathetic activity. Further evidence is the finding of EPSTEIN et al. (1966) that hypercarbia (Pa_{CO_2}, 60 mmHg) during halothane anesthesia increases splanchnic blood flow and decreases vascular resistance. Sympathetic activation, if indeed occurring during hypercarbia, does not have its usual effect on the splanchnic circulation. Instead the direct vasodilating action of carbon dioxide seems to prevail.

Renal vascular resistance increases during halothane anesthesia (MAZZE et al., 1963; DEUTSCH et al., 1966). The effective renal plasma flow decreases 38% and the renal vascular resistance increases 69%. These changes are presumably intrarenal hemodynamic adjustment to the reduced perfusion pressure and elevated vena caval pressure, although increased blood levels of renin or release of vasopressin from the posterior pituitary gland have been suggested as possible mechanisms (GOLDBERG, 1968).

Changes in blood flow and vascular resistance in the skin and muscle have important bearing on the overall hemodynamics because of their relative tissue mass. Clinical observations would certainly indicate that halothane dilates cutaneous vessels. The skin is warm, pink with dilated veins. Measurements in man confirm this. The forearm blood flow increases from 2.6—4 ml/100 ml/min and the resistance decreases from 34—18 units (BLACK and McARDLE, 1962). THOMSON (1967), using a heat clearance technique to measure skin blood flow in man, also found halothane more than doubles the skin blood flow and reduces the calculated skin vascular resistance to 42% of control. Dilation of skin vessels is not limited to arterioles as reflected by change in resistance to inflow. CAFFREY et al. (1965) showed that halothane increases the forearm venous compliance, indicating venous relaxation as well. Question arises as to the basis of cutaneous vasodilation. The data of BLACK and McARDLE (1962) indicate that halothane causes vasodilation through decreased sympathetic discharge as upper arm nerve block increases the blood flow and halothane produces no further change. On the other hand, cross perfusion experiments in dogs show that administration of halothane to the donor, therefore reaching only the limb, increases the venous outflow from the limb (Burn and Epstein, 1959). Emerson and Massion (1967) also found a lowered limb resistance with halothane in dogs whether the limb is innervated or denervated, indicating a direct action of halothane. More recently, Kaijser et al. (1969) showed that in cats as the corneal reflex disappears during halothane inhalation skin vascular resistance averages 51% of control.

Vascular resistance in the skeletal muscle appears to increase with halothane. Lindgren et al. (1965) using skinned hind limbs of cats found a reduction in blood flow. In the isolated gracilis muscle of dogs, perfusion with blood exposed to halothane in a pump oxygenator results in vasodilation [Christoforo and Brody, 1968 (2)]. However, if the muscle is perfused with blood from a donor, administration of halothane to the donor causes vasoconstriction. Christoforo and Brody suggested that halothane may release vasopressin as exclusion of the donor's head from the circulation eliminates the vasoconstriction effect. While plausible, this suggestion needs confirmation in respect to blood levels of vasopressin. In any case, vasopressin release would certainly not explain the decrease in TPR, and specifically, the cutaneous vascular resistance.

At the level of microcirculation, direct visual observation of splanchnic vessels provides the opportunity to study vasomotion, blood flow and vascular response to exogenous epinephrine or other vasoactive substances. Light halothane anesthesia (0.8%, inspired) increases spontaneous vasomotion in the capillaries of dog omentum or rat mesoappendix. Sensitivity to topically applied epinephrine increases. Arteriolar diameter and venule outflow remain unchanged. With increasing halothane concentration (up to 2%) all of these functions are progressively depressed. Pre- and postcapillary vessels dilate and capillary blood flow appears sluggish (Baez and Orkin, 1963).

Changes in mesenteric vascular response to adrenergic transmitters have parallels in other tissues. Garfield et al. (1968) and Price et al. (1968) found in dogs that halothane (0.25—1.5%, inspired) potentiates the response of heart rate to postganglionic sympathetic stimulation. On the other hand, in man the decrease in forearm blood flow during intraarterial infusion of norepinephrine is markedly attenuated by halothane anesthesia (1—4%, inspired) (Black and McArdle, 1962). As mentioned above, hypercarbia caused splanchnic vasodilation instead of the usual vasoconstrictor response (Epstein et al., 1966). In spinal cats halothane reduced the pressor response to stellate ganglion or splanchnic nerve stimulation (Purchase, 1965). These observations would indicate that halothane may interfere with the release of neurotransmitters or the receptor response to neurotransmitters.

Studies on the release and uptake of norepinephrine by peripheral adrenergic nerve gave essentially negative results. The plasma norepinephrine and epinephrine concentrations do not change significantly during light and deep halothane anesthesia (Price et al., 1959; Hamelberg et al., 1960; Elliott et al., 1968). This may be taken as indirect evidence that halothane does not affect the release of these amines. But the normal plasma catecholamine concentration is usually so low (less than 1 µg/l) as to make assessment of these data difficult. Urinary excretion of catecholamines may provide a better index of their release. Again, halothane anesthesia produces no significant changes (Giesecke et al., 1967). In only one isolated report on a patient with pheochromocytoma halothane appeared to suppress the release of norepinephrine and epinephrine from the tumor (Etsten and Shimosato, 1965). Plasma norepinephrine concentration decreased from 1,660 µg/l before anesthesia to 358 and 69 µg/l at 9 and 30 min following induction, respectively. Epinephrine concentrations in the plasma decreased about the same extent.

Attempts have been made to study the effect of halothane on norepinephrine release and uptake by peripheral adrenergic tissues using isotopic technics. In dogs, after pre-labelling the myocardial norepinephrine stores with intracoronary infusion of ^{3}H-norepinephrine (100 μc, 3.4 μg base), radioactivity in the coronary sinus blood and arterio-venous difference across the heart may be taken as a measure of norepinephrine release. Halothane (0.75—1%, inspired) does not appear to change the pattern of norepinephrine release [NGAI et al., 1969 (1)]. The uptake of norepinephrine is not affected by halothane either. In cat ventricular slices incubated in modified Kreb's solution containing ^{3}H-norepinephrine (10 mμg/ml, base) halothane does not change the tissue/medium radioactivity ratio (NAITO and GILLIS, 1968). In rats, after a rapid intravenous injection of 10 μc of ^{3}H-norepinephrine (0.34 μg, base), the specific activities of heart norepinephrine are essentially the same in halothane anesthetized animals as that of controls [NGAI et al., 1969 (1)]. In rats, halothane does not affect the myocardial norepinephrine contents or its turnover rate as measured by the conversion of ^{14}C-tyrosine to ^{14}C-norepinephrine [NGAI et al., 1969 (2)]. All of these findings would indicate that halothane has no significant effect on the peripheral adrenergic system, including biosynthesis, release and uptake of norepinephrine. The effect of halothane on the myocardium, vascular smooth muscle and on their response to sympathetic nerve stimulation or exogenous norepinephrine is most likely due to changes in receptor reactivity, a postsynaptic action. The biochemical bases of this action remain to be elucidated.

Some Other Aspects of Circulation. Halothane in anesthetic concentrations has no measurable effect on the viscosity of blood (BOYAN et al., 1966; BEHAR and ALEXANDER, 1966) or the surface tension of blood and plasma (ARONSON et al., 1967). However, a decrease in blood flow through capillaries and small blood vessels would reduce the shear rate resulting in an apparent increase in viscosity. The contribution of this change to measured vascular resistance is essentially not defined.

Halothane has been reported to increase the blood volume in man. Using Evans blue dye, PAYNE et al. (1959) observed an average increase of 700 ml (14%) 10 min after induction of surgical anethesia. In ten patients GRABLE et al. (1962) found a 10% increase in blood volume after 30 min of halothane anesthesia. Perhaps these changes can be explained on the basis of decreased hydrostatic pressure in the capillaries although the major determinant of hydrostatic pressure, the venous pressure, may increase during halothane anesthesia. MORSE et al. (1963) failed to observe any significant alterations in total blood volume or plasma volume during halothane anesthesia lasting up to 110 min. The reasons for this discrepancy are not clear. PAYNE et al. (1959) and GRABLE et al. (1962) did not measure the venous pressure, whereas MORSE et al. (1963) demonstrated an inverse relationship between central venous pressure and plasma volume.

Drug Interactions. The anesthetic requirement of halothane can be influenced by drugs which change the central catecholamine concentrations (MILLER et al., 1968) as mentioned in the section on the Nervous System. Depletion of peripheral adrenergic stores has been of concern in the past. Some reports suggested that antihypertensive therapy with drugs such as reserpine may represent an added risk during anesthesia (see, for instance, COAKLEY et al., 1956). However, clinical experiences (MUNSON and JENICEK, 1962; MORROW and MORROW, 1963; KATZ et al., 1964) indicate that incidences of hypotension during anesthesia are no greater in patients given reserpine as compared with those not on drug therapy. Hypotension, if it occurs, is usually related to blood loss, depth of anesthesia, surgical manipulation or other factors. Furthermore, as drug depletion of adrenergic stores does not radically alter the receptor response, hypotension usually can be corrected with direct acting vasopressors if this becomes necessary (with due considerations to the halothane induced change in receptor sensitivity and the arrhythmigenic action of catecholamines). OMINSKY and WOLLMAN (1969) expressed the opinion that in hypertensive patients an effective therapeutic regime should not be discontinued before anesthesia. More important is the knowledge of drug action.

Interaction between halothane and digitalis is of interest. In dogs, pretreatment with digitalis attenuates the myocardial depressant and hypotensive actions of halothane (GOLDBERG et al., 1962; SHIMOSATO and ETSTEN, 1963). The toxicity of ouabain as manifested by multiple premature ventricular contractions is reduced considerably by halothane, cumulative toxic doses being 44—46 μg/kg during pentobarbital and 76—78 μg/kg during halothane anesthesia (MORROW and TOWNLEY, 1963). MORROW (1967) also provided data in dogs that during halothane anesthesia concomitant intravenous infusion of norepinephrine (0.017—0.5 μg/kg/ min) reduces the dose of ouabain required to initiate ventricular arrhythmia. Among other action, digitalis may interfere with the uptake of norepinephrine by adrenergic tissues (BOGDANSKI and BRODIE, 1969). Perhaps the arrhythmic effect of digitalis is related to this action. Halothane may attenuate the toxicity of digitalis through changes in receptor sensitivity. Conversely, the negative inotropic effect of halothane is partially antagonized by digitalis, involving contractile elements of the myocardium.

E. Liver

The possible effects of halothane on the liver have been carefully examined by RAVENTÓS (1956) before clinical trials. In various species acute and chronic exposure to anesthetic doses of halothane failed to produce significant functional or morphological changes. Other investigators essentially confirmed RAVENTÓS' original observation. However, in the early 1960s a number of clinical reports cast suspision on halothane as a possible cause of postoperative hepatic damage. These led to re-examination of this problem. In the past few years, the literature is replete with reports concerning toxicology, epidemological surveys, prospective studies in surgical patients and case reports as well as opinions. The Committee on Anesthesia of the National Research Council of the United States conducted an extensive retrospective survey, the National Halothane Study (BUNKER et al., 1969). This and other reports indicate that fatal hepatic necrosis following anesthesia with halothane or other agents occurs rarely. Nevertheless, the problem appears unresolved. LITTLE (1968) reviewed the current state of knowledge. Hepatic effects of anesthesia will be discussed in detail elsewhere in this monograph (Section 4.3). This section will therefore mention only a few pertinent aspects.

Existing evidences indicate that halothane, like other general anesthetics, may affect hepatic function. In man minor and transient abnormalities of hepatic function have been observed. These include changes in serum cholinesterase, cholesterol esterification, alkaline phosphatase, serum bilirubin and serum enzyme activities, glutamic oxaloacetic transaminase (GOT), glutamic pyruvic transaminase (GPT) and ornithine carbamyl transferase (OCT). However, subjects anesthetized with other commonly used anesthetics such as diethyl ether, cyclopropane and nitrous oxide show similar degrees of dysfunction (see LITTLE, 1968). Thus in small clinical series a specific toxic effect of halothane has not been demonstrated. Rather, the stress of general anesthesia and surgery may be contributing factors. Only in one report when the calf liver is being perfused with blood equilibrated with rather high concentrations (3—6%) of halothane, depression of hepatic function has been observed (MIDDLETON et al., 1966). Oxygen consumption and sulfo-bromophthalein excretion fall. The serum GOT activity increases.

It has been speculated that hypotension and hypercarbia during halothane may contribute to transient hepatic dysfunction. MORRIS and FELDMAN (1963) found in man that hypercarbia during halothane anesthesia results in transient hepatic dysfunction of a greater magnitude, suggesting that hypercarbia may compromise hepatic perfusion through splanchnic vasoconstriction. However, whatever action hypercarbia may have on the liver in conjunction with halothane, it seems not mediated through changes in splanchnic circulation (see above, section on Circulatory System).

PRICE et al. (1966) further examined the possible effects of reduced regional blood flow on hepatic function. The ability of the liver to extract indocyanin green is reduced to 66% of control. As hypercarbia increases the splanchnic blood flow, the dye clearance improves slightly to about 73% of control. Interestingly, in spite of the reduced splanchnic blood flow the average oxygen consumption of the splanchnic viscerae does not change significantly. Oxygen consumption is maintained at the expense of a reduced hepatic venous oxygen tension from 53—47 mmHg. If excess lactate can be taken as a measure of tissue hypoxia, halothane anesthesia does not increase excess lactate across the liver. The systemic arterial and venous blood, however, have a small but significant increase in excess lactate.

Morphologically, fatty infiltration and vacuolization of hepatic cells have been observed in various species exposed to halothane. While chloroform always produces necrotic lesions, halothane is notably free of such an effect. Studies of ultra-structures in the hepatic cell also failed to provide evidence for a direct toxic action of halothane in anesthetic concentrations (W. R. BLACKBURN and G. P. HOECH, Jr., personal communication). Changes have been observed only with higher concentrations in perfused liver (MIDDLETON et al., 1966). With 3% halothane vapor added to the perfusate, the smooth endoplasmic reticulum appears to increase. Exposure to 5—6% halothane vapor causes a striking distortion of mitochondrial structure with wrinkling of the outer membrane, loss of cristae and decreased matrix density. In addition, there are vesiculation of rough endoplasmic reticulum and clumping of nuclear chromatin. The significance of these organelle changes is not clear at present because of the high concentration of halothane and nature of the experimental preparation.

Morphologic lesions in man, if they are indeed induced by halothane, are also quite variable in appearance. GALL (1969) summarized the problems involved in determining the etiologic factors for hepatic necrosis after anesthesia and operation. Pre-existing disease, adjuvant treatments and adventitious illness such as viral hepatitis are possibilities not easily ruled out. The National Halothane Study procured protocols of 10,171 autopsies from an estimated total of 856,515 anesthetic exposures, about 30% of which involved halothane. Hepatic necrosis of various degrees was found in 222 cases: 82 massive, 115 intermediate and 25 minor. A multidisciplinary panel reviewed clinical histories and microscopic sections of the liver from cases with massive and intermediate necrosis. The review was carried out without knowledge of the anesthetic used. In the majority causes other than anesthetic have been considered responsible for the hepatic injury. These include shock, prolonged use of vasopressors, overwhelming infection, severe and prolonged congestive heart failure and pre-existing hepatic disease. There remained a small number of cases in which the immediate cause of hepatic injury was unexplained: 9 massive and 10 intermediate necrosis. Of the 9 cases of massive hepatic necrosis, 7 had halothane anesthesia, one each, ether and cyclopropane. Seven of the 10 cases of intermediate necrosis received halothane anesthesia, 2 had ether and 1, nitrous oxide anesthesia (FORREST, 1969).

On the basis of "blind" clinical and pathologic evaluation one might consider that anesthesia may be contributory in some way to the "unexplained" hepatic damage. Yet the panel of pathologists could find no consistent histologic pattern attributable to halothane. The histologic lesions simulate those encountered in fatal viral and some drug-induced forms of hepatitis. The question of concomitant viral infection or direct toxicity of halothane remains unresolved (GALL, 1969). It must be noted that the incidence of post-anesthetic massive hepatic necrosis leading to death is low, about one in 10,000, including that from all causes and involving all commonly used anesthetics.

It would appear that by all criteria halothane is not a direct hepatotoxin. Hepatic lesions are not produced with regularity in animals or in man. The administered dose bears no relationship to the development of hepatic necrosis (except that with exceedingly high concentration in vitro, some secondary effects of unknown mechanism may manifest themselves). The latency of onset of symptoms related to hepatic injury also varies a great deal, from one to as long as 28 days. Thus, none of the prerequisites of a true hepatotoxin as defined by KLATSKIN (1960, 1968) is met in the case of hepatic necrosis associated with halothane anesthesia.

Nevertheless, in the National Halothane Study, most of the "unexplained" cases of hepatic necrosis were associated with halothane anesthesia, often after repeated exposures. The incidence was such that the data could not be analyzed statistically. The possibility still exists, however, that on rare occasions halothane can be the causative factor. Two case reports strongly suggest that halothane can induce hepatitis through sensitization (BELFRAGE et al., 1966; KLATSKIN and KIMBERG, 1969). Both involved anesthetists who were repeatedly exposed to small concentrations of halothane. Deliberate challenge with halothane resulted in chills, fever, headache and myalgia within hours. These symptoms were associated with eosinophilia and other laboratory findings indicative of hepatic injury. Liver biopsy in one subject showed evidence of acute hepatitis. The same subject avoided further exposure to halothane without recurrence of symptoms and signs related to hepatitis (KLATSKIN and KIMBERG, 1969). Thus, halothane-induced hepatitis through this mechanism has been considered an entity (COMBES, 1969).

In perspective, taking all known factors into consideration, hepatic injury through sensitization with halothane appears to be a rare occurrence. Many questions remain unanswered: What are the incidences of fatal and non-fatal hepatic necrosis? If sensitization is indeed the cause, what are the mechanisms? More important, how does one identify the patient at risk? Except for deliberate challenge, can one use some immunologic tests? Are such tests reliable indices? In addition, is it possible that genetic abnormalities involving metabolic pathway of halothane may result in accumulation of toxic metabolites. These are difficult problems awaiting for future studies. It would seem that case reports are not likely to provide answers except to indicate that the problem remains. Clearly, with all the attributes of halothane the rare occurrence of hepatic injury, attributable to halothane or not, should not be taken as a reason to preclude the continued use of halothane. One must also weigh the relative mortality and morbidity of anesthesia from all causes. Again, such comparison between halothane and other common anesthetic practice is not available on sound statistical basis.

F. Other Systems

Kidney. Renal hemodynamics and excretory function are sensitive to many extrarenal influences. The organ also has the capacity of circulatory autoregulation. Changes in renal function during general anesthesia appear stereotyped regardless of the anesthetic administered. The basis for these changes, however, are subject to interpretation and speculation.

In dogs and in man the effects of halothane on renal function have been measured with clearance technics [BLACKMORE et al., 1960; MAZZE et al., 1963; DEUTSCH et al., 1966 (2)]. The study by DEUTSCH et al [1966 (2)] was conducted in young healthy volunteers. The subjects received no other drugs and measurements were carried out without concurrent surgical manipulation. Thus any change in renal function may be interpreted as the effect of halothane. either primarily on the kidney or secondary through some other mechanisms. In addition, adequate hydration before and during the study provided steady urine flow so that data obtained are more likely close estimates of actual values. Under these conditions halothane anesthesia (1.5%, inspired) reduces the estimated renal blood flow (ERBF, 38%) and glomerular filtration rate (GFR, 19%). The filtration fraction increases from 0.21—0.29 with a calculated renal vascular resistance rising from 88—135 arbitrary units. The urine volume falls drastically along with sodium excretion. Urine osmolality increases to a level of about 400% of control. The urine/plasma osmolality ratio also increases. Free water clearance approchesa zero or becomes negative, indicating antidiuresis.

Changes in renal hemodynamics, water and electrolyte clearance may be attributable to the fall in cardiac output and perfusion pressure. The increase in filtration fraction indicates that intrarenal autoregulatory mechanisms may be still operative. Available evidence on the cardiovascular effects of halothane (see above, section on Circulatory System) would suggest that sympathetic nervous activity plays little part in the efferent arteriolar constriction. An interesting observation of DEUTSCH et al. [1966 (2)] is that ethanol, in relatively small amounts (less than 300 ml), initiated a reversal of antidiuresis. As this volume of alcohol is not likely to affect plasma volume or circulatory hemodynamics significantly, its suppressant action on the release of antidiuretic hormone (ADH) strongly favors the possibility that anesthesia causes antidiuresis through ADH activity. Of course, other possibilities cannot be ruled out. These may include the reduced GFR and activation of the renin-angiotensin-aldosterone system through a decreased perfusion pressure.

Under clinical conditions, the use of narcotic premedicant, dehydration, surgical trauma and blood loss would certainly exaggerate the effect of halothane on renal function. The use of osmotic and sustained hydration can attenuate the action of anesthetic and maintain adequate urine flow (BARRY et al., 1964).

Although no data are available, recovery from halothane anesthesia should be accompanied by a restoration of renal function, provided that the state of hydration and circulatory status permit normal renal function. Nevertheless, postoperative suppression of water excretion has been reported, apparently due to ADH release consequent to surgical trauma (MORAN and ZIMMERMAN, 1967). DEUTSCH et al. [1966 (1)] reported a series of 11 elderly patients in whom water retention was more severe and prolonged postoperatively. These authors suggested that inappropriate release of ADH may contribute to the postoperative antidiuresis and hyponatremia. Anesthetic agents per se appear to play little role in the development of this syndrome.

Gastrointestinal Tract. Halothane suppresses salivary and mucous secretion as indicated by clinical experience. Halothane also depresses gastrointestinal motility in concentrations sufficient to maintain light surgical anesthesia in dogs (MARSHALL et al., 1961). Tonus of the gut as well as peristaltic activity decrease within 2—5 min after the administration of halothane. Recovery is equally prompt, requiring 5—10 min. These authors further found that halothane antagonizes the effects of morphine, neostigmine, acetyl-β-methylcholine and barium on intestinal motility, indicating that halothane acts peripherally, probably beyond the neuro-effector junction. An induced change in receptor sensitivity of gastrointestinal smooth muscle agrees well with the action of halothane on other smooth muscles such as the blood vessels and the uterus.

It should be noted that the depressant effects of halothane on the gastro-intestinal tract are not unique but similar to those of other commonly used general anesthetics. An exception is cyclopropane which does not affect the tonus or eliminate rhythmic contraction induced by morphine (WEISEL et al., 1938).

It is not possible to correlate the anesthetic action on gastrointestinal motility and incidences of postanesthetic nausea and vomiting. The reported incidences following halothane vary between 3.4—36% (see PURKIS, 1964). Variables such as sex, age, mental status, nature of operative procedures, as well as the use of narcotics, depth of anesthesia, changes in arterial pressure, occurrence of hyper-carbia and hypoxia, all would have bearings as have been discussed by BELLEVILLE (1961) and PURKIS (1964).

Uterus. In human non-gravid uterine muscle strips in vitro halothane does not change the resting tension but inhibits spontaneous contractions [MUNSON et al., 1968 (2)]. This effect is evident with about 0.37% halothane and virtually complete inhibition occurs with 1.12% halothane. Halothane appears to be a more potent uterine depressant as compared with cyclopropane and nitrous oxide. No significant change in contractility occurs when the muscle strips are exposed to these gases (10% cyclopropane or 50% nitrous oxide). In pregnant women halothane an-esthesia frequently abolishes uterine contraction and the degree of depression relates to the depth of anesthesia (EMBREY et al., 1958; VASICKA and KRETCHMER, 1961). Controversies exist as to the safety of halothane for obstetrical anesthesia. In respect to newborn depression the depth and duration of anesthesia seem important factors as with all general anesthetics. Uterine relaxation and possibility of increased postpartum bleeding are the major objections to halothane. But a number of clinical reports concluded that halothane is safe for obstetrical an-esthesia provided it is administered in the lowest possible concentration (see MOYA and SPICER, 1968). Regardless of the controversy, halothane has been considered an excellent anesthesia to provide prompt uterine relaxation when indicated, as chloroform was used for the same purpose many years ago.

Metabolism. Halothane appears to depress the overall metabolic activity as reflected by total oxygen consumption. According to SEVERINGHAUS and CULLEN (1958) and BERGMAN (1967), oxygen consumption decreases to about 80—85% of the basal level in man. In surgical patients who received premedicants and thiopental as induction agents, halothane (1—2%, inspired) decreases oxygen consumption to the same extent (NUNN and MATTHEWS, 1959). There is a corre-sponding reduction in carbon dioxide production, so that the respiratory quotient remains unchanged at 0.83 (NUNN and MATTHEWS, 1959; BERGMAN, 1967).

The contribution of premedicants and other drugs such as barbiturates and muscle relaxants to the reduced oxygen consumption has been studied by THEYE and TUOHY (1964). These authors compared the observed oxygen consumption with predicted basal values based upon sex, age and body surface area of subjects studied. Possible errors in preanesthetic oxygen consumption measurement from anxiety or other factors are perhaps avoided by this approach. In the absence of permedicant, barbiturate and muscle relaxant oxygen consumption averages 100% of predicted value during halothane anesthesia (1.07%, expired). Oxygen consumption is found to be related to body temperature. Muscle paralysis reduces oxygen consumption (84% of predicted basal value); so does premedication with pentobarbital and meperidine, and induction of anesthesia with thiopental (88 and 84% of predicted vasal values, respectively). Reversal of neuromuscular blockade with neostigmine is followed by an increase in oxygen consumption. Moreover, 2—5 h after premedication and thiopental induction oxygen consumption recovers partially from 88—94% of the predicted value while halothane anesthesia is being maintained (0.75%, expired). It would seem that skeletal muscular activity during anesthesia determines to a large extent the overall oxygen consumption. Changes in oxygen cost of breathing and myocardial work are also expected to influence oxygen consumption.

Changes in oxygen consumption of various vital tissues have been studied in vivo and in vitro. In the dog, oxygen uptake of cerebral cortex decreases from 4.8—2.5 ml/100 gm/min during halothane anesthesia (0.5%, inspired) (McDowall et al., 1963). In normal man WOLLMAN et al. (1964) found that the cerebral oxygen consumption averages 2.8 ml/100 gm/min during halothane anesthesia (1.03%, end-tidal), a slight decrease from that of awake subjects, 3.1 ml/100 gm/min. These authors attributed this change to a fall in body temperature. In vitro studies of HOECH et al. (1966) with rat brain slices showed that 1% halothane depresses oxygen consumption only during the first hour of exposure, but has no significant effect upon continued exposure or after removal of halothane vapor. With cation stimulated brain slices the depressant effect of halothane on oxygen consumption is significantly greater and persists throughout the duration of exposure (2 h).

The myocardial oxygen consumption during halothane anesthesia appears to relate directly with myocardial work (THEYE, 1967). In paralyzed dogs with a right heart bypass providing a steady body perfusion at 2.0 l/min/m², the relationship during halothane inhalation (1%, inspired) can be expressed as $y = 1.4 \pm 2.1$ x, where y is the myocardial oxygen consumption and x, the left ventricular external work. In vitro studies with rat heart slices show that 2% halothane vapor is required to decrease oxygen uptake significantly (HOECH et al., 1966). It would appear, therefore, that in clinically used concentrations the effect of halothane on myocardial oxygen consumption is secondary to decreased myocardial contractility and external work because of reduced cardiac output and arterial pressure.

Changes in oxygen consumption by liver slices exposed to halothane are similar to those observed with heart slices. 1% halothane has no effect and 2% reduces oxygen consumption to about 77% of control (HOECH et al., 1966). In man, halothane anesthesia (1.5%, inspired) produces a slight and insignificant decrease in splanchnic oxygen consumption (PRICE et al., 1966).

The adequacy of tissue oxygenation in the face of depressed circulation is an important consideration. Available evidences indicate that the metabolic demand of vital organs is being met adequately during halothane anesthesia. In dogs and in man halothane anesthesia is not accompanied by biochemical changes indicative of tissue hypoxia. Arterial blood lactate concentration and "excess lactate" show a slight increase but changes are not significant (LOWENSTEIN et al., 1964; PRICE et al., 1966; THEYE and SESSLER, 1967). Cerebral glucose utilization and lactate production (COHEN et al., 1964) as well as arteriovenous difference of lactate and pyruvate across the liver remain unchanged (PRICE et al., 1966).

In dogs, halothane reduces the blood glucose concentration slightly or causes no change (DOBKIN and FEDORUK, 1961; GALLA and WILSON, 1964). In man, however, blood glucose tends to increase to a concentration of about 120 mg/100 ml (KEATING et al., 1959; COHEN et al., 1964; SCHWEIZER et al., 1967). The moderate degree of hyperglycemia apparently results from an inhibited cellular uptake of glucose. Removal of glucose from the plasma after a glucose load is impeded during halothane anesthesia (GALLA and WILSON, 1964). GALLA (1967) further showed in dogs that turnover rate of glucose decreases significantly during halothane anesthesia. In vitro studies with human red blood cells also indicate that halothane interferes with cellular uptake of glucose (GREENE, 1965; GREENE and CERVENKO, 1967). The inhibitory effect of halothane on active transport across cell membrane has also been suggested by studies with tyrosine in rats [NGAI et al., 1969 (2)]. During infusion of ^{14}C-tyrosine at a constant rate the fractional rate constants of plasma tyrosine are 0.047 min^{-1} in control animals and 0.041 min^{-1} in animals under halothane anesthesia (1%, inspired). Expressed differently, the average life time for a tyrosine molecule in the plasma is about 21 min in control animals and 24 min in animals during halothane anesthesia. Perhaps the impeded rate of disappearance of glucose or tyrosine from plasma is related to circulatory depression in that halothane decreases perfusion of tissues which utilize these metabolic substrates. However, the view that halothane inhibits active transport mechanism has some support from the work of ANDERSEN (1966) with toad bladder. With 2% halothane the short-circuited current, an index of active sodium transport, decreases as much as 38%.

Cellular utilization of glucose is most likely not impaired (GALLA, 1967; COHEN et al., 1964). The effect of halothane on the metabolic pathways of amino acids remains to be studied although BRUCE et al. (1968) showed in rats that incorporation of ^{3}H-thymidine into deoxyribonucleic acid is not inhibited by halothane (0.5%, inspired).

Cellular Function. The effect of halothane on mitochondrial function and cellular metabolism has been studied only recently with various preparations in vitro. FINK and KENNY (1968) and FINK et al. (1969) reported that halothane in clinically used concentrations reduces oxygen uptake, inhibits cell growth, increases glucose utilization and lactate production with mouse heteroploid cell culture. The same effects have been observed with mouse ascites tumor cells (Sarcoma Ia) except that these are more sensitive, appreciable effects can be observed with vapor concentrations of halothane as low as 0.05—0.1%. Using rat hepatic mitochondrial suspension COHEN and MARSHALL (1968) found a dose related inhibition of oxygen uptake in the presence of glutamate. This effect is discernible with halothane concentration of 0.7%, reaches a maximum with 3% whereupon the mitochondrial oxygen uptake is 25% of control. It is reversible after exposure of mitochondrial preparations to halothane in concentrations up to 2%, beyond which the reversibility is progressively impaired. These investigators concluded that halothane reversibly inhibits oxidation of reduced nicotinamide adenine dinucleotide (NADH). They further found that halothane interfers with mitochondrial respiratory control.

Halothane in concentrations up to 5% does not affect the anaerobic glycolysis of brain homogenates in vitro (HOECH et al., 1966). The activity of magnesium dependent sodium-potassium activated ATPase in brain homogenates or microsomal preparation is not depressed by halothane either (HOECH and MATTEO, personal communication). UEDA and MIETANI (1967) observed that halothane inhibits this enzyme but only in concentrations exceeding that used clinically. UEDA (1965) also gave evidence from studies on firefly luciferin bioluminescene that halothane may interfere with ATP utilization, an action shared by other anesthetics such as diethyl ether.

An interesting action of halothane on cytoplasmic structure has been observed by ALLISON and NUNN (1968). Microtubules, a highly organized ultrastructure composed of protein lattice and believed to form the scaffold for certain cellular functions, are depolymerized upon exposure to clinical concentrations of halothane (2%). Disruption of orderly arrangement of protein aggregates results in retraction of axopods of *Actinosphaerium*. Mitotic process of plant and mammalian cells stops at the metaphase. Furthermore, halothane makes asters disappear and reduces the birefrigence of mitotic spindles in fertilized *Arbacia* eggs. These effects of halothane are reversible unless cells are exposed to higher halothane concentrations (5—6%) whereupon cellular dissolution occurs. ALLISON and NUNN suggested that anesthetics interact with cellular protein system to bring about such diverse effects. Interaction between anesthetics and protein has been suggested by CLEMENTS and WILSON (1962) and SCHOENBORN et al. (1964). In addition, interference with mitosis has also been shown with halothane in the neural tube of developing chick embryos (SNEGIREFF et al., 1968). On the other hand, BRUCE and TRAURIG (1969) studied the mitotic indices of small intestinal crypt cells in adult rats and found no difference between control animals and those anesthetized with 0.5% halothane.

Teratogenicity of halothane has been reported. In the chick embryo exposure to 2% halothane significantly increases the death rate and incidence of major anomalies (SMITH et al., 1965). In pregnant rats, incidences of fetal resorption, vertebral anomalies and lumbar ribs increase upon exposure to halothane, the vulnerable period being the 8th and 10th days of pregnancy. The degree of damage is related to the halothane concentration and duration of exposure (BASFORD and FINK, 1968).

These recent studies on cellular metabolism and function with anesthetics represent important advances in attempts to understand anesthetic action on a more basic level than organ functions. Although much remains to be elucidated, research along these lines should be expected to provide answers to the mechanisms of anesthetic effects and toxicity. However, at the present the clinical implication of cellular and treatogenetic effects of anesthetics is quite uncertain.

VIII. Clinical Considerations

Halothane is being used under almost all clinical circumstances. Contraindications have been suggested but so far unequivocal supporting evidence is not available. The fact that halothane holds such a widespread popularity among anesthetists does not necessarily mean, however, that it is an ideal anesthetic. An ideal anesthetic should be inexpensive to produce, pure, stable and nonflammable; it should have low solubility coefficients in blood and tissues and an intermediate potency; it should not depress respiration or circulation, or cause major disturbance of other physiologic functions; it should provide adequate muscular relaxation; the induction of anesthesia should be swift and pleasant; and the recovery should be prompt and free from ill effects (SEEVERS and WATERS, 1938; BEECHER and FORD, 1955; ARTUSIO and VAN POZNAK, 1958). Obviously, these considerations change with time, current requirement and state of knowledge. Mancy clinicians believe from personal experience and current available knowledge that halothane is nearly an ideal anesthetic. Nevertheless, the search for a better agent goes on as evidenced by the development of other anesthetics since the introduction of halothane.

The inherent properties and actions of an anesthetic are important but equally relevant are the clinician's training, knowledge and skill in anesthetic management.

Certain pharmacologic actions of halothane are of some concern. The potent cardiovascular depressant effect may lead to extreme hypotension and cardiac arrest. Earlier mishaps in this respect are relatively rare occurrences now, attributable to the use of precision vaporizers and clinicians' awareness of the problem. The common practice of administering halothane in conjunction with other anesthetics and adjuncts with the "balanced" technic would further minimize circulatory depression. According to some authors, moderate hypotension during halothane anesthesia is of no serious consequence. Large experience with deliberate hypotension using halothane appears to support this view.

The problem of hepatic damage through sensitization remains unresolved. In the absence of knowledge regarding its incidence, mechanisms, and suitable means of diagnosis, opinions rendered at present would seem premature. Equally lacking are reliable data on morbidity and mortality attributable to anesthetics per se or to anesthetic management related to the choice of agents. Proper judgement in perspective requires such information.

Pre-existing diseases of the liver and the biliary tract cannot be considered contraindications for the use of halothane. Experience in patients with jaundice of diverse origin, cirrhosis, or biliary tract pathology indicate that postoperative complications and death attributable to hepatic damage are not more frequent with halothane anesthesia (see NGAI, 1969). The National Halothane Study provided further data to refute the notion that halothane anesthesia should not be used for operations on the biliary tract (BUNKER and VANDAM, 1969).

Vasodilation of cerebral vessels and increase in intracranial pressure during halothane anesthesia have been considered hazardous in patients with space-occupying intracranial lesions (JENNETT et al., 1969). However, halothane has been used extensively for neurosurgical procedures, frequently as the drug of choice. As cerebral vessels retain the responsiveness to changes in carbon dioxide tension, hyperventilation together with some degree of hypotension apparently more than compensate for the cerebral vasodilation. Satisfactory operating conditions usually can be achieved.

A. Specific Applications

Halothane is being used to advantage for certain purposes. Deliberate hypotension with halothane anesthesia is readily reversible. As adequate tissue perfusion requires some minimum arterial pressure, guidelines established from past experience should be respected, particularly in patients with cardiovascular diseases.

Halothane facilitates the induction of intentional hypothermia because of cutaneous vasodilation and depression of temperature regulating centers. Indications for hypothermia may include cardiopulmonary by-pass and some intracranial operations, especially when momentary vascular occlusion or elective circulatory arrest is required (CAMPKIN and DALLAS, 1968; GISSEN et al., 1969).

The cerebral vasodilating action of halothane has been suggested to be beneficial under circumstances where cerebral circulation may be compromised by disease or surgical intervention. Definitive data to support this contention are not yet available. Also, there has been no information concerning the value of halothane to relieve cerebral vasospasm.

The use of halothane in pediatric patients may represent one of the more important contributions of this agent to modern anesthesia. Absence of airway irritation by halothane vapor and rapid induction of anesthetic state offer considerable advantages. Infants and children have a relatively small body oxygen store as compared to adults. A smooth and tranquil induction provides an added margin of safety. It also minimizes possible psychic effects of the overall surgical experience. Of importance is the fact that the rate of anesthetic equilibration in infants and children is faster than that in adults (SALANITRE and RACKOW, 1969). "Overpressure" as commonly practiced for induction carries inherent hazards in all patients and particularly in the young.

Current concepts in respect to therapy of shock favor peripheral vasodilation to improve tissue perfusion and oxygenation (see for instance, HERSHEY et al., 1968). DRUCKER et al. (1965) showed in dogs during hypovolemic shock that halothane anesthesia is accompanied by less metabolic disturbances as compared with cyclopropane. Dogs tolerate hemorrhagic shock better with halothane anesthesia than cyclopropane anesthesia (FABIAN et al., 1962). Such controlled comparisons are not possible under clinical conditions. However, one would expect that in the face of significant hypovolemia with compensatory vasoconstriction, halothane anesthesia may well cause decompensation resulting in further fall in the arterial pressure inconsistent with life.

B. Miscellaneous After-effects

Postanesthetic excitement has been correlated with a number of factors (ECKENHOFF et al., 1961). Youth, health, premedication with barbiturate and belladonna, operative procedures, as well as anesthetics influence the incidence of this early postanesthetic complication. The overall incidence of excitement in a large series (14,436 patients) is 5.3%. In 377 patients anesthetized with halothane and nitrous oxide ten developed excitement, an incidence of 2.65%. Other clinical reports also give the impression that recovery from halothane anesthesia is usually tranquil (see for example, JOHNSTONE, 1956; BURNAP et al., 1958).

Shivering occurs frequently following halothane anesthesia. MOIR and DOYLE (1963) reported an incidence of 24% having a significant correlation with decreases in body temperature. Shivering is therefore a response of the temperature regulating centers upon recovery from anesthesia. The generalized muscular activity markedly increases oxygen consumption at a time when the cardiopulmonary functional reserve may be already compromised. Although the majority of patients appear able to cope with the increased oxygen demand by increases in ventilatory volume and cardiac output (BAY et al., 1968), the added strain may well be detrimental in patients with respiratory embarrassment or fixed low cardiac output. Efforts to maintain body temperature during anesthesia and operation, especially in children, would seem beneficial on this account alone. Oxygen inhalation is a readily available therapy to supply the added oxygen needed during shivering.

Postanesthetic *headache* may be attributed to many factors. Halothane anesthesia is associated with a rather high incidence of this complication. In a limited series, TYRRELL and FELDMAN (1968) found that 60% of patients complained of headache following halothane anesthesia with spontaneous respiration (Pa_{CO_2}, 45 mmHg). In patients anesthetized with nitrous oxide, paralyzed with d-tubocurarine and artificially ventilated (Pa_{CO_2}, 33.4 mmHg), only 12% had headache. These observations suggest that headache following halothane anesthesia is probably related to changes in cerebral hemodynamics.

IX. Concluding Remarks

Halothane, designed according to a number of specifications formulated 20 years ago, has been applied to clinical anesthesia with success and wide acceptance. It meets the requirement of a nonflammable and potent anesthetic. The physical and chemical properties and the pharmacologic actions of halothane are such that it can be administered under almost all clinical circumstances. At the same time advances in technology and in sciences related to anesthesiology made possible the thorough and exhaustive study of halothane. Knowledge gained has been applied to clinical practice to advantage. However, much about halothane as well as anesthesia in general remain to be investigated. The continuing search for newer anesthetics reflects the need for a better agent. As the state of anesthesia by definition involves a change in vital functions, at least those of the nervous system, perhaps knowledge and experience are more important considerations.

References

ALLEN, G. D., WARD, R. J., PERRIN, E. B.: Reversal of apnea following artificial ventilation under anesthesia. Anesthesia & Analgesia **46**, 690—697 (1967).

ALLISON, A. C., NUNN, J. F.: Effects of general anaesthetics on microtubules. Lancet **1968 II**, 1326—1329.

ANDERSEN, N. B.: Effect of general anesthetics on sodium transport in the isolated toad bladder. Anesthesiology **27**, 304—310 (1966).

ARONSON, H. B., LAASBERG, H., CHARM, S., ETSTEN, B.: Influence of anaesthetic agents upon plasma electrophoretic mobility and surface tension as related to blood viscosity. Anesthesia & Analgesia **46**, 642—647 (1967).

ARTUSIO, J. F., JR., VAN POZNAK, A.: The concept of intermediate potency. Far East J. Anesth. **21**, 27 (1958).

ASKROG, V. F., PENDER, J. W., SMITH, T. C., ECKENHOFF, J. E.: Change in respiratory dead space during halothane, cyclopropane and nitrous oxide anesthesia. Anesthesiology **25**, 342—352 (1964).

BABAD, A. A., EGER, E. I. II.: The effects of hyperthyroidism and hypothyroidism on halothane and oxygen requirements in dogs. Anesthesiology **29**, 1087—1093 (1968).

BACKMAN, L. E., LÖFSTROM, B., WIDEN, L.: Electro-encephalography in halothane anaesthesia. Acta Anaesth. Scand. 8, 472—474 (1964).

BAEZ, S., ORKIN, L. R.: Effects of anesthetics on the response of the microcirculation to circulaory humors. Anesthesiology **24**, 568—579 (1963).

BARRY, K. G., MAZZE, R. I., SCHWARTZ, F. D.: Prevention of surgical oliguria and renal hemodynamic suppression of sustained hydration. New Engl. J. Med. **270**, 1371—1377 (1964).

BASFORD, A. B., FINK, B. R.: The teratogenicity of halothane in the rat. Anesthesiology **29**, 1167—1173 (1968).

BAY, J., NUNN, J. F., PRYS-ROBERTS, C.: Factors influencing arterial P_{O_2} during recovery from anesthesia. Brit. J. Anaesthesia **40**, 398—407 (1968).

BEECHER, H. K., FORD, C.: Anesthesia: Fifty years of progress. Surg. Gynecol. Obstet. **101**, 105—139 (1955).

BEHAR, M. G., ALEXANDER, S. C.: In vitro effects of inhalational anesthetics on viscosity of human blood. Anesthesiology **27**, 567—573 (1966).

BELFRAGE, S., AHLGREN, I., AXELSON, S.: Halothane hepatitis in an anaesthetist. Lancet **1966 II**, 1466—1467.

BELLEVILLE, J. W.: Postanesthetic nausea and vomiting. Anesthesiology **22**, 773—780 (1961).

BERGMAN, N. A.: Components of the alveolar-arterial oxygen tension difference in anesthetized man. Anesthesiology **28**, 517—527 (1967).

— Properties of passive exhalations in anesthetized subjects. Anesthesiology **30**, 378—387 (1969).

BISCOE, T. J., MILLAR, R. A.: The effect of halothane on carotid sinus baroreceptor activity. J. Physiol. (London) **173**, 24—37 (1964).

— — The effects of cyclopropane, halothane and ether on central baroreceptor pathways. J. Physiol. (London) **184**, 535—559 (1966).

BLACK, G. W.: A review of the pharmacology of halothane. Brit. J. Anaesthesia 37, 688—705 (1965).
— A comparison of cardiac rhythm during halothane and methoxyflurane anaesthesia at normal and elevated levels of Paco₂ Acta Anaesth. Scand. 11, 103—108 (1967).
— McARDLE, L.: The effects of halothane on the peripheral circulation in man. Brit. J. Anaesthesia 34, 2—10 (1962).
BLACKMORE, W. P., ERWIN, K. W., WIEGAND, O. F., LIPSEY, R.: Renal and cardiovascular effects of halothane. Anesthesiology 21, 489—495 (1960).
BLOODWELL, R. D., BROWN, R. C., CHRISTENSON, G. R., GOLDBERG, L. I., MORROW, A. G.: The effect of Fluothane on myocardial contractile force in man. Anesthesia & Analgesia 40, 352—361 (1961).
BOGDANSKI, D. F., BRODIE, B. B.: The effects of inorganic ions on the storage and uptake of H³-nonrepinephrine by rat heart slices. J. Pharmacol. Exptl Therap. 165, 181—189 (1969).
BOTTOMLEY, G. A., SEIFLOW, G. H. F.: Vapour pressure and vapour density of halothane. J. Appl. Chem. (London) 13, 399—402 (1963).
BOYAN, C. P., UNDERWOOD, P. S., HOWLAND, W. S.: The effects of operation, anesthesia and plasma expander on blood viscosity. Anesthesiology 27, 279—283 (1966).
BRANDSTATER, B., EGER, E. I., II, EDELIST, G.: Effects of halothane, ether and cyclopropane on respiration. Brit. J. Anaesthesia 37, 890—897 (1965).
BRENNEN, H. J., HUNTER, A. R., JOHNSTONE, M.: Halothane — a clinical assessment. Lancet 1957 II ,453—457.
BRIDGES, B. E., JR., EGER, E. I., II: The effect of hypocapnia on the level of halothane anesthesia in man. Anesthesiology 27, 634—637 (1966).
BRUCE, D. L., KOEPKE, J. A., TRAURIG, H. H.: Studies of DNA synthesis in the halothane treated rat. In: Toxicity of anesthetics, pp. 123—129. (Fink, B. R., Ed.) Baltimore: Williams and Wilkins 1968.
— TRAURIG, H. H.: The effect of halothane on the cell cycle in rat small intestine. Anesthesiology 30, 401—405 (1969).
BUNKER, J. P., FORREST, W. H., JR., MOSTELLER, F., VANDAM, L. D.: The National Halothane Study — A study of the possible association between halothane anesthesia and postoperative hepatic necrosis. Bethesda: National Institute of General Medical Sciences 1969.
— VANDAM, L. D.: Summary of study of hepatic necrosis. In: The National Halothane Study, pp. 177—182. (Bunker, J. P. et al., Eds.) Bethesda: National Institute of General Medical Sciences 1969.
BURN, J. H., EPSTEIN, H. G.: Hypotension due to halothane. Brit. J. Anaesthesia 31, 199—204 (1959).
— — FEIGAN, G. A., PATON, W. D. M.: Some pharmacologic actions of Fluothane. Brit. Med. J. 2, 479—483 (1957).
BURNAP, T. K., GALLA, S. J., VANDAM, L. D.: Anesthetic, circulatory and respiratory effects of Fluothane. Anesthesiology 19, 307—320 (1958).
BURNS, J., SNOW, G. A.: A modified method for the determination of halothane and other halogen-containing anaesthetics. Brit. J. Anaesthesia 33, 102—103 (1961).
BURTON, P. T. C.: Halothane concentration from a Rowbotham's bottle in a circle absorption system. Brit. J. Anaesthesia 30, 312—316 (1958).
BUTLER, R. A.: Halothane. In: Uptake and distribution of anesthetic agents, pp. 274—288. (PAPPER, E. M., KITZ, R. J., Eds.) New York: McGraw-Hill 1963.
— Pharmacokinetics of halothane and ether. Brit. J. Anaesthesia 36, 193—199 (1964).
— FREEMAN, J.: Gas chromatography as a method for estimating concentrations of volatile anesthetics in blood. Brit. J. Anaesthesia 34, 440—444 (1962).
— KELLY, A. B., ZAPP, J.: The determination of hydrocarbon anesthetics in blood by gas chromatography. Anesthesiology 28, 760—763 (1967).
CAFFREY, J. A., ECKSTEIN, J. W., HAMILTON, W. K., ABBOUD, F. M.: Forearm venous and arterial responses to halothane and cyclopropane. Anesthesiology 26, 786—790 (1965).
CALVERT, J. R., STEINHAUS, J. E., LANGE, S. J., TAYLOR, C. A.: Halothane as a depressant of cough reflex. Anesthesia Analgesia 45, 76—81 (1966).
CAMPKIN, T. V., DALLAS, S. H.: Elective circulatory arrest in neurosurgical operations. Brit. J. Anaesthesia 40, 527—532 (1968). — CESSI, C., MOLINARY, G. A., BARTOT, G.: Effects of ether trichlorethylene and Fluothane on the pulmonary stretch receptors of the cat. Survey Anesthesiol. 7, 617—618 (1963).
CHALAZONITIS, N.: Selective actions of volatile anesthetics on synaptic transmission and autorhythmicity in single identifiable neurons. Anesthesiology 28, 111—123 (1967).
CHATAS, G. J., GOTTLIEB, J. D., SWEET, R. B.: Cardiovascular effects of d-tubocurarine during Fluothane anesthesia. Anesthesia & Analgesia 42, 65—69 (1963).

5*

CHRISTENSEN, M. S., HOEDT-RASMUSSEN, K., LASSEN, N. A.: Cerebral vasodilatation by halothane anesthesia in man and its potentiation by hypotension and hypercapnia. Brit. J. Anaesthesia **39**, 927—934 (1967).

CHRISTOFORO, M. F., BRODY, M. J.: (1) The effects of halothane and cyclopropane on skeletal muscle vessels and baroreceptor reflexes. Anesthesiology **29**, 36—43 (1968).

— — (2) Non-adrenergic vasoconstriction produced by halothane and cyclopropane anesthesia. Anesthesiology **29**, 44—56 (1968).

CLEMENTS, J. A., WILSON, K. H.: Affinity of narcotic agents for interfacial films. Proc. Natl. Acad. Sci. US **48**, 1008—1014 (1962).

COAKLEY, C. S., ALPERT, S., BOLING, J. S.: Circulatory responses during anesthesia of patients on rauwolfia therapy. J. Am. Med. Assoc. **161**, 1143—1144 (1956).

COHEN, P. J., MARSHALL, B. E.: Effects of halothane on respiratory control and oxygen consumption of rat liver mitochondria. In: Toxicity of anesthetics, pp. 24—36. (FINK, B. R., Ed.). Baltimore: Williams and Wilkins 1968.

— WOLLMAN, H., ALEXANDER, S. C., CHASE, P. E., BEHAR, M. G.: Cerebral carbohydrate metabolism in man during halothane anesthesia. Anesthesiology. **25**, 185—191 (1964).

COLERIDGE, H. M., COLERIDGE, J. C. G., LUCK, J. C., NORMAN, J.: The effect of four volatile anesthetic agents on the impulse activity of two types of pulmonary receptors. Brit. J. Anaesthesia **40**, 484—492 (1968).

COLGAN, F. J.: Performance of lungs and bronchi during inhalation anesthesia. Anesthesiology **26**, 778—785 (1965).

—WHANG, T. B.: Anesthesia and atelectasis. Anesthesiology **29**, 917—922 (1968).

COMBES, B.: Halothane induced liver damage — An entity. New Engl. J. Med. **280**, 558—559 (1969).

CRAYTHORNE, N. W. B., HUFFINGTON, P. E.: Effects of propranolol on the cardiovascular response to cyclopropane and halothane. Anesthesiology **27**, 580—583 (1966).

DEUTSCH, S., GOLDBERG, M., DRIPPS, R. D.: (1) Postoperative hyponatremia with the inappropriate release of antidiuretic hormone. Anesthesiology **27**, 250—256 (1966).

— — STEPHEN, G. W., WU, W. H.: (2) Effects of halothane anesthesia on renal function in normal man. Anesthesiology **27**, 793—804 (1966).

— LINDE, H. W., DRIPPS, R. D., PRICE, H. L.: Circulatory and respiratory actions of halothane in normal man. Anesthesiology **23**, 631—638 (1962).

DEVINE, J. C., HAMILTON, W. K., PITTINGER, C. B.: Respiratory studies in man during halothane anesthesia. Anesthesiology **19**, 11—18 (1958).

DOBKIN, A. B., FEDORUK, S.: A comparison of the cardiovascular, respiratory and metabolic effects of methoxyflurane and halothane in dogs. Anesthesiology **22**, 355—362 (1961).

DOMINO, E. F., CORSSEN, G., SWEET, R. B.: Effects of various general anesthetics on the visually evoked response in man. Anesthesia & Analgesia **42**, 735—747 (1963).

DRUCKER, W. R., DAVIS, H. S., BURGET, D., POWERS, A. L., SIEVERDING, E.: Effect of halothane and cyclopropane anesthesia on energy metabolism in hypovolemic animals. J. Trauma **5**, 503—514 (1965).

DUNCAN, W. A. M.: The estimation of halothane in tissues. Brit. J. Anaesthesia **31**, 316—320 (1959).

DUNDEE, J. W., MOORE, J.: Alterations in response to somatic pain associated with anesthesia. IV. The effect of subanaesthetic concentrations of inhalation agents. Brit. J. Anaesthesia **32**, 453—459 (1960).

ECKENHOFF, J. E., KNEALE, D. H., DRIPPS, R. D.: The incidence and etiology of postanesthetic excitement. Anesthesiology **22**, 667—673 (1961).

EGER, E. I., II: A mathematical model of uptake and distribution. In: Uptake and distribution of anesthetic agents, pp. 72—87. (PAPPER, E. M., KITZ, R. J., Eds.). New York: McGraw-Hill 1963.

— Respiratory and circulatory factors in uptake and distribution of volatile anaesthetic agents. Brit. J. Anaesthesia **36**, 155—171 (1964).

— BRANDSTATER, B., SAIDMAN, L. J., REGAN, M. J., SEVERINGHAUS. J. W., MUNSON, E. S.: (1) Equipotent alveolar concentrations of methoxyflurane, halothane, diethyl ether, fluroxene, cyclopropane, xenon and nitrous oxide in the dog. Anesthesiology **26**, 771—777 (1965).

— EPSTEIN, R. M.: Hazards of anesthetic equipment. Anesthesiology **25**, 490—504 (1964).

— ETHANS, C. T.: The effect of inflow, overflow and valve placement on economy of the circle system. Anesthesiology **29**, 93—100 (1968).

— GUADAGNI, N. P.: Halothane uptake in man at constant alveolar concentration. Anesthesiology **24**, 299—304 (1963).

— LARSON, C. P., Jr., SEVERINGHAUS, J. W.: The solubility of halothane in rubber, soda lime and various plastics. Anesthesiology **23**, 356—359 (1962).

— SAIDMAN, L. J., BRANDSTATER, B.: (2) Minimum alveolar anesthetic concentrations: A standard of anesthetic potency. Anesthesiology **26**, 756—763 (1965).

EGER, E. I., II, SMITH, N. T., STOELTING, R. K., WHITAKER, C.: The cardiovascular effects of various alveolar halothane concentrations in man. Anesthesiology 29, 185—186 (1968).

EISELE, J. H., EGER, E. I., II, MUALLEM, M.: Narcotic properties of carbon dioxide in the dog. Anesthesiology 28, 856—865 (1967).

ELLIOTT, J., BLACK, G. W., McCULLOUGH, H.: Catecholamine and acid-base changes during anesthesia and their influence upon the action of propranolol. Brit. J. Anaesthesia 40, 615—623 (1968).

EMBREY, M. P., GARRETT, W. J., PRYER, D. L.: Inhibitory action of halothane on contractility of human pregnant uterus. Lancet 1958 II, 1093—1094.

EMERSON, T. E., JR., MASSION, W. H.: Direct and indirect vascular effects of cyclopropane and halothane in the dog forearm. J. Appl. Physiol. 22, 217—222 (1967).

EPSTEIN, R. A., WANG, H. H., BARTELSTONE, H. J.: The effects of halothane on circulatory reflexes in dog. Anesthesiology 29, 867—876 (1968).

EPSTEIN, R. M., DEUTSCH, S., COOPERMAN, L. H., CLEMENT, A. J., PRICE, H. L.: Splanchnic circulation during halothane anesthesia and hypercapnia in normal man. Anesthesiology 27, 654—661 (1966).

— PAPPER, E. M.: Respiratory factors in the uptake and excretion of anesthetics. Intern. Anesthesiol. Clin. 3, 277—296 (1965).

— RACKOW, H., SALANITRE, E., WOLF, G.: Influence of the concentration effect on the uptake of anesthetic mixtures: The second gas effect. Anesthesiology 25, 364—371 (1964).

ETSTEN, B., SHIMOSATO, S.: Halothane anesthesia and catecholamine levels in a patient with pheochromacytoma. Anesthesiology 26, 688—691 (1965).

FABIAN, L. W., NEWTON, G. W., STEPHEN, C. R.: Simple and accurate Fluothane vaporizer. Anesthesiology 19, 284—287 (1958).

— SMITH, D. P., CARNES, M. A.: Tolerance of acute hypovolemia during cyclopropane and halothane anesthesia. Anesthesia & Analgesia 41, 272—276 (1962).

FERGUSON, J.: The discovery of the anaesthetic halothane — an example of industrial research. Chem. & Ind. (London) 1964, 818—824.

FINK, B. R.: Influence of cerebral activity in wakefulness on regulation of breathing. J. Appl. Physiol. 16, 15—20 (1961).

— KENNY, G. E.: Effects of halothane on cell culture metabolism. In: Toxicity of anesthetics, pp. 37—49. (FINK, B. R., Ed.). Baltimore: Williams and Wilkins 1968.

— — SIMPSON, W. E., III: Depression of oxygen uptake in cell culture by volatile barbiturates and local anesthetics. Anesthesiology 30, 150—155 (1969).

— NGAI, S. H., HANKS, E. C.: The central regulation of respiration during halothane anesthesia. Anesthesiology 23, 200—206 (1962).

FLACKE, W., ALPER, M. H.: Actions of halothane and norepinephrine in the isolated mammalian heart. Anesthesiology 23, 793—801 (1962).

FLETCHER, S. W., Flacke, W., ALPER, M. H.: The actions of general anesthetic agents on tracheal smooth muscle. Anesthesiology 29, 517—522 (1968).

FOLKMAN, J., WINSEY, S., MOGHUL, T.: Anesthesia by diffusion through silicone rubber. Anesthesiology 29, 410—418 (1968).

FORREST, W. H., JR.: Over-all results of the study of hepatic necrosis. In: The National Halothane Study, pp. 91—108. (BUNKER, J. P. et al., Eds.). Bethesda: National Institute of General Medical Sciences 1969.

FREUND, F. G., MARTIN, W. E., HORNBEIN, T. F.: The H-reflex as a measure of anesthetic potency in man. Anesthesiology 30, 642—647 (1969).

FUKUSHIMA, K., FUJITA, T., FUJIWARA, T., OOSHIMA, H., SATO, T.: Effect of propranolol on the ventricular arrhythmias induced by hypercarbia during halothane anesthesia in man. Brit. J. Anaesthesia 40, 53—58 (1968).

GAIN, E. A., PALETZ, S. G.: An attempt to correlate the clinical signs of Fluothane anaesthesia with the electroencephalographic levels. Canad. Anaesth. Soc. J. 4, 289—294 (1957).

GALL, E. A.: Report of the pathology panel. In: The National Halothane Study, pp. 151—161. (Bunker, J. P. et al., Eds.). Bethesda: National Institute of General Medical Sciences 1969.

GALLA, S. J.: Glucose pool size, turnover rate and $C^{14}O_2$ production during halothane anesthesia in dogs. Anesthesiology 28, 251 (1967).

— WILSON, E. P.: Hexose metabolism during halothane anesthesia in dogs. Anesthesiology 25, 96—97 (1964).

GARFIELD, J. M., ALPER, M. H., GILLIS, R. A., FLACKE, W.: A pharmacological analysis of ganglionic actions of some general anesthetics. Anesthesiology 29, 79—92 (1968).

GIESECKE, A. H., JENKINS, M. T., CROUT, J. R., COLLETT, J. M.: Urinary epinephrine and norepinephrine during Innovar-nitrous oxide anesthesia in man. Anesthesiology 28, 701—704 (1967).

GISSEN, A. J., KARIS, J. H., NASTUK, W. L.: The effect of halothane on neuromuscular transmission. J. Am. Med. Assoc. 197, 116—120 (1966).

Gissen, A. J., Matteo, R. S., Housepian, E. M., Bowman, F. O., Jr.: Elective circulatory arrest during neurosurgery for basilar artery aneurysms. J. Am. Med. Assoc. 207, 1315—1318 (1969).
Goldberg, A. H.: Cardiovascular function and halothane. In: Halothane, clinical anesthesia series, pp. 23—60. (Greene, N. M., Ed.). Philadelphia: F. A. Davis 1968.
— Maling, H. M., Gaffney, T. E.: The value of prophylactic digitalization in halothane anesthesia. Anesthesiology 23, 207—212 (1962).
— Phear, W. P. C.: Alteration in mechanical properties of heart muscle produced by halothane. J. Pharmacol. Exptl Therap. 162, 101—108 (1968).
— Ullrick, W. C.: Effects of halothane on isometric contractions of isolated heart muscle. Anesthesiology 28, 838—845 (1967).
Goldman, W.: The Goldman halothane vaporizer Mark II. Anaesthesia 15, 537—539 (1962).
Gottlieb, S. F.: Flammability of halothane, methoxyflurane and fluroxene under hyperbaric conditions. Anesthesiology 27, 195—196 (1966).
Grable, E., Finck, A. J., Abrams, A. L., Williams, J. A.: The effect of cyclopropane and halothane on the blood volume in man. Anesthesiology 23, 828—830 (1962).
Greene, N. M.: Inhalation anesthetics and permeability of human erythrocytes to monosaccharides. Anesthesiology 26, 731—742 (1965).
— Halothane, clinical anesthesia series. Philadelphia: F. A. Davis 1968.
— Cervenko, F. W.: Inhalation anesthetics, carbon dioxide and glucose transport across red cell membrane. Acta Anaesth. Scand. Suppl. 28, 1—28 (1967).
Gregory, G. A., Eger, E. I., II, Munson, E. S.: The relationship between age and halothane requirement in man. Anesthesiology 30, 488—491 (1969).
Hamelberg, W., Sprouse, J. H., Mahaffey, J. E., Richardson, J. A.: Catecholamine levels during light and deep anesthesia. Anesthesiology 21, 297—302 (1960).
Hampton, L. J., Flickinger, H.: Closed circuit anesthesia utilizing known increments of halothane. Anesthesiology 22, 413—418 (1961).
Han, Y. H.: Why do chronic alcoholics require more anesthesia ? Anesthesiology 30, 341—342 (1969).
Harrison, G. A.: The influence of different anaesthetic agents on the response to respiratory tract irritation. Brit. J. Anaesthesia 34, 804—811 (1962).
Hart, W. S.: A simple halothane drip feed. Anaesthesia 13, 458—459 (1958).
Hauswirth, O., Schaer, H.: Effects of halothane on the sino-atrial node. J. Pharmacol. Exptl Therap. 158, 36—59 (1967).
Heisterkamp, D. V., Skovsted, P., Cohen, P. J.: The effects of small increment doses of d-tubocurarine on neuromuscular transmission in anesthetized man. Anesthesiology 30, 500—505 (1969).
Hershey, S. G., Altura, B. M., Orkin, L. R.: Therapy of intestinal ischemic (SMA) shock with vasoactive drugs. Anesthesiology 29, 466—470 (1968).
Hickey, R. F., Graf, P., Nadel, J. A., Larson, C. P., Jr.: The effect of halothane and cyclopropane on total lung resistance in the dog. Anesthesiology 31, 334—343 (1969).
Hill, D. W.: (2) Halothane concentrations obtained with a fluotec vaporizer. Brit. J. Anaesthesia 30, 563—567 (1958).
— Lowe, H. J.: Comparison of concentration of halothane in closed and semi-closed circuits during controlled ventilation. Anesthesiology 23, 291—298 (1962).
Hill, E. F.: (1) Volatile anaesthetics — A method for their controlled administration. Brit. J. Anaesthesia 30, 37—39 (1958).
Hoech, G. P., Jr., Matteo, R. S., Fink, B. R.: Effect of halothane on oxygen consumption of rat brain, liver and heart and anaerobic glycolysis of rat brain. Anesthesiology 27, 770—777 (1966).
Jennett, W. B., Barker, J., Fitch, W., McDowall, D. G.: Effect of anaesthesia on intracranial pressure in patients with space-occupying lesions. Lancet 1969 I, 61—64.
Johnstone, M.: The human cardiovascular response to Fluothane anaesthesia. Brit. J. Anaesthesia 28, 392—410 (1956).
— Halothane-oxygen: A universal anaesthetic. (1) Brit. J. Anaesthesia 33, 29—39 (1961).
— (2) Halothane: The first five years. Anesthesiology 22, 591—614 (1961).
— Beta adrenergic blockade with pronethalol during anaesthesia. Brit. J. Anaesthesia 36, 224—232 (1964).
deJong, R. H., Freund, F. G., Robles, R., Morikawa, K. I.: (1) Anesthetic potency determined by depression of synaptic transmission. Anesthesiology 29, 1139—1144 (1968).
— Hershey, W. N., Wagman, I. H.: Measurement of a spinal reflex response (H-reflex) during general anesthesia in man. Anesthesiology 28, 382—389 (1967).
— Robles, R., Corbin, R. W., Nace, R. A.: (2) Effect of inhalation anesthetics on monosynaptic and polysynaptic transmission in the spinal cord. J. Pharmacol. Exptl. Therap. 162, 326—330 (1968).
Jouvet, M.: Biogenic amines and the state of sleep. Science 163, 32—41 (1969).

Halothane 71

KAIJSER, L., WESTERMARK, L., WÅHLIN, Å.: The influence of depth of halothane anesthesia on cardiac output and skin vascular resistance in the cat. Acta Anaesth. Scand. 13, 39—45 (1969).

KAIN, M. L., NUNN, J. F.: Fresh gas economics of the McGill circuit. Anesthesiology 29, 964—974 (1968).

KALOW, W.: Spectrophotometric determination of fluothane vapor. Canad. Anaesth. Soc. J. 4, 384—387 (1957).

KATZ, R. L.: Epinephrine and PLV-2: Cardiac rhythm and local vasoconstrictor effects. Anesthesiology 26, 619—623 (1965).

— Neuromuscular effects of diethyl ether and its interaction with succinylcholine and d-tubocurarine. Anesthesiology 27, 52—63 (1966).

— EPSTEIN, R. A.: The interaction of anesthetic agents and adrenergic drugs to produce cardiac arrhythmias. Anesthesiology 29, 763—784 (1968).

— GISSEN, A. J.: Neuromuscular and electromyographic effect of halothane and its interaction with d-tubocurarine in man. Anesthesiology 28, 564—567 (1967).

— MATTEO, R. S., PAPPER, E. M.: The injection of epinephrine during general anesthesia with halogenated hydrocarbons and cyclopropane in man. II. Halothane. Anesthesiology 23, 597—600 (1962).

— WEINTRAUB, H. D., PAPPER, E. M.: Anesthesia, surgery and rauwolfia. Anesthesiology 25, 142—147 (1964).

KEATING, V., PATRICK, S. J., ANNAMUNTHODO, H.: Halothane and carbohydrate metabolism. Anaesthesia 14, 268—269 (1959).

KEENEN, R. L.: Prevention of increased pressure in anesthetic vaporizers during controlled ventilation. Anesthesiology 24, 732—734 (1963).

KEET, J. E., VALENTINE, G. W., RICCIO, J. S.: An arrangement to prevent pressure effect on the Vernitrol vaporizer. Anesthesiology 24, 734—737 (1963).

KETY, S. S.: Theory and application of exchange of inert gas at the lungs and tissues. Pharmacol. Revs 3, 1—41 (1951).

KING, E. E., NAQUET, R., MAGOUN, H. W.: Alterations in somatic afferent transmission through the thalamus by central mechanisms and barbiturates. J. Pharmacol. Exptl. Therap. 119, 48—63 (1957).

KITAHATA, L. M.: The effects of halothane and methoxyflurane on recovery cycles of click-evoked potentials from the auditory cortex of the cat. Anesthesiology 29, 523—532 (1968).

KLATSKIN, G.: Symposium on toxic hepatic injury: clinical aspects. Gastroenterology 38, 789—791 (1960).

— Mechanisms of toxic and drug induced hepatic injury. In: Toxicity of anesthetics, pp. 159 to 175. (FINK, B. R., Ed.). Baltimore: Williams and Wilkins 1968.

— KIMBERG, D. V.: Recurrent hepatitis attributable to halothane sensitization in an anesthetist. New Engl. J. Med. 280, 515—522 (1969).

KLEINDORFER, G. B.: The effect of carbon dioxide on ether, ethylene and nitrous oxide anesthesia. J. Pharmacol. Exptl. Therap. 43, 445—448 (1931).

KLIDE, A. M., AVIADO, D. M.: Mechanism for the reduction in pulmonary resistance induced by halothane. J. Pharmacol. Exptl. Therap. 158, 28—35 (1967).

KLINGERSTRÖM, P., WESTERMARK, L.: Local effects of adrenaline and phenylalanyl lysyl-vasopressin in local anesthesia. Acta Anaesth. Scand. 71, 131—137 (1963).

KOPRIVA, C. J., LOWENSTEIN, E.: An anesthetic accident: Cardiovascular collapse from liquid halothane delivery. Anesthesiology 30, 246—247 (1969).

LARSON, C. P., JR., EGER, E. I., II., SEVERINGHAUS, J. W.: The solubility of halothane in blood and tissue homogenates. Anesthesiology 23, 349—355 (1962).

LINDGREN, P., WESTERMARK, L., WÅHLIN, Å.: Blood circulation in skeletal muscles under halothane anaesthesia in the cat. Acta Anaesth. Scand. 9, 83—97 (1965).

LITTLE, D. M., JR.: Effects of halothane on hepatic function. In: Halothane, clinical anesthesia series, pp. 85—138. (GREENE, N. M., Ed.). Philadelphia: F. A. Davis 1968.

LOWE, H. J.: Flame ionization detection of volatile organic anesthetics in blood, gas and tissues. Anesthesiology 25, 808—814 (1964).

LOWENSTEIN, E., CLARK, J. D., VILLAREAL, Y.: Excess lactate production during halothane anesthesia in man. J. Amer. Med. Assoc. 190, 1110—1113 (1964).

MAC DONALD, A. G., McNEILL, R. S.: A comparison of the effect on airway resistance of a new beta blocking drug ICI 50172 and propranolol. Brit. J. Anaesthesia 40, 508—510 (1968).

MAC KAY, I. M.: Clinical evaluations of Fluothane with special reference to a controlled percentage vaporizer. Canad. Anaesth. Soc. J. 4, 235—245 (1957).

MAPLESON, W. W.: An electric analogue for uptake and exchange of inert gases and other agents. J. Appl. Physiol. 18, 197—204 (1963).

MARKELLO, R., KING, B. D.: Practicality of halothane-air anesthesia. N.Y. State J. Med. **64**, 2185—2190 (1964).

MARSHALL, B. E.: Physiological shunting and dead space during spontaneous respiration with halothane-oxygen anaesthesia and the influence of intubation on the physiological dead space. Brit. J. Anaesthesia **38**, 912—922 (1966).

MARSHALL, F. N., PITTINGER, C. B., LONG, J. P.: Effects of halothane on gastrointestinal motility. Anesthesiology **22**, 363—366 (1961).

MARTIN, W. E., FREUND, F. G., HORNBEIN, T. F., BONICA, J. J.: Cardiovascular effects of halothane and halothane-nitrous oxide anesthesia during controlled ventilation. Anesthesiology **30**, 346 (1969).

MARTINEZ, L. R., NORLANDER, O. P.: Arterial oxygen tension during nitrous oxide-oxygen-halothane anaesthesia in patients with cardiovascular and pulmonary disease. Acta Anaesth. Scand. **11**, 353—370 (1967).

MARX, G. F., ANDREWS, I. C., ORKIN, L. R.: Cerebrospinal fluid pressure during halothane anaesthesia. Canad. Anaesth. Soc. J. **9**, 239—245 (1962).

MAZZE, R. I., SCHWARTZ, F. D., SLOCUM, H. C., BARRY, K. G.: Renal function during anesthesia and surgery. Anesthesiology **24**, 279—284 (1963).

McALEAVY, J. C., WAY, W. L., ALSTATT, A. H., GUADAGNI, N. P., SEVERINGHAUS, J. W.: Effect pf P_{CO_2} on the depth of anesthesia. Anesthesiology **22**, 260—264 (1961).

McDOWALL, D. G.: The effects of clinical concentrations of halothane on the blood flow and oxygen uptake of the cerebral cortex. Brit. J. Anaesthesia **39**, 186—196 (1967).

— HARPER A. M., II., JACOBSON, I.: Cerebral blood flow during halothane anaesthesia. Brit. J. Anaesthesia **35**, 394—401 (1963).

McHENRY, L. C., JR., SLOCUM, H. C., BIVENS, H. E., MAYES, H. A., HEYES, G. J.: Hyperventilation in awake and anesthetized man. Arch. Neurol. Psychiat. **12**, 270—277 (1965).

MERKEL, G., EGER, E. I., II.: A comparative study of halothane and halopropane anesthesia. Including method for determining equipotency. Anesthesiology **24**, 346—357 (1963).

MIDDLETON, M. D., ROTH, G. J., SMUCKLER, E. A., NYHUS, L. M.: The effect of high concentrations of halothane on the isolated perfused bovine liver. Surg. Gynecol. Obstet. **122**, 817—825 (1966).

MILLAR, R. A., BISCOE, T. J.: Preganglionic sympathetic activity and the effects of anaesthetics. Brit. J. Anaesthesia **37**, 804—832 (1965).

— — Postganglionic sympathetic discharge and the effects of inhalation anaesthetics. Brit. J. Anaesthesia **38**, 92—114 (1966).

MILLER, R. D., WAY, W. L., EGER, E. I., II.: The effects of alpha-methyldopa, reserpine, guanethidine and iproniazid on minimum alveolar anesthetic requirement (MAC). Anesthesiology **29**, 1153—1158 (1968).

MOIR, D. D., DOYLE, P. M.: Halothane and postoperative shivering. Anesthesia & Analgesia **42**, 423—428 (1963).

MORAN, W. H., JR., ZIMMERMAN, B.: Mechanism of antidiuretic hormone control of importance to the surgical patient. Surgery **62**, 639—644 (1967).

MORI, K., WINTERS, W. D., SPOONER, C. E.: Comparison of reticular and cochlear multiple unit activity with auditory evoked responses during various stages introduced by anesthetic agents. Electroencephalog. and Clin. Neurophysiol. **24**, 242—248 (1968).

MORRIS, L. E.: A new vaporizer for liquid anesthetic agents. Anesthesiology **13**, 587—593 (1952).

— FELDMAN, S. A.: Considerations in the design and function of anesthetic vaporizers. Anesthesiology **19**, 642—649 (1958).

— — Influence of hypercarbia and hypotension upon liver damage following halothane anaesthesia. Anaesthesia **18**, 32—40 (1963).

MORROW, D. H.: Relationship of digitalis tolerance to catecholamines during cyclopropane or halothane anaesthesia. Anaesthesia & Analgesia **46**, 675—687 (1967).

— GAFFNEY, T. E., HOLMAN, J. E.: The chronotropic and inotropic effects of halothane. Anesthesiology **22**, 915—917 (1961).

— MORROW, A. G.: The effects of halothane on myocardial contractile force and vascular resistance. Anesthesiology **22**, 537—541 (1961).

— — The responses to anaesthesia of non-hypertensive patients pretreated with reserpine. Brit. J. Anaesthesia **35**, 313—316 (1963).

— TOWNLEY, N. T.: Effect of anesthetic drugs on digitalis toxicity. Surg. Forum Proc. **14**, 240—242 (1963).

MORSE, H. T., LINDE, H. W., MISHALOVE, R. D., PRICE, H. L.: Relation of blood volume and hemodynamic changes during halothane anesthesia in man. Anesthesiology **24**, 790—795 (1963).

MOTOYAMA, E. K., GLUCK, L., KIKKAWA, Y., KULOVICH, U., SUZUKI, Y. O.: The effects of inhalation anesthetics on pulmonary surfactant. Anesthesiology **30**, 347 (1969).

MOYA, F., SPICER, A. R.: An appraisal of halothane in obstetrics. In: Halothane: Clinical Anesthesia Series, pp. 173—180. (GREENE, N. M., Ed.). Philadelphia: F. A. Davis 1968.

MUNSON, E. S., BOWERS, D. L.: Effects of hyperventilation on the rate of anesthetic equilibration. Anesthesiology 28, 377—381 (1967).

— EGER, E. I., II, BOWERS, D. L.: (1) The effects of changes in cardiac output and distribution on the rate of cerebral anesthetic equilibration. Anesthesiology 29, 533—537 (1968).

— LARSON, C. P., JR., BABAD, A. A., REGAN, M. J., BUECHEL, D. R., EGER, E. I.: The effects of halothane, fluroxene and cyclopropane on ventilation: A comparative study in man. Anesthesiology 27, 716—728 (1966).

— MAIER, W. R., CATON, D.: (2) Effects of halothane, cyclopropane and nitrous oxide on isolated human uterine muscle. Anesthesiology 29, 206 (1968).

MUNSON, W. M., JENICEK, J. A.: Effect of anesthetic agents on patients receiving reserpine therapy. Anesthesiology 23, 741—746 (1962).

NAITO, H., GILLIS, C. N.: Anesthetics and response of atria to sympathetic nerve stimulation. Anesthesiology 29, 259—266 (1968).

NGAI, S. H.: Hepatic effects of halothane. Review of the literature. In: The National Halothane Study, pp. 11—46. (BUNKER, J. P. et al., Eds.). Bethesda: National Institute of General Medical Sciences 1969.

— BOLME, P.: Effects of anesthetics on circulatory mechanisms in the dog. J. Pharmacol. Exptl. Therap. 153, 495—504 (1966).

— DIAZ, P. M., OZER, S.: (1) Uptake and release of norepinephrine: Effects of cyclopropane and halothane. Anesthesiology 31, 45—52 (1969).

— HANKS, E. C., FARHIE, S. E.: (1) Effects of anesthetics on neuromuscular transmission and somatic reflexes. Anesthesiology 26, 162—167 (1965).

— KATZ, R. L., FARHIE, S. E.: (2) Respiratory effects of trichloroethylene, halothane and methoxyflurane in the cat. J. Pharmacol. Exptl. Therap. 148, 123—130 (1965).

— NEFF, N. H., COSTA, E.: (2) The effect of cyclopropane and halothane on the biosynthesis of norepinephrine in vivo: Conversion of ^{14}C-tyrosine to catecholamines. Anesthesiology 31, 53—60 (1969).

NUNN, J. F.: Factors influencing the arterial oxygen tension during halothane anaesthesia with spontaneous respiration. Brit. J. Anaesthesia 36, 327—341 (1964).

— MATTHEWS, R. L.: Gaseous exchange during halothane anaesthesia: the steady respiratory state. Brit. J. Anaesthesia 31, 330—340 (1959).

OMINSKY, A. J., WOLLMAN, H.: Hazards of general anesthesia in the reserpinized patient. Anesthesiology 30, 443—446 (1969).

PAPANTONY, M., LANDMESSER, C. M.: Portable unit for Fluothane-air anesthesia. Anesthesiology 21, 768—773 (1960).

PAPPER, E. M., KITZ, R. J.: Uptake and distribution of anesthetic agents. New York: McGraw-Hill 1963.

PASKIN, S., SKOVSTED, P., SMITH, T. C.: Failure of Hering-Breuer reflex to account for tachypnea in anesthetized man. Anesthesiology 29, 550—558 (1968).

PATTERSON, R. W., SULLIVAN, S. F., MALM, J. R., BOWMAN, F. O., JR., PAPPER, E. M.: The effect of halothane on human airway mechanics. Anesthesiology 29, 900—907 (1968).

PAYNE, J. P., GARDINER, D., VERNER, I. R.: Cardiac output during halothane anaesthesia. Brit. J. Anaesthesia 31, 87—90 (1959).

— SENFIELD, R. M.: Pronethalol in treatment of ventricular arrhythmias during anaesthesia. Brit. Med. J. 1964 I, 603—604.

PENNINGTON, S. N.: The effects of gamma radiation on halothane. Anesthesiology 29, 153—154 (1968).

PERL, W., RACKOW, H., SALANITRE, E., WOLF, G. L., EPSTEIN, R. M.: Intertissue diffusion effect for inert fat-soluble gases. J. Appl. Physiol. 20, 621—627 (1965).

PIERCE, C. E., JR., LAMBERTSEN, C. J., DEUTSCH, S., CHASE, P. E., LINDE, H. W., DRIPPS, R. D., PRICE, H. L.: Cerebral circulation and metabolism during thiopental anesthesia and hyperventilation in man. J. Clin. Invest. 41, 1664—1671 (1962).

PRICE, H. L., DEUTSCH, S., DAVIDSON, I. A., CLEMENT, A. J., BEHAR, M. G., EPSTEIN, R. M.: Can general anesthetics produce splanchnic visceral hypoxia by reducing regional blood flow? Anesthesiology 27, 24—32 (1966).

— LINDE, H. W., JONES, R. E., BLACK, G. W., PRICE, M. L.: Sympathoadrenal responses to general anesthesia in man and their relation to hemodynamics. Anesthesiology 20, 563 to 575 (1959).

— — MORSE, H. T.: Central nervous actions of halothane affecting the systemic circulation. Anesthesiology 24, 770—778 (1963).

— LURIE, A. A., BLACK, G. W., SECHZER, P. H., LINDE, H. W., PRICE, M. L.: Modification by general anesthetics (cyclopropane and halothane) of circulatory and sympathoadrenal responses to respiratory acidosis. Ann. Surg. 152, 1071—1077 (1966).

PRICE, H. L., PRICE, M. L.: Has halothane a predominant circulatory action? Anesthesiology 27, 764—769 (1966).
— — Relative ganglion blocking potency of cyclopropane halothane and nitrous oxide and the interaction of nitrous oxide with halothane. Anesthesiology 28, 349—353 (1967).
— — MORSE, H. T.: Effects of cyclopropane, halothane and procaine on the vasomotor "center" of the dog. Anesthesiology 26, 55—60 (1965).
— WARDEN, J. C., COOPERMAN, L. H., PRICE, M. L.: Enhancement by cyclopropane and halothane of heart rate responses to sympathetic stimulation. Anesthesiology 29, 478 to 483 (1968).
PURCHASE, I. F. H.: The effect of halothane on the sympathetic nerve supply to the myocardium. Brit. J. Anaesthesia 37, 915—928 (1965).
PURKIS, I. E.: Factors that influence postoperative vomiting. Canad. Anaesth. Soc. J. 11, 335—353 (1964).
RACKOW, H., SALANITRE, E., WOLF, G. L.: Quantitative analysis of diethyl ether in blood. Blood/gas distribution coefficient of diethyl ether. Anesthesiology 27, 829—834 (1966).
RAVENTÓS, J.: The action of Fluothane — A new volatile anaesthetic. Brit. J. Pharmacol. 11, 395—410 (1956).
— LEMON, P. G.: Impurities in Fluothane: Their biological properties. Brit. J. Anaesthesia 37, 716—737 (1965).
REGAN, M. J., EGER, E. I., II.: Effect of hypothermia in dogs on anesthetizing and apneic doses of inhalation agents. Anesthesiology 28, 689—700 (1967).
REHDER, K., FORBES, J., ALTER, H., HESSLER, O., STIER, A.: Halothane biotransformation in man. A quantitative study. Anesthesiology 28, 711—715 (1967).
REIN, J., AUSTEN, W. G., MORROW, D. H.: Effects of guanethidine and reserpine of the cardiac responses to halothane. Anesthesiology 24, 672—675 (1963).
ROBINSON, A., DENSON, J. S.: Halothane analyser. Anesthesiology 23. 391—394 (1962). —
ROBSON, J. G., DAVENPORT, H. T., SUGIYAMA, R.: Differentiation of two types of pain by anesthetics. Anesthesiology 26, 31—36 (1965).
RUTLEDGE, C. O., SEIFEN, E., ALPER, M. H., FLACKE, W.: Analysis of halothane in gas and blood by gas chromatography. Anesthesiology 24, 862—867 (1963).
SADOVE, M. S., WALLACE, V. E.: Halothane. Philadelphia: F. A. Davis 1962.
SAIDMAN, L. J.: Physical characteristics of halothane: values and significance. In: Halothane, clinical anesthesia series, pp. 11—22. (GREENE, N. M., Ed.). Philadelphia: F. A. Davis 1968.
— EGER, E. I., II.: Effect of nitrous oxide and of narcotic premedication on the alveolar concentration of halothane required for anesthesia. Anesthesiology 25, 302—306 (1964).
— — MUNSON, E. S., BABAD, A. A., MUALLEM, M.: Minimum alveolar concentrations of methoxyflurane, halothane, ether and cyclopropane in man. Correlation with theories of anesthesia. Anesthesiology 28, 994—1000 (1967).
— — SEVERINGHAUS, J. W.: A method for determining solubility of anesthetics utilizing the Scholander apparatus. Anesthesiology 27, 180—184 (1967)
SALANITRE, E., RACKOW, H.: The pulmonary exchange of nitrous oxide and halothane in infants and children. Anesthesiology 30, 388—394 (1969).
— — WOLF, G. L., EPSTEIN, R. M.: The uptake of ethylene in man. Anesthesiology 26, 305—311 (1965).
SASA, M., NAKAI, Y., TAKAORI, S.: Effects of volatile anesthetics on the evoked potentials and unitary discharges in the central auditory system caused by click stimuli in cats. Japan. J. Pharmacol. 17, 364—380 (1967).
SCHOENBORN, B. P., FEATHERSTONE, R. M., VOGELBUT, P. O., SUSSKIND, C.: Influence of xenon on protein hydration as measured by a microwave absorption technique. Nature 202, 695—696 (1964).
SCHWEIZER, O., HOWLAND, W. S., SULLIVAN, C., VERTES, E.: The effect of ether and halothane on blood levels of glucose, pyruvate, lactate and metabolites of the tricarboxylic acid cycle in normotensive patients during operation. Anesthesiology 28, 814—822 (1967).
SECHZER, P. H.: Discussion on halothane. In: Uptake and distribution of anesthetic agents, pp. 285—288. (PAPPER, E. M., KITZ, R. J., Eds.). New York: McGraw-Hill 1963.
— LINDE, H. W., DRIPPS, R. D., PRICE, H. L.: Uptake of halothane by the human body. Anesthesiology 24, 779—783 (1963).
SEEVERS, M. H., WATERS, R. M.: Pharmacology of anesthetic gases. Physiol. Revs 18, 447 to 479 (1938).
SEVERINGHAUS, J. W., CULLEN, S. C.: Depression of myocardium and body oxygen consumption with Fluothane. Anesthesiology 19, 165—177 (1958).
SHANKS, C. A.: Intravenous octapressin during halothane anaesthesia: a pilot study. Brit. J. Anaesthesia 35, 640—643 (1963).

SHIMOSATO, S., ETSTEN, B.: Performance of digitalized heart during halothane anesthesia. Anesthesiology 24, 41—50 (1963).
SHINOZAKI, T., MAZUZAN, J. E., JR., ABAJIAN, J., JR.: Halothane and the heart. Brit. J. Anaesthesia 40, 79—80 (1968).
SHNIDER, S. M., PAPPER, E. M.: Anesthesia for the asthmatic patient. Anesthesiology 22, 886—892 (1961).
SMITH, B. E., GAUB, M. L., MOYA, F.: Investigations into the teratogenic effects of anesthetic agents. The fluorinated agents. Anesthesiology 26, 260—261 (1965).
SMITH, N. T., CORBASCIO, A. N.: The cardiovascular effects of nitrous oxide during halothane anesthesia in the dog. Anesthesiology 27, 560—566 (1966).
— EGER, E. I., II., WHITAKER, C. E., STEOLTING, R. K., WAYNE, T. F.: The curculatory effects of the addition of nitrous oxide to halothane anesthesia in man. Anesthesiology 29, 212—213 (1968).
SNEGIREFF, S. L., COX, J. R., EASTWOOD, D. W.: The effect of nitrous oxide, cyclopropane or halothane on neural tube mitotic index, weight, mortality and gross anomaly rate in the developing chick embryo. In: Toxicity of anesthetics, pp. 279—293. (FINK, B. R., Ed.). Baltimore: Williams and Wilkins 1968.
STEEN, S. N., LEE, A. S. J.: Prevention of inadvertant excess pressure in closed systems. Anesthesia & Analgesia 39, 264—266 (1960).
STEPHEN, C. R., LITTLE, D. M., JR.: Halothane (Fluothane). Baltimore: Williams and Wilkins 1961.
STIRLING, G. R., MORRIS, K. N., ORTON, R. H., BOAKE, W. C., RACE, D. R., KINROSS, F., THOMSON, J. W., CROSBY, W.: Halothane and circulatory occlusion: some experimental and clinical observations. Brit. J. Anaesthesia 32, 262—272 (1960).
STOELTING, R. K., EGER, E. I., II.: (1) An additional explanation for the second gas effect: A concentrating effect. Anesthesiology 30, 273—277 (1969).
— — (2) Percutaneous loss of nitrous oxide, cyclopropane, ether and halothane in man. Anesthesiology 30, 278—283 (1969).
SUCKLING, C. W.: Some chemical and physical factors in the development of Fluothane. Brit. J. Anaesthesia 29, 466—472 (1957).
— The development of halothane. Part. I. Manchester Univ. Med. School Gazette 37, 53—54 (1958).
THEYE, R. A.: Myocardial and total oxygen consumption with halothane. Anesthesiology 28, 1042—1047 (1967).
— Estimation of partial pressure of halothane in blood. Anesthesiology 29, 101—103 (1968).
— MICHENFELDER, J. D.: The effect of halothane on canine cerebral metabolism. Anesthesiology 29, 1113—1118 (1968).
— SESSLER, A. D.: Effect of halothane anesthesia on rate of canine oxygen consumption. Anesthesiology 28, 661—669 (1969).
— TUOHY, G. F.: Oxygen uptake during light halothane anesthesia in man. Anesthesiology 24, 627—633 (1964).
THOMSON, W. J.: The effect of induction of anaesthesia on peripheral hemodynamics. Brit. J. Anaesthesia 39, 210—214 (1967).
TITEL, J. H., LOWE, H. J.: Rubber gas partition coefficients. Anesthesiology 29, 1215—1216 (1968).
TYRRELL, M., FELDMAN, S. A.: Headache following halothane anaesthesia. Brit. Anaesthesia 40, 99—102 (1968).
UEDA, I.: Effects of diethyl ether and halothane on firefly luciferin bioluminescence. Anesthesiology 26, 603—606 (1965).
— MIETANI, W.: Microcomal ATPase of rabbit brain and effects of general anesthetics. Biochem. Pharmacol. 16, 1370—1374 (1967).
VASICKA, A., KRETCHMER, H.: Effect of conduction and inhalation anesthesia on uterine contractions. Am. J. Obstet. Gynecol. 82, 600—610 (1961).
WALTHER, W. W., SLACK, W. K., CHEW, H. E. R.: The cardiac output under halothane anaesthesia with induced hypotension. Lancet 1964 II, 1266—1267.
WANG, H. H., EPSTEIN, R. A., MARKEE, S. J., BARTELSTONE, H. J.: The effects of halothane on peripheral and central vasomotor control mechanisms of the dog. Anesthesiology 29, 877—886 (1968).
WEISEL, W., YOUMANS, W. B., CASSELS, W. H.: Effect on intestinal motility of cyclopropane anesthesia alone and after morphine-scopolamine premedication. J. Pharmacol. Exptl. Therap. 63, 391—399 (1938).
WOLFSON, B.: Appraisal of the Hook and Tucker halothane meter. Anesthesiology 29, 157—159 (1968).
— CICCARELLI, H. E., SIKER, E. S.: Gas chromatography using an internal standard for the estimation of ether and halothane levels in blood. Brit. J. Anaesthesia 38, 591—595 (1966).

WOLLMAN, H., ALEXANDER, S. C., COHEN, P. J., CHASE, P. E., MELMAN, E., BEHAR, M. G.: Cerebral circulation of man during halothane anesthesia. Anesthesiology **25**, 180—184 (1964).

WOO, S. W., BERLIN, D., HEDLEY-WHYTE, J.: Surfactant function and anesthetic agents. J. Appl. Physiol. **26**, 571—577 (1969).

WOODS, M. A., BROWN, T. A.: A Marrett draw-over inhaler modified for halothane. Brit. J. Anaesthesia **31**, 321—324 (1959).

YAMAMURA, H., WAKSUGI, B., SATO, S., TAKABE, Y.: Gas chromatographic analysis of inhalation anesthetics in whole blood by an equilibration method. Anesthesiology **27**, 311—317 (1966).

3.2. Methoxyflurane and Teflurane

ALAN VAN POZNAK

The story of the synthesis of methoxyflurane and teflurane is different from the usual sequence of events in the synthesis and evaluation of a drug. The usual situation is that a series of chemical compounds is synthesized by a chemist, examined by a pharmacologist for possible useful activity, further examined by a clinical pharmacologist for desirable activity in human beings and then ultimately distributed to the specialist clinicians who will use the drug in their practice.

The development of methoxyflurane and teflurane followed a somewhat different sequence. It began with two practicing anesthesiologists who were hopefully representative of the practitioners who ultimately would use the drugs which were created. Doctor Atusio and I had long felt the need for better non-flammable anesthetics. We had reviewed the characteristics of the agents available to us and had noted, as editiorialized in the Far Eastern Journal of Anesthesia (1958), that those anesthetics which provided the best physiological conditions for the patient, namely diethyl ether and cyclopropane, were flammable. Diethyl ether and cyclopropane had speeds of action and potencies which could be easily handled by the practicing anesthesiologist. The non-flammable agents were either too weak or too strong. Nitrous oxide represented the too weak end of the spectrum and agents such as chloroform and halothane represented the too strong end of the spectrum. It was our hope that a non-flammable agent of approximately twice the potency of nitrous oxide might be synthesized for evaluation and study in animals and eventually in man. We have derived a concept of intermediate potency through which it was hoped the average patient could be lightly anesthetized with 40% of the agent and yet could not be overdosed with as much as 80% of the agent assuming that a safety factor of 2, a not unreasonable requirement, could be expected of the anesthetic.

Our ideal has not yet been realized. Paradoxically, methoxyflurane, which was the first clinically tried anesthetic of all those that we examined, has characteristics entirely different from those which we specified in our concept of intermediate potency. It does not have the rapid onset and offset of action which we hoped to find, nor does it have the limited intermediate potency which we hoped to find. Instead, it is an anesthetic of moderate slowness and extremely high potency so that while our original idea was not realized, an entirely different type of compound was obtained which in its own peculiar way provided much of the safety inherent in diethyl ether but without any of the fire or explosion hazard.

Between the concept of a new anesthetic and its clinical trial, there are many tedious intermediate steps. We were extremely fortunate in having good friends at The Dow Chemical Company in Midland, Michigan and at Abbott Laboratories in North Chicago, Illinois. It was only by a cooperative effort between Dow, ABBOTT and CORNELL that these anesthetics could have been created. The chemistry of organically linked fluorine is a specialty unto itself. The man who provided the technical skill to synthesize the first methoxyflurane for anesthetic purposes and to devise ways to stabilize and purify the compound was Eric R. LARSEN, Ph.D. of The Dow Chemical Company in Midland, Michigan. Doctor LARSEN and his chemical colleagues synthesized numerous compounds for us to evaluate, and with continued exposure to our specialty, Doctor LARSEN demonstrated an increasing knowledge of the field of anesthetics which swept beyond us.

The early evaluation of such compounds has many pitfalls and problems. At such a time it is helpful to have a colleague who has had wide experience in the pharmacology and toxicology of organic solvents and related chemicals. We were particularly fortunate in having as our ally, Doctor MAYNARD CHENOWETH who was pharmacologist to The Dow Chemical Company in Midland, Michigan and a former member of the Pharmacology Department at Cornell University Medical College. Doctor CHENOWETH and his colleagues did the preliminary examinations of methoxyflurane and other compounds, giving us much helpful advice regarding problems that we might reasonably expect in the administration of many of the compounds which they sent to us for evaluation.

Although The Dow Chemical Company has vast facilities for synthesis and testing of chemical substances, at the time that we worked with them, they had little in the way of direct connection with medical consumers. It was at this point that our association with Abbott Laboratories became especially helpful. Abbott Laboratories was already well known to anesthesiologists for their work in developing and marketing sodium Pentothal as well as a large line of intravenous fluids and other materials useful to the practicing anesthesiologist. When it became evident that methoxyflurane was a promising anesthetic for human trial, the medical distribution facilities of Abbott Laboratories were already prepared to take on the task of distributing this agent for trial and ultimately to submit the data to the Food and Drug Administration in Washington so that methoxyflurane could be licensed for distribution as an inhalation anesthetic. Our special thanks are due to Doctors RODNEY GWINN and NORMAN WHEELER who, in the early days of methoxyflurane anesthesia, were instrumental in distributing this compound for investigation and comment and who also had a great deal to do with the submission of the gathered data to the Food and Drug Administration.

Methoxyflurane has been in clinical use for more than 10 years. During this time, many investigators have had the opportunity to explore the usefulness and limitations of this anesthetic agent. Reports have varied from unqualified enthusiasm to outright damnation. Most investigators have concluded that methoxyflurane is a relatively safe anesthetic agent. However, a few have regarded it as highly toxic. A reconciliation of the wide divergence of opinion may be found in the simple and embarrasing explanation that those who are adept in the administration of methoxyflurane are enthusiastic about it and those who do not manage it well are seldom slow to find a reason for condemning this particular anesthetic. Probably the reason for success or failure in the clinical administration of methoxyflurane is effective utilization of certain of the physical and pharmacological characteristics of this anesthetic. The main point to remember is this: although methoxyflurane is the most potent anesthetic in clinical use in terms of the concentration required for maintenance of anesthesia at equilibrium, it is a relatively slow agent to achieve equilibrium with the body. This combination of high potency and prolonged onset of action is somewhat similar to the condition which obtains with diethyl ether. There is however one important difference, methoxyflurane being about ten times as potent as diethyl ether. The third fact which is extremely important to remember with the administration of methoxyflurane is that the saturated vapor pressure of this compound is approximately 25 mmHg at room temperature. For this reason, the maximum precentage which can be achieved from any vaporizer is on the order of 3%. A high flow of gas must pass through the vaporizer if an adequate induction concentration of methoxyflurane is to be obtained.

If the above physical and chemical characteristics of methoxyflurane are kept in mind, this agent may be used in any system which has been found suitable for the administration of diethyl ether. It is not necessary to have a special vaporizer. Methoxyflurane may be administered by the open drop method, similarly to diethyl ether. This is not the recommended procedure but it can be used where a non-flammable anesthetic must be given under emergency conditions or in the absence of sophisticated equipment. Under these conditions, methoxyflurane is given in a manner similar to that for diethyl ether and the dosage is varied according to the response of the patient. The fact that this can be done safely is demonstration of the inherent safety of methoxyflurane. With both of these ether compounds, it is possible to give safe adequate anesthesia by observing the patient. Millions of anesthetics have been given with ethyl ether with no knowledge of the concentration being delivered to the patient. Observation of the patient has been sufficient to guide the administrator in the safe dosage of the anesthetic agent. With the advent of rapid acting agents such as halothane, it became mandatory to provide precision vaporizers since clinical observation of the patient was not sufficient to allow safe administration of the anesthetic. It has become fashionable within recent years to insist upon precision vaporizers for all anesthetic agents. While I believe this is a good practice, it is not essential for such anesthetics as ethyl ether, methoxyflurane and a few others. However, if a precision vaporizer is desired these may be used quite effectively with methoxyflurane. The table below summarizes a few of the important physical characteristics of methoxy-flurane. Familiarity with these will guide the anesthetist in the production of safe satisfactory surgical anesthesia.

Boiling Point, 760 mmHg .... 104.65°
Coefficient, olive oil/water (against 1% methoxyflurane vapor)
    by Wt. at 37 °C 400
Blood/gas 13.0
Latent heat of vaporization .... 58.5 cal/Gm
Molecular Weight 145.979
Specific gravity at 37 °C (with water at 25 °C as 1.000) 1.4006
Vapor Pressures:
    6.27 °C .... 10 mmHg
    17.72 °C .... 20 mmHg
    30.42 °C .... 40 mmHg
    38.51 °C .... 60 mmHg
    49.51 °C .... 100 mmHg
    104.65 °C .... 760 mmHg

I. Pre-Anesthetic Medication

When used prior to an ether induction, the classical purposes of pre-anesthetic medication have been to sedate the patient and to block certain parasympathetic functions which may prove troublesome such as excessive salivation. In 1850 when pre-anesthetic medication was first used, morphine was the only effective hypnoptic medication in common use. Although many other medications superior to morphine for the purpose of the pre-anesthetic medication have appeared in the century following, there is still unnecessary use of morphine and similar narcotic drugs for pre-anesthetic medication for patients who are not in pain. It is our practice not to use narcotics unless our patients are in pain, but for these cases, we do not withhold narcotics, giving whatever dose is sufficient to control the patient's pain within the limits of safety. Pre-anesthetic medication prior to a methoxyflurane anesthesia may only be minimal, since methoxyflurane does not have the pungent irritating odor of diethyl ether nor does it tend to produce excessive salivary secretions. Pentobarbital sodium given intramuscularly 90 min before the patient is to be taken from his room is a satisfactory pre-anesthetic medicant. Adults usually receive 100—200 mg of the drug. Young children may be medicated at a dose of about 5 mg/kg of body weight. Scopolamine is also an excellent pre-anesthetic medication, particularly when amnesia is desired.

We have not routinely used any tranquilizers or phenothiazine drugs in pre-anesthetic medication. There are occasional cases where the use of such drugs is indicated. However, if they are routinely used for all cases, there will be occasional difficulty in maintaining blood pressure while the patient is anesthetized, and there will also be numerous instances of prolonged somnolence in the recovery room.

The previous administration of rauwolfia compounds may lead to sufficient depletion of catecholamines so that the maintenance of an adequate blood pressure during anesthesia may be difficult. For this reason, it is our preference to discontinue rauwolfia compounds at least 2 weeks prior to elective surgery. Emergency cases who have recently received rauwolfia compounds are anesthetized at the lightest possible plane of anesthesia consistent with the surgery to be performed. Several hypertensive patients receiving rauwolfia compounds have been anesthetized with methoxyflurane for neurosurgical treatment of ruptured intracranial aneurysms. These cases were managed without difficulty.

II. Techniques of Administration

A simple and comprehensive statement regarding the administration of methoxyflurane is this: the drug may be administered by any technique suitable for diethyl ether. However, the anesthetist must remember that while the solubilities of methoxyflurane and ether in blood are similar, their vapor pressures and potencies are markedly different. These simple but important facts should be kept in mind throughout the discussion of the various techniques of administration.

A. Open Drop Technique

Open drop administration of methoxyflurane is not recommended for routine clinical practices. However, methoxyflurane may be given by open drop technique is a manner similar to that for diethyl ether. By doing a few cases in this manner, the anesthesiologist can gain valuable practical information regarding the rate at which this anesthetic must be given during induction and maintenance. Although methoxyflurane boils at 103.5 °C and has at 20 °C a saturated vapor pressure of only 25 mmHg, it may be satisfactorily administered by open drop technique because of its relatively low latent heat of vaporization and its high potency.

Any standard type of open drop mask may be used. A few drops of methoxyflurane are placed on the mask and the patient is gradually allowed to become accustomed to the odor and not be frightened by it. Because methoxyflurane does not possess the pungent odor of diethyl ether, patients accept it more readily than they do ether. A few drops of methoxyflurane will be sufficient to saturate the mask. The amount of methoxyflurane will be far less than the amount of diethyl ether used in a similar situation.

The mask is gradually brought closer as the patient indicates that he can tolerate an increased vapor concentration. The rate of dropping is adjusted by the patient's tolerance. The anesthetist must be extremely careful not to saturate the mask since liquid methoxyflurane may drop off the side of the mask and onto the skin or even into the eyes. Methoxyflurane, like diethyl ether, is irritating to mucous membranes and will cause severe, although transient, discomfort.

If a towel is folded around the mask to increase the concentration of methoxyflurane in the inspired mixture, some restriction of respiration of gas exchange will occur. Hypoxia can be lessened by insufflating oxygen under the mask. The stream of oxygen will also help to dilute carbon dioxide which tends to accumulate under the mask. The inability to assist or control respiration during open drop anesthesia is one of the more serious drawbacks to the use of the open drop method, especially for prolonged procedures.

Induction time varies with the individual patient with the degree of preanesthetic medication. About 5—10 min may be required until response to verbal command is lost. However, if the patient is hyperventilating, induction time may be much shorter. The suitability of methoxyflurane for labor and delivery may be related to the maternal hyperventilation which is seen at this time. The experience and skill of the anesthetist is of great importance when this technique is used, since he must rely upon skill and judgment in gaining his patient's confidence, cooperation, and assistance. The intravenous drugs which are so frequently used to obscure the evidence of a poorly managed inhalation anesthetic are not available to the anesthetist who restricts himself to the open drop technique. Under emergency or disaster conditions, and with no more equipment then a rag and a bottle of methoxyflurane, the anesthetist can provide the physiologically safe anesthesia characteristic of diethyl ether, but free from the risk of explosion or fire.

Following the loss of consciousness, there may be a brief excitement stage which is related to the patient's anxiety and the anesthetist's skill rather than any pharmacological characteristic of methoxyflurane. Although methoxyflurane produces profound analgesia, the analgesia takes time to develop and may not be seen during the first 5 min of anesthesia. Painful procedures should therefore be avoided at this time. Surgical anesthesia develops gradually. It is usually evidenced by a slight drop of the systolic blood pressure and a diminution of respiratory tidal volume. The maintenance phase of methoxyflurane anesthesia with open drop technique is similar to that for diethyl ether except that smaller amounts of the anesthetic are required.

In order to avoid prolonged somnolence, the administration of methoxyflurane should be reduced or discontinued well before the end of the operation. Should the patient begin to awaken on the operating table, a very small amount of methoxyflurane will suffice to restore surgical anesthesia.

B. Semi-Closed System

Semi-closed or partial rebreathing systems are extensively used for several reasons. They are ideal for the use of nitrous oxide-oxygen mixtures into which a low percentage of highly potent liquid anesthetic may be vaporized. In addition, respiration may be assisted or controlled as required. Methoxyflurane may be used advantageously in a semi-closed system. The nitrous oxide procides rapid analgesia and some sedation and serves to cover the early minutes of anesthesia while methoxyflurane is being taken into the body. Any type of vaporizer may be used either in the breathing circuit or outside of it. Vaporizers which have been used include Ohio No. 8 and 10 vaporizers, Ohio Verni-Trol vaporizers, Forreger Copper Kettle, Pentec and Pentomatic. The out-of-circle vaporizers have an advantage in that the percentage of methoxyflurane is known. However, the anesthetist should remember that once the mixture is delivered to the breathing circuit, the amount of anesthetic inhaled by the patient will depend on the dynamics of the semiclosed system.

C. Closed System

A standard closed circle may be used for methoxyflurane anesthesia. The anesthetic may be vaporized by any of the vaporizers mentioned above. The closed system works well for maintenance of anesthesia; the induction and washout phases of methoxyflurane anesthesia are often better done utilizing high flow techniques and a semi-closed system.

D. Non-Rebreathing System

Non-rebreathing systems with air have been used for methoxyflurane anesthesia in cardiac catheterization. In this way there is minimum disturbance of the blood gases which the cardio-pulmonary physiologist wishes to measure.

E. Penthrane Analgizer

A single use disposable inhaler has been developed for methoxyflurane analgesia. The patient-held device is charged with 15 ml of methoxyflurane and used for the production of conscious analgesia during labor and delivery. The patient holds the vaporizer in her hand and must close her lips around the tube in order to inhale an analgesic concentration of methoxyflurane. If surgical anesthetic levels are approached, the patient will either lose the ability to close her lips around the tube or allow the vaporizer to slip from her fingers. In either case, inhalation of methoxyflurane will be terminated until the patient recovers sufficiently to hold the vaporizer to her mouth again.

III. Other Drugs Used in Conjunction with Methoxyflurane

Pre-anesthetic medication has been discussed in the previous pages. The hazards of anesthesia in the reserpinized patient have been mentioned. Methoxyflurane appears to have the property of diethyl ether in enhancing the effect of d–tubocurarine. The nature of this mechanism is under investigation. The action of hypotensive drugs appears to be intensified in the presence of methoxyflurane. For this reason, less trimethaphan (Arfonad) is required during methoxyflurane anesthesia. Methoxyflurane has been used with all other drugs common to anesthetic practice and no difficulties have been encountered. Ephinephrine has been safely used with methoxyflurane in many cases and we have no fears about using these two drugs simultaneously. However, Bamforth et al. (1961) have demonstrated that under certain conditions ventribular fibrillation can be produced by the administration of large intravenous doses of ephinephrine in dogs under methoxyflurane anesthesia.

IV. Methoxyflurane and Muscle Relaxants

Methoxyflurane, like diethyl ether, can produce any degree of muscle relaxation needed for surgery. However, in so doing it may depress blood pressure below limits which are considered safe. Therefore, it is considered preferable to use methoxyflurane in a light level of anesthesia and to obtain the needed relaxation with a peripherally acting neuromuscular blocking drug. Usually d-tubocurarine or succinylcholine is used. Because of the relaxant properties of the anesthetic itself, less than the usual amount of neuromuscular blocking drug will be used. The mechanism of action has not been elucidated. Ngai (1961, 1965) has reported that the relaxation seen with methoxyflurane anesthesia comes principally from synaptic interruption at the spinal cord and that peripheral neuromuscular block plays little part. However, other workers have reported a peripheral action of methoxyflurane as well. Van Poznak (1969) has observed that methoxyflurane is extremely potent in its action on the motor nerve terminal which anatomical site is also the primary locus for action of d-tubocurarine as demonstrated by Standaert (1964). Therefore, it seems reasonable to assume that the relaxation obtained when these two agents are used in combination is the result of their additive or potentiating effects at the motor nerve terminal causing failure of the motor nerve terminal to carry high frequency discharge and ultimately, failure of the motor nerve terminal to transmit even single discharge.

V. Induction Techniques

Although methoxyflurane can be used as the sole anesthetic agent, induction is prolonged and to some patients unpleasant. A more rapid and pleasant induction can be obtained by use of intravenous thiobarbiturates. However, children are often frightened by needles and will request inhalation induction in preference to intravenous induction. Drugs which can speed inhalation induction include the following: cyclopropane, nitrous oxide, and halothane. After a cyclopropane induction maintenance of anesthesia with methoxyflurane may not cause any depression of the blood pressure. This is an interesting finding which will receive further investigation.

VI. Types of Surgery Suitable for Methoxyflurane Anesthesia

Methoxyflurane may be used for any patient and any operation but it is better suited for long operations than for short ones. It has been found particularly useful for neurosurgery, plastic surgery, eye surgery, and lengthy procedures about the head and neck such as radical neck dissection and total laryngectomy. Methoxyflurane has also been used successfully for all types of intra-abdominal and intra-thoracic operations including heart surgery with cardio-pulmonary by-pass.

The dynamics of its uptake and distribution make such operations as uterine dilitation and curretage, incision and drainage procedures, dressing changes and rapid tonsillectomies by the guillotine technique less suitable for methoxyflurane anesthesia than for the more rapidly acting agents.

VII. The Use of Methoxyflurane for Obstetrical Analgesia and Anesthesia

Methoxyflurane was well established as a surgical anesthetic before it received trial in labor and delivery. This was done in order to obtain as much information about this drug as possible in surgical patients before methoxyflurane was tried on a healthy young woman who was about to have a healthy baby. The trial of any new drug brings unsuspected and sometimes unpredictable reactions. Since anesthesia for labor and delivery is not essential as it is in most routine surgery, it was felt wise to postpone examination of methoxyflurane in parturient patients until we had learned as much as possible about it in patients whose illnesses required that they receive anesthesia in surgery.

From the slowness of induction and emergence characteristic of methoxyflurane when used as the sole anesthetic agent, one might at first predict that methoxyflurane would not be suitable for labor and delivery. However, early observation soon dispelled this concern. Continued use of methoxyflurane in obstetrics has attested to its safety and efficacy as an analgesic agent superior to any now in use. The slow induction which may be seen in the average surgical patient does not occur in the obstetrical patient, for the reason that the characteristic hyperventilation of labor and delivery raises the respiratory minute volume high enough so that methoxyflurane is brought into the blood stream and brain quite rapidly. Once there, it tends to persist and exerts a profound analgesic and sedative action which persists from one labor pain to the next. Perineal relaxation is usually very good but the progress of labor is not impeded by low doses of methoxyflurane. Because of the marked analgesic action, methoxyflurane may be administered during labor through a patient-held disposable inhaler called the Abbott Analgizer. This device has had enthusiastic acceptance by patients, physicians, and nurses. It has the great advantage that overdose is almost impossible to achieve since the patient will lose the ability to hold the inhaler to her face and will stop the administration of methoxyflurane whenever she becomes markedly sedated by it. Although the device has a number of fail-safe features incorporated in its design, it should nonetheless be used under professional supervision at all times. Studies currently in progress are demonstrating that the analgizer is comparable in safety, reliability and efficacy to two well established draw-over inhalation devices — the Duke Inhaler and the Cyprane Inhaler.

Following the induction of satisfactory analgesia during the first stage of labor, the patient may require additional analgesia for the second and third stages of labor. At this time, when she is transferred to the delivery room, the analgizer-inhaler may simply be plugged into an anesthesia mask since it has a 7/8 inch (23 mm) outside diameter. Alternatively, methoxyflurane with nitrous oxide and oxygen may be given through any standard anesthesia machine. Since the patient is already preloaded with methoxyflurane, the addition of a moderate dose of nitrous oxide will produce intense analgesia very rapidly. Infants delivered this way cry spontaneously and have Apgar Scores which are as good or better than those received by infants delivered by any other technique. Should forceps delivery be required, the addition of more methoxyflurane to the anesthesia mixture will result in the rapid production of sufficient surgical anesthesia to allow for such extraction of the infant. Should cesarean section be required, methoxyflurane may be added to sufficient depth to permit cesarean section. At this time, however, satisfactory operating conditions may be secured more rapidly by the addition of a peripherally acting muscle relaxant so that the surgeon may begin the cesarean section as rapidly as possible. A moderate dose of thiopental sodium may also be used if desired. If an excessive depth of methoxyflurane anesthesia is obtained during cesarean section, the babies will be born sleepy and will be slow to cry and to breathe spontaneously. This is an indication that that the mother has received too much anesthetic prior to the removal of the infant. Once these infants begin to cry, they rapidle ventilate the methoxyflurane out of their system and are in good condition within a few minutes. However, if the initial breaths are unduly prolonged, hyperventilation of the child with oxygen through an endotracheal tube will speed the emergence from methoxyflurane anesthesia. It is my personal preference to keep the anesthesia as light as possible so that instrumentation of the infant's tracheo-broncheal tree will not have to be performed unless absolutely necessary for other indications.

Laboratory studies on isolated strips of human myometrium have demonstrated that methoxyflurane is depressant to uterine contractility and rhythmicity. The dose response and time action relationships are quite similar to those produced by diethyl ether, being consistent from one specimen to another. For both of these anesthetics, there appears to be a similar response with both pregnant and non-pregnant myometrial specimens. The effects produced by these two ethers appear to be quite different from the effect produced by the halogenated hydrocarbon, halothane. Two striking differences are observed when myometrial specimens are exposed to halothane. The first effect is that pregnant specimens are almost twice as sensitive on the average as are non-pregnant specimens. The second effect is that there is a wide variability in response from one specimen to the next, especially in the case of the pregnent specimens. Work is in progress at the New York Hospital-Cornell Medical Center on the effects of anesthetic agents on isolated human myometrial specimens. There is at present very little quantitative information on this subject in the literature.

VIII. Contraindications and Precautions

There are no absolute contraindications to methoxyflurane anesthesia. In the presence of advanced hepatic or renal disease, methoxyflurane like other halogenated anesthetics ought to be avoided until we have learned more about mechanisms of hepatic damage. Because of the known hepato-toxic effects of carbon tetrachloride and chloroform, all halogenated compounds are categorically suspect as liver and kidney poisons until proved otherwise.

Within the last few years, the investigations of VAN DYKE and CHENOWETH (1965) on the metabolic transformations of supposedly inert inhalation anesthetic agents has opened an entirely new field. It is our hope that this pioneer work will elucidate the pathways by which certain halogenated compounds may produce damage to parenchymatous organs. If these pathways can be clearly marked, then the designer of new anesthetics will have had his task much simplified since it will become possible to predict which compounds might be metabolically changed to active fragments that could cause trouble with essential enzyme systems.

Until we have reached this prognostic utopia, we must learn to be content with the simple pedestrian methods currently at our disposal for the evaluation of toxic potential to the liver and kidneys. Examination of post-operative bromsulphalein retention by HUNT and his associates (1959) suggested that methoxyflurane was no more toxic to the liver than ether or cyclopropane as determined in the study of FRENCH and his co-workers (1952). CALE and associates (1962) found that methoxyflurane was not toxic to the kidney of dogs under conditions of repeated exposure, prolonged overdosage, hypoxia, and hypovolemia. The relative hazard of ephinephrine administration during methoxyflurane anesthesia awaits clarification. Until conclusive evidence applicable to human beings is available, it would seem wise not to promulgate the indiscriminate use of ephinephrine during methoxyflurane anesthesia. However, we must confess that although in our writing we suggest caution, it is only because BAMFORTH and co-workers have shown that under certain conditions epinephrine and methoxyflurane may result in ventricular fibrillation in dogs. In our extensive use of methoxyflurane and epinephrine in human beings, we have never had reason to fear the combination, and so we use these two drugs together without undue concern. It is our present feeling that methoxyflurane confers a degree of stability to the cardiovascular system similar to that seen with its nonhalogenated ether counterpart, diethyl ether. No anesthetic can be classified as totally safe in the presence of epinephrine nor can any anesthetic be classified as totally unsafe in the presence of peinephrine. There is a broad spectrum of interaction between various anesthetics and epinephrine with regard to the production of cardiac arrhythmias. We believe that ethers tend to be safer than hydrocarbons in this regard and feel that methoxyflurane confers nearly the same degree of safety which one may see in the presence of diethyl ether anesthesia.

IX. Summary and Critique

We have repeatedly stressed the clinical similarity between the anesthesias produced by methoxyflurane and diethyl ether in terms of analgesia, cardiovascular stability, and muscle relaxation. The major difference is the absence of explosion of fire hazard with methoxyflurane.

We have had methoxyflurane since 1958. In the 12 years that it has been part of our anesthetic armamentarium, we have had ample apportunity to investigate its advantages and disadvantages, its potentialities and its limitations. It has been enthusiastically hailed by some and enthusiastically damned by others. It would seem appropriate at this time to take stock of this anesthetic which we hoped to find in our search for a superior non-flammable anesthetic agent.

In 1958 I said that methoxyflurane was sufficiently interesting in its laboratory studies to warrant a careful clinical trial in man. Though all other opinion may change regarding this anesthetic agent, I believe that that original statement remains true. It is certainly not the ideal anesthetic agent, and I hope that we can do much better than this in years to come. However, cumbersome and clumsy though it may be, it provides many of the essentials of satisfactory anesthesia — analgesia, sedation, unconsciousness, muscle relaxation and cardiovascular stability. Beyond its clinical utility however, it has sparked interest in several areas of research. Because the mechanism of hepato-toxicity, or indeed its very existence, remains an area of much controversy for each individual anesthetic agent, there is need for knowledge about the mechanism of hepato-toxicity. The work of van Dyke and Chenoweth has opened a new chapter in the understanding of parenchymatous toxicity of volatile anesthetic agents. Prior to their work, it was generally believed that with the exception of trichloroethylene, inhalation anesthetics were excreted unchanged. van Dyke and Chenoweth have demonstrated that all commonly used inhalation abesthetics are biotransformed to some degree, and they have further demonstrated that there are different pathways of metabolic breakdown. What remains to be determined is the mechanism whereby metabolic fragments may interfere in essential enzymatic processes and possibly impair renal or hepatic function. The existence of methoxyflurane would be justified even if methoxyflurane did no more than open the pathway of research to a clearer understanding of anesthetic hepato-toxicity. Thus, it might be avoided through synthesis of agents whose metabolic breakdown could be predicted; agents could be designed to that there would be no toxic breakdown products formed.

Methoxyflurane has changed the concept that an anesthetic agent needs to have a high vapor pressure in order to be effective. Methoxyflurane is the first of the clinically used anesthetic agents which has an extremely low vapor pressure. Despite this low vapor pressure, it has the highest biologic potency of any anesthetic agent now in clinical use. In the past when drugs were screened for potential anesthetic value, those of low vapor pressure were discarded. In methoxyflurane we find evidence that agents of low vapor pressure may indeed be extremely effective as an anesthetic. The fact that an anesthetic liquid is difficult to vaporize need not in itself be ground for disqualifying that substance as a potential anesthetic. Indeed, the future may bring us solid compounds which may be of sufficiently high potency to induce analgesia or anesthesia even though they have extremely low vapor pressure. Among the invertebrates, substances such as camphor and naphthalene are capable of exerting profound physiological effects on insects. Perhaps compounds with similar low vapor pressures may be found which will have analgesic or anesthetic effects in animals and man.

Methoxyflurane has contributed to the understanding of the locus of action of anesthetic agents. In common with all other general anesthetic agents, methoxyflurane exerts a profoundly depressant action at the motor nerve terminal preparation of RIKER and associates (1959). This elegant neurophysiological preparation enables us to demonstrate that the motor nerve terminal is exquisitely sensitive to the action of all commonly used general anesthetics. The possibility exists that the central action of general anesthetics may well find its basis in action on nerve terminations rather than cell bodies within the central nervous system.

Methoxyflurane has extended our understanding of ether type anesthetics in comparison with the much more numerous hydrocarbon anesthetics. It is my present belief that when superior non-flammable inhalation anesthetics are synthesized, they will be non-flammable ethers rather than non-flammable hydrocarbons. I would like to believe that methoxyflurane has worthily served as the starting point in our search for superior non-flammable inhalation anesthetics.

X. Teflurane

Teflurane is a non-flammable inhalation anesthetic which in many ways is the counterpart of methoxyflurane. It is a halogenated hydrocarbon rather than an ether as is methoxyflurane. In many ways the pharmacological relationships between teflurane and methoxyflurane are similar to those between cyclopropane and diethyl ether.

Teflurane was originally available to us in 1957 through the synthetic work done at the Dow Chemical Company in Midland, Michigan. Our preliminary trials of this anesthetic in dogs were sufficiently encouraging to allow the extension of its use to man. Our first human anesthesia using teflurane was done in February, 1960. Data on the circulatory system and on liver function indicated that teflurane was essentially non-toxic in man as it was in the laboratory animals. We were joined by three other investigators who reviewed the accumulated results and began clinical use of teflurane in August, 1961. At a conference in September, 1961, the experiences reported by the four investigators were similar. Teflurane performed well as an inhalation anesthetic agent with the exception of cardiac irregularities which were occasionally severe. The conclusions reached at this conference were: 1. that the clinical use of teflurane should continue and 2. that additional laboratory work should be done to enlarge the pharmacologic knowledge. During such investigation, the data of WARNER (1962, 1967) indicated that kidney damage was observed in all the mongrel dogs which had been exposed to a total of 12 h of teflurane anesthesia during a period of one week. These results were contrary to our data and the data of NORTH (1962). However, because of the possibility of nephrotoxicity, c.inical use of teflurane was suspended. When two additional studies by GALINDO and FABIAN were done using pure bred beagles, there was no indication of nephrotoxicity.

With the exception of cardiac irregularities, there has been no dissatisfaction with the performance of teflurane. However, when observed on the cardioscope, these irregularities were so distressing to numerous anesthesiologists that clinical trial of teflurane was abandoned. Personally, I was most sorry to see this happen. It was my belief that this anesthetic agent was as useful as cyclopropane and had in addition the advantage of being non-flammable under operating room conditions. However, I was reluctant to urge my colleagues to use an anesthetic agent which they considered dangerous and so have made little public objection to seeing this anesthetic put on the shelf. It is my belief that it will be rediscovered and that at that time anesthesiologists will wonder why their predecessors had passed it by. When properly used with caution and respect with regard to its speed of action and potency and with appropriate medication to control the occurence of cardiac arrhythmias, teflurane is a thoroughly useful anesthetic agent.

XI. Chemical and Physical Properties

Teflurane is a halogenated ethane: 1,1,1,2-tetrafluro-2-bromoethane. The boiling point is 8.65 °C. Vapor pressure at several temperatures is given in Table 1 on the following page.

Table 1

Temperature 8.65 °C	Pressure 760. mmHg
10.	869.
20.	1240.
30.	1670.
40.	2300.
50.	3060.
65.	4530.

It is stable in the presence of light and does not react with alkali. It is therefore safe for use in the presence of carbon dioxide absorbers. The solubility coefficients in water, oil, and in various human tissues were reported by EDELIST, SINGER and EGER (1964). Water/gas coefficient was 0.32, Blood/gas 0.60, Oil/gas 29.0.

The specific gravity of tefluane is 1.862. The olive oil/water distribution coefficient of teflurane is 423 at 37 °C. The solubility in water at 37° is 0.04 g per 100 g and in olive oil, 30.8 g per 100 g.

Flammability determinations at intervals of 5% up to 70% in oxygen indicate that teflurane is non-flammable.

The water solubility of teflurane compared with other anesthetics is very low, as indicated in Table 2 below.

Table 2. *The water solubility of teflurane and some other inhalation anesthetic agents at 20°C*

Agent	Water solubility (ml gas/100 ml H_2O)
Teflurane	5.
Cyclopropane	30
Halothane	40
Nitrous oxide	68
Chloroform	300
Diethyl Ether	3900

Teflurane can be metered through a cyclopropane flowmeter using the rough calibrations supplied in Table 3 below.

Table 3. *The flow rate of teflurane through cyclopropane flowmeter*

Setting on cyclopropane flowmeter (ml/min)	Teflurane flow (ml/min)
25	16.45
50	36.7
100	80.5
200	119
300	183
400	238
500	311
600	329
700	421
800	476
900	494
1000	548
1100	567
1200	622
1300	731
1400	750
1500	786

XII. Pharmacology

a) Respiratory system — High concentrations of teflurane are depressant to respiration. Lower concentrations cause slight depression of respiration and allow easily assisted and controlled ventilation when required.

b) Heart — In dogs, teflurane produced a stable heart rate and normal sinus rhythm on the electrocardiogram. Rapid intravenous injections of epinephrine in doses from 5—30 micrograms per kilogram caused nodal tachycardia and ventricular premature contractions. One episode of irreversible venrticular standstill occured in one of six dogs following intravenous injection of epinephrine. NORTH (1962) observed that dogs receiving thiopental were more sensitive to the arrhythmogenic action of teflurane. During light anesthesia with teflurane, NORTH found that dogs were more sensitive to epinephrine challenge. During deep anesthesia, intravenous epinephrine even in doses as high as 50 micrograms per kilogram produced no fibrillation.

c) Circulation — In dogs, the blood pressure falls as the level of anesthesia is increased. ARTUSIO et al. (1961) reported that during surgical level of anesthesia in man, the blood pressure decreased on an average of 15% from the controlled values.

d) Liver — The results of liver function tests are quite encouraging. VAN POZNAK (1964) reported that liver function tests performed 3 times each week and biopsy reports every 10 weeks were within normal limits in several dogs repeatedly anesthetized with teflurane from whom liver biopsies were obtained.

WARNER (1967) reported that complete blood counts, blood urea and nitrogen and BSP determinations were all within normal limits. Some of the dogs in his study had received teflurane for 1 h twice weekly for 12 weeks. Others received teflurane for periods of 2—6 h and then repeated to make a total of 12 h exposure in 1 week. NORTH likewise reported no significant change in liver function tests or micriscopic anatomy of liver in dogs exposed for 3 h on successive days for 6 days.

GALINDO reported that all BSP tests were within normal limits in dogs that received 5 weekly exposures of 3—6 h duration.

e) Kidney — The reports of Artusio and van Poznak indicated no evidence of renal pathology following repeated administration of teflurane. The reports of North indicate the same. However, the reports presented by Warner indicated that there were some degenerative processes.

Following the report by Warner, three studies were arranged to investigate further the action of teflurane on the kidney. All three studies used pure bred beagle dogs in order to decrease the incidence of chronic pyelonephritis which is known to occur with considerable frequency in street animals. In all three of the studies, the results contradicted the earlier report of nephrotoxicity of teflurane.

XIII. Miscellaneous Findings

Warner observed that the growth rates of rats were unchanged by exposure to teflurane. Warner also reported that catecholamine determinations obtained from three dogs during plane 2 anesthesia with teflurane showed no deviation from control levels. Smith et al. (1965) reported preliminary studies on several fluorinated anesthetic agents. The concentrations of teflurane; 25% and 40% for 6 h, were sufficiently high to cause a high death rate of chicken embryos and a high rate of fetal anomalies. Organ concentrations of teflurane were determined by Chenoweth in a few dogs; high values of teflurane were found in the superior cervical ganglion and the highest level was found in the adrenal. This is consistent with results obtained by Chenoweth on other anesthetics which had a prediliction for these organs as well. The arterial blood concentration was 15.3 mg/100 g. This was the lowest value obtained — all other tissues had higher values. The highest was in the adrenal which had 326.3 mg/100 g.

XIV. Clinical Use of Teflurane

Artusio, van Poznak and Weingram (1900) reported on 150 administrations of teflurane to patients. Teflurane was given either by closed circle technique or by semi-closed technique. Although either method is suitable, the closed technique can allow repid buildup of toxic concentrations of teflurane. The semi-closed technique was found less likely to allow the buildup of dangerously high concentrations of the anesthetic. Approximately 200 clinical anesthesias were performed in four hospitals. Ages of the patients ranged from 1—89 years. Surgical procedures involved all systems of the body and ranged from brief minor surgical procedures to complicated neurosurgical procedures.

More than 100 patients had a sleep dose of thiopental as part of the induction. No unusual cardiac irregularities were observed. Therefore, North's observation in dogs that thiopental predisposes to arrhythmias does not seem to be borne out in human administration. Complications of teflurane anesthesia have been related to the cardiovascular system and were arrhythmias essentially due to too high a concentration of the anesthetic. Quite satisfactory protection against arrhythmias may be obtained by premedication or treatment of arrhythmias with propranolol.

XV. Summary and Conclusions

Teflurane is in many ways a non-explosive cyclopropane. It has been discontinued for trial in man because many investigators have been fearful of the cardiac irregularities that may be produced by it. However, it is my belief that these same investigators would have rejected cyclopropane had cardioscopes been available during the early days of cyclopropane's trial. It is my belief that when satisfactory premedication to prevent or control arrhythmias is used, teflurane is a safe, reliable and effective anesthetic which deserves reexamination.

References

ARTUSIO, J. F., JR.: Clinical evaluation of methoxyflurane in man. Federation Proc. 19, 272 (1960).
— HUNT, R. E., TIERS, F. M., ALEXANDER, M.: A clinical evaluation of methoxyflurane in man. Anesthesiology 21, 512 (1960).
— VAN POZNAK, A.: The concept of intermediate potency. Far East J. Anesth. 2, 27 (1958).
— — Anesthetic properties of a series of fluorinated compounds. I. Fluorinated hydrocarbons. Toxicol. Appl. Pharmacol. 2, 363—373 (1960).
— — BEIRNE, J. H., MERIN, R. G.: A clinical evaluation of teflurane: A preliminary report. (Presented at 45th Annual Meeting of Federation of American Societies for Experimental Biology, April, 1961.) Abstract in Federation Proc. 20, 312c, Pt. 1.
BAGWELL, E. E., WOODS, E. F.: Cardiovascular effects of methoxyflurane. Anesthesiology 23 51 (1962).
— — GADSDEN, R. H.: Blood levels and cardiovascular dynamics during methoxyflurane inhalation in dogs. Anesthesiology 23, 243 (1962).
— — MAHAFFEY, J.: Cardiovascular effects of methoxyflurane in dogs. Federation Proc. 20, 313 (1961).
BAMFORTH, B. J., SIEBECKER, K. L., KRAEMER, R., ORTH, O. S.: Effect of epinephrine on the dog heart during methoxyflurane anesthesia. Anesthesiology 22, 355 (1961).
CALE, J. O., PARKS, C. R., JENKINS, M. T.: Hepatic and renal effects of methoxyflurane in dogs. Anesthesiology 23, 248 (1962).
CAMPBELL, M. W., HVOLLBOLL, A. P., BRECHNER, V. L.: Penthrane: a clinical evaluation in 50 cases. Anesthesia & Analgesia 41, 134 (1962).
CHENOWETH, M. B., ROBERTSON, D. N., ERLEY, D. S., GOLHKE, R.: Blood and tissue levels of ether, chloroform, halothane and methoxyflurane in dogs. Anesthesiology 23, 101 (1962).
DOBKIN, A. B., FEDORUK, S.: Comparison of the cardiovascular, respiratory, and metabolic effects of methoxyflurane and halothane in dogs. Anesthesiology 22, 344 (1961).
— ISRAEL, J. S.: The effect of SA-97, perphenazine, and hydroxyzine on epinephrine-induced cardiac arrhythmias during methoxyflurane anaesthesia in dogs. Canad. Anaesth. Soc. J. 9, 36 (1962).
EDELIST, G., SINGER, M. M., EGER II., E. I.: Solubility coefficients of teflurane in various biological media. Anesthesiology 25, 223—225 (1964).
FABIAN, L. W.: The effect of three fluorinated compounds on the kidney. (Presented at the Annual Meeting of University Anesthetists, January, 1965.)
FRENCH, A. B., BARSS, T. P., FAIRLIE, C. S., BENGLE, A. L., JR., JONES, C. M., LINTON, R. R., BEECHER, H. K.: Metabolic effects of anesthesia in man. V. A comparison of the effects of ether and cyclopropane anesthesia on the abnormal liver. Ann. Surg. 135, 145 (1952).
GALINDO, A., BRINDLE, F. B., GILBERT, R. G. B.: Renal and hepatic function during teflurane anesthesia.
HUDON, R.: Methoxyflurane. Canad. Anaesth. Soc. J. 8, 544 (1961).
HUNT, R. E., ARTUSIO, J. F., JR., VAN POZNAK, A.: Effect of clinical anesthesia using DA-759 on liver function. Paper presented at Post-graduate Assembly in Anesthesiology, New York, 1959.
ISRAEL, J. S., DOBKIN, A. B., ROBIDOUX, H. J., JR.: The effect of sympathetic blockade of hyperventilation on epinephrine-induced cardiac arrhythmias during anaesthesia with halothane and methoxyflurane. Canad. Anaesth. Sioc. J. 9, 125 (1962).
JUMES, M. G., SIEBECKER, K. L.: Hepatic and respiratory effects of methoxyflurane. Paper presented at Postgraduate Assembly in Anesthesiology. New York, December 1960.
KNOX, P. R., NORTH, W. C., STEPHEN, C. R.: Methoxyflurane — a clinical evaluation. Anesthesiology 23, 238 (1962).
KUZUCU, E.: Methoxyflurane, tetracycline, and renal failure. J. Am. Med. Assoc. 211, 1162 to 1164 (1970).
MEEK, W. J., HATHAWAY, H. R., ORTH, O. S.: Effects of ether, chloroform and cyclopropane on cardiac automaticity. J. Pharmacol. Exptl Therap. 61, 240 (1937).
MILLAR, R. A., MORRIS, M. E.: A study of methoxyflurane anesthesia. Canad. Anaesth. Soc. J. 8, 210 (1961).

Ngai, S. H., Hanks, E. C.: Effect of methoxyflurane on electromyogram, neuromuscular transmission, and spinal reflex. Paper presented at Annual Meeting, American Society of Anesthesiologists, October, 1961.
— — Farhie, S. E.: Effects of anesthetics on neuromuscular transmission and somatic reflexes. Anesthesiology 26, 162—167 (1965).
North, W. C.: Cardiovascular effect of teflurane. Federation Proc. 21, 329c (1962).
— Knox, P. R.: The influence of methoxyflurane upon the cardiovascular response to epinephrine. Federation Proc. 20, 312 (1961).
— — Vartanian, V., Stephen, C. R.: Respiratory, circulatory, and hepatic effects of methoxyflurane in dogs. Anesthesiology 22, 138 (1961).
Power, D. J.: McGill University experiences with methoxyflurane. Canad. Anaesth. Soc. J. 8, 488 (1961).
Riker, W. F., Werner, G., Roberts, J., Kuperman, A.: Pharmacologic evidence for the existence of a presynaptic event in neuromuscular transmission. J. Pharmacol. Exptl Therap. 125, 150—158 (1959).
Siebecker, K. L., Jumes, M. G., Bamforth, B. J., Orth, O. S.: The respiratory effects of methoxyflurane on dog and man. Anesthesiology 22, 143 (1961).
Smith, B. E., Gaub, M. L., Moya, F.: Investigations into the teratogenic effects of anesthetic agents: The fluorinated agents. Anesthesiology 25, 260 (1965).
Standaert, F. G.: The action of d-tubocurarine on the motor nerve terminal. J. Pharmacol. Exptl Therap. 143, 181, 186 (1964).
Thompson, R., Light, G., Holaday, D. A.: Methoxyflurane anesthesia: A clinical appraisal. Anesthesia & Analgesia 41, 225 (1962).
van Dyke, R. A.: On the fate of chloroform (Editorial). Anesthesiology 257.
— Chenoweth, M. B.: Metabolism of volatile anesthetics (Review). Anesthesiology 26, 348 to 357 (1965).
van Poznak, A.: Laboratory and clinical investigations of teflurane. J. Amer. Ass. Nurse Anesthetist 32, 38—42 (1964).
— Artusio, J. F., Jr.: Series of fluorinated ethers. Federation Proc. 19, 273 (1960).
— — Anesthetic properties of a series of fluorinated compounds. I. Fluorinated hydrocarbons. Toxicol. Appl. Pharmacol. 2, 363 (1960).
— — Anesthetic properties of a series of fluorinated compounds. II. Fluorinated ethers. Toxicol. Appl. Pharmacol. 2, 374 (1960).
— Hou, B.: Neuromuscular effects of methoxyflurane. Federation Proc. 28, 419 (1969).
— Ray, B. S., Artusio, J. F., Jr.: Methoxyflurane as an anesthetic for neurological surgery. J. Neurosurg. 17, 477 (1960).
Warner, W. A., Orth, O. S.: Laboratory investigation of teflurane 1,1,1,2-tetrafluoro-2-bromoethane (DA-708). Federation Proc. 21, 325a (1962).
— Weber, D. L., Layton, J. M.: Laboratory investigation of teflurane 1,1,1,2-tetrafluoro-2-bromoethane (DA-708). Anesthesia & Analgesia 46, 32—38 (1967).
Wasmuth, C. E., Greig, J. H., Homi, J., Moraca, J., Isil, N. H., Bitt, E. M., Hale, D. E.: Methoxyflurane — a new anesthetic agent. Cleveland Clinic Quart. 27, 174 (1960).
Wyant, G. M., Chang, C. A., Rapicavoli, E.: Methoxyflurane (Penthrane): a laboratory and clinical study. Canad. Aanseth. Soc. J. 8, 477(1961).

Nota Bene

Professor Morris reports that there has been an explosion with fluroxene. The circumstances involved an anesthetic being given for a tonsillectomy in which the Bovie electrocautery was used as a method of hemostasis during the surgical procedure. Obviously there must have been a fairly high concentration of agent at the time of incident. Detonation occurred in a retrograde fashion so that it involved the anesthetic equipment and not the patient.

3.3. Fluroxene

Lucien E. Morris

Trifluoroethyl-vinyl ether (fluroxene, Fluoromar) introduced as the first volatile anesthetic containing fluorine was prepared by Julius Shukys in 1951 and extensively studied by J. C. Krantz who first anesthetized Dr. M. Sadove with it in 1953 (Krantz, Jr., et al., 1953). It was introduced for clinical trials in 1954 (Orth and Dornette, 1955; Sadove et al., 1956) and accepted by the Food and Drug Administration in 1956, but not marketed then because of the limited facilities for its manufacture and some concern about its high cost. Meantime, the advent of halothane (which came on with a strong advertising campaign) diverted the attention of anesthetists and was enthusiastically received on both sides of the Atlantic. Five years later, largely due to the efforts of Dr. Arthur Neeley, research chemist of the Ohio Chemical and Surgical Equipment Company, who believed it was a unique compound which would stand on its own merits, and supported by the opinion of those who had participated in its clinical trials (Dornette, 1956; Dundee et al., 1957; Gainza et al., 1956; Householder and Morris, 1957; Orth and Dornette, 1955; Sadove et al., 1957; Slater, 1957; Murray Hill Conference, 1956), trifluoroethyl-vinyl ether was placed on the market for use as a general anesthetic.

It received at first only scant and sporadic acceptance because by then it had to compete against not only the well established halothane, but also the subsequently introduced methoxyflurane. Only more recently do its peculiar pharmacological advantages become more apparent and the original faith and enthusiasm expressed by Dr. Neeley appear justified by renewed clinical interest in its special and potential applications, such as the anesthetic management of cardiovascular and other special problems (Joas and Craig, 1969; Miller et al., 1962; Share).

Fluroxene is manufactured from trifluoroethyl alcohol, obtained from interaction of fluorine with tetrachlorethane. The trifluoroethyl alcohol is added to acetylene in the presence of a catalyst and the resultant trifluoroethyl-vinyl ether is purified by fractional distillation.

Fluroxene is a clear, colorless, volatile liquid with a mild etherial odor which is sweet and non-irritant at lower concentrations.

Fluroxene may polymerise and in light may decompose to trifluoroethanol and acetaldehyde. Therefore, a stabilizing agent, 0.01% N-phenyl alpha naphthylamine is used to prevent this decomposition. The dark bottles also prevent the breakdown of the stabilizer by light.

I. Flammability

Over recent years much concern has been expressed about the fire and explosion hazard of agents such as cyclopropane and ether. It is perhaps debatable whether an occasional disastrous consequence should interdict the usage of otherwise highly advantageous agents, but it is nonetheless understandable that the dramatics and notoriety of such an event should sensitize and condition physicians against the usage of flammable agents, even though the incidence of trouble is low when compared with the less dramatic but more frequent hazards of alternative drugs. Evaluation of the problem must carefully differentiate between flammability and explosion. Many things burn which will not explode at ambient pressure. It appears that fluroxene is flammable at or above 4% in anhydrous mixtures with oxygen (4.2% in air) but that the propagation of flame is poor. Therefore, the occurrence of circumstances required for detonation and explosion is unlikely and remote (LAWRENCE and BASTRESS, 1959; MILLER and DORNETTE, 1961). When used with nitrous oxide, and especially when in combination with relaxants, there would be few times that the concentration required for anesthesia need be suffi-

Table 1. *Characteristics of Fluroxene, Trifluoroethyl-vinyl ether* (CF_3-CH_2-O-CH=CH_2)

Molecular weight	126.04
Specific gravity	1.13
Vapor density mol.wt./22.4	5.62 gm/L at 20 °C
Boiling point	43.2 °C
Saturated vapor pressure	
at 20 °C	286 mm
at 25 °C	370 mm
at 37 °C	600 mm
Latent heat of vaporization	7.78 K/mol (61,7 calories/gm)
Partitition coefficients	
water/gas at 37°	0.84
blood/gas at 37°	1.37
brain/gas	1.96
oil/gas at 37°	47.7
oil/H_2O at 37°	91
liver/gas	1.88
muscle/gas	3.11
Solubility in H_2O (30°)	0.4 ml/100 ml
Anesthetic range	2.4—8.0%
Blood levels	15—60 mgm/100 ml
MAC–1 Man	3.4% vapor (15 mgm/100 ml blood)
MAC–1 Dogs	6.0% vapor (32mg/100 ml blood)
MAC–1 Cat	4.0%

cient to ignite, even with an open flame. The presence of water vapor accumulating in a closed system would further elevate the lower limit of percentages at which ignition is possible. MILLER and DORNETTE found the lower limit of flammability of samples taken from circle absorption systems to be $7\frac{1}{2}$%. Other investigators, however (GRAMLING and VOLPITTO, 1963; ZEEDICK et al., 1966), have reported that they were able to explode mixtures of $7\frac{1}{2}$% or less in oxygen. It was also shown that the concentration of samples removed from the closed system were frequently in this same range. It is concluded, therefore, that the technique should be considered potentially flammable. Anhydrous mixtures of fluroxene in the range of 4—8% with oxygen are said to burn feebly because of a high energy requirement for ignition. At 6% the energy needed is not less than 0.3 mJ or to express it in another way, this substance is 30 times as hard to ignite with a spark as is ethyl ether. The decreased flammability is brought about because of the halogenation which achieves oxidation of carbon similar to combination with oxygen.

Unfortunately, the vinyl portion of the molecule is still ready and eager for combination. Despite this controversy it has been suggested that fluroxene is safe to use with electrocautery in cardiac operations (MILLER et al., 1962). This view has not been accepted with any enthusiasm.

The anesthetic range of fluroxene is 2.4—8.0% in air or oxygen. It would be less with augmented respiration because the alveolar concentration would be elevated by the increased alveolar turnover. In dogs and monkeys the anesthetic index is 2.35 (KRANTZ, JR. et al., 1953):

$$\text{anesthetic index} = \frac{\text{concentration required for respiratory arrest}}{\text{concentration for surgical anethesia}} = 2.35.$$

Fluroxene has been measured in arterial blood at levels from 10—60 mgm-% (BAGWELL and WOODS, 1963; DUNDEE et al., 1957; IWATSUKI et al., 1964), and in venous blood from 9—42 mgm-% (HOUSEHOLDER and MORRIS, 1957; SADOVE et al., 1956). It is most reasonable to reduce the concentration of fluroxene required by using it as a supplement to nitrous oxide. 77% nitrous oxide (alveolar concentration 72%) reduced the minimum anesthetic concentration (MAC) in man from 3.4% (fluroxene alone) to only 0.8% (MUNSON et al., 1965). MAC in dogs is 6% (EGER II et al., 1965). This lowers the cost as well as reducing the flammability hazard (MUNSON et al., 1965; VIRTUE and LEVINE, 1964). With nitrous oxide non-flammable concentrations of fluroxene can be maintained for light anesthesia. However, the induction phase may be prolonged unless higher (flammable) concentrations are used.

II. Azeotrope

As a result of the desire to separate the flammability limits from the anesthetic range and with the possibility of also reducing the production costs, studies were made of the azeotrope formed by fluroxene and Freon 113 (1,1,2-trifluoro-2,2,1-trichloroethane) (INAGAKI et al., 1966; KRANTZ, JR. et al., 1960; SARANGI et al., 1962). The lower limit of flammability of this azeotropic mixture was found to be 6.2%, which exceeded the level required for anesthesia in animals (KRANTZ, JR. et al., 1964). Clinical trials were satisfactory and not strikingly different from the use of fluroxene alone but the absolute amount of fluroxene required for clinical anesthesia in man did not seem to be altered (INAGAKI et al., 1966). It is therefore concluded that the azeotrope had little or no advantage over fluroxene alone.

III. Methods of Estimation

Blood and tissue levels of fluroxene have been correlated with the various concentrations and depths of anesthesia used. Earlier estimations followed the technique used for other ethers whereby the volatile compound was removed from blood by aeration or steam distillation or a combination of the two and subsequent bromination (BELL and KRANTZ, JR., 1953; LINDE, 1956). Since fluroxene readily adds bromine to its double bond, the steam distillate can be led to an excess of methanolic bromine solution. At the end of the distillation the excess bromine is reduced with iodide and back titrated with thiosulfate. This method is capable of estimating as little as 1 mgm of fluroxene per 100 ml of blood (LINDE, 1956).

Subsequently, as gas chromatographic methods became more readily available, this technique has become more popular because of its increased sensitivity and the smaller sample required. Anesthetics are either extracted from blood by an organic solvent, such as heptane, or blood is injected directly into the chromato-graph column or into the heated port of a flame ionization detector (BAGWELL and WOODS, 1963; IWATSUKI et al., 1964; LOWE, 1956).

Inspired or end-expiratory concentrations of fluroxene in the mixture of an-esthetic gases can be determined by an infrared detector. The halothane head of the Liston-Becker (Beckman) instrument has been adapted for this purpose (MUNSON et al., 1964, 1965).

IV. Bio-transformation

Fluroxene, like many other inhalation anesthetic agents, is metabolized by the body. Carbon 14 has been used for metabolic studies which indicate that trifluoro-ethyl-vinyl ether is extensively metabolized as evidenced by large amounts of non-volatile organic fluorine containing substances found in the urine. It appears that the vinyl portion of the ether is easily attacked in the biologic system. In animals carbon 14 tagged fluroxene is converted to trifluoroacetic acid and tri-fluoroethanol glucuronide. It has not been ascertained whether this has been the result of an enzymatic action or if this represents a natural instability of the vinyl ether under biological circumstances (BLAKE and CASCORBI, 1970; VAN DYKE and CHENOWETH, 1965).

V. Cardiovascular Effects

In dogs a tachycardia was often seen (KRANTZ, JR. et al., 1953). There was little or no incidence of cardiac arrhythmia even with a challenging dose of epi-nephrine which would routinely produce ventricular tachycardia during cyclo-propane (GAINZA et al., 1956; WHITE, JR. et al., 1956). However, in a subsequent study when approximately twice that dose of epinephrine was used, one animal out of the twelve studied died from ventricular fibrillation (ISRAEL et al., 1962). One clinical group has used epinephrine during fluroxene almost routinely in many hundreds of cases and also have recorded deliberate challenges with intravenous epinephrine in man (1 μg/kg of body weight given in a 15-sec interval). Premature ventricular contractions were seen in three of five patients, but no runs of ventric-ular tachycardia (DORNETTE, 1956; PRICE and DORNETTE, 1965). Since this is the sort of response that might very well occur in awake man with this injection, it appears that trifluoroethyl-vinyl ether, like diethyl ether, does not "sensitize" the conduction system of the heart to the effect of epinephrine, as do cyclopropane, trichloroethylene, and others. Of all the halogenated anesthetics, fluroxene is least likely to exhibit serious arrhythmias with the concomitant use of epinephrine (KATZ and EPSTEIN, 1968).

Initially Virtue noted that in clinical administration of trifluoroethyl-vinyl ether there were sudden and worrisome falls in blood pressure which occurred before other signs of deep anesthesia (GAINZA et al., 1956; Murray Hill Conference, 1956). In a later comparison with halothane when anesthetics with both agents were carefully held to pattern 4 EEG depth, fluroxene was shown to be more stable, have less depression of blood pressure and no change in cardiac output (VIRTUE et al., 1964). Cardiac rhythm is usually undisturbed with minimal changes in the EKG. Indeed, as clinicians have gained experience with this agent they seem to have become more intrigued and satisfied with its usefulness. If blood pressure does fall it should be taken as a sign that the patient is hypovolemic or that the level of anesthesia is momentarily too deep. In this circumstance blood pressure will usually return to near normal levels when the concentration of agent is reduced.

Early reports of cardiovascular responses to fluroxene in dogs (BAGWELL et al., 1966) indicated progressive depression of contractile force, aortic pressure and aortic flow as anesthesia was deepened. This is consistent with the usual findings with most anesthetics. However, more recent studies have shown a higher stroke volume and higher cardiac output at MAC-2 than occur at MAC-1 (MORRIS and STOYKA). This latter observation is consistent with recorded cardiovascular effects of fluroxene in 11 otherwise unmedicated human volunteers at constant temperature and normal $PaCO_2$ (CULLEN et al., 1970). At 5% and 9% fluroxene, cardiac output, heart rate and mean arterial pressure were unchanged from awake control, but at 12% fluroxene the means of cardiac output and heart rate rose by 50% and the mean arterial pressure by nearly 20% in the first 90 min, and a still greater increase occurred after 5 h. In the same study central venous pressure was elevated in the first hour and gradually returned toward normal subsequently. Their data also exhibits some considerable variability with some subjects having a decreased or delayed sympathetic response resulting in an early fall of cardiac output and subsequent compensation. These observations prompted their cautionary warning that despite the overall average of minimal depressant effects that "in a patient with a limited cardiovascular reserve or impaired sympathetic function, a rapid increase in fluroxene could result in severe hypotension."

Interesting information has come from studies with 4, 8, and 12% fluroxene in the cat (SKOVSTED and PRICE, 1970). 4% fluroxene (MAC-1) did not significantly change arterial pressure or cervical sympathetic activity; 8% caused a considerable increase in sympathetic nervous activity (70%) without effect on arterial pressure; 12% caused only slight further change in sympathetic nervous output (87%), but decreased arterial pressure significantly. Baroreceptor denervation during fluroxene was followed by elevation of sympathetic nervous activity to the same degree. It was concluded therefore that fluroxene, like cyclopropane and ether, elevates sympathetic outflow not by reflex barostatic activation but through failure of the reflex by depression of medullary depressor neurons.

Investigation has been made in dogs of the cardiovascular response to deliberately induced acid base changes, including respiratory and metabolic acidosis during fluroxene anesthesia at MAC-1 (STOYKA et al., 1970). Observed cardiac output rose slightly with elevation of $PaCO_2$ but fell in linear fashion as pH declined through the same range following hydrochloric acid infusion or bouts of hypoxia. Similar reductions in pH during fluroxene MAC-2 caused a comparable decline in cardiac output but at a consistently higher level than at MAC-1. Return to MAC-1 caused a fall in cardiac output in the pH range 7.1—7.4 (MORRIS and STOYKA).

VI. Central Nervous System Effects

Fluroxene is credited with an intense analgesia in stage I. The signs of general anesthesia are somewhat different from ether and to some extent resemble those produced by cyclopropane. Consciousness is rapidly lost, anesthesia is quickly achieved and so the incidence of excitement is low and laryngospasm is infrequent. As stage II is entered, there is regular respiration, pupils are small and lateral eyeball movement is quite evident. As depth of surgical anesthesia increases, eyeballs become fixed, the pupils gradually dilate (but not as rapidly as with diethyl ether), tidal volume is decreased and tachypnea frequent.

The electroencephalographic patterns show a progressive change correlated with deepening anesthesia (Dundee et al., 1957; Gainza et al., 1956; House-holder and Morris, 1957). These changes were not always consistent with the clinical signs of anesthesia. It was felt the depth of anesthesia was difficult to judge. Hypotension was said to occur without prior warning of change in depth on the EEG (Gainza et al., 1956). Brechner et al. (1957), identified six EEG patterns with nitrous oxide and trifluoroethyl-vinyl ether anesthesia, while Householder and Morris (1957) correlated four patterns with blood levels of this agent at 9, 15, 18 and 30 mgm-%, the last with burst suppression of the EEG. Iwatsuki et al. (1964), reported nine separate patterns in anesthesia with fluroxene alone and correlated these with arterial blood levels in the range of 10—50 mgm-%. His last two patterns were in deep anesthesia taken beyond the range of burst suppression.

VII. Respiratory Effects

Despite the early and repeated clinical observation (Dundee and Dripps, 1957; Murray Hill Conference, 1956) that in deeper anesthesia respiration tended to become inadequate because of a developing tachypnea, a ventilation study in man found that mean $PaCO_2$ values observed during fluroxene were less than with halothane and the slope of CO_2 response (litres per minute per millilitre of $PaCO_2$) although depressed by anesthesia was greater with fluroxene than with halothane at equipotent anesthetic concentration at multiples of MAC ranging from 1.1—2.5 (Munson et al., 1966).

The tachypnea accompanying deep levels of fluroxene anesthesia was considered to be like that with trichloroethylene, probably due to sensitization of both pulmonary inflation and deflation reflexes (Dundee and Dripps, 1957). A more recent study designed to test this thesis concluded that instead of a sensitization of the Hering-Breuer reflex there is evidence for depression or absence of this control mechanism under general anesthesia so that increased effort does not follow an increased load (Paskin et al., 1968). They further suggest that proper treatment is assistance or control of respiration by mechanical augmentation of respiratory volume. Early laboratory work with dogs mentioned the occurrence of pulmonary edema (Smith, R. M., in Murray Hill Conference, 1956) and this has been seen more recently (Morris and Stoyka; Sawyer) but appears to have been associated with prolonged anesthesia at higher than necessary concentrations (MAC-2 or greater).

VIII. Gastro-intestinal, Hepatic, and Renal Effects

There is a reduction in tone and activity of the smooth muscle of the gastro-intestinal tract during fluroxene. Normal function usually returns shortly upon recovery of consciousness. Nausea and emesis occur less frequently than with diethyl ether, and can be minimized by scrupulous attention to ventilation and avoidance of prolonged anesthesia at deeper levels (Gainza et al., 1956).

In studies made in man, no post-anesthetic derangements of hepatic function have been shown (Brechner et al., 1958; Cannon and Dornette, 1964; Dor-nette, 1956; Morris, 1965; Sadove et al., 1956, 1957). A battery of liver function tests revealed no significantly greater change in liver function after nitrous oxide-Fluoromar than after nitrous oxide-curare (Morris, 1960; Stavney and Morris). After deliberate carbon dioxide challenge during fluroxene anesthesia, there was no deleterious response which is in sharp contrast to the alterations in liver function tests observed following similar challenges during chloroform, halothane, or methoxyflurane (MORRIS, 1962).

No adverse renal effects have been reported. Urea clearance subsequent to fluroxene anesthetics is similar to the findings after most other anesthetic agents in producing minimal or no changes from normal (GAINZA et al., 1956; SADOVE et al., 1957).

IX. Clinical Considerations

The clinical notation that fluroxene is an anesthetic with a rapid onset of action correlates well with its low solubility in blood and other tissues and indicates a low uptake of fluroxene. The relatively low solubility permits the alveolar concentration to rise rapidly and consequently anesthesia is produced quickly. Recovery is also rapid unless the anesthetic has been maintained for a long time. Comparison shows solubility of fluroxene to be intermediate between cyclopropane and halothane, which also is consistent with clinical observations of speeds of induction and recovery.

The frequent complaint of early observers that it was difficult to estimate clinically and be sure of depth of anesthesia reflects not only the rapidity of effect and lability of the fluroxene because of its low solubility, but probably also was contributed to by variable leaks in the anesthetic system as well as some unfamiliarity with the vagaries of the agent itself.

Siallorhea is less than would be expected with diethyl ether but occurs to an extent that routine use of belladonna is useful to keep patients drier and prevent laryngospasm. Pharyngeal reflexes are not very active by the time there is sufficient relaxation of the masseter muscles to allow the jaw to be opened easily. At that point the cords are well abducted so laryngeal intubation is smooth and uneventful.

Relaxation varies directly with depth in young patients but in older adults good surgical conditions for operation in the abdomen seem to require excessively deep levels of anesthesia. In some instances it seems more difficult to attain relaxation of the jaw than relaxation of the abdomen (DUNDEE et al., 1957; ORTH and DORNETTE, 1955).

Respiratory depression appears early, out of proportion to the other signs of deepening anesthesia such as muscle relaxation (Murray Hill Conference, 1956). With overdose there also may be sudden depression of blood pressure with inadequate warning (GAINZA et al., 1956; Murray Hill Conference, 1956). Depression of the respiratory and cardiovascular system can occur before full relaxation. Therefore, this drug is not always suitable as a fully potent anesthetic used alone to provide relaxation in abdominal work. The use of a supplemental intravenous muscle relaxant is indicated in preference to deep anesthesia and the concomitant depression of both respiration and circulation. In our hands the best satisfaction with fluroxene has been as an adjuvant to nitrous oxide utilizing the assistance of additional relaxant drugs as needed. In all but shortest cases intubation is desirable in the interest of reducing the possibility of leaks.

Opiates can be used to combat the tachypnea which is observed in moderate to deep anesthesia. However, it must be recognized that although rate is slowed, tidal excursion is not increased and the ultimate result is decreased ventilation. Because of this tendency assisted ventilation or controlled respiration with maintenance of normal $PaCO_2$ is indicated in all but the lightest plane of anesthesia.

7*

Fluroxene is compatible with sodalime and can be used in all anesthetic systems. However, use of a system with non-rebreathing valves is rather spend-thrift of an expensive agent and requires expert attention to maintain a constant smooth level of anesthesia. On the other hand, apparent changes in depth of anesthesia can occur with extraordinary rapidity no matter what the system used.

Vaporizers which are placed in the patient's rebreathing circuit (V–I–C) allow a rapid increase in concentration of this relatively insoluble agent to potentially dangerous levels of overdosage. For this reason, neither the V–I–C nor the closed system of administration is recommended.

Discrete control over concentration is best obtained in a semiclosed system with the vaporizer placed out of the patient circuit (V–O–C) such as in the design of a Copper Kettle or Vernitrol machine. In these latter systems, the concentration cannot become higher than the diluted mixture provided from the machine.

When the Fluotec vaporizer (V–O–C) is used with fluroxene it provides moderately good control of vapor concentrations up to a maximum of about 5% (at the 4% setting for halothane). An adaptation of this device, called the Fluoromatec, has an empiric scale and provides a range of concentration to approximately 10%.

X. Applications

Trifluoroethyl-vinyl ether is useful in the absence of explosion hazards for procedures which require only light anesthesia. It deserves consideration as an adjuvant to nitrous oxide for dental (HUGHES and DORNETTE, 1961; Murray Hill Conference, 1956; SLATER, 1957), ENT (McCOLLUM, 1966; McCOLLUM and HILDYARD, 1965), orthopedic, gynecologic, urologic and obstetrical procedures, as well as for burn dressings and any other type of operation which requires little relaxation, rapid recovery, or a considerable analgesia. Its compatibility with epinephrine is also of major value.

A number of observers have been enthusiastic about the use of fluroxene in obstetrics (CAVALLARO and DORNETTE, 1961; MARTIN and BOSNAK, 1962; Murray Hill Conference, 1956). This stems partly from its excellent analgesic properties but also from the fact that, in contradistinction to the use of trichloroethylene analgesia, after exposure of the patient to fluroxene the closed absorption system and epinephrine still can be used without concern. Recent work, however, indicates that fluroxene is similar to halothane in respect to the effects upon the uterus and the potential of an increased blood loss, either at delivery or in the circumstance of therapeutic abortions (CULLEN et al., 1970). Since higher concentrations will produce uterine inertia, fluroxene may be useful in circumstances where uterine relaxation is desired.

Recently the suggestion has been made that there may be special merit in the choice of fluroxene for the management of cases for pheochromocytoma removal (JOAS and CRAIG, 1969). Again, the stability of the cardiovascular system and the lack of myocardial sensitization to epinephrine appear to be the primary advantages. However, attainment of normovolemia and avoidance of all causes of autonomic imbalance remain important corollaries of management in these cases.

XI. Conclusion

Although fluroxene is by no means the perfect anesthetic, it does have sufficient attributes to warrant wider usage in selected circumstances and to justify its inclusion in the choices available to all competent anesthesiologists.

References

BAGWELL, E. E., GADSDEN, R. H., RISINGER, K. B. H., WOODS, E. F.: Blood levels and cardiovascular dynamics during fluroxene anaesthesia in dogs. Can. Anaesth. Soc. J. **13**, 378—389 (1966).
— WOODS, E. F.: Federation Proc. **22**, 179, Abstract No. 473 (1963).
BELL, F. K., KRANTZ, J. C., JR.: Anesthesia XVLIII. The estimation of anesthetic trifluor-ethyl vinyl ether in aqueous solution. J. Am. Pharm. Assoc. **42**, 633—634 (1953).
BLAKE, D. A., CASCORBI, H. F.: A note on the biotransformation of fluroxene in two volun-teers. Anesthesiology **32**, 560 (1970).
BRECHNER, V. L., DORNETTE, W. H. L.: Electroencephalographic patterns during nitrous oxide-trifluoro-ethyl vinyl ether anesthesia. Anesthesiology **18**, 321—327 (1957).
— WATANABE, R. S., DORNETTE, W. H. L.: Values for serum glutamic oxalacetic transaminase following anesthesia with fluoromar. Anesthesia & Analgesia **37**, 257—262 (1958).
CANNON, G. M., DORNETTE, W. H. L.: Are all halogens hepatotoxic? Anesthesia & Analgesia **43**, 400—406 (1964).
CAVALLARO, R. J., DORNETTE, W. H. L.: Fluoromar anesthesia in obstetrics; a preliminary report. Obstet. and Gynecol. (U.S.S.R.) **17**, 447—452 (1961).
CULLEN, B. F., EGER, E. I., II, SMITH, N. T., SAWYER, D. C., GREGORY, G. A., JOAS, T. A.: Cardiovascular effects of fluroxene in man. Anesthesiology **32**, 218—230 (1970).
— MARGOLIS, A. J., EGER, E. I., II: The effects of anesthesia and pulmonary ventilation on blood loss during elective therapeutic abortion. Anesthesiology **32**, 108—113 (1970).
DOBKIN, A. B., BYLES, P. H.: The effect of fluroxene (Fluoromar) on acid-base balance in man. Acta Anaesth. Scand. **6**, 115—128 (1962).
DORNETTE, W. H. L.: Trifluoroethylvinyl ether (Fluoromar); a preliminary report on clinical experience and animal experiment. Calif. Med. **85**, 311—313 (1956).
DUNDEE, J. W., DRIPPS, R. D.: The effects of diethyl ether, trichloroethylene, and trifluoro-ethyl vinyl ether on respiration. Anesthesiology **18**, 282—289 (1957).
— LINDE, H. W., DRIPPS, R. D.: Observations on trifluoroethyl vinyl ether. Anesthesiology **18**, 66—72 (1957).
EGER, E. I., II, BRANDSTATER, B., SAIDMAN, L. J., REGAN, M. J., SEVERINGHAUS, J., MUNSON, E. S.: Equipotent alveolar concentrations of methoxyflurane, halothane, diethyl ether, fluroxene, cyclopropane, xenon, and nitrous oxide in the dog. Anesthesiology **26**, 771—777 (1965).
GAINZA, E., HEATON, C. E., WILLCOX, M., VIRTUE, R. W.: Physiological measurements during anaesthesia with fluoromar. Brit. J. Anaesthesia **28**, 411—421 (1956).
GRAMLING, Z. W., VOLPITTO, P. P.: Flammability of fluoromar in the circle absorption system. Anesthesiology **24**, 194—197 (1963).
HUGHES, B. H., DORNETTE, W. H. L.: Trifluoroethyl vinyl ether-nitrous oxide anesthesia for oral surgical operations for ambulatory patients. J. Oral Surg. **19**, 385—391 (1961).
HOUSEHOLDER, J. R., MORRIS, L. E.: Correlations of the electroencephalogram with trifluoro-ethyl vinyl ether (fluoromar) anesthesia. Anesthesiology **18**, 167—168 (1957).
INAGAKI, M., YUSA, T., AOBA, Y., IWATSUKI, K.: Studies on azeotropic mixture of fluoromar and freon 113. Tôhoku J. Exptl Med. **89**, 143—150 (1966).
ISRAEL, J. S., CRISWICK, V. G., DOBKIN, A. B.: Effect of epinephrine on cardiac rhythm during anesthesia with methoxyflurane (penthrane) and trifluoroethyl vinyl ether fluromar). Acta Anaesth. Scand. **6**, 7—11 (1962).
IWATSUKI, K., INAGAKI, M., NISHIOKA, K., TAKAHASHI, H.: Electroencephalographic patterns during anesthesia with fluoromar. Tôhoku J. Exptl Med. **82**, 52—61 (1964).
JOAS, T. A., CRAIG, D.: Fluroxene anesthesia for pheochromocytoma removal. J. Am. Med. Assoc. **209**, 927—929 (1969).
KATZ, R. L., EPSTEIN, R. A.: The interaction of anesthetic agents and adrenergic drugs to produce cardiac arrhytmias. Anesthesiology **29**, 763—784 (1968).
KRANTZ, J. C., JR., CARR, C. J., LU, G., BELL, F. K.: Anesthesia XL. The anesthetic action of trifluoroethyl vinyl ether. J. Pharmacol. Exptl Therap. **108**, 488—495 (1953).
— LING, J. S. L., KOZLER, Z. F.: Anesthesia, LXI: The anesthetic properties of the azeo-tropic mixture of trifluoroethyl vinyl ether (fluoromar) and 112-trifluoro-221-trichloro-ethane (genetron 113). J. Pharmacol. Exptl Therap **130**, 492—496 (1960).
LAWRENCE, J. S., BASTRESS, E. K.: Combustion characteristics of anesthetics. Anesthesiology **20**, 192—197 (1959).
LINDE, H. W.: Estimation of trifluoroethyl vinyl ether (fluoromar) in blood. Anesthesiology **17**, 777—781 (1956).
LOWE, H. J.: Flame ionization detection of volatile organic anesthetics in blood, gases and tissues. Anesthesiology **25**, 808—814 (1964).

McCOLLUM, K. B.: Fluoromar: II. Anesthetic for tonsillectomy and adenoidectomy. Anesthesia & Analgesia 45, 103—105 (1966).
— HILDYARD, V. H.: Fluoromar: I. Anesthetic for otologic surgery. Anesthesia & Analgesia 44, 758—761 (1965).
MARTIN, E. M., BOSNAK, J. N.: Trifluoroethyl vinyl ether (fluroxene, fluoromar) in abstetrics. Can. Anaesth. Soc. J. 9, 419—423 (1962).
MILLER, G. L., DORNETTE, W. H. L.: Flammability studies of fluoromar oxygen mixtures used in anesthesia. Anesthesia & Analgesia 40, 232—237 (1961).
— — CAVALLARO, R. J.: Fluoromar as the anesthetic agent of choice for cardiac operations. Anesthesia & Analgesia 41, 128—133 (1962).
MORRIS, L. E.: Comparison studies of hepatic function following anesthesia with a halogenated agent. Anesthesiology 21, 109—110 (1960).
— Liver function with the fluorinated agents. Proceedings of the First European Congress (Vienna), Varia 242, 1962.
— Liver function with various anesthetic agents. Pacific Med. Surg. 73, 60—62 (1965).
— STOYKA, W.: Unpublished observations.
MUNSON, E. S., LARSON, C. P. JR., BABAD, A. A., REGAN, M. J., BUECHEL, D. R., EGER, E. I. II: The effects of halothane, fluroxene, and cyclopropane on ventilation. A comparative study in man. Anesthesiology 27, 716—728 (1966).
— SAIDMAN, L. J., EGER, E. I. II: Solubility of fluroxene in blood and tissue homogenates. Anesthesiology 25, 638—640 (1964).
— — — Fluroxene: Uptake in man at constant alveolar and constant inspired concentrations. Anesthesiology 26, 8—13 (1965).
— — — The effect of nitrous oxide and morphine on the minimum anesthetic concentration of fluroxene. Anesthesiology 26, 134—139 (1965).
Murray Hill Conference on Fluoromar-Transcript, Ohio Chemical and Surgical Equipment Co., April 1956.
ORTH, O. S., DORNETTE, W. H. L.: Fluoromar as an anesthetic agent. Federation Proc. 14, 376 (Abstract No. 1214) (1955).
PASKIN, S., SKOVSTED, P., SMITH, T. C.: Failure of the Hering-Breuer reflex to account for tachypnea in anesthetized man: A survey of halothane, fluroxene, methoxyflurane and cyclopropane. Anesthesiology 29, 550—558 (1968).
PRICE, H. L.: The significance of catecholamine release during anesthesia. Brit. J. Anaesthesia 38, 707—711 (1966).
PRICE, J. H., DORNETTE, W. H. L.: An assessment of fluroxene-epinephrine compatability in man. Anesthesia & Analgesia 44, 83—88 (1965).
SADOVE, M. S., BALAGOT, R. C., LINDE, H. W.: Trifluoroethylvinyl ether (fluoromar) I. Preliminary clinical and laboratory studies. Anesthesiology 17, 591—600 (1956).
— — — The effect of fluoromar on certain organ functions. Anesthesia & Analgesia 36, 47—51 (1957).
SARANGI, B. K., MORRIS, L. E., HOUSEHOLDER, J. R.: Observations on an azeotrope of fluoromar and freon 113. Anesthesia & Analgesia 41, 702—706 (1962).
SAWYER, D. C.: Personal communication.
SHARE, M.: Personal communication.
SKOVSTED, P., PRICE, H. L.: Central sympathetic excitation caused by fluroxene. Anesthesiology 32, 210—217 (1970).
SLATER, H. M.: The use of trifluoroethyl vinyl ether (fluoromar) in anaesthesia for dentistry. Can. Anaesth. Soc. J. 4, 5—12 (1957).
STAVNEY, L. S., MORRIS, L. E.: Liver function in patients following anesthesia with trifluoroethyl vinyl ether. Unpublished data.
STOYKA, W., MURPHY, P. V., MORRIS, L. E.: Cardiac output variations with acid-base change during trifluoroethyl vinyl ether (fluoromar). Federation Proc. 29, 525 (Abstract No. 1560) (1970).
van DYKE, R. A., CHENOWETH, M. B.: Metabolism of volatile anesthetics. Anesthesiology 26, 348—358 (1965).
VIRTUE, R. W., LEVINE, D.: Cost of anesthesia with fluroxene. Anesthesiology 25, 236—237 (1964).
— VOGEL, J. H. K., PRESS, P., GROVER, R. F.: Respiratory and hemodynamic measurements during anesthesia. J. Am. Med. Assoc. 179, 224—225 (1962).
WHITE, J. M., JR., NATIONS, F. N., STAVNEY, L. S.: Cardiac conduction in the dog during anesthesia with fluoromar. Federation Proc. 15, 499 (1956).
YOUNG, J. A.: New inhalants for dental anesthesia. J. Oral Surg. 23, 503—507 (1965).
ZEEDICK, J. F., THOMAS, G. J., OLIVO, N., JEROSKI, E.: Clinical experience with fluroxene nitrous oxide-oxygen anesthesia as a non-flammable anesthetic. Anesthesia & Analgesia 45, 790—795 (1966).

Section 4.0

Comparative Action on vital System of Man

4.1. Central Nervous System*

ANIBAL GALINDO

With 6 Figures

General anesthesia is a reversible and somewhat selective depression of certain functions of the central nervous system, produced by a variety of structurally dissimilar drugs. The progressive depression of neural functions results in patterns of neurological signs whose characteristics depend on the type of the drug and its concentration in the central nervous system. These neurologic signs, when arranged in stages and planes, are useful to the anesthesiologist as an index of the degree of depression of the central nervous system and as a guide in the administration of anesthesia.

This section is divided into three parts. The first deals with the concept of stages and planes of anesthesia; the second with the physiological basis of the various neurological observations; and the third with the pattern, or combination of clinical signs seen with some of the most commonly used inhalation agents.

A. Stages and Planes of Anesthesia

The concept of stages and planes of anesthesia was originally proposed by SNOW (1847) as a practical guide to anticipate the patient's responses to painful stimuli as well as to prevent fatal overdosage of anesthetics; the graphic arrangement of these stages in horizontal planes was proposed by GUEDEL in 1920. This arrangement is based on a progressive and predictable depression of reflex responses, and on an equally predictable sequence of changes in vital signs, observed during the administration of an anesthetic.

The scheme described by GUEDEL (1951) (Fig. 1), long accepted as a classic model of the progression of ether anesthesia, is inadequate for classifying the levels of anesthesia with other agents. Furthermore, the use of premedication, muscle relaxants, and the combination of various agents have reduced its usefulness in clinical practice. The need for a universal scheme, applicable to all anesthetics, has stimulated several authors to propose various modifications of GUEDEL's description (GILLESPIE, 1943; MUSHIN, 1948; LAYCOCK, 1953; WOODBRIDGE, 1957; DORNETTE, 1964). The various planes of anesthesia have been reduced to two stages; the first is called "light" or "superficial" anesthesia and is characterized by minimal analgesia and muscular relaxation. The second is called "deep" or "profound" anesthesia and is characterized by greater CNS depression. The transition from superficial to deep anesthesia is not sharp and varies

* Supported by NIH PHS Grant GM 15991-03

from one anesthetic to the other. Changes in respiratory pattern are useful with ether, the degree of hypotension may be useful with halothane, while lack of motor responses to peripheral stimuli marks the presence of "deep" barbiturate sleep.

The fact that the pattern of depression changes with different agents suggests that the general phenomenon known as anesthesia involves multiple mechanisms.

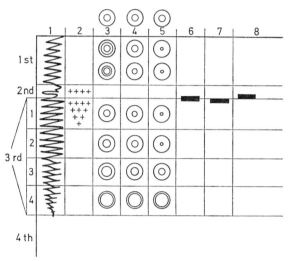

Column 1. Respiration   Column 6. Eyelid reflex
Column 2. Eyeball activity   Column 7. Area of swallowing
Columns 3, 4, 5. Pupils   Column 8. Area of vomiting

Fig. 1. Guedel's scheme describes the gradual onset of ether anesthesia. Muscular relaxation is satisfactory for abdominal surgery in the third stage planes 2—3, while at the same level ventilation and arterial blood pressure are little depressed. The sequence observed with other anesthetics is different. During halothane anesthesia, the pupils tend to remain constricted; ventilation, blood pressure, and heart rate are depressed from the beginning of surgical anesthesia (third stage), relaxation of the abdominal muscles parallels this depression. With methoxyflurane anesthesia the respiratory system is more depressed than the cardiovascular; satisfactory relaxation of abdominal muscles is obtained with less arterial hypotension than with halothane. Cyclopropane, like ether, has little effect on the cardiovascular system but strongly depresses pulmonary ventilation; the pupils dilate somewhat sooner and muscular relaxation is similar to that produced by ether. Nitrous oxide induces unconsciousness and analgesia with most reflexes and homeostatic mechanisms undepressed; similarly there is no muscular relaxation. From GUEDEL, 1951, by courtesy of the Editor of Inhalation Anesthesia: A Fundamental Guide, editor The Macmillan Company

It is now clear that the neuropharmacology of anesthetics is too complex. Rather than searching for a universal scheme of stages and planes of anesthesia, we must understand the neurophysiological basis behind the various patterns of CNS depression.

The pattern of neurological signs observed with ether anesthesia was at one time thought to follow a "standard sequence of neuronal depression" (HARRIS, 1951); an explanation strongly influenced by the concept of "levels of function" proposed by Hughlings Jackson. The stratification of stages and planes of anesthesia was correlated with a horizontal localization of functions; it was assumed that the sequential depression was based on precise anatomical localization. The central nervous system was thought to consist of various separate "centers" each one with a different function; thus, according to the sequential hypothesis, amnesia was produced by a preferential depression of cells in the frontal association area, stupor indicated suppression of remaining areas of the cortex, hyper-reflexia was caused by a release of hypothalamic control from the cortex; and loss of temperature-regulation indicated complete hypothalamic depression. It was reasoned that the newest neurological structures (neopallium) were more susceptible to the effect of anesthetics than the older formations (archipallium and paleopallium).

We cannot discard the correlation between function and precise anatomical localization, but must also take into account that the CNS appears to function as an integrated whole rather than as a rigidly departmentalized structure (SHERRINGTON, 1906). It is more reasonable for the understanding of the mode of action of anesthetics to localize preferential sites of action in a functional manner, or in terms of common neurotransmitters, or of specific membrane characteristics, than to postulate a sequence of effects on hypothetical "centers". Recent hypotheses correlate anesthesia with a selective depression of the brain stem "activating system" (FRENCH et al., 1953) or, alternatively with a specific depression of cholinergic pathways (KRNJEVIC, 1967; PHILLIS, 1968). While these ideas advocate a functional organization of the mechanism of anesthesia, they fail to explain the varied patterns of CNS depression normally observed with the different anesthetic agents.

There is no single hypothesis at the present time that could explain the various patterns of neurological depression observed with different anesthetics, but if we accept the existence of multiple mechanisms and sites of action it is necessary to investigate the reasons for these differences; as well as determining which structure, if any, needs to be selectively depressed to induce general anesthesia.

The discussion of neurological observations which follows in the next two parts of this section, is oriented to the preferential effects of a given anesthetic. It is granted that these effects increase with increasing concentration of anesthetic in the blood, and that they can be modified by combination of drugs, or by pre-existent conditions (e.g. acid-base disturbances).

B. Clinical Observations

Analgesia. Depression, or complete suppression of pain perception represents the main reason for the clinical use of anesthetics. Unfortunately, the understanding of the mechanisms involved in this perception, and consequently the manner in which they can be depressed, is poor at the present time.

For some investigators pain is just another sensorial modality with its own specific receptors and neuronal pathways. Recent findings of nerve fibres responding only to noxious stimuli (BURGESS and PERL, 1967; PERL, 1968) gives support to this hypothesis. Other investigators (WEDDELL, 1955; SINCLAIR, 1955) believe that pain is the subjective accompaniment of a high frequency discharge of impulses at one extreme of the sensorial spectrum. MELZACK and WALL (1965) have recently proposed a theory that could accommodate both hypotheses; for them pain is described as a specific input signal carried only by small nerve fibres, transmission of which is modulated by a gate-like arrangement in the spinal cord. This "gate" — which actually consists of one or more spinal synapses — would be opened or closed by several inputs converging from the periphery through larger nerve fibres, and descending inputs from higher structures in the CNS.

It is reasonable to assume that anesthetics could block noxious stimuli at different points along their pathway; either by interfering with the pattern of transmission, or by depressing the excitability of the neuronal pathway. The manner in which anesthetics produce analgesia is not known, but it must be related to either a specific drug structure or to some peculiarity of the neuronal pathway, or to both of them.

There is no common physicochemical characteristic identifiable conclusively with the ability of a drug to produce anesthesia. The inhalation agents show a suggestive correlation between lipid solubility and analgesic potency (Fig. 2), as defined by the so-called minimal alveolar concentration (MAC) needed to prevent the reaction of the patient to a skin incision (SAIDMAN, et al. 1967).

Limited knowledge of the functioning of afferent pathways is another reason for avoiding conclusions on the mechanisms responsible for their functional im-

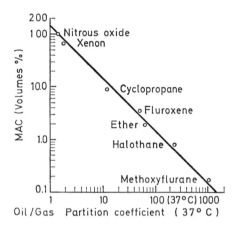

Fig. 2. Relation between MAC and oil/gas partition coefficient. The line through the points satisfies the equation, MAC times oil/gas partition coefficient equals 143—143 being the average of all multiplications of MAC and oil/gas partition coefficient from experimental data. From SAIDMAN et al., 1967, by courtesy of the Editor of Anesthesiology

pairment by anesthetics. Incoming messages can be blocked at the pre- or post-synaptic structures. LØYNING et al. (1964) found that thiamylal depressed pre-synaptic terminals; SHAPOVALOV (1964) and SOMJEN and GILL (1965) on the other hand, found that ether and pentobarbital depressed the post-synaptic membrane. Synaptic depression has been described in both, nonspecific (pain) (DAVIS et al., 1957) and specific pathways (DOMINO et al., 1963). It is argued that the depression of the former is greater or "more effective" (DAVIS et al., 1961), but this pre-supposes knowledge of the functional importance of electrical signals in the CNS which is as yet only beginning to emerge (MOUNTCASTLE et al., 1966). As discussed previously, the existence of multiple mechanisms of action could accommodate dissimilar drugs, as well as dissimilar patterns of action [GALINDO, 1968 (1, 2), 1969].

The results obtained with the methods used to test the "potency" of an analgesic drug are difficult to interpret since they are based on subjective responses to a "painful" stimulation not always reproducible. Furthermore, a patient may be fully conscious of these stimuli, yet be tolerant to them, while an unconscious subject may respond violently to even innocuous stimulation. Subject to these limitations we can accept that some general anesthetic agents are powerful analgesics, e.g. ether, and other weak analgesics, e.g. halothane (DUNDEE and MOORE, 1960), as judged by the state of consciousness of the patient and his response to painful stimulation. With a potent agent analgesia can be produced in conscious patients, but with weak agents, unconsciousness is needed. If we compare the drugs (Fig. 2) on the basis of minimal alveolar concentration (MAC), weak analgesics such as halothane, appear more powerful than excellent analgesics such as ether or nitrous oxide (ARTUSIO, 1954; DUNDEE and MOORE, 1960).

The minimal alveolar concentration (MAC) is a useful guide for the level of anesthesia needed to start a surgical operation. The MAC concept is also useful for comparing the degree of cardiovascular depression at doses of anesthetic agents equipotent with respect to depression of motor responses. Similar correlations have been made in the past for the purpose of determining the depth of anesthesia; however, with MAC this correlation appears more practical and accurate, but limited to a single point, all or none, on a reflex response.

The MAC does not give information about the overall depression of the central nervous system since other responses of this system can be affected sooner or more intensively. MAC is not an index of analgesia since loss of pain perception may coexist with motor responses to peripheral stimulation, as discussed previously. Finally, it is erroneous to apply multiples of MAC by extrapolation. Doubling the concentration of a given anesthetic does not double its depressant action, as recently demonstrated in the cat by DE JONG et al. (1968).

Unconsciousness. Reversible unconsciousness characterizes general anesthesia. Commonly we identify this state with sleep; a related phenomenon though involving a different mechanism. Normal physiological sleep can be interrupted by stimulation, has two defined phases, and is frequently accompanied by dreaming (JOUVET, 1967); these three characteristics are absent from anesthetic "sleep".

Destruction of the activating system in the brain stem reticular formation induces a state of sleep and coma with disappearance of the arousal response in the EEG (LINDSLEY et al., 1949). Preferential depression of this system by anesthetics — mainly barbiturates — (MAGNI et al., 1961; KING, 1955; RANDT et al., 1958; RANDT and COLLINS, 1959) is considered to be the cause of anesthesia; the effect is thought to be related to the multisynaptic nature of the pathway (MORUZZI and MAGOUN, 1949; FRENCH et al., 1953), as previously envisaged by SHERRINGTON (1906) and BREMER (1937). However, other multisynaptic structures located in the same area are not affected by anesthetics (PRINCE and SHANZER, 1966). Furthermore activation, and not depression, of some caudally located nuclei induces some strong inhibitory effects such as physiological sleep (JOUVET, 1967). It should be added that depression of the brain stem activating system by anesthetics does not constitute a proof that they act by a selective depression of this area, nor that this depression is required to produce general anesthesia.

An alternative to this precise anatomical localization of anesthetic action is the pharmacological localization proposed by KRNJEVIC (1967) and PHILLIS (1968). They suggest a correlation between the conscious state and the diffuse multisynaptic cholinergic system involving the brain stem, striatum and deeper cortical layers. Preferential depression of cholinergic systems could explain the anesthetic state, as proposed by MATTHEWS and QUILLIAM (1964). This subject is discussed by FINK in the section on Biochemistry of Anesthetics in this same book.

Excitation. A period of uncoordinated movements and delirium is observed during the administration of ether. This period is interpreted as a normal excitement stage of the CNS before the onset of true surgical anesthesia, and is designated as one of the stages of anethesia. However, this excitement period is absent or minimal during the administration of those anesthetics that do not irritate the respiratory mucosa. Furthermore, if both trigeminal nerves are divided, ether does not produce excitement (ROSSI and ZIRONDOLI, 1955; ROGER et al., 1956), suggesting that this stage may be produced by a local activation of the reticular formation which in turn induces an exaggerated response of the CNS.

Muscular relaxation. During surgical anesthesia the patient is unconscious and unresponsive to painful stimulation. The degree of muscular relaxation serves to indicate the "plane" of anesthesia, and it is accepted that a progressive loss of muscular tone parallels a respiratory depression. The mechanism of this muscular relaxation is not clear, but it appears to be mediated by a central depression that may, or may not produce a simultaneous respiratory impairment. However, these effects are not uniform and they vary according to the anesthetic, e.g. ether anesthesia produces good relaxation of abdominal muscles with little changes in blood pressure or respiration; the same muscular relaxation with halothane induces a marked cardiorespiratory depression. The muscular contracture observed in response to surgical maneuvers is a reflex response and its disappearance is related to the loss of spinal reflexes (NGAI et al., 1964; DE JONG et al., 1967; FREUND et al., 1967). It must be kept in mind that the presence of this response does not imply conscious perception of the stimulus by the patient.

In light planes of anesthesia, the expiratory muscles undergo active contraction (FINK, 1960; FREUND et al., 1964), probably related to a central stimulation of γ motoneurons (DIETE-SPIFF et al., 1962) or to an increase in the resistance to expiration (BISHOP, 1968). At high concentrations various anesthetics potentiate the action of curare (WATLAND et al., 1957), but only ether is depressant of the myoneural junction at the concentrations normally used to produce surgical anesthesia (NGAI et al., 1964).

Electroencephalogram. Not all anesthetics have a similar effect on the encephalogram (EEG) nor is the loss of consciousness associated with a standard EEG pattern. This lack of uniformity, during the initial stages of anesthesia, once more suggests the existence of various mechanisms responsible for the depression of the central nervous system.

Regardless of the initial EEG pattern, a progressive increase in the anesthetic concentration leads to higher voltages and slower frequencies, in other words to a synchronization of the EEG (FAULCONER and BICKFORD, 1960; MARSHALL et al., 1965). Under deep levels of anesthesia, all cortical electrical activity is suppressed (Fig. 3). High arterial tension of CO_2, in the presence of cyclopropane, accelerates this suppression (CLOWES et al., 1953), while the opposite effect is observed with halothane (BACKMAN et al., 1964). During the periods of uptake and elimination of anesthetics there exists a "lag" between a given EEG level and the clinical signs normally seen under steady state conditions. During uptake, the EEG corresponds to a deeper plane of anesthesia than expected from clinical observations; the converse is observed during recovery (GALLA et al., 1958).

The disappearance of highly variable and individual patterns in favor of a uniform tracing characterizes the effect of anesthetics on the EEG (BEECHER and McDONOUGH, 1939). These patterns may differ during the initial periods, when e.g. barbiturate anesthesia induces a high voltage fast frequency pattern rarely seen with inhalation agents (FORBES et al., 1956), but upon deepening of anesthesia they tend to be uniform for all agents.

From a practical point of view (MARSHALL et al., 1965), we can differentiate three EEG patterns, light (predominance of fast frequency 15—30 c/s and low voltage less than 50 μV) deep (slow frequency 3/4 c/s high voltage 75—100 μV and very deep (slow frequency 1—4 c/s or burst suppression, voltage over 100 μV).

The EEG waves represent potential differences between the dendrites of cortical cells, and their frequency appears directly related to the number of units involved (HILL and PARR, 1963). The electroencephalogram of adults has some characteristic patterns of rhythms: Alpha rhythm with a frequency of 8—13 cps observed under resting conditions over the temporal-parietal-occipital areas. It is by far the most common and at one time was believed to be the only rhythm. The amplitude varies between 5—50 μV. Advancing age brings slower rhythms (OBRIST, 1954). Beta rhythm is the next most common rhythm with a frequency

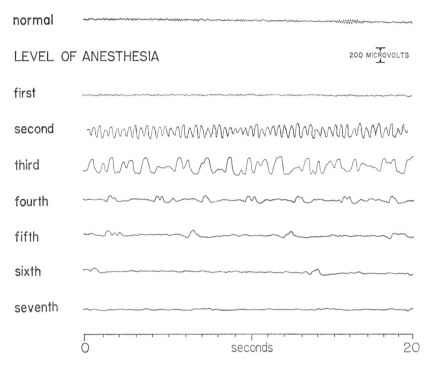

Fig. 3. Electroencephalographic patterns characteristic of successive EEG levels of ether — N₂O anesthesia. From COURTIN et al., 1950, by courtesy of the Editor of Proc. Staff Meet. Mayo Clinic

between 18—30 cps and a maximum amplitude of 20 μV, observed mostly on the posterior part of the brain. Delta rhythm has a frequency of less than 4 cps, and is not found under normal circumstances in awake adults. Theta rhythm: 4—7 cps frequency, observed mainly in the fronto-temporal area, normally found in children.

Some anesthetics (e.g. ether) depress, in addition to transmission across non-specific multisynaptic pathways (pain), transmission along specific afferent systems as shown by their effect on visually and auditory evoked (Fig. 6) potentials recorded on the somato-sensory cortex. These effects vary depending on the drug being administered (HERTZ et al., 1967). Other anesthetics (e.g. halothane) have little effect on these potentials (DOMINO et al., 1963; KITAHATA, 1968). However, when functional studies on the recovery cycle of paired stimuli are made, they unveil a consistent depression previously undetected (Fig. 4) (KITAHATA, 1968).

Other Central Effects of Anesthetics. There are several reflexes and homeostatic mechanisms that depend on the normal functioning of a chain of neurons. They can be divided into exteroceptor initiated reflexes, such as pupillary reaction to light and eye movements; and interoceptor initiated reflexes including mechano-receptor mediated reflexes; chemoreceptor mediated reflexes, and homeostatic mechanisms.

Pupillary reflex to light: This is a multisynaptic reflex which starts at the rods and cones on the retinal surface, synapses with the bipolar and ganglion cells,

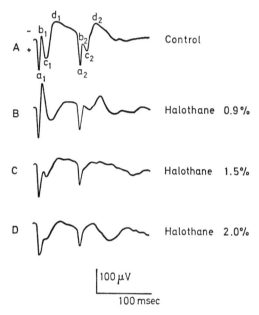

Fig. 4. Typical computer-averaged evoked responses from the A-one (Al) auditory cortex of Cat 1 following paired click stimuli with 70 msec interval, formed by computer summation of 32 responses. Note the progressive depression of amplitude of a_2 relative to that of a_1 as the concentration of halothane is progressively increased. From KITAHATA, 1968, by courtesy of the Editor of Anesthesiology

and runs centripetally with the optic nerve to the pretectal region. Axons from these cells end in the Edinger-Westphal nucleus bilaterally. The efferent limb leaves the central nervous system via the III nerve to the ciliary ganglion from which a final postganglionic fiber ends in the sphincter of the iris. Pupillary dilation is under sympathetic control from the superior cervical ganglion, acting on the dilator muscle of the iris. Sympathetic stimulation, deep anesthesia and hypoxia enlarge the diameter of the pupils. Constriction in response to light is lost in the latter two circumstances. Because of their extreme sensitivity to numerous drugs and hormones, the light reflex as well as the size of the pupils are of only moderate value in the determination of depth of anesthesia, but in general the disappearance of pupillary contraction in response to light can be considered as one of the signs indicating that anesthesia has become "deep".

Eye Movements: Involuntary eye movements indicate "light" anesthesia and the existence of a centrally mediated activity. Removal of the brain above the mesocephalon does not affect ocular rotation because lower centers are involved in their origin. Eye movements are prominent during the administration of barbiturates and normally characterize light anesthesia (SPIEGEL and COLLINS, 1940). It is interesting to note the correlation between abnormal eye movements and the loss of recent memory. MAZZIA and RANDT (1966) consistently found amnesia in those patients unable to center their eyes under very light anesthesia (mostly halothane); otherwise, these patients appeared well oriented and able to follow simple intructions and mental operations.

Mechanoreceptor Mediated Reflexes: In this category are the carotid sinus reflex, and possibly the reflexes involved in postural vasoconstriction. Despite their importance, there is a paucity of information on their comparative depression by various anesthetics in man. Barbiturates are known to impair postural vasoconstriction in the dog (ABEL et al., 1968). The receptors themselves are sensitized, or little affected by volatile agents (WHITTERIDGE, 1958; BISCOE and MILLAR, 1964; ROBERTSON et al., 1956). However, the reflex arc is centrally depressed (PRICE et al., 1959; BROWN and HILTON, 1956; BISCOE and MILLAR, 1966).

Chemoreceptor mediated reflexes: The chemoreceptor mediated reflexes of interest in anesthesia are the cardiovascular and respiratory responses to high P_aCO_2 and pH and low P_aO_2. Because of the multiple mechanisms involved in these responses, a clear effect of anesthetics on the central end of these reflex arcs is difficult to demonstrate. Furthermore, the uptake of some anesthetics (barbiturates) by the CNS is increased under hypercarbia (GOLDBERG et al., 1961). Moreover changes in acid-base balance are known to reduce the stimulation produced by high P_aCO_2 in the CNS; this factor, in addition to the depth of anesthesia, may change a pressor into a depressor response (CARSON et al., 1965). It is reasonable to suspect the existence of similar interactions in man during the administration of inhalation agents; it is also likely that these agents depress the central end of chemoreceptor mediated reflexes even in the presence of sensitization of their peripheral receptors (BISCOE and MILLAR, 1968).

The cardiovascular response to high P_aCO_2 represents the integration of peripheral depression and central stimulation (DOWING et al., 1963). Under normal conditions high CO_2 induces a peripheral vasoconstriction, arterial hypertension and tachycardia, but under anesthesia these responses decrease progressively until the only effect seen is peripheral vasodilation, hypotension and bradycardia. There are only a few studies on the correlation between the systemic response to increased P_aCO_2 and the inspired concentration of a given anesthetic. High P_aCO_2 during anesthesia with 1% halothane in man induces cardiovascular stimulation (PRYS-ROBERTS et al., 1968) the magnitude of this response is reduced when the inspired concentrations of this anesthetic is increased to 2% (MARTIN et al., 1968). There are no comparative studies on the cardiorespiratory responses to various P_aCO_2 levels during the administration of different anesthetic agents. Responses to hypoxia and catecholamines are still present at deep planes of anesthesia, and their disappearance marks the state of maximal depression of the CNS.

Temperature regulation: Central core temperature is homeostatically regulated by adjusting the balance between heat production and heat loss. This mechanism involves complex neuronal pathways in which the hypothalamus plays a central role. Skin, as well as internal, changes in temperature are detected by thermoreceptors that induce a series of responses involving hormonal secretions, vascular reflexes, respiratory responses, and muscular activity. Similar to other reflex arcs, the response to environmental temperature changes is depressed under anesthesia

(HEMINGWAY, 1941; GOLDBERG and ROE, 1960). Only few experimental studies have been made with anesthetics on thermosensitive cells in the hypothalamus and their results are not conclusive (MURAKAMI et al., 1967).

Anesthetized patients do not respond to environmental, or internal temperature changes. This is important when dealing with children, septicemic patients, patients with sustained muscle contraction, and when the operating room temperature is either too low or too high (BURFORD, 1940; SAIDMAN et al., 1964; HOGG and RENWICK, 1966; GOLDBERG and ROE, 1966). Following halothane nitrous oxide-oxygen anesthesia patients shivering had a consistent temperature drop (1.2 °C) according to JONES and McLAREN (1965). However, it has been suggested, without adequate evidence, that anesthetic agents (halothane, ether) may increase temperature by uncoupling phosphorylation (WILSON et al., 1966).

Apart from the above considerations there are clinical as well as experimental reports of a not well understood malignant hyperpyrexic syndrome (HARRISON et al., 1969; KATZ, 1970; BERMAN et al., 1970). This syndrome has been associated with the administration of halothane, succinylcholine and chloroform. These drugs may trigger an unknown mechanism in a genetically predisposed individual to induce a lethal rise in temperature (HARRISON et al., 1969).

ADH Production: Anesthetic agents seem to increase the production of antidiuretic hormone (PAPPER and PAPPER, 1964) and by this mechanism decrease urine formation as well as by a vasoconstrictor effect on the renal artery bed (MILES and WARDENER, 1952). They may also have a direct effect on the permeability of the tubular epithelium to water and electrolytes (CRANDELL et al., 1966).

C. Anesthetic Agents

1. Ethers — Diethyl Ether (Ether)

The pattern of depression of the central nervous system observed during diethyl ether anesthesia is the best known and serves as a reference for other anesthetics. Its slow onset permits a clear demarcation of the various stages of anesthesia (Fig. 1). Ether anesthesia is characterized by marked analgesia and minimal cardiorespiratory (autonomic) depression. (KATZ and NGAI, 1962) Muscular relaxation appears related to depression of synaptic transmission in the spinal cord as shown by experiments in man with the H reflex (DE JONG et al., 1967). In cat NGAI et al. (1964) demonstrated both depression of the myoneural junction and, predominantly, a depression of the spinal, corneal, and masseteric reflexes.

ARTUSIO (1954) made clinical observations with analgesic concentrations of ether. He further divided the stage of analgesia in three planes. The first was considered preanalgesia and preanesthesia; the second, partial analgesia and total amnesia, and the third, total analgesia and amnesia. These planes could be obtained at inspired concentrations (partial pressures) between 1 and 2% of an atmosphere. The patients were first induced with a barbiturate and then intubated using topical anesthesia. No excitation was observed upon awakening or reanesthetization, an observation consistent with experimental studies on the mechanisms of excitation during ether induction previously discussed. DUNDEE and MOORE (1960), on the other hand, found that even if ether is a good analgesic at these concentrations, patients did not tolerate the vapors unless they were heavily premedicated (or intubated). The MAC for ether is 1.92% (SAIDMAN et al., 1967), a figure close to the analgesic concentrations found by ARTUSIO and DUNDEE.

COURTIN et al. (1950) and FAULCONER (1952) describe seven electroencephalographic levels with ether anesthesia (Fig. 3). Level I corresponds to analgesia, the

concentration of ether in the blood is 52 mg/100 cc (7 mM/l). This level is characterized by fast activity and slow voltage. Similar to other anesthetics, deepening
of anesthesia increases the voltage and reduces the frequency. Level III corresponds
to stage III plane I of the Guedel scheme, blood concentration is 84 mg/100 cc
(11.4 mM/l). Fast frequency and slow voltage co-exist with slow waves (3—5 cycles/
sec) and high voltage. At level V the blood concentration is approximately 120 mg/
100 cc (16.2 mM/l) and only slow waves of high voltage are present. Flattening
of the EEG characterizes level VII.

Diethyl ether anesthesia is effective in reducing the amplitude of visually
evoked responses in the cerebral cortex (DOMINO et al., 1963). This finding supports
the idea that ether not only depresses transmission along the nonspecific pathway,
but also acts on the classic specific afferent systems thought to be resistant to
anesthetics (DAVIS et al., 1957; HAUGEN and MELZACK, 1958). The irritant properties of ether may stimulate ventilation at superficial planes of anesthesia (KATZ
and NGAI, 1962), a property shared with several other vapors; ventilation is
finally depressed under deep anesthesia. Blood pressure and cardiac output are
relatively well maintained during its administration.

As discussed before, muscular relaxation under ether is centrally mediated and
possibly related to its depressant affect upon spinal synaptic transmission (AUSTIN
and PASK, 1952; NGAI et al., 1964). However, during induction of anesthesia the
expiratory muscles undergo a period of increased activity (FREUND et al., 1964).

In summary the pattern of ether anesthesia is one of: a) good analgesia and
muscular relaxation, b) depression of synaptic transmission on afferent pathways
and, c) minimal depression of autonomic functions at the inspired concentrations
normally used in clinical anesthesia.

Other ethers share these three characteristics, but because of explosive mixtures with oxygen (trifluro-ethyl vinyl ether: Fluroxene, divinyl ether: Vinethene,
ethyl vinyl ether: Vinemar) or liver toxicity (divinyl ether), are not widely used
in clinical practice. An exception is methoxyflurane (Penthrane) also a powerful
analgesic (BOISVERT and HUDON, 1962), nonflammable at normal operating room
temperature, but with intermediate depressant action on autonomic functions.

A new ether, difluoromethyl 1,1,2-trifluoro-2-chloroethyl ether, known as
Ēthrane, is presently undergoing clinical tests. This is a stable, volatile, non-
explosive anesthetic agent with the muscle relaxant properties of ethers, and
apparently without the cardiorespiratory depressant effects of halogenated agents
(DOBKIN et al., 1968; LEBOWITZ et al., 1970). There are, associated with the administration of this anesthetic, neurological signs of central nervous system excitation manifested in the EEG by spiking activity, and peripherally by transient
tonic-clonic movements and muscular twitching.

2. Halogenated Agents

Halothane — Bromochlorotrifluoroethane: This anesthetic is a poor analgesic
(DUNDEE and MOORE, 1960); however, the inspired concentration needed to
prevent movements of the patient upon surgical stimulation, as determined by
MAC (0.77%) is less than that required with ether (SAIDMAN et al., 1967). Muscular
relaxation during halothane anesthesia lags behind other neurological or cardiorespiratory depressions.

Heat loss under halothane is greatly increased due to peripheral vasodilation;
this fact, in addition to the loss of temperature regulation normally present during
anesthesia, may account for the consistent temperature drop reported during it-
administration (JONES and McLAREN, 1965). Cardiovascular depression is a sub-

ject of controversy. In addition to a direct depression of the myocardium (Gold-BERG, 1968) halothane depresses autonomic reflexes (Biscoe and Millar, 1966) possibly by direct effect on the CNS (Price et al., 1963).

Halothane has a minimal effect on cortically evoked potentials (Domino et al., 1963), but if two auditory stimuli are delivered at various time intervals and the recovery of the second is studied as a function of their temporal separation, halothane depresses the second stimulus by increasing the "recovery time" (Kitahata, 1968) (Fig. 4).

The electroencephalographic patterns observed during halothane anesthesia appear similar to the patterns described with ether. Gain and Paletz (1957) described seven EEG levels. Level I is characterized by fast activity and low voltage. In subsequent levels the frequency is reduced and the voltage increased. Muscular relaxation is said to be satisfactory at level III. Beyond level III, halothane is a powerful depressant of cardiorespiratory functions. Backman et al. (1964) disagree with this description. They considered that thiopental induction, nitrous oxide, or low P_aCO_2, each one by itself, or their combination, could account for the slowing of the EEG (Fig. 5); for them halothane, when given as the only anesthetic, had no significant effect on the frequency, but increased the voltage of the EEG waves; an effect different from the common slowing of the EEG observed with other inhalation agents. Arterial hypotension had no effect on the EEG of healthy patients under halothane, but if present in elderly subjects slowed the EEG and increased the voltage, as previously described in all patients in whom arterial hypotension and anesthesia were combined (Beecher et al., 1938).

In summary the pattern of halothane anesthesia is characterized by: a) relatively poor analgesia and muscular relaxation, b) little effect on cortically evoked potentials or the EEG, and c) greater depression of autonomic functions when analgesia and muscular relaxation are present.

Chloroform. Objective data on the effects of chloroform in the central nervous system of man are few. It is a powerful analgesic, but the only comparative study comes from experiments on rabbits (Pittinger et al., 1960); however, long clinical experience confirms its analgesic properties in man (Waters, 1951). Chloroform is a powerful depressant of cardiorespiratory functions, but it is not known to what extent this is a central action. Six electroencephalographic levels have been described (Thomas et al., 1961). The sequence is similar to that described for ether. In level I the mean blood concentration is 4.8 mg/100 cc (0.4 mM/l). This level presents bursts of 8—10 cycles/sec waves with a voltage of 50 μmV. In level II the blood concentration is 9.6 mg/100 cc (0.8 mM/l). It has a frequency of 7 to 10 cycles/sec and a higher voltage. Level III corresponds to stage III of Guedel's scheme, blood concentration is 22.4 mg/100 cc (1.9 mM/l) and the frequency 2 to 3 cycles/sec. From levels IV to VI the EEG becomes slower without presenting the burst suppression characteristic of ether and methoxyflurane.

Methoxyflurane — 2,2-dichloro-1,1-difluroethyl methyl ether (Penthrane). This anesthetic combines the analgesic properties of ethers with the autonomic depression — both respiratory and cardiovascular — of halogenated agents. Because of its physical characteristics, deep planes of anesthesia are slow and difficult to obtain, therefore it is commonly used in clinical practice in combination with barbiturates or nitrous oxide. The MAC of methoxyflurane is 0.16% (Saidman et al., 1967).

Four electroencephalographic levels of anesthesia have been described during the administration of methoxyflurane in man (Wolfson et al., 1967). There is also a lag between a given EEG level and the expected neurological depression and/or blood concentration. Stage (level) I is characterized by fast activity and low voltage. In stage II the frequency is slower (Theta waves), 4—7 cycles/sec, and the voltage higher. Blood concentration in this stage varies from 8.5 to 18.9 mg/100 cc (0.51—1.1 mM/l), depending on whether methoxyflurane is combined with nitrous oxide or thiopental. Still slower frequency (delta waves) and higher voltage is present in stage III at blood levels between 12.5—27.5 mg/100 cc

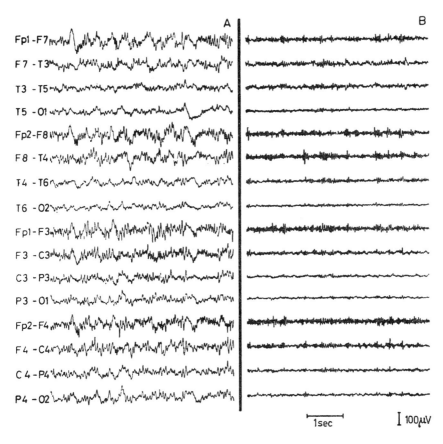

Fig. 5. Effects of low P_aCO_2 during halothane anesthesia. A. EEG during anaesthesia with 2% halothane in oxygen and artificial respiration with a ventilation of 12 l per min. P_eCO_2, 28 mmHg. The EEG is dominated by irregular slow activity. B. 4 min after discontinuation of artificial respiration. P_aCO_2, 49 mmHg. The slow activity has disappeared and is replaced by fast halothane activity. From BACKMAN et al., 1964, by courtesy of the Editor of Acta Anaesth. Scand

(0.75—1.7 mM/l). Intermittent EEG suppression (burst suppression) is observed in stage IV at blood levels between 17.5 and 30.5 mg/100 cc (1.06—1.9 mM/l). It is possible that this EEG pattern would be different if methoxyflurane were administered alone (only with oxygen) and under constant P_aCO_2 levels, but presently no such study has been performed. Methoxyflurane, like halothane, has little effect on cortically evoked potentials (Fig. 6) (DOMINO et al., 1963) but it affects the recovery cycle of paired stimuli (KITAHATA, 1968).

Trichloroethylene. This is a powerful analgesic in both animals (PITTINGER et al., 1960) and man (ATKINSON, 1960; DUNDEE and MOORE, 1960). Similar to the other halogenated agents, trichloroethylene is also a powerful depressant of auto-

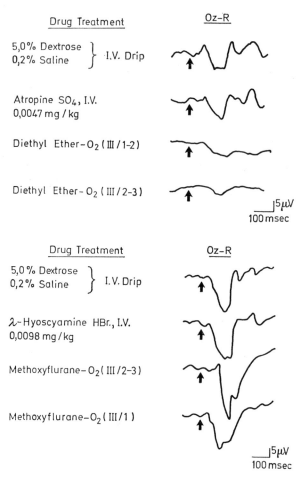

Fig. 6. Effects of methoxyflurane-oxygen and diethyl ether-oxygen anesthesia on the visually evoked response in man. The light stimulus was presented at the arrow every second for 200 flashes to the subject whose eyes were closed. The voltage calibration represents that of the average evoked response. Negativity is upwards. The recordings during the various drug treatments are as designated. Note that in spite of deep methoxyflurane-oxygen anesthesia, as evidenced by marked hypotension, the visual response is not depressed. Unlike methoxyflurane, diethyl ether-oxygen anesthesia markedly alters the evoked response. From DOMINO, 1963, by courtesy of the Editor of Anesthesia and Analgesia Current Researches

nomic functions (PARKHOUSE, 1965). Toxic products produced by decomposition of this anesthetic, when used in circle circuit with soda lime, have been considered the cause of cranial nerve palsies (OSTLERE, 1953). Coincidentally this agent is known to produce a selective relaxation of the mandibular muscles (BRITTAIN, 1948).

3. Other Anesthetics

Nitrous Oxide. The anesthetic properties of this gas were clearly demonstrated by FAULCONER et al. (1949). They administered 50% nitrous oxide in oxygen at two atmospheres of pressure. Under these conditions loss of consciousness occurred in 2 min and surgical anesthesia in 5. Disappearance of alpha rhythm coincided with unconsciousness, while delta rhythm of high amplitude characterized clinical anesthesia. In other observations, HENRIE et al. (1961) could not find electro-encephalographic changes with 30% N_2O despite impaired performances on verbal and visual retention tests. The analgesic properties of nitrous oxide are well known clinically (DUNDEE and MOORE, 1960) and are applied in the obstetric and dental fields. However, its main use is as a coadjunct in general anesthesia. It potentiates the effect of barbiturates in animal experiments (PITTINGER et al., 1960) and increases the depth of anesthesia when combined with other agents in man (FAULCONER, 1952). The extrapolated MAC of nitrous oxide is 101%. At analgesic concentrations it has little effect on autonomic functions, except in the presence of hypoxia or CO_2 retention.

Cyclopropane. Cyclopropane is a potent analgesic agent (DUNDEE and MOORE, 1960), but an intermediate inspired concentration is required to prevent motor responses to surgical stimulations (MAC 9.2%) (SAIDMAN et al., 1967). It depresses respiration and has little effect on the cardiovascular system. The latter has been interpreted differently. PRICE et al. (1965) consider that cyclopropane spares the "pressor" areas of the brain stem, while depressing "depressor" sites. NGAI and BALME (1966) on the other hand, found that cyclopropane depressed also the "pressor" center, but had no significant action on sympathetic cholinergic responses. The peripheral effects of this anesthetic on the cardiovascular system antagonize any central depressant properties that may it have. Cyclopropane is known to induce renal vasoconstriction (MILES and WARDENER, 1952), and to increase resistance in the mesenteric vascular bed (PRICE et al., (1966) and the hepatic artery (GALINDO 1965).

POSSATI et al. (1953) described six electroencephalographic levels during cyclopropane anesthesia in man. Similar to the other inhalation agents, level I showed a fast frequency and a low voltage; from level II to VI, the trend was toward slower frequencies and high voltages with periods of burst suppression appearing at level IV; there are periods of silence lasting no more than 3 sec and appearing between groups of waves of 4—6 cycles/sec. Blood concentrations of cyclopropane varied from 2—17 mg/100 cc (0.5—4 mM/l) in levels I and V respectively. These values are in agreement with COHEN and BEECHER's (1951) data on the concentration of cyclopropane needed to produce surgical anesthesia — 6—24 mg/100 cc (1.4—5.7 mM/l). Cyclopropane is also effective in reducing the amplitude of visually evoked cortical potentials (DOMINO et al., 1963).

Summary

The concept of stages and planes of anesthesia is useful as a guide in the administration of general anesthetic agents. It is based on a predictable sequence of neurological observations and changes in vital signs seen with a given anesthetic agent. The grouping of these observations forms characteristic patterns of drug action; the best known being associated with ether and originally described by GUEDEL. The reason for the existence of different patterns is not known, it could be explained by differences in the mechanisms and sites of action of the various drugs.

According to the effect of anesthetics on three broad areas: a) analgesia and muscular relaxation, b) EEG and evoked potentials, and c) autonomic functions (cardiovascular and respiratory systems), they can be divided into three groups. Group one is formed by most ethers. They are potent analgesics and depressants of the EEG and evoked potentials, having relatively little effect on autonomic functions. Group two comprises some halogenated agents (e.g. halothane). They are poor analgesics and have little effect on evoked potentials or the EEG; on the other hand, these agents are powerful depressants of autonomic functions. Group three, an intermediate group, includes cyclopropane, methoxyflurane and chloroform. They are potent analgesics with variable effects on the EEG, evoked potentials, or autonomic functions. These three groups are presented for convenience. A classification of anesthetic agents, according to their mechanisms of action is not possible at the present time. However, with the growth of knowledge we can forsee a classification based on pre- and post-synaptic effects (sites of action) where anesthetics alter the permeability of excitable membranes to various ions (mechanisms of action).

References

ABEL, F. L., WALDHAUSEN, J. A.: Influence of posture and passive tilting on venous return and cardiac output. Am. J. Physiol. 215, 1058—1066 (1968).

ARTUSIO, J. F.: Di-ethyl ether analgesia: a detailed description of the first stage of ether anesthesia in man. J. Pharmacol. Exptl. Therap. 111, 343—348 (1954).

ATKINSON, R. S.: Trichloroethylene anesthesia. Anesthesiology 21, 67—77 (1960).

AUSTIN, G. M., PASK, E. A.: Effect of ether inhalation upon spinal cord and root action potentials. J. Physiol. (London) 118, 405—411 (1952).

BACKMAN, L. E., LÖFSTROM, B., WIDÉN, L.: Electroencephalography in halothane anesthesia. Acta Anaesth. Scand. 8, 115—130 (1964).

BEECHER, H. K., MCDONOUGH, F. K.: Cortical action potentials during anesthesia. J. Neurophysiol. 2, 289—307 (1939).

— — FORBES, A.: Effects of blood pressure changes on cortical potentials during anesthesia. J. Neurophysiol. 1, 324—331 (1938).

BERMAN, M. C., HARRISON, G. G., BULL, A. B., KENCH, J. E.: Changes underlying halothane-induced malignant hyperpyrexia in landrace pigs. Nature 225, 653—655 (1970).

BISCOE, T. J., MILLAR, R. A.: The effect of halothane on carotid sinus baroreceptor activity. J. Physiol. (London) 173, 24—37 (1964).

— — The effects of cyclopropane, halothane and ether on central baroreceptor pathways. J. Physiol. (London) 184, 535—559 (1966).

— — Effects of inhalation anaesthetics on carotid body chemoreceptor activity. Brit. J. Anaesthesia 40, 2—12 (1968).

BISHOP, B.: Diaphragm and abdominal muscle activity during induced hypotension. J. Appl. Physiol. 25, 73—79 (1968).

BOISVERT, M., Hudon, F.: Clinical evaluation of methoxyflurane in obstetrical anesthesia: A report on 500 cases. Canad. Anaesth. Soc. J. 9, 325—330 (1962).

BRECHNER, V. L., BAUER, R. O., BENSTON, G. E., BETHUNE, R. M., MAISEL, G., DILLON, J. B.: Electroencephalographic effect of hypercarbia during nitrous oxide-oxygen-thiamylal-demerol anesthesia. Anesthesia & Analgesia 41, 91—104 (1962).

— DORNETTE, W. H. L.: Electroencephalographic patterns during nitrous oxide-trifluoroethyl vinyl ether anesthesia. Anesthesiology 18, 321—327 (1957).

BREMER, F.: Différence d'action de la narcose étherique et du sommeil barbiturique sur les réactions sensorielles acoustiques du cortex cérébral: significance de cette différence en ce qui concerne le méchanisme du sommeil. Compt. renal. soc. biol 124, 848—852.

BRITTAIN, G. J. C.: Trichloroethylene (Trilene) as an anaesthetic in neurosurgery. Anesthesia & Analgesia 27, 145—152 (1948).

BROWN, R. V., HILTON, J. G.: Effectiveness of baroreceptor reflexes under different anesthetics. J. Pharmacol. Exptl. Therap. 118, 198—203 (1950).

BURFORD, G. E.: Hyperthermia following anesthesia. Anesthesiology 1, 208—215 (1940).

BURGESS, P. R., PERL, E. R.: Myelinated afferent fibres responding specifically to noxious stimulation of the skin. J. Physiol. (London) 190, 541—562 (1967).

CARSON, S. A. S., CHORLEY, G. E., HAMILTON, F. N., LEE, D. C., MORRIS, L. E.: Variation in cardiac output with acid-base changes in the anesthetized dog. J. Appl. Physiol. **20**, 948—953 (1965).

CLOWES, G. H. A., JR., KRETCHMER, H. E., MCBURNEY, R. W., SIMEONE, F. A.: The electro-encephalogram in the evaluation of the effects of anesthetic agents and carbon dioxide accumulation during surgery. Ann. Surg. **138**, 558—568 (1953).

COHEN, E. N., BEECHER, H. K.: Narcotics in preanesthetic medication. A controlled study. J. Am. Med. Assoc. **147**, 1664—1668 (1951).

COURTIN, R. F., BICKFORD, R. G., FAULCONER, A., JR.: The classification and significance of electroencephalographic patterns produced by nitrous oxide-ether anesthesia during surgical operations. Proc. Staff Meetings Mayo Clinic **25**, 197—206 (1950).

CRANDELL, W. B., PAPPAS, S. G., MAC DONALD, A.: Nephrotoxicity associated with methoxy-flurane. Anesthesiology **27**, 591—607 (1966).

DAVIS, H. S., COLLINS, W. F., RANDT, C. T., DILLON, W. H.: Effect of anesthetic agents on evoked central nervous system responses: Gaseous agents. Anesthesiology **18**, 634—642 (1957).

— QUITMEYER, V. E., COLLINS, W. F.: The effect of halothane (Fluothane) on the thalamus and midbrain reticular formation. Anaesthesia **16**, 32—49 (1961).

DE JONG, R. H., FREUND, F. G., ROBLES, R., MORIKAWA, K.-I.: Anesthetic potency determined by depression of synaptic transmission. Anesthesiology **29**, 1139—1144 (1968).

— HERSHEY, W. N., WAGMAN, I. H.: Measurement of a spinal reflex response (H-reflex) during general anesthesia in man. Anesthesiology **28**, 382—389 (1967).

DIETE-SPIFF, K., DODSWORTH, H., PASCOE, J. E.: An analysis of the effect of ether and ethyl-chloride on the discharge frequency of gastrocnemius fusimotor neurones in the rabbit. Symposium on muscle receptors, pp. 43—47. Hong Kong: University Press 1962.

DOBKIN, A. B., HEINRICH, R. G., ISRAEL, J. S., LEVY, A. A., NEVILLE, J. F., JR., OUNKASEM, K.: Clinical and laboratory evaluation of a new inhalation agent: compound 347 (CHF$_2$-O-CF$_2$-CHF Cl). Anesthesiology **29**, 275—287 (1968).

DOMINO, E. F., CORSSEN, G., SWEET, R. B.: Effects of various general anesthetics on the visually evoked response in man. Anesthesia & Analgesia **42**, 735—747 (1963).

DORNETTE, W. H. L.: The anatomic basis of the signs of anesthesia. Anesthesia & Analgesia **43**, 71—81 (1964).

DOWING, S. E., MITCHELL, J. H., WALLACE, A. G.: Cardiovascular responses to ischaemia, hypoxia, and hypercarbia of the central nervous system. Am. J. Physiol. **204**, 881—887 (1963).

DUNDEE, J. W., MOORE, J.: Alterations in response to somatic pain associated with anesthesia. IV: The effects of sub-anaesthetic concentrations of inhalation agents. Brit. J. Anaesthesia **32**, 453—459 (1960).

EPSTEIN, R. A., WANG, H. H., BARTELSTONE, H. J.: The effects of halothane on circulatory reflexes of the dog. Anesthesiology **29**, 867—876 (1968).

FAULCONER, A., JR.: Correlation of concentrations of ether in arterial blood with electroence-phalographic patterns occurring during ether-oxygen and during nitrous oxide, oxygen and ether anesthesia of human surgical patients. Anesthesiology **13**, 361—369 (1952).

— BICKFORD, R. G.: Electroencephalography in anesthesiology. Springfield: Charles C. Thomas 1960.

— PENDER, J. W., BICKFORD, R. G.: The influence of partial pressure of nitrous oxide on the depth of anesthesia and the electroencephalogram in man. Anesthesiology **10**, 601—609 (1949).

FINK, B. R.: A method of monitoring muscular relaxation by the integrated abdominal electromyogram. Anesthesiology **21**, 178—185 (1960).

FORBES, A., MERLIS, J. K., HENRIKSEN, G. F., BURLEIGH, S., JIUSTO, G. L.: Measurement of the depth of barbiturate narcosis. Electroencephalog. and Clin. Neurophysiol. **8**, 541—558 (1956).

FRANK, G. B.: Drugs which modify membrane excitability. Federation Proc. **27**, 132—136 (1968).

FRENCH, J. D., VERZEANO, M., MAGOUN, H. W.: A neural basis of the anesthetic state. Arch. Neurol. Psychiat. **69**, 519—529 (1953).

FREUND, F., ROOS, A., DODD, R. B.: Expiratory activity of the abdominal muscles in man during general anesthesia. J. Appl. Physiol. **19**, 693—697 (1964).

FREUND, F. G., HORNBEIN, T. F., MARTIN, W. E., PARMENTIER, P.: Effect of halothane and halothane nitrous oxide on the H-reflex in man (Abst.) Anesthesiology **29**, 191 (1968).

GAIN, E. A., PALETZ, S. G.: An attempt to correlate the clinical signs of fluothane anesthesia with the electroencephalographic levels. Canad. Anaesth. Soc. J. **4**, 289—294 (1957).

GALINDO, A.: Hepatic circulation and hepatic function during anaesthesia and surgery. II. The effect of various anaesthetic agents. Canad. Anaesth. Soc. J. **12**, 337—348 (1965).

GALINDO, A.: (1) Mechanisms of anaesthesia and some observations on synaptic inhibition. Ph. D. Thesis, McGill Univ., Montreal 1968.
— (2) Electrophysiological methods in anaesthesia research. Canad. Anaesth. Soc. J. **15**, 528—538 (1968).
— Effects of procaine, pentobarbital and halothane on synaptic transmission in the central nervous system. J. Pharmacol. Exptl. Therap. **169**, 185—195 (1969).
GALLA, S. J., ROCCO, A. G., VANDAM, L. D.: Evaluation of the traditional signs and stages of anesthesia: An electroencephalographic and clinical study. Anesthesiology **19**, 328—338 (1958).
GILLESPIE, N. A.: The signs of anesthesia. Current Researches Anesthesia & Analgesia **22**, 275—282 (1943).
GOLDBERG, A. H.: Cardiovascular function and halothane. In: Halothane — Clinical anesthesia series. (GREEN, N. M., Ed.). Philadelphia: F. A. Davis Co 1968.
GOLDBERG, M. A., BARLOW, C. F., ROTH, L. J.: The effect of carbon dioxide on the entry and accumulation of drugs in the central nervous system. J. Pharmacol. Exptl. Therap. **131**, 308—318 (1961).
GOLDBERG, M. J., ROE, F. C.: Temperature changes during anesthesia and operations. Arch. Surg. **93**, 365—367 (1966).
GUEDEL, A. E.: Inhalation Anesthesia: a fundamental guide, 2nd ed. New York: The Macmillan Co. 1951.
HARRIS, T. A. B.: The mode of action of anaesthetics. Edinburgh: E. & S Livingstone Ltd. 1951.
HARRISON, G. G., SAUNDERS, S. J., BIEBUYCK, J. F., HICKMAN, R., DENT, D. M., WEAVER, V., TERBLANCHE, J.: Anaesthetic-induced malignant hyperpyrexia and a method for its prediction. Brit. J. Anaesthesia **41**, 844—855 (1969).
HAUGEN, F. P., COOPPOCK, W. J., BERQUIST, H. C.: Nitrous oxide hypalgesia in trained subjects. Anesthesiology **20**, 321—324 (1959).
— MELZACK, R.: The effects of nitrous oxide on responses evoked in the brain stem by tooth stimulation. Anesthesiology **18**, 183—195 (1957).
HEMINGWAY, A.: The effect of barbital anesthesia on temperature regulation. Am. J. Physiol. **134**, 350—358 (1941).
HENRIE, J. R., PARKHOUSE, J., BICKFORD, R. G.: Alteration of human consciousness by nitrous oxide as assessed by electroencephalography and psychological tests. Anesthesiology **22**, 247—259 (1961).
HERTZ, A., FRALING, F., NIEDNER, I., FARBER, G.: Pharmacologically induced alterations of cortical and subcortical evoked potentials compared with physiological changes during the awake-sleep cycle in cat. In: The evoked potentials, pp. 164—176. New York: Cobb W. & Marocutti 1967.
HILL, J. D. N., PARR, G.: Electroencephalography. New York: MacMillan 1963.
HOGG, S., RENWICK, W.: Hyperpyrexia during anesthesia. Canad. Anaesth. Soc. J. **13**, 429—436 (1966).
HUGHES, J. R., KING, B. D., CUTTER, J. A., MARKELLO, R.: The EEG in hyperventilated, lightly anesthetized patients. Electroencephalog. and Clin. Neurophysiol. **14**, 274—277 (1962).
JONES, H. D., McLAREN, A. B.: Postoperative shivering and hypoxemia after halothane, nitrous oxide and oxygen anesthesia. Brit. J. Anaesthesia **37**, 35—41 (1965).
JOUVET, M.: Neurophysiology of the states of sleep. Physiol. Rev. **47**, 117—177 (1967).
KATZ, D.: Recurrent malignant hyperpyrexia during anesthesia. Anesthesia & Analgesia **49**, 225—230 (1970).
KATZ, R. L., NGAI, S. H.: Respiratory effects of diethyl ether in the cat. J. Pharmacol. Exptl. Therap. **138**, 329—336 (1962).
KING, E. E.: Differential action of anesthetics, and interneurone depressants upon EEG arousal and recruitment responses. J. Pharmacol. Exptl. Therap. **116**, 404—417 (1956).
— NAQUET, R., MAGOUN, H. W.: Action of pentobarbital on somatic afferent conduction in the cat with special reference to the thalamic relay (Abstr.) J. Pharmacol. Exptl. Therap. **113**, 31 (1955).
KITAHATA, L. M.: The effects of halothane and methoxyflurane on recovery cycles of click-evoked potentials from the auditory cortex of the cat. Anesthesiology **29**, 523—532 (1968).
KRNJEVIĆ, K.: Chemical transmission and cortical arousal. Anesthesiology **28**, 100—105 (1967).
LAYCOCK, J. D.: Signs and stages of anaesthesia a restatement. Anaesthesia **8**, 15—20 (1953).
LEBOWITZ, M. H., BLITT, C. D., DILLON, J. B.: Clinical investigation of compound 347 (Ethrane). Anesthesia & Analgesia **49**, 1—10 (1970).
LEWY, F. H., GAMMON, G. D.: Influence of sensory system on spontaneous activity of cerebral cortex. J. Neurophysiol. **3**, 387—395 (1940).

LILJESTRAND, G.: Effects of ethyl alcohol and some selected substances on baroreceptor and chemoreceptor activity. Acta. Physiol. Scand. **29**, 74—82 (1953).

LINDSLEY, D. B., BOWDEN, J. W., MAGOUN, H. W.: Effect upon the EEG of acute injury to the brain stem activating system. Electroencephalog. and Clin. Neurophysiol. **1**, 475—486 (1949).

LØYNING, Y., OSHIMA, T., YOKOTA, T.: Site of action of thiamylal sodium on the monosynaptic spinal reflex pathways in cats. J. Neurophysiol. **27**, 408—428 (1964).

MAGNI, R., MORUZZI, G., ROSSI, G. F., ZANCHETTI, A.: EEG arousal following inactivation of the lower brain stem by selective injection of barbiturate into the vertebral circulation. Arch. ital. biol. **99**, 33—71 (1961).

MARSHALL, M., LONGLEY, B. P., STANTON, W. H.: Electroencephalography in anesthetic practice. Brit. J. Anaesthesia **37**, 845—857 (1965).

MARTIN, W. E., FREUND, F. G., HORNBEIN, T. F.: Cardiovascular effects of hypo- und hypercarbia during halothane and halothane-nitrous oxide anesthesia (unpublished).

MATTHEWS, E. K., QUILLIAM, J. P.: Effects of central depressant drugs upon acetylcholine release. Brit. J. Pharmacol. **22**, 415—440 (1964).

MAZZIA, V. D. B., RANDT, C.: Amnesia and eye movements in first stage anesthesia. Arch. Neurol. (Psychiat.) **14**, 522—525 (1966).

MELZACK, R., WALL, P. D.: Pain mechanisms: a new theory. Science **150**, 971—979 (1965).

MILES, B. E., DE WARDENER, H. E.: Renal vasoconstriction produced by ether and cyclopropane anaesthesia. J. Physiol. (London) **118**, 140—144 (1952).

MORUZZI, G., MAGOUN, H. W.: Brain stem reticular formation and activation of the EEG. Electroencephalog. and Clin. Neurophysiol. **1**, 455—473 (1949).

MOUNTCASTLE, V. B., TALBOT, W. H., KORNHUBER, H. H.: The neuronal transformation of mechanical stimuli delivered to the monkey's hand. In: Touch, Heat and Pain, pp. 325 to 351, (DE REUCK, A. V. S., KNIGHT, J., Eds.). London: J. and A. Churchill 1966.

MURAKAMI, N., STOLWIJK, A. J., HARDY, J. D.: Responses of preoptic neurons to anesthetics and peripheral stimulation. Am. J. Physiol. **213**, 1015—1024 (1967).

MUSHIN, W. W.: The signs of anaesthesia. Anaesthesia **3**, 154—159 (1948).

NGAI, S. H., BOLME, P.: Effects of anesthetics on circulatory mechanisms in the dog. J. Pharmacol. and Exptl. Therap. **153**, 495—504 (1966).

— HANKS, E. C., FARHIE, S. E.: Effects of anesthetics on neuromuscular transmission and somatic reflexes. Anesthesiology **26**, 162—167 (1964).

— TSENG, D. T. C., WANG, S. C.: Effect of Diazepam and other central nervous system depressants on spinal reflexes in cats: A study of site of action. J. Pharmacol. Exptl. Therap. **153**, 344—351 (1966).

OBRIST, W. D.: The electroencephalogram of normal aged adults. Electroencephalog. and Clin. Neurophysiol. **6**, 235—244 (1954).

OSTLERE, G.: Trichloroethylene Anesthesia. Edinburgh: E & S Livingstone 1953.

PAPPER, S., PAPPER, E. M.: The effects of preanesthetic, anesthetic and postoperative drugs on renal function. Clin. Pharmacol. and Therap. **5**, 205—215 (1964).

PARKHOUSE, J.: Trichloroethylene. Brit. J. Anaesthesia **37**, 681—687 (1965).

PERL, E. R.: Myelinated afferent fibres innervating the primate skin and their response to noxious stimuli. J. Physiol. (London) **197**, 593—615 (1968).

PHILLIS, J. W.: Acetylcholine release from the cerebral cortex: its role in cortical arousal. Brain Res. **7**, 378—389 (1968).

PITTINGER, C. B., KEASLING, H. H., WESTERLUND, R. L.: Comparative effects of anesthetics agents on tooth pulp thresholds in rabbits. Anesthesiology **21**, 112—113 (1960).

POSSATI, S., FAULCONER, A., Jr., BICKFORD, R. G., HUNTER, R. C.: Electroencephalographic patterns during anesthesia with cyclopropane: correlation with concentration of cyclopropane in arterial blood. Anesthesia & Analgesia **32**, 130—135 (1953).

PRICE, H. L., DEUTSCH, S., DAVIDSON, I. A., CLEMENT, A. J., BEHAR, M. G.: Can general anesthetics produce splanchnic visceral hypoxia by reducing regional blood flow? Anesthesiology **27**, 24—32 (1966).

— LINDE, H. W., JONES, R. E., BLACK, G. W., PRICE, M. L.: Sympatho-adrenal responses to general anesthesia in man and their relation to hemodynamics. Anesthesiology **20**, 563—575 (1959).

— — MORSE, H. T.: Central nervous actions of halothane affecting the systemic circulation. Anesthesiology **24**, 778—780 (1963).

— LURIE, A. A., BLACK, G. W., SECHZER, P. H., LINDE, H. W., PRICE, M. L.: Modification by general anesthetics (cyclopropane and halothane) of circulatory and sympathoadrenal responses to respiratory acidosis. Ann. Surg. **152**, 1071—1077 (1960).

— PRICE, M. L., MORSE, H. T.: Effects of cyclopropane, halothane and procaine on the vasomotor "center" of the dog. Anesthesiology **26**, 55—60 (1965).

PRINCE, D. A., SHANZER, S.: Effects of anesthetics upon the EEG response to reticular stimulation. Patterns of slow synchrony 21, 578—588 (1966).
PRYS-ROBERTS, C., KELMAN, G. R., GREENBAUM, R., KAIN, M. L., BAY, J.: Hemodynamics and alveolar-arterial PO$_2$ differences at varying P$_a$CO$_2$ in anesthetized man. J. Appl. Physiol. 25, 80—87 (1968).
RANDT, C. T., COLLINS, W. F., DAVIS, H. S., DILLON, W. H.: Differential susceptibility of afferent pathways to anesthetic agents in the cat. Am. J. Physiol. 192, 305—310 (1958).
— — Effect of anesthetic agents on spinal cord of cat. Am. J. Physiol. 196, 340—342 (1959).
ROBERTSON, J. D., SWAN, A. A. B., WHITTERIDGE, D.: Effect of anesthetics on systemic baroreceptors. J. Physiol. (London) 131, 463—472 (1956).
ROGER, A., ROSSI, G. F., ZIRONDOLI, A.: Le rôle des afférences des nerfs crâniens dans le maintien de l'état vigile de la préparation encéphale isolé. Electroencephalog. and Clin. Neurophysiol. 8, 1—13 (1956).
ROSSI, G. F., ZIRONDOLI, A.: On the mechanism of cortical desynchronization elicited by volatile anesthetics. Electroencephalog. and Clin. Neurophysiol. 7, 383—390 (1955).
RUBIN, M. A., FREEMAN, H.: Brain potential changes in man during cyclopropane anesthesia. J. Neurophysiol. 3, 33—42 (1940).
SAIDMAN, L. J., EGER II, E. I., MUNSON, E. S., BAGAD, A. A., MUALLEM, M.: Minimum alveolar concentrations of methoxyflurane, halothane, ether and cyclopropane in man: Correlation with theories of anesthesia. Anesthesiology 28, 994—1002 (1967).
— HARVARD, E. S., EGER II, E. I.: Hyperthermia during anesthesia. J. Am. Med. Assoc. 190, 1029—1032 (1964).
SHANES, A. M.: Electrochemical aspects of physiological and pharmacological action in excitable cells. Pharmacol. Revs. 10, 59—164 (1958).
SHAPOVALOV, A. I.: Intracellular microelectrode investigation of effect of anesthetic on transmission of excitation in the spinal cord. Federation Proc. Trans. Suppl. 23, T, 113—116 (1964).
SHERRINGTON, C. S.: The integrative action of the nervous system. 1947 ed., Oxford: University Press 1906.
SINCLAIR, D. C.: Cutaneous sensation and the doctrine of specific energy. Brain 78, 584—614 (1955).
SNOW, J.: The inhalation of vapors of ether in surgical operations. London: John Churchill 1847.
SOMJEN, G., GILL, M.: The mechanism of the blockade of synaptic transmission in the mammalian spinal cord by ether and thiopental. J. Pharmacol. 140, 19—30 (1963).
SPIEGEL, E. A., COLLINS, D. A.: Ocular rotation in anesthesia and under the influence of supranuclear centers. J. Neurophysiol. 3, 59—65 (1940).
THOMAS, D. M., MAC KRELL, T. H., CONNER, E. H.: The electroencephalogram during chloroform anesthesia. Anesthesiology 22, 542—547 (1961).
WATERS, R. M., (Ed.): Chloroform — a study after 100 years. Madison: The University of Wisconsin press 1951.
WATLAND, D. C., LONG, J. P., PITTINGER, C. B., CULLEN, S. C.: Neuromuscular effects of ether, cyclopropane, chloroform and Fluothane. Anesthesiology 18, 883—890 (1957).
WEDDELL, G.: Somesthesis and the chemical senses. Ann. Rev. Psychol. 6, 119—136 (1955).
WHITTERIDGE, D.: Effect of anaesthetics on mechanical receptors. Brit. Med. Bull. 14, 5—7 (1958).
WILSON, R. D., NICHOLS, R. J., DENT, T. E., ALLEN, C. R.: Disturbances of oxidative phosphorylation mechanism as a possible etiological factor in sudden unexplained hyperthermia occurring during anesthesia. Anesthesiology 27, 231—232 (1966).
WOLFSON, B., SIKER, E. S., CICCARELLI, H. E., GRAY, G. H., JONES, L.: The electroencephalogram as a monitor of arterial blood levels of methoxyflurane. Anesthesiology 28, 1003—1009 (1967).
WOODBRIDGE, P. D.: Changing concepts concerning depth of anesthesia. Anesthesiology 18, 536—550 (1957).

4.2. Autonomic Nervous System

Robert W. Gardier

With 5 Figures

I. Introduction

In considering drug effects on the autonomic nervous system, acknowledgement must be made, at the outset, that changes in autonomic nervous activity produced by pharmacological means are not necessarily a result of the direct action of the agent on the receptors of this essentially efferent system. Anesthetic agents probably alter autonomic function by effects on afferent receptors or on some select sites in the central nervous system. However, drug effects on the final common pathway of autonomic outflow will have precedence in determining organ and organ system pharmacodynamics. It is not the intention of the author to present an encyclopedic approach to the subject material of this chapter, but rather to exploit concepts that are explicit or implied in the data presently available from the experimental pharmacology of anesthetic drugs. Rather than consider each agent as a pharmacological entity, the presentation will be in the mode of systems analyses and dissections of these will be carried out only so far as they complement the whole and expose the problems and voids therein.

II. Afferent Nervous System

1. Baroreceptor Effects

The vast amount of research conducted on baroreceptor function until most recent times has been presented in the monumental treatise by Heymans and Neil (1958). These authors indicate that even the most direct appraisal of drug effects on baroreceptor function, by recording impulse traffic in the appropriate nerve, such as the sinus branch of the glossopharyngeal nerve arising from the carotid baroreceptors, can still present equivocal results in terms of contaminating chemoreceptor fibers, sympathetic nervous effects on the sinus vascular smooth muscle and humoral substances originating from sites quite remote from these afferent receptors. Resetting of the barostat (McCubbin et al., 1956; McCubbin and Page, 1963) is a poorly understood phenomenon which may involve one or both of the last two modulating influences. With apt consideration of the problems involved, especially in terms of the mechanical aspects and arterial pulse, Robertson et al. (1956) found that diethyl ether, chloroform, and trichloroethylene, but not cyclopropane, increased the sensitivity of the carotid and aortic baroreceptors. With chloroform and trichloroethylene, this sensitivity was most apparent as a reduction in baroreceptor sensing threshold since the most marked increments in afferent activity occurred at reduced arterial pressures. With diethyl ether, the increased sensitivity of the baroreceptors held over a wider range of arterial pressures. These authors pointed out, however, that the results were obtained over transient periods of anesthetic inhalation and that prolonged exposure to these agents, especially the halogenated hydrocarbons, could reduce the frequency response maximum similar to that observed on pulmonary stretch receptors (Whitteridge and Bulbring, 1944; Liljestrand, 1953). Landgren et al. (1953) likewise performing experiments in cats, determined that intra-carotid injections of diethyl ether and chloroform decreased or abolished baro-receptor activity. The incompatibility of the results from these two laboratories may be resolved simply on the basis of anesthetic concentrations. The earlier data on cyclopropane, however, does not conform with the more recent work of Price and Widdicombe (1962) wherein cyclopropane increased baroreceptor activity in the presence of pulsatile and static intra-sinus pressure. It is somewhat difficult to resolve this conflict especially since the sinus preparation of Price and Widdi-combe needed the necessarily poorer perfusion in the experiment for the imposition of a static pressure. Under the conditions of a circulatorily isolated carotid sinus, decreased responsiveness of the baroreceptors is a more likely phenomenon. Yet, such conditions prevailed when these investigators demonstrated increased sinus nerve activity under cyclopropane. Biscoe and Millar (1964) have demonstrated a sensitization of baroreceptors with the newer halogenated hydrocarbon, halo-thane, in a variety of animal species. Much earlier, Hering (1927) had indicated that anesthetic concentrations of chloroform stimulated carotid sinus mechanisms.

Biscoe and Millar (1964) provided a comprehensive discussion of possible mechanisms responsible for the sensitization process with halothane. Speculations could be based on the distensibility of the arterial wall. By relaxing vascular smooth muscle, halothane should enhance distension of the carotid sinus and provide a greater change in geometry of this area with each pressure pulse. Thus, a potentially greater distortion of the baroreceptor may be invoked as the cause of sensitization. Such an explanation should receive adequate consideration even though it does not conform with deductions based on other drug effects. Con-versely, the sensitization with cyclopropane is probably provoked by increased tension in the sinus wall (Price and Price, 1962). Additional evidence nullifying a theory of increased distensibility as an etiologic factor resides in the work of Heymans and Delaunois (1953) and Heymans et al. (1953). These authors concluded from topical application of such drugs as norepinephrine and tolazoline that agents causing smooth muscle contraction, thereby lowering the distensibility of the sinus wall, will increase baroreceptor excitability. A simple explanation of baroreceptor sensitization, however classic it may be, will border on naiveté when the deliberations of Landgren et al. (1952) regarding small and large baroreceptors are taken into account. Finally, Paintal (1964) has localized the action of volatile anesthetics, in producing sensitization of baroreceptors, to the regenerative region of the afferent sensory nerve ending (Fig. 1). For an in depth presentation of the pharmacology of mechanoreceptors, the reader is referred to that review.

2. Chemoreceptor Effects

Modification of chemoreceptor activity by general anesthetics has not been studied so extensively as the effects of these agents on baroreceptors. This relative void may result from the knowledge that respiratory drive from chemoreceptors remains, even when the respiratory center is severely inhibited by drugs classified as central nervous system depressants. The pertinence of anesthetic effects on chemoreceptor function relates, herein, to the reflex effects on autonomic outflow. Evidence for anesthetic-induced alterations in autonomic activity via chemo-receptors is limited and the pharmacologist should be aware of the experimental needs in this area. For a comprehensive treatment of the anatomy, histology,

physiology, and biochemistry of chemoreceptors, reference is made again to
HEYMANS and NEIL (1958), to the presentation by ANICHKOV and BELENKII (1963),
and a more recent review of the pharmacology by SMITH (1967). Usually, chemoreceptor function is studied as an aside to the larger and apparently more interesting problem of baroreceptor control. The publication by PRICE and WID-
DICOMBE may be cited as an example wherein may be found the cryptic report
that cyclopropane had no effect on the chemoreceptor responses to nicotine,
cyanide, and asphyxia.

An important pharmacological relationship between modern anesthetics and
chemoreceptors is suggested indirectly in the original publication on halothane.
RAVENTÓS (1956) demonstrated a reversal of the pressor response to large doses
of acetylcholine in the atropinized dog under anesthesia with halothane. This
effect was interpreted as ganglionic blockade and was supported by displaying a
reduction in the pressor response to electrical stimulation of the greater splanchnic

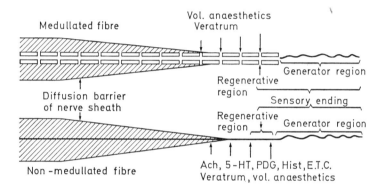

Fig. 1. Schematic diagrams of sensory endings of medullated and non-medullated nerve
fibres showing the two parts of an ending and the probable site of action of drugs at the
regenerative region, where there is no diffusion barrier. A greater variety of drugs affects the
endings of non-medullated fibres because the fibres themselves are more susceptible to these
drugs (PAINTAL, 1964)

nerve. Such a conclusion is one of many in this area that indicate how stubbornly
classical concepts may be held despite evidence to the contrary.

ATANACKOVIC and DALGAARD-MIKKELSEN (1950) demonstrated that the pressor response to small doses of acetylcholine was mediated through chemoreceptor
stimulation. The biphasic pressor effect to large doses was a combination of chemoreceptor excitation and direct stimulation of the adrenal medulla. In a sequel to
much earlier studies, COMROE and MORTIMER (1964) separated the responses to
aortic body stimulation from carotid body stimulation by the simple but ingenious
method of prolonging the circulation time between these areas. Generally, pharmacological stimulation of the aortic body gave lesser respiratory stimulation but
was responsible for the pressor response. Carotid body stimulation usually produced bradycardia and hypotension. Even though it is difficult to refute the
clearly demarcated evidence presented by COMROE and MORTIMER, there are considerable data that do not conform to their results. In addition to ATANACKOVIC
and DALGAARD-MIKKELSEN, more recently ABIKO and ITO (1967) and ABIKO et al.
(1967) have indicated that the initial component of the acetylcholine pressor

response originates in the carotid bodies. The reason for differences in results from those of COMROE and MORTIMER may reside in the agonists tested, i.e., nicotine versus acetylcholine, in the drugs used for anesthesia, or, most likely, whether atropine was part of the experimental protocol. Nevertheless, the data are convincing that carotid body stimulation does have a significant reflex sympathetic component.

When the chemoreceptors are denervated, the pressor response to acetylcholine is changed to a depressor one. Such a pressor reversal produced by an alkyl-substituted urea was thought to result solely from a blockade at the adrenal medulla (GARDIER et al., 1960) and the same selective blockade was considered for halothane. However, no evidence for an adrenal medullary blocking action by halothane could be found by these authors. They therefore concluded that the hypotensive response to acetylcholine (pressor reversal) under halothane was explicable on the basis of myocardial depression (GARDIER et al., 1963). In pursuing the mechanism of the pressor reversal further, GARDIER and TRABER (1965) belatedly realized the involvement of the chemoreceptors in the pressor response. On this basis, CARTER et al. (1967) confirmed an earlier impression that acetylcholine given intravenously to produce the arterial pressor response, i.e., the nicotinic effect, had no direct stimulant effect in sympathetic ganglia.

Apparently unaware of the attack on the classical concept of the mechanism for the "nicotinic" response to acetylcholine, given intravenously, GEBBER (1969) obtained evidence that nicotine, in the intravenous doses used to produce chemoreceptor stimulation, also does not directly initiate propagated impulses in postganglionic sympathetic nerves. Thus, investigators determining anesthetic effects on the autonomic nervous system by measuring responses to "ganglionic" drugs can ill afford to be poorly informed on the total pharmacology.

The pragmatic aspects of the influence of anesthetic agents on chemoreceptors may have clinical importance in the patient with a history of asthma. The anesthesiologist is acutely aware of the potential complications in such patients under anesthesia and exercises appropriate caution in their pharmacological management. These patients seldom present a problem, usually doing better under anesthesia than in the conscious state. The anesthesiological and ventilatory care, with its chemoreceptor overlay, could be responsible for the uneventful nature of the procedure. Glomectomy (carotid body ablation) has been a recommended surgical treatment for the asthmatic patient (NAKAYAMA, 1961; OVERHOLT, 1963). Thus, a depressant action on chemoreceptors by anesthetics may prevent the initiation or continuation of an asthmatic attack. Nevertheless, the final common pathway cannot be ignored when ascribing a therapeutic effect in so complicated an experiment as the anesthetic state. For example, pre-anesthetic atropine could have a prophylactic effect that might erroneously be ascribed to the general anesthetic. Yet, the time lag between the administration of this small dose of atropine and the induction of anesthesia is often sufficient to dissipate the muscarinic blockade (GARDIER, 1961).

In addition to the indirect evidence for chemoreceptor depression by halothane as suggested by the reversal of the pressor response to acetylcholine, other earlier studies by DRIPPS and DUMKE (1943) clearly indicated that diethyl ether and cyclopropane inhibited chemoreceptor activity. The cause of the discrepancy between these data and the later results of PRICE and WIDDICOMBE is not apparent.

The teleological aspects of chemoreceptor function, referrable to reflex stimulation of selective portions of sympathetic outflow needs to be studied with renewed and imaginative vigor. Past investigative approaches can be categorized as physiological or pharmacological depending on whether drugs were used as the explanative tools. Subtle differences do exist for the afferent limb. Ganglionic blocking agents will prevent or reduce chemoreceptor stimulation to such drugs as nicotine and acetylcholine while enhancing that to cyanide or hypoxia. MOE et al. (1948) were the first to demonstrate this dichotomy which was later confirmed by DONTAS and NICKERSON (1956) by neuroelectrical recordings from the carotid branch of the glossopharyngeal nerve. Nevertheless, physiological or pharmacological stimulation of these afferent sites results in cardiovascular patterns which are directed toward increasing the supply of oxygen to vital tissues. This implies a reflex excitation of only certain portions of the sympathetic nervous system. The Russian investigators have been keenly aware of this selectivity as indicated in the publications of BELENKII and STROIKOV (1950) and especially that of FEDORCHUK (1954). She found that the increase in blood pressure associated with carotid chemoreceptor stimulation by small doses of nicotine was due mainly to an increase in adrenomedullary secretion; the direct vascular reflex being of lesser importance. ARMITAGE (1965) reaches a contrary conclusion relative to the adrenal participation in the pressor response, but the published data by this author appear not to support his contention too strongly. In our own laboratory (ROWE et al.), the initial pressor phase of the response to acetylcholine in the dog was reduced by more than one half, simply by bilateral section of the greater splanchnic nerve. When this was combined with splenectomy, the secondary pressor phase, i.e., that phase resulting from stimulation of the adrenal medulla, both directly by the drug and reflexly through the nerve, was also significantly reduced. This gives credence to the possibility of a select or discrete pathway between chemoreceptors and splanchnic sympathetic outflow. It would be expedient for chemoreceptor activation through hypoxia to constrict abdominal visceral arterioles, to contract the spleen for the infusion of oxygen-carrying red cells, to discharge epinephrine from the adrenal, which supplements the nervous activity and provides a beta stimulant to increase cardiac output and dilate bronchioles. Support for such a discrete pathway may be derived cautiously from the publication by KAHN and MILLS (1967). Complementing this are the studies of ABIKO and ITO (1967) with acetylcholine in which they noted that the rise in blood pressure preceded an increase in myocardial contractile force. Splanchnic nerve stimulation could increase cardiac output merely by increasing venous return through contraction of the venous reservoir and combined with elevated splanchnic arteriovascular resistance will affect blood pressure prior to any change in cardiac inotropy.

For a limited but critical study of the pharmacology of chemoreception, the reader is referred to the work of EYZAQUIRRE and KOYANO (1965). Furthermore, whatever the potential for anesthetics to affect autonomic activity by a primary action on chemoreceptors, the complexities attending the pharmacological approach to discriminate these areas as sites of action can be amply appreciated.

III. Central Nervous System

Following a series of preliminary investigations, LEVY (1913) published a treatise on the production of ventricular arrhythmias in the cat under chloroform anesthesia. From one aspect of his work, LEVY concluded, "... a sensory stimulation under light chloroform anesthesia may, through one or more reflex mechanisms, throw the ventricles of the heart into a condition of permanent and fatal fibrillation, or may initiate irregularities which may terminate later in ventricular fibrillation. Under fully established chloroform anesthesia such an event never happens." Sensory stimulation consisted of electrical shocks to the central ends of the cut sciatic and splanchnic nerves. Although all the evidence presented in this and a subsequent publication (LEVY, 1914) indicated a local action of chloroform on the heart, it also clearly demonstrated that no measurable depression of central sympathetic activity was produced by the anesthetic.

Experiments, contemporary to LEVY's, actually had incriminated a central sympathetic excitation in the activities of both diethyl ether and chloroform. In cats anesthetized with these agents, innervated adrenal glands had "adrenalin" contents lower than the denervated glands of the opposite side (ELLIOTT, 1912). Additionally, electrical stimulation of somatic afferent nerves served to enhance the depletion of amines in the adrenal caused by diethyl ether. Through surgical ablation, the reflex centers, as possible sites of drug action, were located between the corpora quadrigemina and the first thoracic segment of the spinal cord. It is impossible to discern from ELLIOTT's work whether the anesthetics stimulated pressor centers or inhibited depressor centers — a present day matter of controversy (vide infra). However, from his surgical description, it is reasonable to assume that autonomic diencephalic centers were spared. Therefore, the enhancement of adrenal amine depletion by afferent nerve stimulation may have occurred through reflex brain stem augmentation of anesthetic dependent sympathetic hyperactivity originating in the hypothalamus. About two decades later, a group of Canadian workers made the chance observation that decerebration (sectioning between the superior colliculus and vestibular nucleus) affected the production of arrhythmias under chloroform (BEATTIE et al., 1930). Essentially, these investigators located a sympathetic center in the posterior hypothalamus that was stimulated by chloroform. Thus, a sophisticated neuropharmacological approach had confirmed the action of at least one inhalation anesthetic on central autonomic function.

By the succeeding decade, neurophysiologists knew that sympathetic tone was a function of at least three central components: hypothalamus, medullary vasomotor center, and baroreceptors (BRONK et al., 1940), all potential targets for anesthetic effects. Furthermore, subtle species variations may exist among experimental animals that will have a bearing on the loci of anesthetic action as explained for man. For example, PEISS (1960) suggests that an afferent path extends rostrally from the dorsal medulla to the hypothalamus in the cat because latent cardioacceleration resulting from stimulation of the dorsal medulla is abolished by lesions caudal to the hypothalamus. Adrenalectomy also prevents this response and lends further weight to the argument (vide supra) favoring a selective pathway between chemoreceptors and adrenal medulla. Stimulation of the ventrolateral medulla produced immediate pressor and cardioaccelerator effects which were unaffected by either procedure. From this report and the work of others (CHEN et al., 1937) there is a suggestion that reflex cardioacceleration may be represented at higher levels in the cat than in the dog. However, it is hoped that such erudite differences do not invalidate comparisons of data between species when such generally accepted neurophysiological techniques as classical decerebration are used to define central anesthetic actions.

If interest in the effect of inhalation anesthetics on central autonomic function had waned since those early days, it was renewed vigorously by the previously cited results of PRICE and WIDDECOMBE regarding the sensitizing effect of cyclopropane on baroreceptors. This was incompatible with increased sympathetic activity as the suspected mechanism of cardiovascular action of this agent. The paradox was resolved by demonstrating a selective inhibition of a depressor center in the canine medulla. Moreover, the central representation of cyclopropane activity was confined strictly to the medulla as determined by surgical sectioning of the brain stem (PRICE et al., 1963). From this beginning to the present time, the literature reflects the spirited research that has been conducted to answer the many questions that have been posed in this area.

PRICE and coworkers subsequently turned their attention to the central effect of halothane, using the circulatorily isolated head of the dog. They came to the conclusion [PRICE et al., 1963 (1)] that this halogenated hydrocarbon decreased central sympathetic and, to a much lesser extent, central parasympathetic activity. Later, by employing anesthetic solutions infiltrated into medullary pressor and depressor areas, halothane was found to inhibit both functions whereas cyclopropane was disproportionately less effective on the pressor center [PRICE et al., 1965 (1)]. Further studies demonstrated reductions in preganglionic sympathetic activity with halothane in the normal, decerebrate, and spinal cat (SKOVSTED et al., 1969). Inhibition of hypothalamic centers by halothane certainly was not indicated and neither was unequivocal inhibition of a medullary depressor center, since decrements in activity still were recorded with depressor nerve stimulation. Inhibition of the medullary pressor center was a reasonable conclusion to be derived from the data, but it would have been extremely more informative if the center's susceptibility to further suppression by baroreceptor activity were tested in the decerebrate preparation. The lateral horn cells appear to have some intrinsic tone, when blood pressure is supported, that can be reduced by halothane. Methoxyflurane had very little of the central autonomic depressant properties described for halothane. Evidence for a suppression of brain stem mediated pressor activity could be demonstrated only in baroreceptor denervated animals (SKOVSTED and PRICE, 1969).

The rabbit responds to cyclopropane, halothane, and diethyl ether with an increase in sympathetic activity while simultaneously displaying a circulatory depressor response to the last two. Presumably this stimulation was central in origin since baroreceptor denervation had no effect on the qualitative nature of the response (MILLAR and BISCOE, 1965). Continued exploration for the site of this sympathetic stimulation in the rabbit [BISCOE and MILLAR, 1966 (1)] pointed to an inhibition of the depressor pathway, with a decreasing order of potency: cyclopropane, diethyl ether, halothane. Such data conformed to the denoted action of cyclopropane on the canine medullary depressor center, but a similar conclusion relative to halothane is circumspect (vide supra). Stimulation of sympathetic activity by cyclopropane centrally, also has been confirmed in man (PRICE et al., 1965).

Conversely, numerous other investigators have published data demonstrating an inhibition of the medullary pressor function by cyclopropane. MARKEE et al. (1966) using the cross-perfusion technique to the heads of dogs, found that the pressor response to central stimulation in the recipient was more susceptible to cyclopropane than was the depressor response. Some inhibition of the depressor effect was noted in single animal experiments. This occurred at the high concentration (20%) and was suggestive of a cord effect. Confirmation of the "pressor inhibition" concept came in rapid succession from several related laboratories. In one series of experiments, cyclopropane, in concentrations of 20% and above, decreased pressor and spared depressor responses to afferent nerve stimulation during major vessel occlusion (BARTLESTONE et al., 1966) while in another series this agent raised the threshold for pressor responses resulting from hypothalamic stimulation (NGAI and BOLME, 1966). This last may merely reflect a depression of the medullary center if the descending pathway from the hypothalamus forms a junction there. However, a lack of effect on the carotid occlusion response makes such an explanation questionable. Both halothane and cyclopropane spared the vasodepressor pathway that was excited by mesencephalic stimulation.

A very interesting and extremely provocative study was published during this time by Katz (1966). This author, by means of decerebration, was able to abolish cardiac arrhythmias generated by halopropane ($CHF_2CF_2CH_2Br$). Halopropane-carbon dioxide arrhythmias did not respond to decerebration but responded to spinal cord transection at C-1. The evidence indicated that the anesthetic *per se* increased sympathetic activity through stimulation of a supra-pontine site, whereas carbon dioxide stimulates in the brain stem probably at the level of the

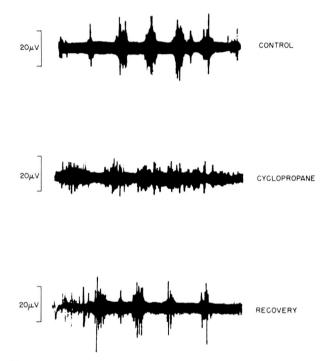

Fig. 2. Sympathetic nerve activity as observed in absence of cocaine. Typical effect of cyclopropane in changing pattern of sympathetic activity is presented. Each display is a 2-second sweep on the cathode-ray oscilloscope [Gardier et al., 1967 (1)]

vasomotor center. Increased sympathetic tone induced by carbon dioxide appears as better defined, exaggerated, and more synchronized action-potentials than recorded in a sympathetic nerve trunk under normocarbia (Millar and Biscoe, 1965, 1966). Conversely, all anesthetics used in those experiments where spontaneous activity has been recorded (Millar and Biscoe, 1965; Skovsted and Price, 1969), produced an asynchronous sympathetic rhythm with poorly defined pulses of activity. This change in pattern (Fig. 2) is disconcerting when quantitative comparisons with the pre-anesthetic state are needed (Gardier et al., 1967), since it could dictate the peak titer of neurohumor present at the receptor site. Although asynchronous firing from a population of sympathetic nerves has gained additional attention more recently (Skovsted and Price, 1969), no categorical evidence for its origin is available. Nevertheless, could the anesthetics be stimulating the sympathetic center in the posterior hypothalamus (KATZ, 1966), or an associated ascending medullary-pontine pathway producing tonic activity while concomitantly depressing the medullary coordinating center that provides the summation necessary for the synchronized pulsatile phenomena ? Several arguments against this generalization may be proposed. Firstly, neither cyclopropane nor halothane has been shown to inhibit the sympathetic stimulation induced by carbon dioxide (PRICE et al., 1959; MILLAR and MORRIS, 1960) which acts at the medullary level (vide supra). Secondly, this University of Pennsylvania group has found that the increased preganglionic sympathetic activity under cyclopropane was not inhibited by decerebration (PRICE et al., 1969). However, presented therein was the first faint evidence from that laboratory supporting a central pressor inhibitory property of cyclopropane. Specifically, 20% cyclopropane depressed sympathetic activity in the baroreceptor decompensated cat, whereas 30% was required to produce an increment. Thirdly, the threshold for hypothalamic stimulation was elevated by cyclopropane (NGAI and BOLME, 1966). However, this effect is ambiguous because of lower center susceptibility and thus may not necessarily oppose the hypothesis.

In attempting to resolve the continuing controversy surrounding the central autonomic effects, CHRISTOFORO and BRODY (1968) provided further evidence for suppresion of the medullary pressor site by cyclopropane and halothane. More importantly, however, was the introduction of another central phenomenon relative to these agents — that of releasing vasopressin in vasoactive quantities from the posterior pituitary [CHRISTOFORO and BRODY, 1968 (1)]. Halothane stimulates the release of antidiuretic hormone (BLACKMORE et al., 1960) as does cyclopropane (HABIF et al., 1951). This effect prudently may be ascribed to a direct releasing property. Yet, anesthetics also could modulate hormone release by elevating titers of adrenergic and, less likely, cholinergic amines through increased autonomic nervous system activity. The intimate association between neurohypophysial secretion and autonomic nervous system neurohumors has received due attention (DUKE and PICKFORD, 1951; GIERE and EVERSOLE, 1954; KIVALO and ARKO, 1957; FUJITA and HARTMANN, 1961). Since adrenergic amines are inhibitors of posterior pituitary secretion, opposing functions may be incorporated in the total activity of a single anesthetic agent. However, the well-known "blood-brain barrier" to circulating biogenic amines must be anticipated in any feedback regulation of posterior pituitary secretion. The reverse relationship, i.e., neurohypophysial stimulation of central autonomic activity would involve a contrived link between anterior and posterior hypothalamus.

Enhanced vascular reactivity to posterior pituitary pressor principle has been demonstrated when sympathetic function is compromised in either an obvious [NASH, 1962; GARDIER et al., 1965, 1965 (1); BARTLESTONE and NASMYTH, 1965] or subtle manner (CHENOWETH et al., 1958). In the baroreceptor denervated dog, an osmotic challenge (VERNEY, 1947) will produce a pressor effect having a sympathetic component that is amenable to autonomic blocking agents (TRABER et al., 1968). A similar effect in the rabbit has been ascribed, totally, to sympathetic stimulation originating in the hind brain, since it persisted after sectioning caudal to the diencephalon and was abolished by high cord trans-section and by an alpha adrenergic blocking agent (HOLLAND et al., 1958, 1959). Obviously, the complete versus the partial participation of the sympathetic nervous system in the above events could be species dependent.

The osmotic challenge in both dog and rabbit could be expected to release antidiuretic hormone by stimulation of osmoreceptors in the anterior hypothalamus (JEWELL and VERNEY, 1957). The studies in the rabbit argue against the probability of vasopressin being a central sympathetic stimulant and thus mediating increases in sympathetic activity. However, any inflexibility in autonomic activity induced by inhalation anesthetics (vide infra) could allow the vasoconstrictor properties of an enhanced serum titer of antidiuretic hormone to become evident. Additional information on stimulation of neurohypophysial secretion by anesthetic and other agents may be found in the recent review in this Handbook (GINSBURG, 1968).

IV. Peripheral Nervous System

1. Preganglionic Effects

In the previous section, a cursory acknowledgement was made of a spinal cord depressant action for halothane (SKOVSTED et al., 1969). Since the preganglionic sympathetic nerves were those involved, this prologue will be concerned with the limited evidence favoring an insidious cord effect for this and other agents.

By splenic plethysmography and intestinal activity recordings, BHATIA and BURN (1933) found that diethyl ether and chloroform stimulated sympathetic activity in the spinal but not totally pithed cat. More recently, BURN and EPSTEIN (1959) described a qualitatively similar but quantitatively lesser activity for halothane. However, pithing of the spinal cord was not accomplished in these later day experiments. GRAVENSTEIN et al. (1960) related their observations of nictitating membrane contractions in the spinal animal to a possible stimulating action by cyclopropane in the spinal cord. Thus, it is not unreasonable to consider a stimulation of lateral horn cells as a potential property of inhalation anethetics. Furthermore, this "would be" effect on the preganglionic neuron appears to be the only "evidence" available for an excitatory action of this group of agents on efferent sympathetic neurones.

2. Ganglionic Effects

Because KOBACKER and RIGLER (1929) felt that the presence of anesthesia made liable the misinterpretation of certain cardiac research data, they possibly were the first to plan an experiment for the sole purpose of studying the autonomic properties of an anesthetic agent. These investigators demonstrated vagal ganglionic blockade with diethyl ether, but were unable to draw so categorical a conclusion for the stellate ganglion. From later investigations on the perfused stellate ganglion of the cat, LARRABEE and POSTERNAK (1952) described a preferential depression of synaptic transmission versus axonal conduction by diethyl ether and chloroform. In the same year, LARRABEE and HOLADAY published a classical reference (1952) on ganglionic depression by diethyl ether and chloroform. These volatile liquids produced greater depression of postganglionic action potentials resulting from high frequency rather than low frequency stimulation of the preganglionic superior cervical nerve in cats. Further, the initial fast component of the compound postganglionic action-potential was more susceptible to suppression than the secondary slow component. Depression of ganglionic transmission by diethyl ether has been confirmed by other investigators (NORMANN and LÖFSTRÖM, 1955; BISCOE and MILLAR, 1966) and probably is the site for the depressing action of diethyl ether on the carotid occlusion response in dogs (BROWN and HILTON, 1956).

Despite all the evidence favoring a ganglionic blocking action in both parasympathetic and sympathetic limbs, a desirable attribute of ether anesthesia involves increased sympathetic activity (CATTELL, 1923). Furthermore, neuropharmacological recordings of spontaneous postganglionic activity appear to be faithful reproductions of elevated preganglionic tone produced by this agent (MILLAR and BISCOE, 1966). Removal of sympathetic nervous influence unmasks a remarkably potent direct depressant effect (McALLISTER and ROOT, 1941; BREWSTER et al., 1953).

Historically, the autonomic activity of cyclopropane has a number of similarities to that of diethyl ether. In the experiments conducted by MILLAR and BISCOE (1966), there was no evidence that cyclopropane reduced ganglionic transmission since the increased spontaneous preganglionic activity was accurately represented in the postganglionic fibers. The fact that sympathectomy from the stellate to the 6th thoracic paravertebral ganglion did not prevent ventricular arrhythmias in response to hypercarbia in the cat under cyclopropane indicates that the sympathetic junction at the adrenal medulla also remains functional to physiological stimulation (ROBBINS and THOMAS, 1960).

Postganglionic recordings obtained by artificial (electrical) stimulation of preganglionic nerves show that cyclopropane is a weak but definite ganglionic blocking agent whether the parameter is the conducted action-potential (NORMANN and LÖFSTRÖM, 1955; BISCOE and MILLAR, 1966) or an end organ response (PRICE and PRICE, 1967). It is of some merit to point out here that the presence of atropine or possibly gallamine in experiments on ganglionic function will have a definite influence on the results. An abbreviated explanation of this statement will be given later.

The original publication by RAVENTÓS (1956) describing the pharmacology of halothane presented data that justifiably could be interpreted as a selective ganglionic blocking capability for this drug. An alternative explanation based on a suppression of chemoreceptor sensitivity plus a direct depressant effect on the heart by halothane has been argued and the pharmacological analogy between chemoreceptors and autonomic ganglia has been presented (vide supra). The heritage that RAVENTÓS gave succeeding researchers was the privilege to confirm or deny the conclusions drawn from his original study. Both possibilities have been accomplished.

PRICE and PRICE (1966) demonstrated a ganglionic blocking action for halothane, in the presence of atropine, which was not dependent on stimulation frequency. These workers also were able to show a small blocking action of nitrous oxide which added to the effect of halothane (PRICE and PRICE, 1967). The independence from stimulation frequency suggests a mechanism of blockade different from that of known competitive antagonists (PATON, 1954; RIKER and KOMALA-HIRANYA, 1962; TRABER et al., 1967). Depression of ganglionic function with halothane has been recorded with single electrical shocks to preganglionic fibers at low frequency (BISCOE and MILLAR, 1966), inconsistently to spontaneous activity MILLAR and BISCOE, 1966) and probably not at all to elevated activity induced by hypercarbia (MILLAR and MORRIS, 1960). Although additional evidence favoring ganglionic suppression exists (PURCHASE, 1965; EPSTEIN et al., 1966), there are sufficient data available to refute such claims.

A classical pharmacological approach has indicated that halothane alone has no effect on vagal or superior cervical ganglia but will enhance the ganglionic blocking action of d-tubocurarine or hexamethonium at the latter site (BURN et al., 1957). By somewhat complex indirect methods, SEVERINGHAUS and CULLEN (1958) also were forced to conclude that ganglionic blockade could not be justified as a mechanism for the circulatory depression produced by this halogenated hydrocarbon. Additional testimony against autonomic blockade has been provided for true ganglionic sites (LI et al., 1968) and for the adrenal neuromedullary junction (GARDIER et al., 1963).

Most recently the ganglionic effect of inhalation agents has been reported in terms of blockade of nicotinic and muscarinic receptors. Halothane, diethyl ether, and cyclopropane have an inhibitory action on both receptor sites whereas no effect was demonstrable for nitrous oxide (GARFIELD et al., 1968). Halothane appeared to be a more effective ganglionic muscarinic blocking agent than diethyl ether and the nature of the total blockade may be described as competitive according to PATON's criterion (1954) of a waning response to repetitive stimulation. A subsequent study from the same laboratory indicated that nicotinic sites,

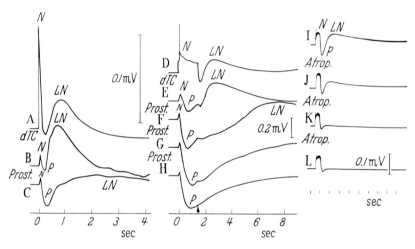

Fig. 3. A—L. Postganglionic potentials set up by preganglionic volleys and recorded between the ganglion and the postganglionic trunk of the isolated superior cervical ganglion of rabbit. A—C potentials evoked by single preganglionic volleys in concentrations of dTC of 2.5 × 10⁻⁵ M in A, and 8×10⁻⁵ M for B, C, with also 3 × 10⁻⁶ M prostigmine in C. D—H similar series but with repetitive stimulation, 20/sec for 1.4 sec, end of tetanus being marked by arrow below: D and E in dTC 1.6 × 10⁻⁵ M and 8 × 10⁻⁵ M respectively: in addition progressive prostigmine in F—H, 3×10⁻⁷ M, 3×10⁻⁶ M and 6×10⁻⁶ M. I—L, similarly evoked potentials, but for repetitive stimulation of 40/sec for 0.5 sec, and with ganglion curarized by 10 μg/ml of dihydro-β-erythroidine. Atropine concentrations were 0.1 μg/ml, 0.5 μg/ml, and 8.0 μg/ml for J, K and L respectively. Many N, P and LN waves are labelled. (J. C. ECCLES, 1964, taken from R. M. ECCLES, 1952 and R. M. ECCLES and LIBET, 1961)

only, were loci for ganglionic blockade with halothane (ALPER et al., 1969). This work has opened up the pharmacology of anesthesia to a new and complex challenge.

The autonomic activity of acetylcholine was stated by DALE (1914) to be muscarinic if it were blocked by atropine and nicotinic if it were still observed in the presence of atropine but were paralyzed by excess nicotine. The pharmacology of the autonomic nervous system developed in DALE's long shadow and therefore, was inclined to appoint postganglionic cholinergic nerve post-junctional sites as "muscarinic" and preganglionic cholinergic nerve post-junctional sites (ganglionic) as "nicotinic". Some indication that ganglionic receptors were not solely confined to the category of "nicotinic" became available from KOPPANYI's work (1932) with muscarinic drugs. Two decades later, ROSAMOND ECCLES (1952) provided experimental proof for at least two pharmacologically distinct ganglionic receptor sites. This was accomplished by recording, under special conditions, the peculiar electrical potentials that develop between the isolated (rabbit) superior cervical ganglion and the distal end of the cut postganglionic nerve upon stimulation of the preganglionic nerve. Continued application of this technique broadened and extended the scope of ganglionic neuropharmacology (ECCLES and LIBET, 1961).

In the presence of sufficient d-tubocurarine (dTC) to inhibit the postganglionic spike, preganglionic stimulation (volley) produced an initial rapid negative wave followed by a positive deflection and then a longer lasting (late) negative wave. This sequence occurred over a period of approximately 2 sec and the respective waves were labeled "N", "P", and "LN" in chronological order (Fig. 3) and were of known postsynaptic origin. Additional dTC or some other competitive blocking agent will depress the N wave. Reserpine, alpha adrenergic blocking agents or atropine will attenuate the P wave. High doses of anticholinesterases or small doses of atropine will depress the LN wave. Botulinum toxin, which prevents the

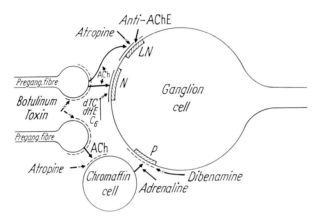

Fig. 4. Diagrammatic representation of the postulated production of the N, P and LN waves of ganglion cells by transmitter released by preganglionic impulses. The receptor sites are shown on the surface of the ganglion cell. The postulated pathways of the transmitter substances, ACh and adrenaline, are shown by arrows and the postulated sites of action of the various pharmacological agents are indicated by arrows, the arrows with crosses signifying depressant actions. (J. C. ECCLES, 1964, modified from R. M. ECCLES and LIBET, 1961)

release of acetylcholine from nerve terminals, will prevent all phases of the response. A schematic representation of the receptors and events is presented in Fig. 4. Thus, according to classical terminology, the N site is considered "nicotinic", P-"adrenergic", and LN-"muscarinic". For a lucid and more extensive tabulation of the contributions to this esoteric area and the interpretations to be made therefrom, the reader is referred to ECCLES' book (1964) on the physiology of synapses.

Complementary pharmacological data were soon available to substantiate the presence of muscarinic and nicotinic sites in sympathetic ganglia. TAKESHIGE and VOLLE (1962) were able to show a bimodal postganglionic effect when acetylcholine was injected intra-arterially to suitably conditioned ganglia. There occurred an early brief discharge of relatively large action-potentials that was susceptible to

curare. The early discharge was followed by a more prolonged low amplitude
asynchronous discharge which had a lower threshold for activation by acetylcholine and was abolished by atropine (Fig. 5). Moreover, responses of organ
systems to sympathetic stimulation despite the presence of competitive ganglionic
blockade were found to be abolished by atropine (Hilton, 1961; Long and
Eckstein, 1961; Hilton and Steinberg, 1966; Steinberg and Hilton, 1967).
The involvement of ganglionic muscarinic receptors in the excitation of the nictitating membrane following stimulation of the preganglionic superior cervical
nerve has been reported (Trendelenburg, 1966). Confirmation of such ganglionic
receptors in the sympathetic pathway to another organ (Flacke and Gillis, 1968)
and organ system followed, even to relating the responses to asynchronous low

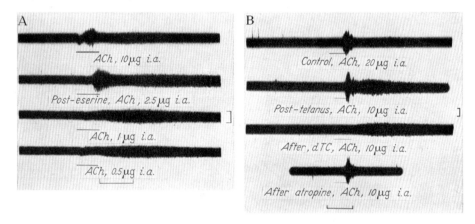

Fig. 5a—b. Postganglionic discharges of cat superior cervical ganglion in response to intra-
arterial injections of acetylcholine in the quantities indicated and at the times shown by the
horizontal lines. In (a) an intra-arterial injection of 100 μg of eserine greatly increases the
effectiveness of ACh in evoking a delayed discharge. In (b) after conditioning by a tetanus (60 per
sec for 10 sec) there is in the second record an increase in the delayed discharge. The third and
fourth records show selective depression of the early and delayed discharges by dTC and
atropine respectively. Time scales 1 sec; Voltage scales, 10 μV. (J. C. Eccles, 1964, taken
from Takeshige and Volle, 1962)

amplitude action-potentials in the postganglionic fibers (Brown, 1967). All these
modern-day experiments simply served to vindicate the earlier conclusion that all
autonomic pathways could not be interrupted by a classical ganglionic blocking
agent (Moe and Freyburger, 1950).

It is appropriate to conclude that separate receptor sites exist on a single
postganglionic neurone, yet it is equally important to point out that a postganglionic (at least sympathetic) trunk is not composed of a uniform population of
fibers. Different histological and conduction characteristics have been associated
with innervation of specific structures (Bishop and Heinbecker, 1932; Eccles,
1935). The compound action potential, arising from such dishomogeneity, is almost distinctive for postganglionic sympathetic extracellular recordings and its
alteration may be a useful indicator of discrete sympathetic function (Fernandez
de Molina and Perl, 1965). Pharmacologically distinct *cell types* in sympathetic
ganglia have been suggested (Shaw et al., 1948; Shaw and MacCallum, 1949;

MAINLAND and SHAW, 1952) and the diverse agents that affect ganglionic function have been aptly reviewed (TRENDELENBURG, 1967). Moreover, much evidence has accumulated now to indicate that sympathetic ganglia are not catholic even within a specie (VOGT, 1964) and a similar variation may apply to parasympathetic ganglia (JACOBOWITZ, 1965; MARKS et al., 1962).

Presently, little consideration has been given to the effect of inhalation anesthetics in terms of such aforementioned fundamental neuropharmacology. The artificiality of the experimental conditions discourages the application of that sort of data to pragmatic problems. However, it is common practice in modern anesthesia to expose the patient to a multiplicity of pharmacodynamic actions influencing the anesthetic state, which are no less complicated than most of the contrived laboratory experiments.

The studies by GARFIELD et al. (1968) and ALPER et al. (1969) wherein cardiac chronotropy was measured to preganglionic accelerator nerve stimulation have introduced to the field of anesthesia an awareness of ganglionic nicotinic and muscarinic receptors. But, there is a great need to correlate the pertinent nervous activity with end organ responses. This was the intention of LI et al. (1968) who were probably dealing with compound action potentials from a mixed fiber population and not with ganglionic muscarinic receptors. Apparently, LARRABEE and HOLADAY (1952) also were contending only with nicotinic receptor sites when determining the blocking potency of diethyl ether and chloroform as a function of stimulation frequency. Despite attempts to implicate a physiological role for muscarinic receptors in ganglia (LIBET, 1964), some reconciliation still is needed as to what constitutes an appropriate stimulus for autonomic nervous system and effector organ function (FOLKOW, 1952; ECCLES, 1955; BLACKMAN and PURVES, 1969). Conversely, the pharmacological ramifications are quite real. Treatment of organophosphorus poisoning (GILLIS et al., 1968) and overcoming the tolerance developed to ganglionic blocking agents (VOLLE, 1966) are examples of problems that will benefit from the added knowledge. A more extensive coverage of the pharmacology of autonomic ganglia can be found in the International Encyclopedia of Pharmacology and Therapeutics [VOLLE, 1966 (1)].

There is a paucity of information concerning the effects of newer inhalation anesthetics on autonomic ganglia. Two pioneering studies have indicated that methoxyflurane does not compromise the integrity of the sympathetic nervous system [BAGWELL and WOODS, 1962; MILLAR and MORRIS, 1960 (1)]. Meanwhile, a recent investigation makes suspect some blockade by this agent at the adrenal medulla [LI et al., 1968 (1)].

3. Nerve Ending

The ability to stimulate release (KOPIN, 1964) or inhibit uptake (TITUS and DENGLER, 1966) of catecholamines by nervous tissue has not been a prime objective of anesthesia research. One or both mechanisms could be considered for halothane and cyclopropane (PRICE et al., 1959, 1960, 1968; GARFIELD et al., 1968). However, a comparison with cocaine as the prototypic compound for inhibiting amine uptake (WHITBY et al., 1960) has provided circumstantial evidence that in addition to cyclopropane [GARDIER et al., 1967 (1); GARDIER and HAMELBERG, 1968), halothane, methoxyflurane, and diethyl ether do not influence this property of adrenergic tissue (NAITO and GILLIS, 1968). Actual measurements of cardiac uptake of norepinephrine have provided confirmation for the lack of such an effect by halothane and cyclopropane (PRICE et al., 1968). Neither cyclopropane nor halothane influence the synthesis and release of catecholamines [NGAI et al., 1969, 1969 (1)]. Although several anesthetics are known cholinergic stimulants

(JONES et al., 1961) no studies are known to this reviewer that incriminate the sympathetic cholinergic-link hypothesis of BURN and RAND (1959, 1960) in the sympathetic profile of anesthesia.

V. Effector Sites

Classical pharmacological methods for studying the actions of inhalation anesthetics on adrenergic receptors are seriously impeded by the phenomenon common to most of these agents, i.e., sensitization to the production of cardiac ventricular arrhythmias. The nature of the problem is such that a standardized approach has been submitted for determining this sensitizing property (MEEK et al., 1937). This is not to say that responsiveness to catecholamine cannot be tested *in vivo* under anesthesia. This has been done even in man (MATTEO et al., 1962, 1963; KATZ et al., 1962; PRICE et al., 1958, 1959). However, because of compromised dosing and marginal effects, conclusions referrable to receptor function are difficult. Furthermore, dose-effect variations exist relative to arrhythmia development. This is exemplified by the difference in susceptibility between halothane and cyclopropane, being greater during light anesthesia with the former and during deep anesthesia with the latter.

Diethyl ether does not sensitize the heart for the production of ventricular arrhythmias and thus allows the employment of suitable pharmacodynamic doses of catecholamines. Alteration of receptor function by this agent appears unlikely. The direct cardiovascular depressant properties of diethyl ether are countered by a functioning sympathetic nervous system (MCALLISTER and ROOT, 1941; BREWSTER et al., 1953; BHATIA and BURN, 1933; CATTELL, 1923) which, happily, is partly responsible for its clinical safety. In view of this, it is surprising to find that reserpine treatment did not quantitatively alter the depressant properties of diethyl ether [BAGWELL et al., 1964 (1)] unless the explanation resides in a resistance to depletion on the part of the adrenal medulla (MUSCHOLL and VOGT, 1958). Diethyl ether is without effect on the responses of isolated tissues to endogenous (NAITO and GILLIS, 1968) or exogenous adrenergic amines (PRICE and PRICE, 1962) and yet may produce a profile of beta receptor stimulation *in vivo* (JONES et al., 1962).

The irritant properties of diethyl ether mimic certain cholinergic responses, but it cannot be said that ether is either a postganglionic muscarinic agonist or antagonist although a non-specific blockade of acetylcholine has been demonstrated (FLETCHER et al., 1968). Cholinergic stimulation produced by halothane and cyclopropane is sensitive to inhibition by atropine (JONES et al., 1961).

Generally, the actions of volatile liquids on vital organ function must be termed "depressant". With halothane, chloroform, methoxyflurane, ethrane, and teflurane, the evidence is overwhelmingly in favor of either a direct effect on the heart [BHATIA and BURN, 1933; BURN et al., 1957; CRAYTHORNE and HUFFINGTON, 1966; LI et al., 1968; MORROW and MORROW, 1961; NAITO and GILLIS, 1968; NAYLOR, 1959; PURCHASE, 1965; SEVERINGHAUS and CULLEN, 1958; SHIMOSATO et al., 1968, 1969, 1969 (1); WARNER et al., 1967) or blockade of the physiological response of the heart to endogenous or exogenous catecholamines (NAYLOR, 1959; GARDIER et al., 1963; PRICE and PRICE, 1966). Neither reserpine treatment (FLACKE and ALPER, 1962; REIN et al., 1963) nor denervation significantly alters the decrement in cardiac function produced by halothane (MORROW et al., 1961). Although norepinephrine can partially antagonize the effects of halothane on the heart, FLACKE and ALPER (1962) feel that a common receptor is not involved. Additional findings with halothane include direct relaxation of vascular and intestinal smooth muscle (McArdle and Black, 1963), reduction of the vascular smooth muscle response to reflex stimulation (Epstein et al., 1968) or to norepinephrine (Price and Price, 1962; Christoforo and Brody, 1968) and relaxation of the spleen (Burn and Epstein, 1959). The results of Epstein et al. (1966) offer a choice between a direct depressant or a catecholamine antagonizing action for halothane. Conversely, chloroform has been found to augment the contraction of the aortic strip of the rabbit to norepinephrine (Price and Price, 1962).

Klide and coworkers (1967, 1969) have raised the exciting possibility that halothane has direct or indirect beta receptor stimulating properties. This could explain the exaggerated chronotropic response registered by Garfield et al. (1968) and Price et al. (1968) upon stimulation of the postganglionic cardiac accelerator nerve in animals under halothane anesthesia. Previously, in experiments under halothane anesthesia, Craythorne and Huffington (1966) had described a negative chronotropic response to propranolol, a beta receptor blocking agent. Other investigators (Fletcher et al., 1968) have not been able to ascribe a tracheal smooth muscle relaxing property of halothane to beta receptor stimulation but have proposed a non-specific anticholinergic effect.

Most of the evidence disclosing a suppression of organ function by anesthetic agents favors a mechanism that is outside of the receptor and is non-specific. Sensitizing the myocardium for the production of arrhythmias to catecholamines argues against alpha adrenergic blockade as a remote mechanism of action (Nickerson, 1959). Abolition of such an arrhythmia by beta blocking agents (Artusio et al., 1967) is not proof that the anesthetic is a beta receptor stimulant. Finally, there is little apparent information regarding a direct action, by any of the volatile anesthetics, on postganglionic muscarinic receptors.

The pharmacological activity of cyclopropane in the vicinity of the receptor is a mixed one. This drug has been shown to increase cardiac output at low inspiratory concentrations and to depress this parameter in high inspiratory concentrations (Jones et al., 1960). No depression was evident in the transplanted human heart (Keats, 1969). Myocardial depression has been reported *in vitro* (Naito and Gillis, 1968) and in the normal and reserpine treated animal *in vivo* (Bagwell et al., 1964). Despite causing a decreased cardiac output, cyclopropane, interestingly enough, increased blood pressure and heart rate in the dog treated with reserpine (Rusy et al., 1965). This is suggestive of increased central sympathetic activity operating on a nervous or adrenal medullary amine pool that was resistant to depletion. Apropos to the latter, is the description of the dog under cyclopropane as an adrenal medullary responding animal (Deutsch et al., 1962).

Increased sympathetic activity counters both the direct negative inotropy and the vagal mediated negative chronotropy produced by cyclopropane (Price et al., 1962). Moreover, several examples of enhancement of local adrenergic function by this agent are available (Gravenstein et al., 1960; Price et al., 1968) although in at least one case, there may be a question of specificity (Price and Price, 1962). Nitrous oxide has also been found to enhance the response to norepinephrine (Price and Price, 1962). Beta blockade will counteract the cardiac effects of cyclopropane (Craythorne and Huffington, 1966).

VI. Biochemistry

Encouraged by the speculations of certain investigators that the elevated catecholamine levels (Price et al., 1960) or enhanced effector organ responses (Gravenstein et al., 1960) under cyclopropane anesthesia could be a product of reduced amine biotransformation, enzymatic studies were initiated to investigate these problems as well as to search for a biochemical lesion in arrhythmia production. Only cyclopropane, of four agents examined (diethyl ether, halothane, and chloroform) inhibited catechol-o-methyl transferase activity *in vitro* (GARDIER et al., 1967; GARDIER and HAMELBERG, 1968). Whether this effect can be demonstrated *in vivo* and have clinical significance is dubious [GARDIER et al., 1967 (1); PRICE et al., 1968]. Other investigators have concluded that cyclopropane, halothane, and diethyl ether have no effect on monoamine oxidase (MAO) in rat brains *in vivo* despite an increased serotonin turnover produced by diethyl ether and the production of increased 5 hydroxy-indole acetic acid levels (5HIAA) by all three (DIAZ et al., 1968). When tested on rat liver, mitochondrial MAO *in vitro*, cyclopropane, and diethyl ether were found to have a low order of inhibition, whereas the halogenated hydrocarbons, methoxyflurane, halothane, and chloroform produced a high order of inhibition (SCHNEIDER and GARDIER, 1969). LINEWEAVER-BURKE plots have indicated that the inhibition by all of these agents could best be described as competitive inhibition (SCHNEIDER and GARDIER). Conversely, all of the agents so far examined (halothane, methoxyflurane, cyclopropane, and diethyl ether) significantly stimulate monoamine oxidase activity in the cat heart *in situ* and in the isolated guinea pig heart (SCHNEIDER and GARDIER). Nevertheless, any alteration in catecholamine biotransformation is only of subtle pharmacological significance (CROUT, 1961) and may not have clinical application.

VII. Concluding Remarks

The autonomic pharmacology of inhalation anesthetic agents may have been made unduly complex by the inattention of many investigators to the cardinal rule of drug testing, i.e., the need for dose-effect relationships. Certainly, the application of this principle was inferred in the early work of LEVY when he related arrhythmia development to the level of chloroform anesthesia. In modern times, HAMELBERG et al. (1960) demonstrated that serum catecholamine titers were a function of anesthetic depth. Thus, much more clarity can be brought to the field by appropriate consideration of this aspect in future research protocols.

In addition to dose-dependent activities, more recognition must be paid to the pitfalls of species difference. If the animal studies are to be applied to man, then species must be selected which demonstrate a particular action in a way similar to man. In the case of adrenal medullary secretion stimulated by diethyl ether, the dog responds like infant man but not like adult man (BUNKER et al., 1962). Thus, discrimination in terms of age must also be distinguished concomitantly with species variation. Another pertinent example relates to the production of ventricular arrhythmias. This author has experienced an inability to produce arrhythmias by stimulating the cardiac accelerator nerve in the dog under anesthesia with sensitizing agents; whereas the arrhythmic response to this stimulus is present in the cat (HARRIS and GARDIER). Fortunately or unfortunately, as the case may be, the dog appears to be the most widely used species for evaluating the cardiac properties of anesthetic agents.

Finally, the concept of discrete sympathetic nervous system function as opposed to the whole system functioning as a single unit, derives a good measure of support from the pharmacology of anesthetic agents. Reference may be made again to diethyl ether (BUNKER et al., 1962) which produces a metabolic acidosis in the infant human and the dog by a selective stimulation of the adrenal medulla, and release of epinephrine. No adrenal medullary participation appears in adult man (PRICE, 1957). Application of this knowledge to the newer agents which have a hyperglycemic potential, such as methoxyflurane (WASMUTH et al., 1960), should be made. Therefore, the property of anesthetics to act upon distinct groups of sympathetic neurones must be recognized. By giving greater consideration to dose-response relationships, species differences and discrete stimulation or inhibition of sympathetic activity when devising new approaches to the study of anesthetic effects on autonomic activity, we can look forward to more meaningful and continued contributions to the pharmacology of anesthesia.

Summary

With few exceptions, inhalation anesthetics have been found to enhance baroreceptor activity and suppress chemoreceptor activity. The paucity of work devoted to such studies on chemoreceptors is in sharp contrast to the considerable effort expended on the apparently more relevant baroreceptor function.

Stimulation of central sympathetic and parasympathetic centers by general anesthetics undoubtedly occurs. Supra-pontine, medullary and cord sites have been incriminated in both excitation and inhibition of sympathetic outflow. Cardiac ventricular arrhythmias produced by halogenated hydrocarbons have a central component residing in the area of the posterior hypothalamus. Increased sympathetic tone under cyclopropane anesthesia appears to result from a selective depression of a medullary depressor center, although this conclusion is highly controversial.

Autonomic ganglionic blockade has been proposed for all inhalation anesthetics studied, with the possible exception of methoxyflurane. Most recent investigations of ganglionic function have involved the influence of these agents on sympathetic muscarinic and nicotinic receptors. For many, the degree of blockade probably is of minor pharmacological significance. Moreover, considerable evidence exists in opposition to ganglionic blockade as the mechanism for the cardiovascular depression from halothane.

Generally, the volatile liquids are direct effector-organ depressants and reduce responsiveness to catecholamines without being alpha adrenergic blocking agents. Data favoring beta receptor stimulation are available for diethyl ether, cyclopropane, and, most recently, for halothane. Certain anesthetics have been reported to be without influence on uptake or release of catecholamines while effects by the various agents on amine biotransformation are mixed and of questionable significance.

Acknowledgements

The author acknowledges support of his own work by USPHS grants H-7306, HE-08808 and the Central Ohio Heart Association.

References

ABIKO, Y., ITO, G.: The effect of propranolol on the pressor response to acetylcholine in atropinized dogs. Arch. intern. pharmacodynamie 167, 413—419 (1967).
— — HIGUCHI, I., KANEKO, Y., ISHIKAWA, H., ITO, M.: The inhibitory effect of procaine on the initial pressor response to acetylcholine in atropinized dogs. Arch. intern. Pharmacodynamie 170, 445—452 (1967).
ALPER, M. H., FLEISCH, J. H., FLACKE, W.: The effects of halothane on the responses of cardiac sympathetic ganglia to various stimulants. Anesthesiology 31, 429—436 (1969).
ANICHKOV, S. V., BELENKII, M. L.: Pharmacology of the carotid body chemoreceptors. Oxford: Pergamon Press Ltd.; Distributed by The Macmillan Co., New York, New York 1963.

Armitage, A. K.: Effects of nicotine and tobacco smoke on blood pressure and release of catecholamines from the adrenal glands. Brit. J. Pharmacol. 25, 515—526 (1965).

Artusio, J. R., Jr., van Poznak, A. A., Weingram, J., Sohn, Y. J.: Teflurane — a non-explosive gas for clinical anesthesia. Anesthesia & Analgesia 46, 657—664 (1967).

Atanackovic, D., Dalgaard-Mikkelsen, S.: Chemoreceptors and acetylcholine hypertension. Arch. intern. Pharmacodynamie 84, 308—316 (1950).

Bagwell, E. E., Durst, G. G.: Influence of reserpine on cardiovascular and sympatho-adrenal responses to cyclopropane anesthesia in the dog. Anesthesiology 25, 148—155 (1964).

— — Linker, R. P.: (1) Influence of reserpine on cardiovascular and sympatho-adrenal responses to ether anesthesia in the dog. Anesthesiology 25, 15—24 (1964).

— Woods, E. F.: Cardiovascular effects of methoxyflurane. Anesthesiology 23, 51—57 (1962).

Bartelstone, H. J., Katz, R. L., Ngai, S. H.: Effect of cyclopropane on reflexly induced circulatory responses in the dog. Anesthesiology 27, 756—763 (1966).

— Nasmyth, P. A.: Vasopressin potentiation of catecholamine actions in dog, rat, cat, and rat aortic strip. Am. J. Physiol. 208, 754—762 (1965).

Beattie, J., Brow, G. R., Long, C. N. H.: Physiological and anatomical evidence for the existence of nerve tracts connecting the hypothalamus with spinal sympathetic centers. Proc. Roy. Soc. (London) B 106, 253—275 (1930).

Belenkii, M. L., Stroikov, Yu. N.: Bull. Exp. Biol. Med. U.S.S.R.) 30, 358 (1950), as cited in Pharmacology of the carotid body chemoreceptors by Anichkov, S. V., Belenkii, M. L., p. 31. Oxford: Pergamon Press, Ltd. 1963.

Bhatia, B. B., Burn, J. H.: The action of ether on the sympathetic system. J. Physiol. (London) 78, 257—270 (1933).

Biscoe, T. J., Millar, R. A.: The effect of halothane on carotid sinus baroreceptor activity. J. Physiol. (London) 173, 24—37 (1964).

— — The effect of cyclopropane, halothane, and ether on sympathetic ganglionic transmission. Brit. J. Anaesthesia 38, 3—12 (1966).

— — Effect of cyclopropane, halothane, and ether on central baroreceptor pathways. (1) J. Physiol. (London) 184, 535—559 (1966).

Bishop, G. H., Heinbecker, P.: A functional analysis of the cervical sympathetic nerve supply to the eye. Am. J. Physiol. 100, 519—532 (1932).

Blackman, J. G., Purves, R. D.: Intracellular recordings from ganglia of the thoracic sympathetic chain of the guinea pig. J. Physiol. (London) 203, 173—198 (1969).

Blackmore, W. P., Erwin, K. W., Wiegand, O. F., Lipsey, R.: Renal and cardiovascular effects of halothane. Anesthesiology 21, 489—495 (1960).

Brewster, W. R., Jr., Isaacs, J. P., Wainø-Andersen, T.: Depressant effect of ether on myocardium of the dog and its modification by reflex release of epinephrine and norepinephrine. Am. J. Physiol. 175, 399—414 (1953).

Bronk, D. W., Pitts, R. F., Larrabee, M. G.: Role of hypothalamus in cardiovascular regulation. Research Publs. Assoc. Nervous Mental Disease 20, 323—341 (1940).

Brown, A. M.: Cardiac sympathetic adrenergic pathways in which synaptic transmission is blocked by atropine sulphate. J. Physiol. (London) 191, 271—288 (1967).

Brown, R. V., Hilton, J. G.: The effectiveness of the baroreceptor reflexes under different anesthetics. J. Pharmacol. Exptl. Therap. 118, 198—203 (1956).

Bunker, J. P.: Metabolic acidosis during anesthesia and surgery. Anesthesiology 23, 107—122 (1962).

Burn, J. H., Epstein, H. G.: Hypotension due to halothane. Brit. J. Anaesthesia 31, 199—204 (1959).

— — Feigan, G. A., Paton, W. D. M.: Some pharmacological actions of fluothane. Brit. Med. J. II, 479—483 (1957).

— Rand, M. J.: Sympathetic postganglionic mechanism. Nature 184, 163—165 (1959).

— — Sympathetic postganglionic cholinergic fibers. Brit. J. Pharmacol. 15, 56—66 (1960).

Carter, V. L., Jr., Traber, D. L., Gardier, R. W.: Investigation of sympathetic activity resulting from a dose of acetylcholine producing a hypertensive response. J. Pharmacol. Exptl. Therap. 156, 232—237 (1967).

Chen, M. P., Lim, R. K. S., Wang, S. C., Yi, C. L.: On the question of a myelencephalic sympathetic centre. 2. Experimental evidence for a reflex sympathetic centre in the medulla. Chinese J. Physiol. 11, 355—366 (1937).

Chenoweth, M. B., Ellman, G. L., Reynolds, R. C., Shea, P. J.: A secondary response to pressor stimuli caused by sensitization to an endogenous pituitary hormone. Circulation Research. 6, 334—342 (1958).

Christoforo, M. F., Brody, M. J.: Effects of halothane and cyclopropane on skeletal muscle vessels and baroreceptor reflexes. Anesthesiology 29, 36—43 (1968).

— — (1) Non-adrenergic vasoconstriction produced by halothane and cyclopropane anesthesia. Anesthesiology 29, 44—56 (1968).

COMROE, J. H., MORTIMER, L.: The respiratory and cardiovascular responses of temporally separated aortic and carotid bodies to cyanide, nicotine, phenyldiguanide, and serotonin. J. Pharmacol. Exptl. Therap. 146, 33—41 (1964).

CATTEL, McK.: Studies in experimental traumatic shock. VI. The action of ether on the circulation in traumatic shock. Arch. Surg. 6, 41—84 (1923).

CRAYTHORNE, N. W. B., HUFFINGTON, P. E.: Effects of propranolol on the cardiovascular response to cyclopropane and halothane. Anesthesiology 27, 580—583 (1966).

CROUT, J. R.: Effect of inhibiting both catechol-0-methyl transferase and monoamine oxidase on cardiovascular responses to norepinephrine. Proc. Soc. exp. Biol. Med. 108, 482—484 (1961).

DALE, H. H.: The action of certain esters and ethers of choline and their relation to muscarine. J. Pharmacol. Exptl. Therap. 6, 147—190 (1914).

DEUTSCH, S., LINDE, H. W., PRICE, H. L.: Circulatory and sympathoadrenal responses to cyclopropane in the dog. J. Pharmacol. Exptl. Therap. 135, 354—357 (1962).

DIAZ, P. M., NGAI, S. H., COSTA, E.: The effects of cyclopropane, halothane, and diethyl ether on the cerebral metabolism of serotonin in the rat. Anesthesiology 29, 959—963 (1968).

DONTAS, A. S., NICKERSON, M.: Effects of stimulants and of ganglionic blocking agents on carotid body chemoreceptors. Arch. intern. Pharmacodynamie 106, 312—331 (1956).

DRIPPS, R. D., DUMKE, P. R.: The effects of narcotics on the balance between central and chemoreceptor control of respiration. J. Pharmacol. Exptl. Therap. 77, 290—300 (1943).

DUKE, H. N., PICKFORD, M.: Observations on the action of acetylcholine and adrenalin on the hypothalamus. J. Physiol. (London) 114, 325—332 (1951).

ECCLES, J. C.: The action potential of the superior cervical ganglion. J. Physiol. (London) 85, 179—206 (1935).

— The physiology of synapses, pp. 131—137. Berlin-Göttingen-Heidelberg: Springer 1964.

ECCLES, R. M.: Responses of isolated curarized sympathetic ganglia. J. Physiol. (London) 117, 196—217 (1952).

— Intracellular potentials recorded from an mammalian sympathetic ganglion. J. Physiol. (London) 130, 572—584 (1955).

— LIBET, B.: Origin and blockade of the synaptic responses of curarized sympathetic ganglia. J. Physiol. (London) 157, 484—503 (1961).

ELLIOTT, T. R.: The control of the suprarenal glands by the splanchnic nerves. J. Physiol. (London) 44, 374—409 (1912).

EPSTEIN, R. A., WANG, H., BARTELSTONE, H. J.: The effects of halothane on circulatory reflexes of the dog. Anesthesiology 29, 867—876 (1968).

EPSTEIN, R. M., DEUTSCH, S., COOPERMAN, L. H., CLEMENT, A. J., PRICE, H. L.: Splanchnic circulation during halothane anesthesia and hypercapnia in normal man. Anesthesiology 27, 654—661 (1966).

EYZAQUIRRE, C., KOYANO, H.: Effects of some pharmacological agents on chemoreceptor discharges. J. Physiol. (London) 178, 410—437 (1965).

FEDORCHUK, YE. S.: Bull. Exp. Biol. Med. (U.S.S.R) 6, 7 (1954), as cited in Pharmacology of the carotid body chemoreceptors by ANICHKOV, S. V., BELENKII, M. L., pp. 55 and 197. Oxford: Pergamon Press, Ltd. 1963.

FERDANEZ DE MOLINA, A., PERL, E. R.: Sympathetic activity and the systemic circulation in the spinal cat. J. Physiol. (London) 181, 82—102 (1965).

FLACKE, W., ALPER, M. H.: Actions of halothane and norepinephrine in the isolated mammalian heart. Anesthesiology 23, 793—801 (1962).

— GILLIS, R. A.: Impulse transmission via nicotinic and muscarinic pathways in the stellate ganglion of the dog. J. Pharmacol. Exptl. Therap. 163, 266—276 (1968).

FLETCHER, S. W., FLACKE, W., ALPER, M. H.: The actions of general anesthetic agents on tracheal smooth muscle. Anesthesiology 29, 517—522 (1968).

FOLKOW, B.: Impulse frequency in sympathetic vasomotor fibres correlated to the release and elimination of the transmitter. Acta Physiol. Scand. 25, 49—76 (1952).

FUJITA, H., HARTMANN, J. F.: Electron microscopy of neurohypophysis in normal, adrenalin-treated, and pilocarpine-treated rabbits. Z. Zellforsch. 54, 734—763 (1961).

GARDIER, R. W.: Vasodepression to intravenous acetylcholine with attendant vagal blockade — A study of atropine resistance. Arch. exptl. Pathol. Pharmakol., Naunyn-Schmiedebergs 241, 433—441 (1961).

— ABREU, B. E., RICHARDS, A. B., HERRLICH, H. C.: Specific blockade of the adrenal medulla. J. Pharmacol. Exptl. Therap. 130, 340—345 (1960).

— ENDAHL, G. L., HAMELBERG, W.: Cyclopropane: Effect on catecholamine biotransformation. Anesthesiology 28, 677—679 (1967).

— HAMELBERG, W.: Effect of anesthetics on catecholamine biotransformation. In: Toxicity of anesthetics, pp. 209—219. Baltimore (Maryland): The Williams and Wilkins Co. 1968.

Gardier, R. W., Reier, C. E., Traber, D. L., Rowe, H. M., Hamelberg, W.: (1) Elevated plasma norepinephrine during cyclopropane anesthesia as a possible function of decreased amine metabolism. Anesthesia & Analgesia **46**, 800—805 (1967).

— Richards, A. B., Stoelting, V. K., White, N.: The mechanism whereby halothane reverses the pressor responses to acetylcholine. Brit. J. Pharmacol. **20**, 586—591 (1963).

— — James, E. A., Jr., Wheeler, J. E.: Vasopressin vasodynamics I. The Pharmacology of tachyphylaxis. Arch. intern. Pharmacodynamie **153**, 232—239 (1965).

— Traber, D. L.: Activity of the splanchnic nerve and carotid chemoreceptors in the origin of the pressor responses to acetylcholine. J. Pharmacol. Exptl. Therap. **150**, 75—83 (1965).

— Wheeler, J. E., James, E. A., Jr.: (1) Vasopressin vasodynamics II. The Pathophysiology of hypertension. Arch. intern. Pharmacodynamie **153**, 240—248 (1965).

Garfield, J. M., Alper, M. H., Gillis, R. A., Flacke, W.: A pharmacological analysis of ganglionic actions of some general anesthetics. Anesthesiology **29**, 79—92 (1968).

Gebber, G. L.: Neurogenic basis for the rise in blood pressure evoked by nicotine in the cat. J. Pharmacol. Exptl. Therap. **166**, 255—263 (1969).

Giere, F. A., Eversole, W. J.: Effects of adrenal medullary hormones on antidiuretic substances in blood serum. Science **120**, 395—396 (1954).

Gillis, R. A., Flacke, W., Garfield, J. M., Alper, M. H.: Actions of anticholinesterase agents upon ganglionic transmission in the dog. J. Pharmacol. Exptl. Therap. **163**, 277—286 (1968).

Ginsburg, M.: Production, release, transportation and elimination of the neurohypophysial hormones — neurohypophysial hormones and similar polypeptides, Heffter's Handbuch der experimentellen Pharmakologie. Vol. 23, pp. 286—371. Berlin-Heidelberg-New York: Springer 1968.

Gravenstein, J. S., Sherman, E. T., Andersen, T. W.: Cyclopropane-epinephrine interaction on the nictitating membrane of the spinal cat. J. Pharmacol. Exptl. Therap. **129**, 428—432 (1960).

Habif, D. V., Papper, E. M., Fitzpatrick, H. F., Lawrance, P., Smythe, C. Mc C., Bradley, S. E.: Renal and hepatic blood flow, glomerular filtration rate and urinary output of electrolytes during cyclopropane, ether, and thiopental anesthesia, operation and immediate postoperative period. Surgery **30**, 241—255 (1951).

Hamelberg, W., Sprouse, J. H., Mahaffey, J. E., Richardson, J. A.: Catecholamine levels during light and deep anesthesia. Anesthesiology **21**, 297—302 (1960).

Harris, S. G., Gardier, R. W. Unpublished results.

Heymans, C., Delaunois, A. L.: Action of drugs on pressure-response and distensibility of carotid sinus arterial wall. Arch. intern. Pharmacodynamie **96**, 99—104 (1953).

— — van den Heuvel-Heymans, G.: Tension and distensibility of carotid sinus wall; pressoceptors and blood pressure regulation. Circulation Research **1**, 3—7 (1953).

— Neil, E.: Reflexogenic areas of the cardiovascular system. Boston: Little, Brown, and Comp. 1958.

Hering, H. E.: Die Karotissinus-Reflexe auf Herz und Gefäße. Dresden u. Leipzig: Steinkopff 1927.

Hilton, J. G., Steinberg, M.: Effects of ganglion and parasympathetic blocking drugs upon the pressor response elicited by elevation of the intracranial fluid pressure. J. Pharmacol. Exptl. Therap. **153**, 285—291 (1966).

Holland, R. C., Sundsten, J. W., Sawyer, C. H.: Blood pressure changes induced by "osmoreceptor" activation. Anat. Record **130**, 316 (1958).

— — — Effects of intracarotid injections of hypertonic solutions on arterial pressure in the rabbit. Circulation Research **7**, 712—720 (1959).

Jacobowitz, D.: Histochemical studies of the autonomic innervation of the gut. J. Pharmacol. Exptl. Therap. **149**, 358—364 (1965).

Jewell, P. A., Verney, E. B.: An experimental attempt to determine the site of the neurohypophysial osmoreceptors in the dog. Phil. Trans. Roy. Soc. London Ser. B **240**, 197—324 (1957).

Jones, R. E., Deutsch, S., Turndorf, H.: Effects of atropine on cardiac rhythm in conscious and anesthetized man. Anesthesiology **22**, 67—73 (1961).

— Guldmann, N., Linde, H. W., Dripps, R. D., Price, H. L.: Cyclopropane anesthesia. III. Effects of cyclopropane on respiration and circulation in normal man. Anesthesiology **21**, 380—393 (1960).

— Linde, H. W., Deutsch, S., Dripps, R. D., Price, H. L.: Hemodynamic actions of diethylether in normal man. Anesthesiology **23**, 299—305 (1962).

Kahn, N., Mills, E.: Centrally evoked sympathetic discharge: a functional study of medullary vasomotor areas. J. Physiol. (London) **191**, 339—352 (1967).

Katz, R. L.: Neural factors affecting cardiac arrhythmias induced by halopropane. J. Pharmacol. Exptl. Therap. **152**, 88—94 (1966).

KATZ, R. L., MATTEO, R. S., PAPPER, E. M.: Injection of epinephrine during general anesthesia with halogenated hydrocarbons and cyclopropane in man. Halothane. Anesthesiology **23**, 597—600 (1962).

KEATS, A. S., STRONG, M. J., GIRGIS, K. Z., GOLDSTEIN, A., JR.: Observations during anesthesia for cardiac homotransplantation in ten patients. Anesthesiology **20**, 192—198 (1969).

KIVALO, E., ARKO, H.: The effect of noradrenalin and acetylcholine on water diuresis and neurosecretory substance of the rat. Ann. Med. exp. Fenn. **35**, 398—403 (1957).

KLIDE, A. M., AVIADO, D. M.: Mechanism for the reduction in pulmonary resistance induced by halothane. J. Pharmacol. Exptl. Therap. **158**, 28—35 (1967).

— PENNA, M., AVIADO, D. M.: Stimulation of adrenergic beta receptors by halothane and its antagonism by two new drugs. Anesthesia & Analgesia **48**, 58—65 (1969).

KOBACKER, J. L., RIGLER, R.: Behavior of extra-cardiac nerves of cat under ether — a potential source of error. J. Pharmacol. Exptl. Therap. **37**, 161—175 (1929).

KOPIN, I. J.: Storage and metabolism of catecholamines: the role of monoamine oxidase. Pharmacol. Revs. **16**, 179—191 (1964).

KOPPANYI, T.: Studies on the synergism and antagonism of drugs. I. The non-parasympathetic antagonism between atropine and the miotic alkaloids. J. Pharmacol. Exptl. Therap. **46**, 395—405 (1932).

LANDGREN, S., LILJESTRAND, G., ZOTTERMAN, Y.: Wirkung von Alkohol, Aceton, Äther und Chloroform auf die Chemoreceptoren des Glomus Caroticum. Arch. Exptl. Pathol. Pharmakol, Naunyn-Schmiedebergs **219**, 185—191 (1953).

LARRABEE, M. G., HOLADAY, D. A.: Depression of transmission through sympathetic ganglia during general anesthesia. J. Pharmacol. Exptl. Therap. **105**, 400—408 (1952).

— POSTERNAK, J. M.: Selective action of anesthetics on synapses and axons in mammalian sympathetic ganglia. J. Neurophysiol. **15**, 91—114 (1952).

LEVY, A. G.: The exciting causes of ventricular fibrillation in animals under chloroform anesthesia. Heart **4**, 319—378 (1913).

— The genesis of ventricular extrasystoles under chloroform with special reference to consecutive ventricular fibrillation. Heart **5**, 299—334 (1914).

LI, T. H., GAMBLE, C., ETSTEN, B. E.: Stellate ganglionic transmission and myocardial contractile force during halothane anesthesia. Anesthesiology **29**, 444—455 (1968).

— SHAUL, M. S., ETSTEN, B. E.: (1) Decreased adrenal venous catecholamine concentrations during methoxyflurane anesthesia. Anesthesiology **29**, 1145—1152 (1968).

LIBET, B.: Slow synaptic responses and excitatory changes in sympathetic ganglia. J. Physiol. (London) **174**, 1—25 (1964).

LILJESTRAND, G.: The effects of ethyl alcohol and some related substances on baroreceptor and chemoreceptor activity. Acta Physiol. Scand. **29**, 74—82 (1953).

LONG, J. P., ECKSTEIN, J. W.: Ganglionic actions of neostigmine methylsulfate. J. Pharmacol. Exptl. Therap. **133**, 216—222 (1961).

MAINLAND, J. F., SHAW, F. H.: Comparison of ganglionic blocking agents. Nature **170**, 418—419 (1952).

MARKEE, S. J., WANG, H. H., WANG, S. C.: Effects of cyclopropane on central vasomotor mechanism of the dog. Anesthesiology **27**, 742—755 (1966).

MARKS, B. H., SAMORAJSKI, T., WEBSTER, E. J.: Radiautographic localization of norepinephrine H³ in the tissues of mice. J. Pharmacol. Exptl. Therap. **138**, 376—381 (1962).

MATTEO, R. S., KATZ, R. L., PAPPER, E. M.: The injection of epinephrine during general anesthesia with halogenated hydrocarbons and cyclopropane in man. Trichloroethylene. Anesthesiology **23**, 360—364 (1962).

— — — The injection of epinephrine during general anesthesia with halogenated hydrocarbons and cyclopropane in man. Cyclopropane. Anesthesiology **24**, 327—330 (1963).

McALLISTER, F. F., ROOT, W. S.: The circulatory responses of normal and sympathectomized dogs to ether anesthesia. Am. J. Physiol. **133**, 70—78 (1941).

McARDLE, L., BLACK, G. W.: Effects of cyclopropane on peripheral circulation in man. Brit. J. Anaesthesia **35**, 352—357 (1963).

McCUBBIN, J. W., PAGE, I. H.: Neurogenic component of chronic renal hypertension. Science **139**, 210—215 (1963).

— GREEN, J. H., PAGE, I. H.: Baroreceptor function in chronic renal hypertension. Circulation Research **4**, 205—210 (1956).

MEEK, W. J., HATHAWAY, H. R., ORTH, O. S.: Effects of ether, chloroform, and cyclopropane on cardiac automaticity. J. Pharmacol. Exptl. Therap. **61**, 240—252 (1937).

MILLAR, R. A.: Postganglionic sympathetic discharge and the effect of inhalation anesthetics. Brit. J. Anaesthesia **38**, 92—113 (1966).

— BISCOE, T. J.: Preganglionic sympathetic activity and the effects of anesthetics. Brit. J. Anaesthesia **37**, 804—832 (1965).

MILLAR, R. A., MORRIS, M. E.: Induced sympathetic stimulation during halothane anesthesia. Canad. Anaesth. Soc. J. 7, 423—428 (1960).
— — (1) A study of methoxyflurane anaesthesia. Canad. Anaesth. Soc. J. 8, 210—215 (1960).
MOE, G. K., CAPO, L. R., PERALTA, R. B.: Action of tetraethylammonium on chemoreceptor and stretch receptor mechanisms. Am. J. Physiol. 153, 601—605 (1948).
— FREYBURGER, W. A.: Ganglionic blocking agents. Pharmacol. Revs. 2, 61—95 (1950).
MORROW, D. H., GAFFNEY, T. E., HOLMAN, J. E.: The chronotropic and inotropic effects of halothane — A comparison of effects in normal and chronically cardiac denervated dogs. Anesthesiology 22, 915—917 (1961).
— MORROW, A. G.: The effects of halothane on myocardial contractile force and vascular resistance. Direct observations made in patients during cardiopulmonary bypass. Anesthesiology 22, 537—541 (1961).
MUSCHOLL, E., VOGT, M.: The action of reserpine on the peripheral sympathetic system. J. Physiol. (London) 141, 132—155 (1958).
NAKAYAMA, K.: Surgical removal of the carotid body for bronchial asthma. Diseases of Chest 40, 595—604 (1961).
NAITO, H., GILLIS, C. N.: Anesthetics and response of atria to sympathetic nerve stimulation. Anesthesiology 29, 259—266 (1968).
NASH, C. B.: Vasopressin tachyphylaxis and reserpine pretreatment. Pharmacologist 4, 150 (1962).
NAYLOR, W. G.: The action of fluothane, chloroform, and hypothermia on the heart. Australian J. Exptl. Biol. Med. Sci. 37, 279—288 (1959).
NGAI, S. H., BOLME, P.: Effects of anesthetics on circulatory regulatory mechanisms in the dog. J. Pharmacol Exptl. Therap. 153, 495—504 (1966).
— DIAZ, P. M., OZER, S.: The uptake and release of norepinephrine. Effects of cyclopropane and halothane. Anesthesiology 31, 45—52 (1969).
— NEFF, N. H., COSTA, E.: (1) The effects of cyclopropane and halothane on the biosynthesis of Norepinephrine in vivo. Anesthesiology 31, 53—60 (1969).
NICKERSON, M.: Blockade of the actions of adrenaline and noradrenaline. Pharmacol. Revs. 11, 443—461 (1959).
NORMANN, N., LÖFSTRÖM, B.: Interaction of d-tubocurarine, ether, cyclopropane, and thiopental on ganglionic transmission. J. Pharmacol. Exptl. Therap. 114, 231—239 (1955).
OVERHOLT, H.: Resection of carotid body (cervical glomectomy) for asthma. J. Am. Med. Assoc. 180, 809—812 (1962).
PAINTAL, A. S.: Effects of drugs on vertebrate mechanoreceptors. Pharmacol. Revs. 16, 341—380 (1964).
PATON, W. D. M.: Transmission and block in autonomic ganglia. Pharmacol. Revs. 6, 59—67 (1954).
PEISS, C. N.: Central control of sympathetic cardioacceleration in the cat. J. Physiol. (London) 151, 224—237 (1960).
PRICE, H. L.: Circulating adrenaline and noradrenaline during diethyl ether anesthesia in man. Clin. Sci. 16, 377—387 (1957).
— COOK, W. A., JR., DEUTSCH, S., LINDE, H. W., MISHALOVE, R. D., MORSE, H. T.: Hemodynamic and central nervous actions of cyclopropane in the dog. Anesthesiology 24, 1—10 (1963).
— DEUTSCH, S., COOPERMAN, L. H., CLEMENT, A. J., EPSTEIN, R. M.: Splanchnic circulation during cyclopropane anesthesia in normal man. Anesthesiology 26, 312—319 (1965).
— JONES, R. E., DEUTSCH, S., LINDE, H. W.: Ventricular function and autonomic nervous activity during cyclopropane anesthesia in man. J. Clin. Invest. 41, 604—610 (1962).
— LINDE, H. W., JONES, R. E., BLACK, G. W., PRICE, M. L.: Sympathoadrenal Responses to general anesthesia in man and their relation to hemodynamics. Anesthesiology 20, 563—575 (1959).
— — MORSE, H. T.: (1) Central nervous actions of halothane affecting the systemic circulation. Anesthesiology 24, 770—778 (1963).
— LURIE, A. A., BLACK, G. W., SECHZER, P. H., LINDE, H. W., PRICE, M. L.: Modification by general anesthetics (cyclopropane and halothane) of circulatory and sympathoadrenal responses to respirarory acidosis. Ann. Surg. 152, 1071—1077 (1960).
— — JONES, R. E., PRICE, M. L., LINDE, H. W.: Cyclopropane anesthesia: II. Epinephrine and norepinephrine in initiation of ventricular arrhythmias by carbon dioxide inhalation. Anesthesiology 19, 619—630 (1958).
— PRICE, M. L.: Has halothane a predominant circulatory action? Anesthesiology 27, 764—769 (1966).
— — Relative ganglion-blocking potencies of cyclopropane, halothane, and nitrous oxide with halothane. Anesthesiology 28, 349—353 (1967).

PRICE, H. L., PRICE, M. L., MORSE, H. T.: (1) Effects of cyclopropane, halothane, and procaine on the vasomotor "center" of the dog. Anesthesiology **26**, 55—60 (1965).
— WARDEN, J. C., COOPERMAN, L. H., MILLAR, R. A.: Central sympathetic excitation caused by cyclopropane. Anesthesiology **30**, 426—438 (1969).
— — — PRICE, M. L.: Enhancement by cyclopropane and halothane of heart rate responses to sympathetic stimulation. Anesthesiology **29**, 478—483 (1968).
— WIDDICOMBE, J.: Actions of cyclopropane on carotid sinus baroreceptors and carotid body chemoreceptors. J. Pharmacol. Exptl. Therap. **135**, 233—239 (1962).
PRICE, M. L., PRICE, H. L.: Effects of general anesthetics on contractile responses of rabbit aortic strips. Anesthesiology **23**, 16—20 (1962).
PURCHASE, I. F. H.: The effect of halothane on the sympathetic nerve supply to the myocardium. Brit. J. Anaesthesia **37**, 915—928 (1965).
RAVENTÓS, J.: The action of fluothane — a new volatile anesthetic. Brit. J. Pharmacol. **11**, 394—410 (1956).
REIN, J., AUSTEN, W. G., MORROW, D. H.: Effects of guanethidine and reserpine on the cardiac responses to halothane. Anesthesiology **24**, 672—675 (1963).
RIKER, W. K., KOMALAHIRANYA, A.: Observations on the frequency dependence of sympathetic ganglion blockade. J. Pharmacol. Exptl. Therap. **137**, 267—274 (1962).
ROBERTSON, J. D., SWAN, A. A. B., WHITTERIDGE, D.: Effect of anesthetics on systemic baroreceptors. J. Physiol. (London) **131**, 463—472 (1956).
ROBBINS, B. H., THOMAS, J. D.: Cyclopropane arrhythmias in the cat. Their cause, prevention, and correction. Anesthesiology **21**, 163—170 (1960).
ROWE, H. M., GASPAR, L., BARKER, W., GARDIER, R. W.: Unpublished results.
RUSY, B. F., WHITHERSPOON, C. D., MONTANER, C. G., FREEMAN, E., MACHADO, R. A., WESTER, M. R., KRUMPERMAN, L. W.: Effect of reserpine on cardiac function during thiopental-cyclopropane anesthesia in the dog. Anesthesiology **26**, 14—20 (1965).
SCHNEIDER, D. R., GARDIER, R. W.: Monoamine oxidase inhibition produced by general anesthetics. Pharmacologist **11**, 237 (1969).
— — Unpublished results.
SEVERINGHAUS, J. W., CULLEN, S. C.: Depression of myocardium and body oxygen consumption with fluothane. Anesthesiology **19**, 167—177 (1958).
SHAW, F. H., KEOGH, P., McCALLUM, M.: The possibility of the dual nature of sympathetic ganglion cells. Australian J. Exptl. Biol. Med. Sci. **26**, 139—152 (1948).
— McCALLUM, M.: The possibility of the dual nature of sympathetic ganglion cells. II. Australian J. Exptl. Biol. Med. Sci. **27**, 289—296 (1949).
SHIMOSATO, S., SHANKS, C., ETSTEN, B. E.: Effects of methoxyflurane and sympathetic nerve stimulation on myocardial mechanics. Anesthesiology **29**, 538—549 (1968).
— SUGAI, N., ETSTEN, B. E.: Effect of methoxyflurane on the inotropic state of myocardial muscle. Anesthesiology **30**, 506—512 (1969).
— — IWATSUKI, N., ETSTEN, B. E.: (1) The effect of ēthrane on cardiac. muscle mechanics. Anesthesiology **30**, 513—518 (1969).
SKOVSTED, P., PRICE, H. L.: The effects of methoxyflurane on arterial pressure, preganglionic sympathetic activity and barostatic reflexes. Anesthesiology **31**, 515—521 (1969).
— PRICE, M. L., PRICE, H. L.: The effects of halothane on arterial pressure, preganglionic sympathetic activity and barostatic reflexes. Anesthesiology **31**, 507—514 (1969).
SMITH, C. M.: Effect of drugs on the afferent nervous system. In: Drugs affecting the peripheral nervous system, Vol. 1., pp. 521—573. New York: Marcel Dekker, Inc. 1967.
STEINBERG, M., HILTON, J. G.: Effect of sympathectomy and adrenalectomy upon ganglion blockade. J. Pharmacol. Exptl. Therap. **156**, 215—220 (1967).
TAKESHIGE, C., VOLLE, R. L.: Bimodal response of sympathetic ganglia to acetylcholine following eserine or repetitive preganglionic stimulation. J. Pharmacol. Exptl. Therap. **138**, 66—73 (1962).
TRABER, D. L., CARTER, V. L., JR., GARDIER, R. W.: Regarding a necessary condition for ganglionic blockade with competitive agents. Arch. intern. Pharmacodynamie **168**, 339 to 343 (1967).
— WILSON, R. D., GARDIER, R. W.: A pressor response produced by the endogenous release of vasopressin. Arch. intern. Pharmacodynamie **176**, 360—366 (1968).
TITUS, E., DENGLER, H. J.: The mechanism of uptake of norepinephrine. Pharmacol. Revs. 18, 525—535 (1966).
TRENDELENBURG, U.: Transmission of preganglionic impulses through the muscarinic receptors of the superior cervical ganglion of the cat. J. Pharmacol. Exptl. Therap. **154**, 426—440 (1966).
— Some aspects of the pharmacology of autonomic ganglion cells. Ergebn. Physiol., biol. Chem. u. exptl. Pharmakol. **59**, 1—85 (1967).

VERNEY, E. B.: The antidiuretic hormone and the factors which determine its release. Proc. Roy. Soc. (London) B. **135**, 25—106 (1947).

VOGT, M.: Sources of noradrenaline in the immunosympathectomized rat. Nature **204**, 1315 to 1316 (1964).

VOLLE, R. L.: Modification by drugs of synaptic mechanisms in autonomic ganglia. Pharmacol. Revs. **18**, 839—869 (1966).

— (1) Muscarinic and nicotinic stimulant actions at autonomic ganglia. Vol. 1, Sect. 12. International Encyclopedia of Pharmacology and Therapeutics. Braunschweig: Pergamon Press (1966).

WARNER, W. A., ORTH, O. S., WEBER, D. L., LAYTON, J. M.: Laboratory investigation of teflurane. Anesthesia & Analgesia **46**, 32—38 (1967).

WASMUTH, C. E., GREIG, J. H., HOMI, J., MORACA, J., ISIL, N. H., BITTE, E. M., HALE, D. E.: Methoxyflurane — a new anesthetic agent. Cleveland Clinic. Quart. **27**, 174—183 (1960).

WHITBY, L. G., HERTTING, G., AXELROD, J.: Effect of cocaine on the disposition of noradrenalin labelled with tritium. Nature **187**, 604—605 (1960).

WHITTERIDGE, D., BULBRING, E.: Changes in activity of pulmonary recpetors in anesthesia and their influence on respiratory behavior. J. Pharmacol. Exptl. Therap. **81**, 340—359 (1944).

4.3. Circulatory Effects of Modern Inhalation Anesthetic Agents

N. Ty Smith* and Penelope Smith**

With 7 Figures

I. Introduction

This chapter describes the circulatory effects of newer inhalation anesthetics. Some excellent reviews have appeared on the subject, the earliest being the classic review by PRICE (1960). A collection of papers presented at a National Academy of Sciences Symposium (PRICE and COHEN, 1964), discusses basic circulatory physiology as a preliminary to the effects of anesthetic agents. A more recent monograph by PRICE (1967) is useful to those seeking to understand, as well as to know, the circulatory effects of anesthetics. Articles by BLACK (1965), TOMLIN (1965), and DUNDEE (1966) are also noteworthy. ETSTEN and SHIMOSATO (1964) have described their extensive work on halothane, methoxyflurane, and other agents. Theirs was probably the first review on anesthesia and the "new" physiology of myocardial mechanics. Finally, GOLDBERG's [1968 (2)] thorough account of the effects of halothane on the cardiovascular system should be read by all.

Halothane is certainly the most widely used anesthetic agent in the United States. To match this clinical preponderance, the majority of the articles published in the past 10 years on anesthesia and the cardiovascular system include halothane. Although halothane is the only agent for which the circulatory picture is anywhere nearly complete, many gaps are apparent. Methoxyflurane is the second most thoroughly studied agent. Examination of other modern inhalation agents has either just begun, or was discontinued early when it became apparent that clinical acceptance of the agent was unlikely.

Our original intent was to compare agents quantitatively and qualitatively. However, the problems of making such a comparison from the available literature are insurmountable. In order to relieve the reader of the temptation of comparing agents, we shall discuss the anesthetic agents separately.

The dangers of comparing agents too closely include: (1) species variations, (2) lack of proper control values, (3) time factors, (4) selection of variables to measure, (5) equipotency, (6) ventilation, (7) use of other anesthetic agents, and (8) concomitant surgery. Some of these problems are common to the investigation of all pharmacologic agents; others are nearly unique to the study of the circulatory effects of anesthetics.

_____

* Recipient of National Institutes of Health Career Development Award No. 1K3-GM-31757.
** The authors are supported by Research Grant No. GM-12527 from the Institute of General Medical Science, United States Public Health Service and Grant No. FR 70 from the General Clinical Research Center Branch, Division of Research Facilities Resources.

1. *Species variations* are actually less marked among inhalation anesthetic agents than among most other pharmacologic agents, at least as far as therapeutic potency is concerned. The variation among several species of mammals in the minimum alveolar concentration (MAC) required to prevent reaction to a standard stimulus, is only 20—30% (Eger, personal communication). Most anesthetic agents, particularly the modern inhalation agents, appear to be non-specific depressants, although the response of the sympathoadrenal system to them varies considerably among both species and agents.

Man is probably the most commonly used experimental subject for anesthetic agents. In fact, many of the present day anesthetic techniques used in experimental animal pharmacology and physiology were first acquired and perfected in man. Until recently, only brief preliminary animal investigations preceded the use of an agent in the operating room. The differences between the techniques of administration of different anesthetic agents are often only of degree, and the anesthetist feels that he can rely on his background of thousands of cases to "try out" a new agent. More recently, thanks to the excellent work of Eger and others, a knowledge of the physical properties of an inhalation agent has allowed us to predict the action of an agent even before its trial in animals or man.

2. *Control Values.* The preparation of an animal for cardiovascular measurements usually eliminates any chance of obtaining true normal values. Procedures which can easily be done in a conscious human subject, for example the placement of catheters, are usually done under anesthesia in animals. The measurement of certain variables requires a thoracotomy, either several weeks or a few hours prior to the study. To circumvent these problems, atraumatic techniques, such as the ballistocardiogram, have been introduced. In addition, one may train animals for several weeks by daily brief exposures to an agent (Eisele, 1969).

Even in man it may be difficult to obtain a satisfactory control state, for the subject may be apprehensive from insertion of catheters and from anticipation of losing consciousness and receiving potent drugs. If major surgery is to follow the study, preanesthetic apprehension is increased. The investigator is thus faced with the dilemma of whether or not to contaminate an investigation pharmacologically by administering a sedative drug to relieve this anxiety. Some of the most striking cardiovascular responses to anesthetics may be the result of allaying apprehension by inducing sleep.

3. *Time Factors.* During the time that equilibration of an anesthetic agent takes place, a circulatory adaptation to the agent may also be occurring. For example, several studies (Deutsch et al., 1962; Wenthe et al., 1962; Eger et al., 1968) have indicated that during 2—3 h of halothane anesthesia, certain circulatory variables return towards normal. The adaptation to ether and fluroxene is even more rapid. Thus, some of the observed differences between agents may be due to differences of time between induction and measurement of the variables.

4. *Selection of Variables.* Often no agreement exists on which variables should be used to characterize a particular function of the cardiovascular system. In fact, we often do not know if a variable accurately describes the physical variable (work, power, energy) it is intended to. This is best demonstrated by the current controversy over "myocardial contractility" (see section on myocardial function). In addition, a choice is often necessary between measuring a variable directly and using a traumatic or invasive procedure, such as a thoracotomy or left heart catheterization, or measuring the variable indirectly and sacrificing accuracy for gentleness. The invasive technique may change the variable, the system, and the animal. Noninvasive techniques such as the ballistocardiogram, pulse waves, heart

sounds, and transcutaneous Doppler show great promise, but validation of the information obtained from them is necessary.

5. *Equipotency.* Even when an investigator compares anesthetic agents in the same study using the same species, variables, laboratory, equipment, and technicians, rarely does he attempt to use comparable depths of anesthesia. And most of the attempts have relied on blood levels of anesthetics or the electroencephalogram. The therapeutic actions of anesthetics are so varied, that it may never be possible to compare agents at equipotent levels. The concept of MAC, the minimal alveolar concentration of an agent which can prevent a response to a standard painful stimulus in 50% of the subjects, may serve as a useful tool in this regard. However, the only concentrations of anesthetics which are equipotent are at MAC itself. Multiples of MAC do not necessarily represent equipotent depths, that is, twice halothane MAC may not be construed as equal in potency to twice fluroxene MAC. In fact, herein lies the importance of MAC: we expect to find differences in circulatory effects of anesthetics at different MAC multiples. Such differences permit a comparison of the relative ranges of safety between anesthetics. The use of MAC as a dose yardstick also allows us to graph the relative course of depression or stimulation within the ranges of safety.

6. *Ventilation.* Here is another quandary. Should one allow ventilation to proceed spontaneously with possible carbon dioxide accumulation, acidosis, and altered intrathoracic pressure patterns, each affecting the circulation? Or should ventilation be controlled, with a resultant increase in mean central venous pressure, or mean right atrial pressure, and decrease in venous return, cardiac output and arterial pressure? Controlling ventilation during pre-anesthetic measurements is a partial answer, but circulatory compensatory mechanisms that are quite active during the awake stage are often obtunded by anesthesia.

7. *Other Anesthetic Agents.* In man and in animals, anesthetic agents other than those under study are often used. Barbiturates may be employed during surgical preparation of an animal or for induction in a human. Nitrous oxide, thought of usually as a diluent gas without any actions of its own, is used casually. However, several investigators [SMITH, 1966 (1), 1968, 1969, 1970; HORNBEIN, 1969; JOHNSTONE, 1959, 1961] have shown that nitrous oxide can markedly influence the circulatory response to several agents.

8. *Surgery.* Too often measurements of anesthetic effect take place during surgery. Sugery imposes such an array of imponderables in the course of the same procedure, that comparisons rarely hold true. The study of anesthetic versus surgical effects is essentially an open-ended one, requiring a careful discrimination of the pharmacodynamic effect of the anesthetic *per se*, the physiological derangement imposed by surgery and the nonlinear interaction of both.

Individual agents will be described under separate headings, as listed in Table 1. A brief background for their evaluation will be provided in the pages that follow.

A. Hemodynamics

Arterial Pressure. This is the most frequently measured variable, mainly because it is exceptionally easy to record. It, along with heart rate, has been measured routinely during anesthesia since the early part of the century. If anything, the importance of arterial pressure has been greatly overemphasized. One of the first questions we ask of a new agent is "Does it decrease arterial pressure"? If it does, it is a dangerous agent. If it does not, it is a safe agent. Or is it? Norepinephrine can by itself produce shock, myocardial necrosis, and/or pulmonary edema. Phenoxybenzamine, under proper circumstances, protects against shock. A patient

Table 1. *Outline of topics used to describe the inhalation anesthetic agents*

I. *Hemodynamics*
   a) Cardiac Output
      1. General
      2. Extra-anesthetic factors
      3. Adaptation
      4. Induction
      5. Oxygen consumption
      6. Hemorrhage
   b) Arterial Pressure
      1. General
      2. Extra-anesthetic factors
      3. Adaptation
      4. Induction
   c) Heart Rate
      1. General
      2. Extra-anesthetic factors
      3. Adaptation
      4. Induction
      5. Mechanisms
   d) Stroke Volume
      1. General
      2. Adaptation
      3. Induction
   e) Total Peripheral Resistance
   f) Central Venous Pressure or Right Atrial Pressure

II. *Regional Circulation*
   a) Pulmonary
   b) Coronary
   c) Renal
   d) Splanchnic
   e) Cerebral
   f) Limb
   g) Microcirculation

III. *Myocardial Function*

IV. *Arrhythmias*
   a) Incidence and types
   b) Hemodynamic effects of atrial arrhythmias
   c) Effect of CO_2
   d) Administration of epinephrine and other agents
   e) Adrenergic block
   f) Mechanism of arrhythmias

V. *Catecholamines*
   a) Plasma and tissue catecholamine levels
   b) Norepinephrine release and disposition
   c) Response to catecholamines
   d) Adrenergic blockade

---

can have increased arterial pressure with poor tissue perfusion or decreased arterial pressure with adequate tissue perfusion. Our concern with arterial blood pressure, however, has led to some important investigations. It became apparent that an elaborate combination of factors influences arterial pressure. The attempt to separate and define these factors has contributed much to the study of effects of anesthetics on the circulation and the autonomic nervous system.

The regulation of arterial pressure can be described by the equation: Mean arterial pressure = cardiac output x total peripheral resistance. Thus, a change in either cardiac output or total peripheral resistance can affect arterial pressure. Total peripheral resistance is influenced mainly by changes in arteriolar radius. The factors regulating cardiac output are described below.

Cardiac Output. Much investigation has focused on the measurement of cardiac output. The function of the heart, after all, is to pump blood. Another reason for the popularity of cardiac output is that several other variables can be derived from it.

Cardiac output is controlled by the blood volume, the tone of the blood vessels, and the state of the myocardium. There are several types of vessels in the vascular bed. Constriction or dilation of each type imposes a different influence on cardiac output and arterial pressure. Constriction of capacitance vessels returns more blood to the heart, which is thus primed to eject more blood. Arteriolar constriction, by increasing resistance, increases arterial pressure but often decreases cardiac output. Postcapillary constriction increases capillary hydrostatic pressure, causing a gradual loss of fluid from the vascular space and in turn a decrease in venous return, cardiac output, and arterial pressure. Precapillary constriction may have the opposite effect. Constriction of some vascular beds and dilation of others can exaggerate or diminish the overall effects.

The heart itself can influence its own output by increasing its frequency and/or strength of contraction. The latter increases the "vis a tergo" and decreases the end-systolic volume from any given end-diastolic volume.

Central Venous Pressure and Right Atrial Pressure. These measurements are assumed to be approximately equivalent. Claims have been made that they reflect the performance of the heart, the blood volume, or the effective blood volume. Unfortunately, pressures in the right atrium may not mirror events in the systemic circulation. In particular, false negatives are often seen with this measurement. For example, PRICE (personal communication) has reported a series of patients developing frank pulmonary edema; central venous pressure was normal in one-half of the patients in whom it was recorded. Furthermore, the error in absolute measurement can be considerable, since the proper zero level is difficult to locate.

Calculated Variables. Arterial pressure, cardiac output, heart rate, and right atrial pressure are the basic measurements. Most other hemodynamic variables are calculated from these. The calculated values add no new information. However, they do help the investigator and his readers to understand the action of an agent. Some of the calculated variables to which we shall refer are: stroke volume, total peripheral resistance, left ventricular minute work, and left ventricular stroke work.

Particularly in man, total peripheral resistance (the quotient of mean arterial pressure minus right atrial pressure divided by cardiac output) is usually measured erroneously. Although *total* flow ("cardiac output") is measured, only regional arterial pressure is measured, that is, pressure is measured in a peripheral artery. Thus the state of the vessels in that limb plays an exaggerated role in the calculated "total" peripheral resistance. For true systemic vascular resistance, aortic pressure must be used.

B. Regional Blood Flow

The study of regional blood flow is important for two reasons. First, some investigators (GUYTON, 1968) believe that the sum of the regional blood flows *is* the cardiac output, in other words, that cardiac output is solely determined by the needs and the vascular reactivity of the various organs and tissues. Second, flow to some regions is more important than that to others, due to differences in metabolic demands. Thus, cerebral and coronary blood flows must be sustained from minute to minute; renal, hepatic, and mesenteric blood flows may be interrupted for short periods; and fat, bone, and tendons can survive without blood flow for a long time. It is beyond the scope of this chapter to evaluate the significance of the change in regional blood flow produced by an anesthetic agent, since this significance varies with the clinical situation. For example, increased cerebral blood flow is to be avoided when an elevated cerebral spinal fluid pressure is undesirable, such as with a brain tumor, while a decrease in flow can be disastrous during surgery for cerebral vascular occlusive disease. A diminution in coronary blood flow with certain agents may mean that myocardial oxygen requirements have decreased or that perfusion pressure is inadequate.

Local as well as sytemic actions induced by the anesthetic can affect regional flow. Probably the most important factors in the control of all regional circulations are the perfusing (arterial) pressure and the available cardiac output. The effects of other factors vary among the regions. Hypoxia dilates most vascular beds, but constricts pulmonary vessels. Coronary circulation is acutely sensitive to hypoxia, and the cerebral circulation to hypercarbia. Cerebral circulation is capable of autoregulation, but is not controlled by the sympathetic nervous system, while splanchnic flow is occasionally too sensitive to sympathetic stimulation. Other factors, such as central vasomotor influences or ganglionic transmission, are unknown.

There are two particularly neglected areas in this field: pulmonary circulation and the microcirculation. The anesthetic importance of the pulmonary bed is vastly underestimated, in view of the fact that this bed is an obligatory path for most of the cardiac output. The tiny vessels of the microcirculation control the flow of blood to an organ, and the distribution of blood within the organ itself. Their importance has long been recognized in shock, but not until recently have investigators focused on the influence of anesthetic agents: their direct action on the vessels and their modification of the response to vasomotor influences.

C. Cardiac Arrhythmias

Considerable emphasis has been placed on the effect of anesthetics on cardiac rhythm. Cardiac asystole and ventricular fibrillation are often preceded by ventricular tachycardia or multifocal ventricular extrasystoles in patients with organic heart disease. It has been assumed that the same sequence occurs during anesthesia in man. For this reason, ventricular arrhythmias are of concern to both anesthetist and surgeon. The advent of routine continuous electrocardiographic monitoring has accomplished several things. It has revealed the high incidence of arrhythmias during anesthesia, thereby replacing the ignorant bliss of premonitoring days with constant anxiety. It has demonstrated that anesthetic agents by themselves are often less important a precipitating factor than hypoxia, hypercarbia, and release of epinephrine. Finally, it has shown that ventricular arrhythmias are not necessarily followed by ventricular fibrillation. In fact, this sequence has rarely been documented during anesthesia in man. One would like to know from the mass of data accumulated from electrocardiographic studies during anesthesia: (1) how often ventricular fibrillation is preceded by ventricular arrhythmias in man, (2) what type and what sequence of arrhythmias are followed by fibrillation, and (3) how important is the timing of an arrhythmia in relation to the vulnerable period of the ventricle. These questions are difficult to investigate in clinical anesthesia, much less in animal studies, because of the large number of factors influencing the incidence and character of arrhythmias during anesthesia: (1) species; (2) heart rate; (3) arterial pressure; (4) depth and type of anesthesia; (5) sensory stimulation; (6) vagal tone; (7) sympathetic tone; (8) ventilation, including pH_a and $PaCO_2$; (9) arterial oxygen tension; (10) ionic milieu (other than H^+); (11) body temperature; (12) exogenous catecholamines; and (13) other drugs given previously or simultaneously (digitalis, reserpine, atropine). It seems probable that the human heart is much less susceptible to ventricular fibrillation than is the canine heart. Also, we have evidence that ventricular arrhythmias produce much less hemodynamic distress than do certain supraventricular arrhythmias, such as atrio-ventricular dissociation (see halothane, arrhythmias).

D. Catecholamines

The classic investigation of BREWSTER (1953) demonstrated the importance of the sympathetic nervous system in the circulatory response to anesthetic agents. Although ether, a known myocardial depressant, decreases cardiac output and increases right atrial pressure when administered to a heart-lung preparation, it produces the opposite effects in the intact dog. BREWSTER showed indirectly that release of catecholamines counteracted the direct myocardial depressant effects of ether. Since then, much emphasis has been placed on this area of anesthetic action. From a deceptively simple statement on the influence of an agent on serum catecholamine levels, the subject has evolved to a systematic analysis of the components of the autonomic nervous system: baroreceptor sensitivity, medullary vasomotor center; neuronal transmission; ganglionic transmission, both pressor and depressor; catecholamine release from peripheral nerve endings and the adrenal gland; re-uptake, synthesis, and metabolism of catecholamines; altered sensitivity to catecholamines, including adrenergic block or supersensitivity. Most of the factors directly concerned with the autonomic nervous system are discussed by GARDIER in chapter 4.2. Our chapter will comment on those factors related directly to catecholamines.

E. Myocardial Function

Next to arterial pressure, myocardial function is of the most concern to anesthetists. Although we cannot yet measure a depression of myocardial contractility, we often attribute cardiovascular disasters in the operating room to this effect. Until 10—15 years ago, certain anesthetic agents were considered unsafe because they were myocardial depressants. It then became apparent that *all* anesthetic agents depress the myocardium as part of their nonspecific depression of excitable tissue. Investigations were then centered on the relative myocardial depressant actions of each agent. These actions are extremely difficult to evalute. There are at least three major problems in assessing myocardial function: (1) choosing the variable by which to measure function, (2) measuring function as atraumatically as possible, and (3) either compensating for, eliminating, or calculating the changes in contractility caused by factors other than the drug itself.

Myocardial function is usually measured in terms of myocardial "contractility". However, no single measurement has been universally accepted as the true expression of myocardial contractility. This uncertainty is rendered more obvious by the vast number of variables claimed to reflect contractility. Table 2 lists some of these variables.

Unfortunately, most proposed measurements of myocardial contractility require destructive procedures, that is the preparation necessary for the measurement causes profound changes in the variable measured, as well as the animal

Table 2. *Some proposed indicators of myocardial function*

Cardiac output
Stroke volume
Arterial pressure
Pulse pressure
Left ventricular minute work
Left ventricular stroke work
Left ventricular stroke power

Ejection time index
Isovolumic contraction time
Pre-ejection period
The interval between onset of systole and peak force of contraction
The interval between onset of electrical systole and peak rate of rise of left ventricular pressure

Ventricular function curves
Area under ventricular function curves

Left ventricular pressure
Maximum rate of rise of left ventricular pressure (dP/dt_{max})
Peak aortic flow
Peak aortic acceleration
Vibrocardiogram
Apex cardiogram
Ultralow frequency acceleration ballistocardiogram
Acceleration pneumocardiogram
Myocardial contractile force measured by a Brodie-Walton strain gauge

Peak force of contraction in an isolated heart
Peak displacement of isotonic contraction in an isolated heart
Peak rapidity of change of length of isotonic contraction
Change of force in relation to time

Force-velocity curve
Maximum velocity of myocardial fiber at zero load (V_{max})
Maximum force generated at zero velocity of myocardial contractile element (P_0)

The isometric time tension index (ITT)

$$\frac{dP/dt}{\text{Maximum left ventricular pressure}}$$

$$\frac{\text{Pre-ejection period}}{\text{Aortic diastolic pressure}}$$

$$\frac{1}{(\text{Pre-ejection period})^2}$$

The maximum mean force during ejection

itself. Particularly destructive are those requiring thoracotomy or isolation of the heart. The measurements obtained from these radical techniques are admittedly more direct. Although nondestructive measurements, such as the ballistocardiogram or heart sounds, do not measure contractility in terms familiar to physiologists or pharmacologists, they do allow the subject to be in a normal state.

The performance of the heart as determined by most measurements is affected by several physiological factors. Among these are heart rate; preload, or end diastolic fiber length; afterload, or mean aortic pressure; and the tone of the autonomic nervous system. In isolated preparations, these can be easily controlled. However, in intact animals it is almost impossible to control anything except heart rate, or to measure end diastolic volume accurately with a nondestructive technique. Changes in these physiological factors may mask the effect of an anesthetic on contractility.

With these problems in mind, we shall discuss some currently accepted measurements used to describe the performance of the heart.

Ventricular Function Curves. The FRANK-STARLING law of the heart states that the strength of contraction of a segment of myocardial muscle is directly related to the length of the segment just before contraction (the initial fiber length).

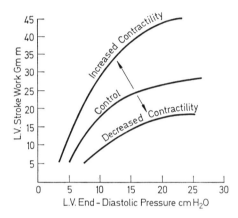

Fig. 1. Schematic representation of ventricular function curves obtained under control conditions, during the administration of a positive inotropic agent (increased contractility) and during a negative inotropic state (decreased contractility). LV = left ventricular

In the heart-lung preparation, it was shown that stroke work is a function of diastolic fiber length (PATTERSON and STARLING, 1914). Later the concept of measuring stroke work over a range of ventricular end-diastolic pressures was elaborated by SARNOFF and his collaborators (1962). They assumed that during diastole the ventricles act as passive bags; therefore, the pressure in these bags is directly proportional to the volume and hence the fiber length. They concluded that the relationship between the mean ventricular end-diastolic pressure and the stroke work of the corresponding ventricle (the ventricular function curve, Fig. 1) defines the contractile state of the ventricle. Significant increases in ventricular contraction are accompanied by shifts of the ventricular function curve upward and to the left, whereas a depression of contractility is identified by displacement of the curve to the right and downward (Fig. 1). The original concept of STARLING has been expanded beyond recognition, with end-diastolic fiber length being replaced by ventricular end-diastolic pressure, mean atrial pressure, central venous pressure, and even peripheral venous pressure. Either strength of contraction or stroke work in the heart-lung preparation has been replaced by stroke volume, stroke power, left ventricular minute work, cardiac output, dP/dt, etc.

The examination of ventricular function curves has provided considerable useful information on the effects of anesthetic agents, particularly through the excellent work of the group from Tufts. However, there have been several objections to this technique. Rushmer (1962) found in intact, unanesthetized animals, that activities, such as exercise or eating, produced little change in stroke work, particularly if the kinetic component of work was excluded from the calculation, as has been customary. Therefore, diastolic fiber length, measured directly, was held to be of trivial importance in the control of performance, since during the adrenergic stimulation accompanying a stress such as exercise, no change or an actual decrease in ventricular diameter occurred, while aortic flow velocity and rate of ventricular pressure development increased (Rushmer, 1962). Braunwald and his associates (1965) showed later that if heart rate was maintained constant, the Frank-Starling mechanism could be shown to be operative in conscious animals and in man.

However, the sensitivity of ventricular function curves is less than some of the methods discussed below (Covell et al., 1966). Fortunately, for pharmacologists, anesthetic agents are such marked depressants of myocardial function that a sensitive method is not required to demonstrate depression; a sensitive one is required, however, if depression is to be quantitated, or if one agent is to be compared with another.

There are several objections to the use of stroke work in the construction of ventricular function curves. The appeal of stroke work probably arises from the fact that it combines in a single measurement, the two most distinctive aspects of muscular contraction — tension development and shortening. That these two variables tend to vary in opposite directions when the load on a muscle is changed, lends a further superficial plausibility to the use of stroke work as an index of contractility. The condemning fact, however, is that the relation between tension and shortening is not a simple inverse proportion, and for these reasons (as well as others) ventricular stroke work does not remain constant as ejection pressure is varied (Blinks, 1969).

Rate of Rise of Ventricular Pressure (dP/dt). Wiggers (1927) proposed several decades ago that the rate of myocardial fiber shortening was clearly a function of myocardial performance. This concept was revised by Gleason and Braunwald (1962) in the measurement of the left ventricular dP/dt. After the initial enthusiasm, Wallace et al. (1963) pointed out that the maximum dP/dt is influenced by changes in end diastolic volume, aortic pressure, and heart rate, independently of any change in contractility. Changes in dP/dt_{max} can reflect changes in "contractility" if no changes or opposite changes occur in aortic pressure, heart rate, and end diastolic volume. This can be a difficult set of conditions to attain in an intact animal.

Myocardial Contractile Force. Another proposed indicator of myocardial contractility is the force of contraction of a segment of myocardium as recorded by a strain gauge arch sutured to the ventricular wall (Walton and Houck, 1966). The influence of changes in pre- and afterload are eliminated by stretching the segment under the arch 50% above its resting length. The strain gauge arch is allowed to shorten only a very small distance, so that nearly isometric tension is recorded. It would seem that the maximum force measured by this technique is the maximal load (force) at zero velocity (P_0) as shown on the lower right of the force-velocity curve (Fig. 2). However, P_0, as envisioned by Hill (1938) was the maximum force generated by skeletal muscle during the *tetanic* state. This state cannot be achieved in the heart and hence myocardial contractile force (MCF) does not measure P_0. Even if we were able to measure P_0 directly, we would have to view the data with some skepticism. BRAUNWALD et al. (1967) have shown that inotropic interventions change V_{max} with or without a change in P_0. An advantage of the strain-gauge technique to pharmacologists is that MCF is not sensitive to heart rate, at least in human subjects (SONNENBLICK et al., 1965, 1966). Thus changes in heart rate do not complicate the interpretation of the data.

Peak Aortic Acceleration. Of all the data to be obtained from flowmeter measurements, the most significant is aortic flow acceleration (RUSHMER, 1964; NOBLE et al., 1966). RUSHMER (1964) has described the "initial ventricular impulse", the initial rapid push given by the ventricle to the blood being ejected into the aorta. He feels that this reflects the events of isometric contraction and thus may be a very sensitive indicator of myocardial performance. Indeed, STARR (1950), in his

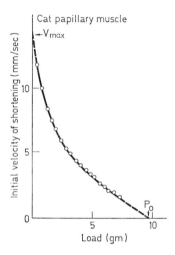

Fig. 2. The inverse relation between the initial velocity of isotonic shortening and increasing afterload: the *force-velocity relation*. From BRAUNWALD, E., ROSS, J. JR., SONNENBLICK, E. H.: Mechanisms of contraction of the normal and failing heart; Little, Brown and Co. Boston: 1968. By permission

classic studies on cadavers, noted that a normal force ballistocardiogram could be produced only when a sharp blow was imparted by a mallet to a syringe injecting blood into the aorta and the pulmonary artery — the hand alone could not simulate normal ejection.

An analogy to illustrate the importance of aortic acceleration in assessing the performance of the heart compares the function of the heart to that of an automobile engine. We can describe the function of the engine by stating how far the automobile travels in a trip, that is the displacement of the automobile; this is equivalent to stroke volume or cardiac output. A second way would be to measure the maximum velocity of the automobile, equivalent to peak aortic flow. A third description is to calculate its acceleration, equivalent to ventricular dP/dt or peak aortic acceleration. It is obvious that the third variable is by far the most important, for the automobile as well as the heart. Acceleration is the first function to be impaired if the performance of either is diminished.

An indirect noninvasive method of measuring peak aortic acceleration exists. The high frequency force ballistocardiogram or the ultra-low frequency acceleration ballistocardiogram has shown a remarkable correlation with aortic acceleration under various conditions (WINTER et al., 1966, 1967; SMITH et al., 1969) of circulatory stimulation or depression.

What is the influence of changes in aortic pressure or end diastolic volume on aortic acceleration? Studies of NOBLE et al. (1966) have shown in dogs that passive changes in position (lying to standing, etc.) produced little change in aortic acceleration, although changes in stroke volume and peak aortic flow were quite large, and reflected changes in end diastolic volume. Subsequent reports (SUTHERLAND et al., 1969) demonstrate that aortic flow acceleration does not respond to rapidly induced changes in blood volume. Furthermore, cutting the aorta suddenly,

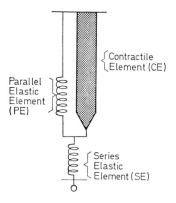

Fig. 3. The Hill model for muscle (1938). At rest the CE is freely extensible, suggesting that the resting tension is supported entirely by the PE. Note that some of the force generated by the CE will expend itself into the SE. From BRAUNWALD, E., ROSS, J. JR., SONNENBLICK, E. H.: Mechanisms of contraction of the normal and failing heart; Little, Brown and Co. Boston: 1968. By permission

so that the succeeding stroke volume is ejected against zero resistance, does not change the peak aortic acceleration of that beat. Thus, the influence of pre- and afterload is probably quite small.

Myocardial Mechanics. Present concepts of myocardial mechanics derive from the recent extension of the studies of HILL (1938) in skeletal muscle to isolated cardiac muscle (PODOLSKY, 1961; WILKIE, 1954, 1956) and, thence, to an attempted analysis of the intact ventricle (SONNENBLICK et al., 1965). The model that HILL (1938) proposed to explain the mechanical activity of muscle serves as a framework for viewing experimental findings in the heart and as a background for theoretical extension of current concepts. In HILL's model (Fig. 3) a contractile element (CE) is arranged in series with a passive elastic component (SE). Arranged in parallel with these two components is another passive element, the parallel elastic component (PE). At rest, the CE is thought to be quite extensible, so that resting tension is not supported by the CE-SE complex, but rather by the PE. The relation between muscle length and resting tension therefore describes the length-resting tension curve of the PE. Upon activation of the muscle, the CE acquires the ability to shorten and to develop force. Since the CE is attached to the external environment only through the SE, the manner in which force is developed depends on the interaction of the shortening CE with the spring-like SE. Thus, during an isometric contraction (Fig. 4), in which the ends of the muscle are fixed, the CE shortens, stretches the spring-like SE, and builds up force at the ends of the system. The manner in which this force increases is determined by three factors: (1) the shortening properties of the CE, defined by the force-velocity relation at any given instant during contraction; (2) the elastic properties of the SE, defined by the load-extension curve of this internal spring; and (3) the time allowed for the interaction between this shortening CE and the lengthening SE, that is, the duration of the active state. Thus, the CE and SE are both altered by load (or force) and demonstrate their properties within limits of time.

Viscous elements should also be considered in this model. HILL (1938) has shown that these viscous elements do not exist in the CE. However, viscous

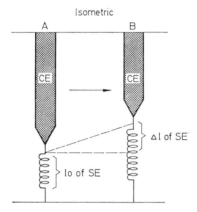

Fig. 4. Rearranged Hill Model (without PE): Isometric Contraction. A is the initial resting state, B an instant during active contraction. lo = initial length; Δl = change in length. From BRAUNWALD, E., Ross, J., JR., SONNENBLICK, E. H.: Mechanisms of contraction of the normal and failing heart. Little, Brown and Co. Boston: 1968. By permission

elements are present in the PE, as indicated by the observation that stress relaxation — that is, a fall in tension following a sustained extension — occurs after stretch of the heart muscle to a fixed length. Nevertheless, viscous elements in the PE are appreciable only at abnormally high resting tensions. Recently SONNENBLICK et al. (1966) found viscosity in the SE of heart muscle as well. Viscosity in the SE results in a slight fall in resting tension at a constant muscle length, associated with an increase in the force of contraction, regardless of how this increase in force is brought about.

The active state or the activity of the CE was initially defined by HILL (1949) for skeletal muscle as the force-generating potential of the CE at any instant. The maximum intensity of active state is said to be present when this force-generating capacity is greatest. To measure the maximum intensity of active state within this definition, the CE must be neither shortening nor lengthening, a condition provided by imposition of quick stretches on the muscle. PODOLSKY (1961) has expanded this definition to consider the active state as a mechanical measure of the chemical processes in the CE that generate force and shortening. Within this broader definition, force and velocity are both considered, and the mechanical definition of the active state becomes the capacity of the CE to shorten in accordance with the force-velocity relation (Jewell and Wilkie, 1960).

Since the manner in which the CE shortens is intimately dependent on load, the latter must be carefully controlled to segregate CE performance from overall muscle contraction. By study of an isotonic contraction — that is, a contraction with constant load — the activity of the CE could possibly be characterized in a mechanical experiment independently of the characteristics of the SE, that is, the SE remains constant. In Fig. 5 the Hill model has been arranged for an afterloaded isotonic contraction. The system is fixed at its upper end. The lower end rests upon a support that determines its initial length. The small load that establishes its resting length is termed the preload. A load (P) has been added to the end of the system but rests on the support and is felt by the CE only after the

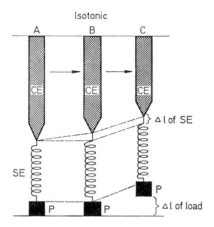

Fig. 5. Rearranged Hill Model (without PE): Isotonic Contraction. A is the initial resting state, B the instant during active isometric contraction just before isotonic contraction, and C an instant during afterloaded isotonic contraction. P = load, Δl = change in length, From Braunwald, E., Ross, J., Jr., Sonnenblick, E. H.: Mechanisms of contraction of the normal and failing heart. Little, Brown and Co. Boston: 1968. By permission

onset of contraction. Hence this load is termed an afterload. The preload and the afterload comprise the total load. With activation of the muscle, the CE starts to shorten and to stretch the SE, thus building up force. When the force built up in stretching the SE equals the load (P), the muscle will begin to shorten and to lift the load (point B). Once the load moves, the force that is stretching the SE remains constant and the shortening of the overall system will reflect only the shortening of the CE. Thus, by study of the afterloaded isotonic contraction, the shortening of the CE may be analyzed.

By studying the relation between load and velocity of shortening, Hill (1938) described what has been termed the most fundamental property of the CE, the force-velocity relation. In Fig. 6, the afterload has been progressively increased while the preload, which determines initial muscle length, has been kept constant. As the afterload is augmented, the initial velocity of shortening decreases, as noted by the dashed lines. If the initial velocity of shortening is then plotted as a function of total load, (preload plus afterload), a characteristic inverse relation between force and velocity is found, which represents the force-velocity relation

(Fig. 2). When the load (P) approaches zero, velocity of shortening is maximum and termed V_{max}. V_{max} has been proposed as an extremely sensitive indicator of contractility, one which is not dependent on preload. As the load is increased, both the velocity and the extent of shortening progressively decrease, until external shortening cannot occur and a maximum isometric force ($\sim P_0$) is developed.

As HILL (1938) has noted, the nature of this curve can be characterized mathematically as a displaced hyperbola:

$$(P + a)\,(V + b) = (P_0 + a)\,b,$$

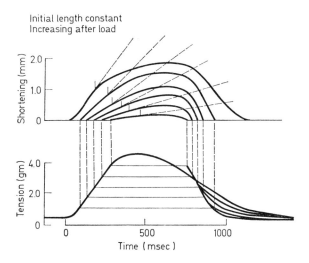

Fig. 6. Relation between tension development and shortening of the cat papillary muscle. As contraction begins, tension rises, as shown in the bottom tracing. As soon as the muscle lifts the afterload, it shortens, as shown in the top tracings. The dashed lines in the top tracings represent the initial velocity of shortening. Both the extent and the velocity of shortening diminish as afterloads are increased. From BRAUNWALD, E., ROSS, J., JR., SONNENBLICK, E. H.: Mechanisms of contraction of the normal and failing heart; Little, Brown and Co. Boston: 1968. By permission

where P = load; V = velocity of shortening at that load; P_0 = the maximum isometric force, and a and b are constants representing the displacement of the hyperbola. In this form this expression comprises the well-known Hill equation (HILL, 1938). When the muscle is operating on this inverse P-V curve, the maximum intensity of active state may be said to be present. During the process of activation, which has been shown to be time-dependent and relatively slow in heart muscle (SONNENBLICK, 1965; BRADY, 1965), this curve will gradually be approached. Then during relaxation, as the active state declines, the relation between force and velocity will move away from this curve. In this manner the active state expresses the extent to which the contractile machinery is turned on at any time, regardless of whether or not the muscle is shortening or developing force.

Objections have been raised even to the beautifully structured investigations described above. JEWELL and BLINKS (1968) and BRADY (1968) have summarized evidence that the model proposed (Fig. 3) cannot explain certain findings and that the model shown in Fig. 7 has not been eliminated as a possibility. A careful look at the model in Fig. 7 reveals that force of the force-velocity curve cannot be calculated simply by subtracting resting tension from peak developed tension, since part of the resting tension may reside in the SE. Furthermore, V_{max} must be extrapolated from the force-velocity curve. Since there is an internal load for the heart to overcome, V_{max}, that is the velocity of shortening against zero-load, can never be directly measured, and it may be that it can never be correctly extrapolated.

Taken together, three fundamental relationships (length-active tension, force-velocity, and time course of the intensity of the active state) provide a fairly complete description of the mechanical behavior of muscle and a reasonable framework for understanding it. Four variables (force, velocity, length and time) are

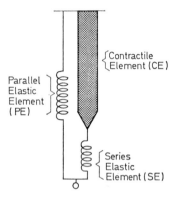

Fig. 7. An alternate to the Hill Model. Although the CE is freely extensible, the amount of the resting tension supported by the PE and SE is not measurable

involved, all of which may be changing simultaneously during the course of contraction. FRY (1962) has proposed that a change in myocardial contractility be defined as a change in the performance of the heart that results from the change in the relationships among these four variables during the active state. This definition does not simplify the measurement of contractility, but it does provide an objective criterion for deciding whether a given change should be attributed to a change in myocardial contractility. However, it is only a first step to decide whether or not a given agent produces a true change in myocardial contractility. As RUSHMER (1962) has pointed out, it is a dangerous over-simplication to describe a given change in the performance of the heart only as an increase or decrease in contractility. To do so is to lose sight of important differences between the mechanisms for the altered contractility produced by different interventions, any of which may lead to this change. One must go on to provide a complete description of the changes produced; this is inescapable, whether one describes the changes in the terminology of hemodynamics, or of muscle physiology.

The best suggestion comes from RUSHMER (1961) who proposes that instead of trying to define myocardial contractility in terms of a single measurement, it is better to characterize the performance of the heart in engineering terms, such as acceleration, work, power, dimensional changes, etc. He would discard the often misused and misleading term "contractility". One must remember that in the intact heart, a large complex muscle, other features than contractility affect its performance. The first factor is excitation, or the distribution and speed with which the bioelectric impulse is conducted to all parts of the muscle. In isolated thin strips of muscle in a bath, massive field stimulation assures a uniform delivery of excitation that does not ordinarily occur in the intact heart. The second consideration is synergy of contraction (STARR, 1962; GORLIN and SONNENBLICK, 1968). Normally, there is an orderly sequence of contraction. Even if the contractile state of two zones of muscle are similar, the local changes in effective tension and velocity can vary widely because of differences in time of activation, thickness of muscle, elasticity and other factors. Cardiac action can also be altered by the following factors discussed in detail above. (1) Change in initial or end diastolic volume (preload); (2) change in impedance to injection (afterload); and (3) change in frequency of contraction or rate.

II. Halothane

A. Hemodynamics

1. Cardiac Output

The effect of halothane anesthesia on cardiac output has been measured in heart-lung preparations, intact animals, and humans.

In heart-lung preparations of various animals, halothane decreases cardiac output. The decrease in cardiac output is generally proportional to the concentration of halothane and is usually due to a decrease in stroke volume.

In animals halothane usually decreases cardiac output. However, in an early study, RAVENTOS (1956) failed to note any change in cardiac output in two dogs given an unspecified concentration of halothane after an unspecified amount of morphine. In dogs, ETSTEN and LI (1960) and STIRLING and his co-workers (1960) showed that lower concentrations did not change cardiac output, while higher concentrations of halothane markedly decreased it. SAITO et al. (1965), in dogs with previously performed thoracotomies, observed a decrease in cardiac output which was enhanced with increasing depth of halothane. In another study [1966 (1)], they observed a 25% decrease in cardiac output after 19 min in dogs spontaneously breathing 2% inspired halothane. The same concentration of halothane produced no change in cardiac output when ventilation was assisted. However, control values in the dogs during assisted ventilation were as low as halothane-induced cardiac output levels in the spontaneously breathing animals. THEYE and SESSLER (1967) studied unpremedicated dogs paralyzed with an infusion of succinylcholine. When the inspired concentration of halothane was changed from 0.8—2.5%, cardiac output decreased 58%. In another study (SESSLER and THEYE, 1966), they noted a 30—60% decrease in cardiac output when inspired halothane concentration was changed from 0.8—3.2%. DOBKIN et al. (1962) in dogs with assisted ventilation, observed a decrease in cardiac output from 3.17—1.95 l/min. HAMILTON et al. (1966) observed a 37% decrease in cardiac output in dogs anesthetized with halothane-oxygen down to MAC 3 (2.7% endtidal halothane concentration). SMITH and CORBASCIO (1966) induced dogs with thiopental and maintained them with succinylcholine. Plotting arterial concentration of halothane against cardiac output, they noted an exponential decrease with both halothane-oxygen and halothane-nitrous oxide-oxygen. Blood levels of 24 mg-% (1.32%

endtidal) produced a decrease of 35—40%. No essential difference in the curves was seen.

In horses (Eberly et al., 1968) cardiac output was 40% lower in anesthetized recumbent animals than in awake standing ones. The authors noted no difference in cardiac output changes between animals induced with thiopental (3 g) plus pentobarbital (1 g), and those receiving no barbiturates for induction.

As might be anticipated, cardiac output has been studied more frequently in man than in animals. Eger and Hügin (1961) noted a decrease in cardiac output in patients premedicated with meperidine and scopolamine and ventilated mechanically. Cardiac output was measured by the ultra-low frequently displacement ballistocardiogram. Tuohy and Theye (1964) measured cardiac output in ten patients subjected to 6 h of anesthesia, surgery, and unreplaced blood loss. The patients had received pentobarbital, meperidine and atropine for pre-anesthetic medication and thiopental-succinylcholine for induction. Anesthesia was maintained with 0.5—1% halothane in nitrous oxide (65%)-oxygen. Ventilation was controlled. During the 6 h interval, cardiac output decreased from 1.96—1.82 l/min, a significant change. The slight decrease in cardiac output could be explained by the unreplaced blood loss.

Lundborg et al. (1967) observed a 16% decrease in cardiac output in spontaneously breathing patients undergoing cardiac catheterization procedures. The patients had been premedicated with a lytic cocktail — a mixture of meperidine, chlorpromazine, and promethazine. Severinghaus and Cullen (1958) administered 1.5% halothane to patients premedicated with morphine and scopolamine. Anesthesia was induced with 200—300 mg thiopental plus succinylcholine. Nitrous oxide (75%) in oxygen was given and ventilation was controlled. After 15 min of steady-state anesthesia, cardiac output had decreased 31% from the control level. Payne et al. (1959), after premedication with pentobarbital 200 mg and atropine 0.65 mg, induced anesthesia in 12 normal patients with up to 5% inspired halothane. Observations of cardiac output were made 15 min after induction. They noted an increase in cardiac output in seven and a decrease in five patients, each ventilating spontaneously an inspired halothane concentration of 2%.

McGregor and associates (1958) anesthetized 12 children with 1% halothane and 50% nitrous oxide in oxygen, noting a 16.4% decrease in cardiac output. These children were premedicated with pentobarbital, morphine sulfate, and scopolamine. In another series of 16 children, administration of 0.25% halothane did not significantly change cardiac output, but 2—3% halothane produced a 15—23% decrease. Kubota and Vandam (1962) in normal patients premedicated with pentobarbital and atropine or scopolamine and induced with thiopental observed a 23% decrease in cardiac output when halothane was administered in 75% nitrous oxide. Ventilation was controlled. Yoshida et al. (1965) anesthetized patients with halothane in 75% nitrous oxide. They compared decreases in cardiac output with halothane concentration in the blood. No depression of cardiac output was seen when concentration was less than 5 mg-%; cardiac output was decreased about 15% at 10 mg-% (0.55% end-tidal) and 30% at a level of 15 mg-%. When blood concentration was greater than 20 mg-%, cardiac output was reduced by 40%.

Walker et al. [1962 (1, 2)] noted a drop in cardiac index from 2.65 to 2.43 l/min/m² in five spontaneously ventilating normal volunteer subjects induced with thiopental-succinylcholine and maintained with 1.5% halothane. Virtue et al. (1962) measured cardiac output in ten normal volunteer subjects premedicated with intravenous atropine or scopolamine. Fluroxene had been given 42 min prior to the halothane as part of the same study. Sufficient halothane in air was given to maintain electroencephalographic level 4. Cardiac output went from 4.94 to 5.17 l/min, not a significant difference. WYANT et al. (1958) studied unpremedicated normal volunteer subjects. After induction with an intravenous barbiturate, halothane was administered in a closed-system during spontaneous ventilation until the arterial pressure was as low as considered safe. Cardiac output and systolic blood pressure fell in a parallel fashion until the pressure reached a plateau. This hypotension produced by high concentrations was accomplished by a severe decrease in cardiac output to as low as 40% of control.

a) Extra-Anesthetic Factors

TOMLIN et al. (1966) noted a progressive decrease in cardiac output when the concentration of halothane in oxygen was increased. Cardiac output increased at a given concentration of halothane when respiratory acidosis was induced. THEYE et al. (1966) carried out hemodynamic and blood gas studies during halothane anesthesia and surgery in seven premedicated patients induced with thiopental and succinylcholine. Without exception, cardiac output was greater during normocapnia than during hypocapnia ($PaCO_2$ = about 27 torr). They suggested that altered activity of the sympathetic nervous system produced these changes, although withdrawal of the vasodilating effects of carbon dioxide could also have played a part. PRYS-ROBERTS et al. (1967) observed the relationship between cardiac output and $PaCO_2$ in patients. Whether these patients received premedication, thiobarbiturates, or other drugs was not stated. The investigators calculated a slope of 0.03 l/min/70 kg/torr $PaCO_2$ and a resting value of 3.21 l/min/kg at an inspired concentration of 1%. In contrast, HORNBEIN et al. (1969) observed nearly twice the values in unpremedicated normal subjects: 0.062 l/min/70 kg/torr $PaCO_2$ and 5.63 l/min/70 kg. The $PaCO_2$ at resting cardiac outputs was similar in the two studies, eliminating one explanation for a difference in results. In addition to premedication, possible explanations are a difference in elapsed time after induction and a nonlinearity in the CO_2-cardiac output response curve. PRYS-ROBERTS et al., fit their curve between 23.5—70 torr $PaCO_2$, HORNBEIN et al., only upward from a $PaCO_2$ of 49 torr.

TOMLIN et al. (1966) measured the response of cardiac output in the dog to changes in pH, $PaCO_2$, and body temperature during halothane anesthesia. A decrease in body temperature decreased cardiac output by 10% per degree C. Decreased pH or increased $PaCO_2$ also decreased cardiac output.

SHIMOSATO and ETSTEN (1963) observed a 50% decrease in cardiac output in dogs receiving 1% halothane and a 67% decrease in dogs receiving 2% halothane. Halothane administered to digitalized animals increased cardiac output. The control cardiac output, however, was lower in these animals than in non-digitalized ones.

CRAYTHORNE and HUFFINGTON (1966) observed that propranolol, a beta-adrenergic blocking agent, administered to dogs during halothane anesthesia produced no further depression of cardiac output.

In open-chest dogs (MAHAFFEY et al., 1966) after induction with halothane-nitrous oxide, halothane consistently decreased mean aortic flow (cardiac output minus coronary blood flow) as measured by an electromagnetic flowmeter. After chemical sympathectomy (epidural with tetracaine), this depression was even more marked.

FARMAN (1967) anesthetized patients with halothane in 50% N_2O after premedication with scopolamine or atropine. Cardiac output increased 48% after the intravenous injection of 0.6 mg atropine during anesthesia. The studies were performed during surgery, and no preanesthetic values were measured.

Halothane administered to 22 patients decreased cardiac output by 30%
(Walther et al., 1964). A further decrease in arterial pressure produced by intravenous hexamethonium resulted in a variable response in cardiac output, which
remained stable or increased when the systemic pressure was greater than
65 torr. On the other hand, hypotension produced by a lumbar peridural
(1.5% lidocaine) during anesthesia, consistently decreased cardiac output, by a
mean of 22%. Lidocaine absorbed into the bloodstream may have influenced these
results. We have produced a decrease in cardiac output and arterial pressure in
normal volunteer subjects merely by injecting 80—100 mg of lidocaine to block
the sympathetic nerves in the axilla of one arm (unpublished data).

b) Adaptation

Deutsch et al. (1962) examined the response to halothane as a function of
time in spontaneously ventilating unpremedicated subjects, each exposed to a constant inspired (not end-tidal) concentration of halothane. Absolute concentrations
differed in each subject. A 15% decrease in cardiac output was observed after
44 min, but cardiac output returned almost to normal 30 min later. Eger et al.
(1968) studied twelve young normal volunteer subjects under the same circumstances, except for control of ventilation and maintenance of a constant *alveolar*
halothane concentration during steady-states. A dose-response curve was constructed for each subject after 35 min, 100 min, and 300 min of anesthesia. After
the initial decrease, cardiac output returned to normal more slowly than in
Deutsch's (1962) study and could not reach control values if end tidal halothane
concentration was greater than 1.6%. Both investigators felt that an increase in
blood volume was not the cause of the adaptation. They suggested that either
increasing painful stimulus from prolonged immobilization (Deutsch et al., 1962)
or increased release of or sensitivity to catecholamines (Eger et al., 1968) was
responsible. Wenthe et al. (1962) studied premedicated patients induced with
100 mg thiopental and anesthetized with 50% nitrous oxide-halothane via a mask.
Ventilation was spontaneous or controlled. They noted a decrease of 24, 31, and
12% during light, deep and subsequent light anesthesia when ventilation was
spontaneous. The corresponding reductions during controlled ventilation were
37%, 48%, and 47%. The first set of figures shows an adaptation of cardiac
output with time, the second measurement of cardiac output under light anesthesia
being higher than the first. This adaptation was not apparent under controlled
ventilation, probably because the sequence of observation had varied among
patients. Adaptation was also seen by Smith et al. [1968 (1)] who observed the
response to sudden changes of 0.5—1.7% in halothane concentration in eight
normal unpremedicated subjects. Ventilation was controlled. The resulting changes
in cardiac output were delayed in time and decreased in magnitude late, as compared to early in the course of halothane administration (1.5—2.3 vs. 0.3 to
0.9 l/min maximum changes).

c) Effects of Induction

Recent development of techniques for measuring cardiac output under dynamic
conditions have made possible the study of the effects on cardiac output of induction with halothane. Eisele et al. (1969) gave ten breaths of 3% halothane in
oxygen to meticulously trained dogs, and noted a slight (8%) decrease in cardiac
output during the first 40 sec. Smith et al. [1968 (1)] in studying unpremedicated
human volunteers noted a mean peak 37% increase in cardiac output during
the first 3 min of induction. Apprehension and the odor of halothane could have
played a role in the latter responses.

d) Oxygen Consumption

GUYTON (1968) has suggested that the metabolic needs of the peripheral tissues control cardiac output. Does some of the decrease in cardiac output during halothane anethesia, therefore, reflect a decreased oxygen demand by the tissues? THEYE and SESSLER (1967) noted a 17% decrease in $\dot{V}_{O_2}$ when halothane was increased from 0.8—2.5% (mean expired). Cardiac output, as noted before, was approximately halved. They suggested that the decrease in $\dot{V}_{O_2}$ might be an indirect effect mediated by halothane-induced circulatory changes, although they could not rule out direct metabolic depressant effects of halothane per se. Payment of an oxygen debt was not observed when the concentration of halothane was returned to 0.8%. Later, THEYE (1967) investigated paralyzed dogs in which constant systemic blood flow rates were assured by a right heart by-pass. They determined $\dot{V}_{O_2}$ for the heart and for the rest of the body. $\dot{V}_{O_2}$ for the latter decreased with an increase of halothane from 0.1—0.9%. This was felt to be a direct depressant effect of halothane. Decreases in myocardial $\dot{V}_{O_2}$ were related to decreases in external work of the heart and were considered to represent indirect depressant effects of halothane. BABAD (1968) noted in hyperthyroid, euthyroid, and hypothyroid dogs no correlation between metabolic state and halothane requirement as evaluated by determination of MAC, except at the extremes of $\dot{V}_{O_2}$ range. However, deepening anesthesia decreased oxygen requirement, the decrease being most pronounced in the hypermetabolic animals. DEUTSCH et al. (1962) in four normal volunteer subjects noticed a decrease in oxygen consumption of 26—43%. Similar results were seen by SEVERINGHAUS and CULLEN (1958).

SHINOZAKI et al. (1968) and MAZUZAN et al. (1962) measured a 26—29% decrease in cardiac output in volunteer patients with halothane-oxygen or halothane-air anesthesia. If atropine was administered with halothane-oxygen only a 6% decrease was seen. Atropine added during halothane-oxygen anesthesia increased cardiac output by 26%. After halothane-oxygen was changed to halothane-air, a 25% decrease in cardiac output was noted. They concluded that the decrease in cardiac output observed with halothane-oxygen anesthesia represents an adjustment to greater oxygen extraction per unit volume of blood. SMITH et al. [1968 (2)] found no change in cardiac output when halothane-oxygen was switched to halothane-air, plus enough O_2 to maintain a normal Pa_{O_2}. Ventilation was controlled in the latter study, spontaneous in the former. The Pa_{O_2}'s in SHINOZAKI's (1968) study ranged from 42—65 torr; in SMITH's they ranged from 100—110 torr. Hypoxia to the level observed in the former study usually increases cardiac output (CULLEN and EGER, unpublished data).

GREIFENSTEIN (1966) provided indirect evidence as to whether the decrease in cardiac output produced deprivation of oxygen to cells, as estimated by measurement of excess lactate (HUCKABEE, 1958). In premedicated patients undergoing surgery, halothane with 50% nitrous oxide did not produce excess lactate. Halothane-oxygen anesthesia under surgical conditions did show an excess lactate production, comparable to that obtained with cyclopropane.

e) Hemorrhage

Since halothane usually decreases cardiac output, it could be dangerous to administer it during hemorrhage when cardiac output and blood volume already are depressed. FREEMAN (1962) in dogs could detect no difference in the mortality produced by hemorrhage when halothane at an inspired concentration of 1.5% was compared to light ether. ANDREWS et al. (1966), comparing halothane with methoxyflurane, observed that survival after controlled hemorrhage was greater with methoxyflurane.

f) Halothane-Ether Azeotrope

In an effort to counteract the cardiovascular and ventilatory depression seen with halothane, Hudon et al. (1958) introduced a mixture of halothane-ether in 2:1 proportions. This is a true azeotrope. Dechêne et al. (1962), without comparing this azeotropic mixture to controls, stated that the azeotrope did not change cardiac output in dogs. Wyant et al. (1960), using an ether-halothane mixture, detected a fall in cardiac output only when arterial pressure was severely depressed by overdosage. Déry (1964) observed an increased cardiac output in premedicated (meperidine-atropine) patients with this type of mixture. However, his observations were made during surgery.

2. Arterial Pressure

Since arterial pressure is easier to measure than cardiac output, more data are available on the response of arterial pressure to halothane. Unfortunately, the surgical stimulus present during many measurements makes interpretation and comparison of results difficult. Undoubtedly, hypotension does occur with halothane administration, but disagreement exists among investigators as to the amount, significance, and cause.

Arterial pressure levels have been studied in dogs, cats, rabbits, and horses. Raventos (1956) showed that halothane produced hypotension in the first three species. He recorded systolic arterial pressures of 60—80 torr at the time that spontaneous ventilation ceased. Blackmore et al. (1960) noted hypotension in unpremedicated dogs given halothane-oxygen anesthesia. Philippart (1963) reported a decrease of 62.3% in mean arterial pressure in dogs, but these animals had already undergone extensive surgery for bypass measurement of coronary flow. Ngai and Bolme [1966 (1)] demonstrated that light and deep halothane in oxygen (1% and 1.5—1.8% inspired concentration) decreased mean arterial pressure 31 and 47%, respectively. Hamilton et al. (1966) in dogs noted an 18, 48 and 66 mmHg decrease in mean arterial pressure at 1, 2 and 3 times MAC (0.9% alveolar concentration). Price and Price (1966) noted a 70 and 90 torr decrease at 1 and 2%, while 0.5% had little effect in dogs prepared under pentobarbital anesthesia.

Smith and Corbascio [1966 (1)] plotted percent change in arterial pressure against mg-% halothane concentration in arterial blood. They observed a somewhat less marked negative slope when halothane-nitrous oxide-oxygen was administered as compared to halothane-oxygen. At a blood concentration of 24 mg-%, arterial pressure decreased 40—50%.

Dobkin and Fedoruk (1961) noted a 50 torr drop in mean arterial pressure in dogs breathing 2% halothane-oxygen spontaneously and a 37 torr decrease in animals with controlled ventilation. Dobkin et al. (1962) assisted ventilation in dogs premedicated with perphenazine and induced with thiopental. They noted a drop in arterial pressure from 138/94 to 121/82 after 90 min of 2% halothane in oxygen. In dogs prepared with thiopental-succinylcholine anesthesia, Galindo and Baldwin (1963) noted a 47% decrease in mean arterial pressure during deep anesthesia, defined as a frequency in the frontal-occipital electroencephalogram recording of 30% less than control value. Rein et al. (1963), in open-chest dogs, recorded during control periods and subsequent administration of 0.5, 1.0, 1.5, and 2.0% halothane in oxygen, mean arterial pressures of 142, 135, 130, 124, and 85. Mahaffey et al. (1961) noted a 59% decrease in mean arterial pressure in open-chest dogs prepared with halothane, stabilized with 67% nitrous oxide in oxygen, and re-anesthetized with 3% halothane. Li et al. (1968) in open-chest dogs prepared under pentobarbital, chloralose or both, measured a decrease in arterial pressure from 124—89 torr. In unpremedicated dogs (THEYE and SESSLER, 1967) mean arterial pressure decreased 48 torr (40%) when the mean-expired concentration of halothane was changed from 0.8—2.5%.

EBERLY et al. (1968) reported decreases in mean and systolic arterial pressure in horses anesthetized with halothane-oxygen. Control values were recorded while the horses were standing. HALL (1957) observed decreases in arterial pressure in horses, followed by increases after 30 min of anesthesia.

Results in man show little qualitative differences from those seen in animals. JOHNSTONE (1956) observed hypotension with halothane anesthesia in the first clinical report. Several early investigators [SEVERINGHAUS and CULLEN; HUDON et al., 1957 (2); STEPHEN et al., 1957] suggested that depth of anesthesia was contributory to the amount of hypotension. Later it was demonstrated that the rate of induction was also important.

CARSON et al. (1959) in 500 anesthetics, and HANSEN et al. (1959) in 1000 anesthetics, both described consistent hypotension. They often used uncalibrated vaporizers, and profound hypotension was frequent. In an analysis of 162 patients receiving halothane during surgery (CHATAS et al., 1963), hypotension of greater than 20% was noted in 8% of the patients receiving 0.2—1.0% halothane and 15% of patients receiving 1.1—1.5% halothane, as measured by a vaporizer. In a retrospective study, MOYERS and PITTINGER (1959) noted a 16.1% decrease in arterial pressure in 50 patients receiving halothane. COPPOLINO (1963), in another retrospective study, reported a mean decrease of 24 torr during halothane anesthesia in 200 patients. In 603 administrations of halothane in children, aged from newborn to 13 years (BREAKSTONE, 1962), halothane was claimed to have caused mild hypotension, with no morbidity. The stimulation of surgery may have influenced these results. In an interesting double-blind (but not "double-sniff") study of patients receiving either halothane or chloroform (BAMFORTH et al., 1960) a slightly greater incidence of hypotension was noted in patients receiving halothane, although hypertensive episodes matched hypotensive ones in number. The incidence of hypotension was greatest 15 min after the onset of administration of either agent. BOURGEOIS-GAVARDIN (1959) noted a decrease of more than 40 torr during induction in 12 of 100 patients. DOBKIN (1958), in 100 patients induced with barbiturate-succinylcholine and maintained with 0.5% halothane in nitrous oxide-oxygen, observed moderate decreases (less than 10 to 15%) in only 15% of the patients, no falls in the others.

MAZUZAN et al. (1962), in three patients with fixed heart rate resulting from A-V block or implanted pacemakers, noted no decrease in arterial pressure from administration of 1—2% halothane in oxygen. LUNDBORG et al. (1967), in patients undergoing heart catheterization after premedication with lytic cocktail, described a 21% decrease in arterial pressure with 1.0—1.5% halothane in oxygen or in nitrous oxide-oxygen. EGER and HÜGIN (1961) observed a mean 20 torr decrease in 12 patients premedicated with meperidine and 1-hyoscyamine and given halothane in oxygen or nitrous oxide-oxygen. SUMMERS et al. (1962), in 16 healthy premedicated patients induced with thiopental noted a decrease of 25 torr systolic arterial pressure.

ELLIOTT et al. (1968) induced ten normal subjects with thiopental-succinylcholine. Ventilation was spontaneous and the subjects were intubated. After 25 min of 2% halothane, vaporizer concentration, mean arterial pressure, measured by auscultation, decreased from 89.0—65.5 torr. VIRTUE et al. (1962) measured direct arterial pressure in ten normal volunteer subjects premedicated with intravenously administered atropine or scopolamine. Fluroxene had been given 42 min prior to the halothane as part of the same study. Sufficient halothane in air to maintain electroencephalographic level 4 decreased arterial pressure from 119 to 89. Mean arterial pressure fell from 85.6—64.9 in five spontaneously ventilating normal volunteer patients induced with thiopental-succinylcholine and maintained with 1.5% halothane [Walker et al., 1962 (1); Fabian, 1966]. The trachea was sprayed with 6% cocaine. Measurements were taken after 35 min of steady-state anesthesia. Wyant et al. (1958) deliberately induced severe hypotension in normal volunteer subjects induced with thiamylal and breathing spontaneously. This was early in the investigation of halothane, and the authors observed the remarkable property of a rapid recovery of arterial pressure upon discontinuation of halothane, even after levels as low as 25 torr systolic.

Halothane-oxygen produced similar decreases (16—20%) in mean arterial pressure whether halothane-oxygen was administered after air or after 100% oxygen (Shinozaki et al., 1968). Air or oxygen changed to halothane-oxygen plus atropine produced only a 6—8% decrease in arterial pressure.

Neill and Nixon (1965) administered halothane to patients induced with 200—500 mg thiopental plus 25—45 mg d-tubocurarine. The decrease in arterial pressure following this induction sequence was no different than that seen after induction with thiopental-succinylcholine.

a) Extra-Anesthetic Factors

Black et al. (1959) noted a consistent drop in arterial pressure when halothane was given to normal unpremedicated patients. Changes in arterial pressure during inhalation of carbon dioxide were inconsistent. Theye et al. (1966) observed the effects of hypocapnia achieved by over-ventilation of patients breathing halothane in oxygen or in nitrous oxide-oxygen during surgery. No significant change was noticed in arterial pressure.

In dogs studied by Craythorne and Huffington (1966), addition of 0.2 mg/kg propranolol intravenously produced no significant change in the hypotension existing under halothane anesthesia. Elliott et al. (1968) induced ten normal subjects with thiopental-succinylcholine. Ventilation was spontaneous and the subjects were intubated. Administration of propranolol, 1 mg intravenously after 25 min of 2% halothane vaporizer concentration, resulted in a drop in mean arterial pressure from 68.4—58.0, with no change in heart rate. The changes in arterial pressure were not seen in ten subjects given ether. Since pH was normal in these latter subjects, and depressed in the ten subjects receiving halothane due to hypercarbia, the authors concluded that the H^+ level was more important than the norepinephrine level in determining the effects of propranolol.

Walther et al. (1964) noted a 28% decrease in arterial pressure in patients induced with thiopental-succinylcholine and maintained with nitrous oxide-oxygen-halothane. A further decrease of about 40% was seen upon administration of hexamethonium or of 1.5% lidocaine into the peridural space.

In spontaneously breathing dogs, Fabian et al. (1962) noted a decrease from 118/76 to 87/58 during administration of an unspecified amount of halothane to dogs prepared with thiamylal. Bleeding of 30% of the animal's blood volume resulted in a further decrease in arterial pressure to 47/32. Duration of hemorrhage or interval between hemorrhage and measurements were not stated.

Shimosato and Etsten (1963) noted approximately 35 and 80 torr decreases in arterial pressure with 1 and 2% halothane in unpremedicated dogs prepared with succinylcholine and local anesthesia. Preanesthetic administration of 0.03 to 0.05 mg/kg ouabain intravenously did not prevent these decreases.

b) Adaptation

EGER et al. (1968) reported in normal unpremedicated subjects a 22—25% decrease in mean arterial pressure at MAC 1—2 (0.8—1.6% alveolar halothane concentration) and a 32—49% decrease at MAC 2—2.5. "Recovery" of arterial pressure occurred at deep levels, while a further decrease occurred at light levels. In their premedicated patients, WENTHE et al. (1962) noted an 11, 31 and 12% decrease during change from light to deep to light anesthesia with spontaneous ventilation. The equivalent figures for controlled ventilation were 28, 41, and 22%. These values do not indicate an adaptation in arterial pressure.

The subjects studied by DEUTSCH et al. (1962) did exhibit a slight trend to recovery of arterial pressure values, from 27% below control at 44 min to 17% less than control at 112 min. MORSE et al. (1963) noted a decrease of 22 torr in young normal volunteer subjects anesthetized with 1—1.5% endexpired halothane in oxygen. The arterial pressure rose 9 torr from its nadir after 90 min of anesthesia.

Changes in arterial pressure following sudden changes in halothane were studied in normal subjects early and late in anesthesia (SMITH et al., 1968). The maximum change early in anesthesia was 16—24 torr, compared to 10 torr late in anesthesia.

c) Effects of Induction

EISELE et al. (1969) noted a slight decrease in arterial pressure during the first ten breaths of halothane administered to trained dogs. SMITH (1968) noted no change in mean arterial pressure during the first 3 min of halothane administered to unpremedicated human volunteer subjects, although cardiac output, stroke volume, and heart rate increased.

d) Halothane-Ether Azeotrope

In dogs, DECHÊNE et al. (1962) noted hypertension from 130 up to 160 to 180 torr during very light azeotrope anesthesia. During observations in 6000 unselected cases receiving the halothane-azetropic mixture, WYANT (1963) observed hypotension, defined as a 25% decrease from pressures recorded immediately prior to the onset of hypotension, in 40% of patients during induction and 10% during maintenance.

DÉRY et al. (1964) detected a "very slight" (17 torr) decrease in arterial pressure during azeotrope anesthesia in 20 spontaneously ventilating unpremedicated patients undergoing surgery. Anesthesia was delivered by mask. WYANT (1960) in seven normal volunteer subjects felt that the azeotrope mixture had less of an effect on arterial pressure than did halothane alone. Light anesthesia produced no changes in mean arterial pressure, while deep surgical anesthesia decreased arterial pressure to 70—80 torr. JOHNSTONE et al. (1961) noted a further decline in arterial pressure when azeotrope was substituted for halothane-oxygen in patients. RAVENTOS and DEE (1959) observed no difference in arterial pressure response between halothane and halothane-ether. In both of these studies, the concentration of halothane in the halothane-ether mixture was equivalent to that when halothane alone was given. For a rigid comparison of these two agents, equipotent levels would have to be determined for the azeotrope and halothane. This is impossible for the azetrope with present techniques, since the uptake characteristics of ether and halothane are disparate. Thus, except for extremely long anesthesia, no constant ratio of alveolar or arterial concentrations could be obtained. Therefore, an azeotrope "MAC" either cannot be determined or cannot be applied.

3. Heart Rate

Changes in heart rate are not so consistent as changes in arterial pressure or cardiac output. The effect of anesthetics on heart rate seems more dependent on initial values, which in the animals studied have ranged from 40 to over 200.

ASHER and FREDERICKSON (1962) noted that the effect of halothane on the isolated perfused (LANGENDORF) rabbit heart was unpredictable except at very high concentrations, when depression of heart rate always occurred. BURN et al. (1957), using the heart-lung preparation, found that 1% halothane increased the rate from 150—160; 2% brought it back to 148.

RAVENTOS (1956) noted in premedicated monkeys, dogs, cats and rabbits a decrease in heart rate from 130—170 beats per minute down to 120—140 beats per minute. The premedicated horse shows no decrease in heart rate during administration of halothane-oxygen (EBERLY et al., 1968), but has a control heart rate of only 40. NGAI and BOLME [1966 (1)] observed a decrease from 126 down to 90 and 89 at light and deep halothane-oxygen anesthesia in dogs. HAMILTON et al. (1966) found a lesser change in dogs previously anesthetized with thiopental-succinylcholine. The rates for control and MAC 1, 2, and 3 were 146, 146, 132, and 131. SMITH and CORBASCIO [1966 (1)] observed a biphasic response in heart rate to halothane-oxygen and to halothane-nitrous oxide-oxygen in unpremedicated dogs induced with thiopental. Heart rate increased at lower concentrations and decreased at higher concentrations. However, the changes were only ±10% and were not significant.

In spontaneously breathing unpremedicated dogs, 2% halothane decreased heart rate from 135 down to 103; in dogs with controlled ventilation, the change was 124 down to 81. Trained, unpremedicated dogs (BLACKMORE et al., 1960) induced with halothane showed no change in heart rate at 1.5—2% halothane. Halothane produced no change in heart rate in dogs induced with thiopental-succinylcholine (GALINDO and BALDWIN, 1963). In open-chest dogs (REIN et al., 1963) under chloralose anesthesia, values for heart rate at control and 0.5, 1.0, 1.5 and 2.0% halothane were 167, 161, 148, 140 and 134. Increasing halothane to 2.5% in dogs already anesthetized with 0.8% halothane increased heart rate from 95—119 (THEYE and SESSLER, 1967). LI et al. (1968) in open-chest dogs, prepared during pentobarbital anesthesia, chloralose anesthesia, or both, noted a decrease in heart rate from 170 to 142 beats per minute under halothane anesthesia. DOBKIN et al. (1962) in dogs premedicated with perphenazine and induced with thiopental noted a decreased heart rate after 90 min of 2% halothane in oxygen.

Bradycardia was noted almost exclusively in the early reports on humans (JOHNSTONE, 1956; BRYCE-SMITH and O'BRIEN, 1956; BURNS et al., 1957). The considerably lower incidence of bradycardia reported in later papers and in studies on normal subjects suggests either that atropine premedication has successfully antagonized halothane bradycardia, that lower and more predictable concentrations of halothane are being used with the advent of precision vaporizers, and/or that induction has not been so rapid. The last two would tend to avoid excessively high concentrations of halothane.

Heart rate did not change in patients with heart disease, premedicated with a lytic cocktail, and given halothane-nitrous oxide-oxygen, halothane-oxygen, or halothane-air (LUNDBORG et al., 1967). Fifteen unpremedicated patients studied by BLACK et al. (1959) showed no change in heart rate under halothane anesthesia. In 16 patients premedicated with meperidine-scopolamine, halothane decreased heart rate by ten beats per minute. ALLARIA et al. (1967) noted no decrease in heart rate in six patients induced with thiopental-succinylcholine. Fifty pre-medicated patients who received halothane (BAMFORTH et al., 1960) showed a tendency towards a slight bradycardia, but this was not so pronounced as in 50 similar patients receiving chloroform. In two retrospective studies (MOYERS and PITTINGER, 1959; COPPOLINO, 1963), 250 patients receiving halothane showed no overall change in heart rate.

Ten volunteer unpremedicated subjects (MORSE et al., 1963) spontaneously breathing 1.5—2.0% halothane showed no change in heart rate. Heart rate showed a variable response in normal volunteer subjects anesthetized with halothane-oxygen, after breathing 100% oxygen. Ventilation was controlled (EGER et al., 1968). Heart rate rose from 65 to 80 in ten normal volunteer subjects premedicated with intravenous atropine or scopolamine and given halothane in air (VIRTUE et al., 1962). Fluroxene had been given 42 min prior to the halothane as part of the same study. ELLIOTT et al. (1968) induced ten normal subjects with thiopental-succinylcholine. Ventilation was spontaneous and the subjects were intubated. After 25 min of 2% halothane vaporizer concentration, heart rate had decreased from 86.8 to 64.0. WALKER et al. [1962 (1, 2)] noted a slight decrease in heart rate from 68 to 65 in five normal volunteer spontaneously ventilating patients induced with thiopental-succinylcholine and maintained with 1.5% halothane. The trachea was sprayed with 6% cocaine. Measurements were taken after 35 min of steady-state anesthesia. Bradycardia was observed in WYANT's normal volunteer subjects (1958) induced with thiopental. Hypotension in these studies was greater than that usually seen in clinical anesthesia, arterial pressure decreasing to 25 torr. Transition from air or 100% oxygen to halothane-oxygen in normal patients produced a decrease in heart rate of 10—12% (SHINOZAKI et al., 1968).

a) Extra-Anesthetic Factors

Heart rate went down from 164 to 151 upon administration of halothane to dogs induced with thiamylal (FABIAN et al., 1962). Bleeding of 30% of the blood volume increased heart rate to 178.

MUNCHOW and DENSON (1965) constructed a dose-response curve for the effect of atropine on heart rate in human adults, using a cumulative 15-min infusion. Regression equations for both negative and positive chronotropic sections of the dose-response curve were calculated. Halothane-nitrous oxide shifted the acce-leration part of the curve to the left, while almost eliminating the deceleration part. The presence of nitrous oxide may have contributed to the tachycardia: we have observed a striking tachycardia in subjects receiving hexamethonium and halothane-oxygen when nitrous oxide was added to the inspired mixture.

b) Adaptation

Heart rate did not change in spontaneously ventilating subjects given halo-thane-oxygen for 44 min. After 73 min, it had increased 10%, accounting for all the recovery of cardiac output described above (DEUTSCH et al., 1962). In WENTHE's study (1962), light-deep-light halothane anesthesia was administered. Heart rate decreased 20, 17, and 14% in succession. Thus the same heart rate compensation with time is seen. EGER et al. (1968) found either no change or a slight increase in rate with time at any given end-tidal halothane concentration.

c) Induction

EISELE (1969) observed a decrease in heart rate during the first ten breaths of halothane-oxygen administered to trained dogs. Heart rate increased during the first 3 min of halothane-oxygen administered to unpremedicated human volunteers

[Smith et al., 1968 (1)]. The maximum increase was 27%. Maruyama et al. (1966) noted a 24 beat-per-minute drop in heart rate during the first 9 min of induction with halothane in five infants and children.

d) Mechanisms

The causes of the changes in heart rate observed with halothane are still open to question. Many investigators and clinicians have been able to reverse brady-cardia associated with halothane by using atropine (Breakstone, 1962; Shinozaki et al., 1968; Wyant et al., 1958; Farman, 1967) or gallamine (Smith et al., 1967). Atropine administered before halothane-oxygen induction completely prevented bradycardia in normal volunteer patients (Farman, 1967).

Yet halothane decreased heart rate in the spinal vagotomized dog (Kohli et al., 1966) and in the spontaneously beating perfused frog (Krantz et al., 1958), toad (Nayler, 1959) or cat heart [Purchase, 1966 (2)]. The heart rate was lowered in heart-lung preparations, taken either from normal or from reserpine-pretreated dogs (Flacke and Alper, 1962) and in cardiac denervated dogs (Morrow et al., 1961). High doses of atropine had no effect in this situation. Pretreatment with reserpine or guanethidine (Rein et al., 1963) produced a consistently greater degree of negative chronotropy in dogs, and addition of propranolol during halothane anesthesia in dogs (Craythorne and Huffington, 1966) decreased heart rate by 13 beats. These data are consistent with a direct negative chronotropic action of halothane on the sino-atrial pacemaker tissue.

Information gleaned from isolated perfused cat heart preparations [Purchase, 1966 (2)] indicates that halothane may produce the following sequence of events: (1) sinus bradycardia, (2) atrio-ventricular nodal rhythm, (3) complete antegrade and retrograde atrio-ventricular nodal block, (4) atrio-ventricular dissociation, and (5) asystole. Hauswirth and Shaer (1967), studying membrane potentials from isolated sino-atrial tissue of rabbits, observed that halothane decreased velocity of diastolic depolarization as well as maximal diastolic potential. The former effect would tend to decrease atrial rate, the latter to increase it. Depending on which of these mechanisms prevailed, acceleration or deceleration of individual isolated atria occurred in this study. These observations may in part explain the diverse responses seen in intact animals.

e) Halothane-Ether Azeotrope

The azeotropic mixture appeared to induce bradycardia in all of the studies in which heart rate was recorded (Raventos and Dee, 1959; Déry et al., 1964; Wyant et al., 1963).

4. Stroke Volume

Surprisingly, few of the investigators who took the trouble to measure cardiac output, went further to make the simple calculation of stroke volume. The majority of those who did saw that most of the decrease in cardiac output was due to a decrease in stroke volume [Eger and Hügin, 1961; Deutsch et al., 1962; Eger et al., 1968; Lundborg et al., 1966; Theye and Sessler, 1967; Allaria et al., 1967; Eberly et al., 1968; Severinghaus and Cullen, 1958; Smith and Corbascio, 1966 (1)] in the horse, dog and human. Shinozaki et al. (1968) saw an equal influence of heart rate and stroke volume on cardiac output during halothane anesthesia and felt that much of the decrease in stroke volume was due to the high concentration of oxygen usually used with halothane. Switching from air to 100% oxygen in awake subjects will, of course, produce a slight bradycardia.

WENTHE et al. (1962) in subjects, and HAMILTON et al. (1966) in dogs, detected an influence of heart rate on cardiac output at deeper levels of halothane.

WALKER et al. [1962 (1, 2)], noted no change in stroke volume in five normal spontaneously ventilating patients induced with thiopental-succinylcholine and maintained with 1.5% halothane, although there was a decrease in cardiac output.

a) Adaptation

The increase in cardiac output seen by DEUTSCH et al. (1962) with continued administration of halothane-oxygen was not influenced by stroke volume. However, in EGER's subjects (1968) part of the cardiac output adaptation was due to an increase in this variable.

b) Induction

EISELE (1969) detected a slight decrease in stroke volume during the first ten breaths of 3% halothane in oxygen administered to trained dogs. SMITH (1968) noted an increase of 17% during the first 3 min of halothane in unpremedicated human volunteers.

5. Total Peripheral Resistance

Total peripheral resistance is obtained by dividing cardiac output into the difference between mean arterial and right atrial pressures. As might be expected, since halothane usually decreases both arterial pressure and cardiac output, changes in total peripheral resistance are not so pronounced. In fact, increases (McGREGOR et al., 1958; SHIMOSATO and ETSTEN, 1963; SEVERINGHAUS and CULLEN, 1958; KUBOTA, 1962), decreases [WYANT et al., 1958; EGER et al., 1968; DEUTSCH et al.,1962; SMITH, 1968; THEYE, 1967; MORROW and MORROW, 1961; WALKER et al., 1962 (1, 2); PAYNE, 1959; WALKER, 1962] and no change [SHINO-ZAKI et al., 1968; LUNDBORG et al., 1966; WENTHE et al., 1962; EGER and HÜGIN, 1961; SMITH, 1968 (1); THEYE and SESSLER, 1967; VIRTUE et al., 1962] have all been reported.

The concomitant use of nitrous oxide seems to be an important factor in determining the influence of halothane on total peripheral resistance. With one exception (THEYE and SESSLER, 1967) those investigators who used halothane-oxygen noted a decrease in total peripheral resistance. In this exception, the comparison was made between 0.8 and 2.5% halothane, rather than between no halothane and halothane. This distinction may be important, since EGER et al. (1968), in comparing different levels of halothane anesthesia in man, noted a slight increase in total peripheral resistance as concentration increased, although total peripheral resistance at low concentrations was significantly less than control. Furthermore, the same investigators (THEYE, 1967) who had observed the one exception, in a later study noted a decrease when halothane-oxygen was used.

When nitrous oxide was used in the anesthetic mixture, total peripheral resistance either increased or did not change. SMITH and CORBASCIO [1966 (1)] in comparing the effects of halothane-oxygen with halothane nitrous oxide-oxygen in dogs, noted a decrease in total peripheral resistance when halothane-oxygen was administered, but no change when halothane-nitrous oxide-oxygen was administered on a different occasion to the same animals. Later, in studies on volunteer subjects, SMITH et al. [1968 (2)] showed that the addition of nitrous oxide to halothane-oxygen produced an increase in total peripheral resistance; subsequent withdrawal of nitrous oxide returned the total peripheral resistance to its level just prior to the addition of nitrous oxide. Serum norepinephrine levels were increased by the addition of nitrous oxide, indicating that much of the effect of the nitrous oxide could have been due to the release of catecholamines.

6. Central Venous Pressure

Virtue et al. (1962) measured central venous pressure in ten normal volunteer subjects premedicated with intravenoulsy administered atropine or scopolamine. Fluroxene had been given 42 min prior to the halothane as part of the same study. Sufficient halothane in air was given to maintain electroencephalographic level 4. Central venous pressure went from 7.7 to 9.0 torr, not a significant difference. Eger et al. (1968) in normal subjects found a rise in right atrial pressure which was linearly related to end-tidal halothane concentrations. At any given concentration, the pressure remained constant or fell slightly with time.

Morrow and Pierce (1968) studied the acute effects of halothane on systemic venous reflex reactivity in dogs. The venous bed was isolated in ten dogs by simultaneously occluding the pulmonary artery, aorta, and each vena cava, and by opening an aortic cannula into a heparinized reservoir. Changes in caval pressure were measured during 56 episodes of total circulatory arrest, and used as control values for comparison with the changes seen after the addition of an inspired halothane concentration of 2% for 2 min. Caval pressure rose abruptly with the onset of total circulatory arrest. A secondary pressure rise occurred after 10—12 sec and continued until circulatory arrest was stopped. The mean control plateau pressures were 6.95 torr in the inferior vena cava, and 8.32 torr in the superior vena cava; during halothane they were 6.25 and 7.19, respectively. The decrease in inferior vena caval pressure during halothane was significant. The decrease in secondary pressure rise in the inferior vena cava was significant, but the change in the pressure rise in the superior vena cava was not. These changes in venous tone are part of the etiology of the hypotensive response to halothane in patients, particularly those with hypovolemia. It is noteworthy that they took place to such an extent within 2 min from the onset of anesthesia.

B. Regional Blood Flow

1. Pulmonary Circulation

Stirling et al. (1960) measured mean pulmonary artery pressure in three dogs submitted to a constant rate of cardiac inflow (100 ml/kg/min). Pulmonary artery pressure rose from 20 to 30 torr after 30 min of 2% halothane vaporizer concentration. Since right atrial (and hence probably left atrial) pressure rose by the same amount, some of the increase in pulmonary artery pressure could have reflected that of the left atrium.

Wyant et al. (1958) measured pulmonary artery pressures in five normal unpremedicated subjects induced with thiamylal. Pulmonary artery pressure and vascular resistance remained stable until extreme systemic hypotension (down to 25 torr systolic) was produced. At this time, pressure fell slightly, while resistance rose markedly from 60—140 up to 130—150 dyne-sec-cm^{-5}.

2. Coronary Blood Flow

Long and Pittinger (1958) observed that in the isolated rabbit heart, halothane increased coronary blood flow, an effect which they interpreted as being a direct favorable action of halothane on coronary smooth muscle. A transient (20—30 min) increase in coronary blood flow has been noted in the isolated cat heart at a constant perfusing pressure of 40 torr [Purchase, 1966 (2)]. In the canine heart-lung preparation, halothane increased coronary blood flow at a time when cardiac work remained unchanged (ALPER et al., 1967; FLACKE et al., 1963).

In intact dogs, on the other hand [BAGWELL, 1965; ALPER et al., 1967; PHILIPPART, 1963; MERIN and ROSENBLUM, 1967; SAITO, 1965; SAITO et al., 1966 (2)] coronary flow decreased during halothane anesthesia. BAGWELL (1965), using an electromagnetic flowmeter, noted a decrease in coronary flow, *pari passu* with a decrease in arterial pressure. GOLDBERG [1968 (2)] and MERIN and ROSENBLUM (1967) have observed a concomitant decrease in coronary flow and myocardial oxygen consumption.

On the basis of excess lactate studies (BAGWELL, 1965), it has been suggested that, although coronary blood flow is diminished, it is adequate for the needs of the myocardium. THEYE (1967) measured myocardial minute oxygen consumption in dogs. When halothane was changed from 0.1—0.9%, $\dot{V}_{O_2}$ decreased 5%. This decrease was directly related to the degree of decrease in cardiac output and arterial pressure and was considered to represent an indirect depressant effect. MERIN (1969) measured oxygen and substrate uptake, as well as myocardial blood flow (Kr 85) in the *in situ* dog heart. Myocardial blood flow, oxygen uptake, and left ventricular stroke work decreased significantly when very light halothane was changed to very deep halothane. He observed no evidence of myocardial hypoxia: myocardial excess lactate changed from positive in the control period to negative in the depressed state. There was very little glucose uptake in either state, and an elevated myocardial threshold for glucose was demonstrated. Fatty acid and pyruvate uptake decreased, while lactate uptake remained unchanged. He concluded that no deleterious effect of deep halothane was seen on the heart itself. In an attempt to investigate the apparent block of myocardial glucose uptake by halothane, MERIN (1970) induced hyperglycemia in a further series of eight dogs. In spite of a blood glucose level of 150—450 mg-%, there was little glucose uptake during either light or deep halothane anesthesia. The cause-effect relationship between this phenomenon and the myocardial depression seen with halothane could not be established by these investigations.

3. Renal Circulation

Multiple factors have been implicated in attempting to explain the effects of general anesthesia on renal function. These include the secretion of antidiuretic hormone (ADH), aldosterone, and catecholamines (BACHMAN, 1955; LLAURADO, 1957; NELSON et al., 1961); decreased cardiac output, systolic and renal arterial pressure, and total peripheral resistance (SHIPLEY and STUDY, 1950, 1951; THOMPSON and PITTS, 1952; BERNE and LEVY, 1950, 1952; LYNN and SHACKMAN, 1951); peripheral shunting of systemic blood volume with renal vasoconstriction (PAPPER and NGAI, 1956); changes in body temperature and acid-base balance (SEGAR et al., 1956; HUTCHIN et al., 1961); and underhydration (MAZZE et al., 1963).

FABIAN et al. (1962) measured renal blood flow with an electromagnetic flowmeter in dogs anesthetized with thiamylal. Neither cyclopropane nor halothane produced a significant decrease in renal blood flow. Hemorrhage of 30% of the blood volume caused a 50% decrease in renal blood flow at a lower arterial pressure than does cyclopropane. BOSOMWORTH et al. (1963) studied dogs under cyclopropane and halothane anesthesia. No control values were given. Renal blood flow was measured with an electromagnetic flowmeter. They observed that 10% cyclopropane produced a significantly lower renal blood flow than did 0.6% halothane. They could not detect a significant difference in the influence of either agent on renal blood flow when blood volume was decreased by 30%, nor on the per cent blood volume remaining when renal blood flow ceased. BLACKMORE et al. (1960), in trained, unpremedicated, well-hydrated dogs observed a significant decrease in glomerular filtration rate, renal plasma flow, and urine flow during 1 h of 2% halothane. During the following hour at 1.5% halothane, glomerular filtration rate and renal plasma flow returned towards control values. They concluded that there was a correlation between the cardiovascular and renal responses to halothane, and that, in sufficient concentration, halothane has a significant but reversible action on renal function.

MILLER et al. (1965), in anesthetized patients during surgery, concluded that the depression of glomerular filtration rate by halothane bore no obvious direct relationship to arterial pressure. In a later study (MILLER et al., 1966) they investigated unpremedicated patients during surgery. Although no statistics were given, the authors suggested that glomerular filtration rate did have a direct relation to arterial pressure. MAZZE et al. (1963) investigated premedicated (morphine and scopolamine) patients during halothane anesthesia and surgery. They felt that the decrease in urinary volume and sodium excretion during halothane anesthesia may be entirely due to the decrease in glomerular filtration rate and renal plasma flow. They suggested that these changes may be prevented by the prophylactic administration of saline or hypertonic mannitol. BARRY et al. (1964) in patients premedicated with morphine and scopolamine and observed during surgery, noted that hydration with 0.3% saline solution did, in fact, allow effective renal plasma flow and glomerular filtration to be maintained during light (0.5 to 1.0% vaporizer concentration) halothane anesthesia. Deeper anesthesia (1.2—3.0% halothane) abolished the differences between the two groups, that is, the same depression of renal plasma flow and glomerular filtration rate occurred with and without hydration.

The most useful report to date is that by DEUTSCH et al. (1966). In studies on normal, unpremedicated volunteer subjects, halothane decreased glomerular filtration rate 19% and effective renal plasma flow 38%. Renal vascular resistance and filtration fraction were increased 69 and 39%, respectively. These results suggest that some renal vasoconstriction occurred, particularly in the efferent arterioles. During a water diuresis produced with 4% fructose, the inhalation of 1.5% halothane decreased urine volume by more than 90%, decreased free water clearance to negative values, and cut sodium excretion to 40% of control. Ethanol administration markedly increased urine volume and restored free water clearance, but did not significantly affect sodium clearance. These data strongly suggest ADH liberation during administration of halothane, a finding in agreement with that of CRISTOFORO and BRODY [1968 (2); see Peripheral (Limb) Circulation].

4. Splanchnic Circulation

MIDDLETON et al. (1966) studied the effects of a high concentration of halothane on the isolated, perfused, bovine liver. Exposure to 3% halothane for 3 h produced no demonstrable biochemical change, except for a temporary decrease in oxygen uptake by the liver. The administration of 5—6% halothane was associated with a further decrease in oxygen consumption, manifested by an even greater increase in venous oxygen pressure.

BOETTNER et al. (1965) studied dogs placed on cardiopulmonary bypass after administration of pentobarbital-gallamine. They noted a parallel decrease in systemic and splanchnic blood flows. There was no apparent shift of flow to or from the splanchnic circulation.

AHLGREN et al. (1966, 1967) estimated hepatic blood flow in dogs by calculating the disappearance rate of Xenon 132 injected into the portal vein. The administration of 1—3% halothane, under conditions of adequate alveolar ventilation, minimal changes in Pa_{CO_2}, and no hypoxia, produced a decrease in hepatic blood flow paralleling the changes in cardiac output. If Pa_{CO_2} was allowed to increase during deep halothane anesthesia, an even more pronounced decrease in hepatic blood flow occurred. GALINDO (1965) noted a decrease in canine hepatic blood flow and hepatic arterial vascular resistance with most anesthetic agents studied, including halothane. He also confirmed the relation between systemic circulatory changes and hepatic flow. In another study, GALINDO et al. (1963) stated that halothane anesthesia under normal conditions decreased hepatic blood flow, as measured by electromagnetic flowmeters. Inhalation of carbon dioxide increased hepatic artery and portal vein flow during halothane anesthesia, but produced a further decrease in hepatic blood flow during chloroform. Metabolic acidosis played an important role in decreasing hepatic blood flow in all experimental conditions.

Studies in man have essentially confirmed the above results. EPSTEIN (1966) and EPSTEIN et al. (1966) observed in normal unpremedicated subjects that halothane decreased splanchnic blood flow as measured by the Fick principle, using indocyanine green. In contrast to that produced by cyclopropane, this decrease in blood flow was due to arterial hypotension rather than to an increase in vascular resistance. Indeed, there was some evidence for a decrease in vascular tone. Respiratory acidosis, instead of increasing vascular resistance, decreased it. They therefore felt that hepatic ischemia (MORRIS and FELDMAN, 1963) should not be invoked to explain the increased incidence of hepatic damage after respiratory acidosis incurred during halothane inhalation. In another phase of this study, it was found that the institution of controlled ventilation produced a significant decrease in flow and a significant increase in vascular resistance. They thought that this effect might have been mechanical, that is, due to active compression of the liver by the diaphragm.

PRICE et al. (1966), in normal unpremedicated subjects, determined that this decrease in hepatic flow did not cause a critical decrease in the availability of oxygen to the splanchnic viscera. Splanchnic oxygen utilization was not consistently affected, and restoration of flow to initial levels gave no clear evidence that an oxygen debt had been incurred during the period of decreased flow. Excess lactate was produced by the splanchnic viscera during cyclopropane, but not during halothane anesthesia.

5. Cerebral Circulation

GALINDO and BALDWIN (1963) studied dogs induced with thiopental and paralyzed with succinylcholine. Internal carotid blood flow was measured with an electromagnetic flowmeter. During administration of halothane through a non-calibrated vaporizer, vessel blood flow increased 25.8%, vascular resistance decreased 56.4%, and cerebral spinal fluid pressure increased 79.2%. McDOWALL et al. (1966) used the Kr 85 clearance rate from exposed cerebral cortex to measure local cortical blood flow in dogs prepared under thiopental-nitrous oxide-succinyl-choline. They noted a mean decrease of 46% in cerebral blood flow (CBF), an increase in cerebral vascular resistance (CVR) of 50% and a decrease in cerebral oxygen uptake ($CMRO_2$) of 49%. The changes in flow and resistance were felt to be secondary to the decrease in $CMRO_2$. In later studies, on the other hand, McDOWALL (1967) observed a dose-related vasodilating effect of halothane. CBF increased in spite of decreases in perfusion pressure. Reductions in CVR were thought to be due both to autoregulation, which tended to prevent a decrease in

flow when perfusion pressure dropped, and to direct vasodilating effects of halothane, which tended to increase flow above control levels. Although these mechanisms achieved their maximum with 4% halothane, flow was not increased at
this concentration because of the large decrease in perfusion pressure. Using
chronically implanted heat conductivity probes, Schmahl (1965) detected an
increase in blood flow to the thalamus or hypothalamus with 1.9% halothane,
in spite of decreased perfusion pressure.

Indirect evidence for a decrease in cerebral circulatory perfusing pressure in
man was noted by Farmati et al. (1967), who observed that retinal systolic and
diastolic pressures decreased in children at the same time that systemic arterial
pressure was constant.

Wollman et al. (1964), in an excellent study, used Kr 85 for the inert gas
method in normal unpremedicated volunteer subjects. With 1.2% halothane in
oxygen (nonrebreathing system) at normocarbia, mean total CBF was 50.8 ml/
100 g/min, an increase of 14% over control measurements obtained in the awake
state. Perfusion pressure decreased 32% and cerebral vascular resistance decreased
42%. A modification of the inert gas technique also has been used to study humans.
(McHenry et al., 1965). Blood isotope concentrations were measured during the
period of desaturation, that is, after cessation of isotope inhalation. Compared to
control measurements taken while the subjects were breathing room air, 1% halothane plus 50% nitrous oxide in oxygen (semi-closed circle system) lowered cerebral
vascular resistance 43%, from 1.68 to 0.95 torr/ml/100 g/min. Mean arterial
pressure fell 13% (to 76 mmHg) and cerebral blood flow increased 64%. The
Pa_{CO_2}, however, had increased to 47.4 torr.

Alexander et al. (1964) studied the effects on CBF of changing Pa_{CO_2} during
halothane anesthesia in unpremedicated volunteer subjects. Mean end-tidal halothane concentration for all subjects was 0.98%. Alveolar minute volume was
maintained constant, while inhaled CO_2 concentration was varied so that Pa_{CO_2}
ranged between 19 and 56 torr. Cerebral blood flow varied linearly with Pa_{CO_2}
under the conditions of this study. In comparing their results with others obtained
during the awake state, they noted that the shape of the Pa_{CO_2} response curve
was altered by the vasodilation which occurred during halothane.

Christensen et al. (1967) studied unpremedicated subjects induced and maintained with halothane. The mean cerebral blood flow was 54.4 ml/100 g/min
during 1% halothane in oxygen, compared with a control value of 43. Cerebral
vascular resistance decreased 26%, a-v O_2 difference 40%, and cerebral cortical
oxygen uptake 26%. Ten additional subjects were studied during anesthesia plus
induced hypotension (up to 62% decrease below control values), hypercapnia (up
to 57 torr), or both. Cerebral blood flow increased slightly with the combination
of all three, while cerebral vascular resistance decreased by a mean of 55%.
Maintenance of normocapnia with hypotension did not alter the decrease in cerebral vascular resistance. Maintenance of normotension with hypercapnia produced
a marked increase in cerebral blood flow to 192% of the control level. However,
in two subjects with clinical evidence of cerebral vascular disease, cerebral vascular
resistance decreased to the same low level present during hypotension.

6. Peripheral (Limb) Circulation

One of the earliest studies on limb circulation was performed by Burn and
Epstein (1959) who perfused the canine hind limb with blood from a donor animal.
When the lungs of the donor dog were ventilated with a mixture containing halothane, blood pressure in the recipient's iliac artery decreased and venous outflow
from the limb increased. This suggests that halothane caused a nonneurogenically

mediated vasodilation. LINDGREN et al. (1964) studied skinned cat limbs, the paws of which were ligated. They observed a decrease in muscle blood flow (both arterial and venous) and a slight, but consistent increase in vascular resistance. Later, these same investigators (LINDGREN et al., 1965) noted in cats increased skin flow and a decreased cutaneous vascular resistance. NGAI and BOLME [1966 (1)], measuring flow and resistance in the external iliac artery during chronic dog experiments, found that halothane could increase, and certainly did not decrease, vascular resistance in the limb.

The above observations contrast with those of EMERSON and MASSION (1967), who found that with the head included in the circulation, and with nervous and arterial connections intact, total limb flow would always increase, in spite of the large decrease in perfusion pressure. Conceivably, such findings may be related to either a reduction (BLACK and MCARDLE, 1962; LINDGREN et al., 1965) or absence (AKESTER and BRODY, 1967) of change in vascular resistance. EMERSON and MASSION (1967) studied the effects of halothane on the vascular resistance of the dog forelimb, both innervated and denervated, with natural (varying) or pump-controlled (constant) flow. They found that the decrease in limb resistance resulted primarily from a decrease in prevenous resistance. Similar results were found in denervated limbs; therefore, this vasodilation may not have been entirely dependent on limb vasomotor nerves, and may have been due in part to a direct relaxing effect of halothane. However, since blood which had been equilibrated with halothane in an *in vitro* (blood oxygenator) system did not affect vascular resistance, and since constant vasodilation was not achieved with a dog heart-lung-limb system, the effect of this agent on vascular smooth muscle may be primarily indirect. The data of EMERSON and MASSION still do not allow a direct effect of halothane, and in somewhat similar studies, CRISTOFORO and BRODY (1967), working with a totally isolated gracilis muscle preparation perfused with blood from a blood oxygenator, found that halothane produced vasodilation. However, when the head was included in the circulation, halothane produced vasoconstriction, even with all connections severed. This vasoconstriction was unaffected by the *alpha*-adrenergic blockade produced by the intra-arterial injection of phentolamine. In the same preparation these authors [CRISTOFORO and BRODY, 1968 (1)] subsequently noted that vasoconstrictor responses to local injection of norepinephrine were depressed significantly by halothane. Reflex vasoconstriction was depressed, while reflex vasodilation was unaffected. The use of pentobarbital, which is known to depress reflexes, and gallamine, which has some ganglionic blocking action in areas other than the cardiovagal junction, could have influenced their results. The authors believe that halothane caused liberation of vasopressin, which in turn produced vasoconstriction. The release of ADH by halothane in large quantities to produce limb vasoconstriction, if it occurred in man, could be cause for concern, since vasopressin is also a potent coronary vasoconstrictor.

Since neither CRISTOFORO and BRODY nor EMERSON and MASSION reported blood content of halothane, it is not possible to make meaningful comparisons of their results. Perhaps the most plausible conclusion at present is that halothane can decrease limb vascular resistance, probably by a combination of a direct effect at a prevenous site in both skin and muscle and by lowering normal vasoconstrictor tone. However, under certain circumstances vasopressin may be released, resulting in limb vasoconstriction. The nature of these special circumstances, however, remain to be elucidated.

BLACK and MCARDLE (1962) induced unpremedicated patients with thiopental and maintained them with nitrous oxide 75% plus oxygen. They obtained control readings after administration of thiopental. A decrease in forearm blood flow (venous occlusion plethysmograph) and vascular resistance occurred with halothane. Vasodilation was thought to be neurogenic, since it was abolished by nerve block. Halothane also interfered with the ability of norepinephrine to constrict peripheral vessels. Atropine administered intravenously produced a reversal of bradycardia and hypotension, an increase in forearm blood flow, and little alteration in vascular resistance. Atropine injected intra-arterially had no effect on forearm blood flow. Pauca and Sykes (1967) used a Whitney strain gauge plethysmogram to study forearm blood flow in patients. They tried to separate the influence of endotracheal intubation, surgery, premedication, and nitrous oxide. Thiopental-halothane decreased blood flow to the forearm. The other factors did not seem to exert any influence on forearm flow. Caffrey et al. (1965) noted that 1.2% inspired halothane reduced forearm blood flow, while 2—3.5% increased it. Readings were made before surgery in unpremedicated patients. No thiopental was used and ventilation was controlled to the degree necessary to maintain a normal P_{CO_2}. Forearm blood flow increased during induction with halothane (Taylor and Denson, 1967) (2.5 to 3.2 ml/100 ml tissue/min), fell (3.2 to 2.5) during deep anesthesia, and then steadily increased to 5.2 and remained at this level until and during emergence. Since the patients were studied before and during surgery, the influence of surgery and halothane on the later changes cannot be differentiated.

7. Microcirculation

Baez and Orkin studied the capillaries of the omentum of the dog and the mesoappendix of the rat (Murray et al., 1963). The administration of 0.8% halothane resulted in an increase both in spontaneous vasomotion and in sensitivity to topical epinephrine in the region of the precapillary sphincter and the metarterioles. There were no changes in either venular or arteriolar luminal diameter. With increasing halothane concentrations ranging from 0.8—2.0%, vascular activity, vasomotion, sensitivity to topical epinephrine, and venular blood flow were depressed in proportion to the anesthetic depth. Dilation of precapillary and postcapillary vessels, including small arteries and large collecting venules, also occurred. These results indicate that deep halothane anesthesia is associated with sluggish capillary blood flow and impairment of venous return.

In studying the ability of anesthetics to modify the microcirculatory hemodynamics of shock, Baez and Orkin (1964) subjected unanesthetized rats to rotating drum trauma. Following termination of the trauma, control data were obtained after tracheostomy, femoral artery cannulation, and exposure of the mesoappendix had been performed under pentobarbital and local anesthesia. During the next hour, the rats were exposed to halothane and additional observations were made. The administration of 0.7—1.0% halothane resulted in increased vascular reactivity to topically applied epinephrine. Vasomotion was enhanced initially, but began to decline towards the end of the experimental period. Venular hyperreactivity was also present but was not sustained. Initial arterial constriction returned towards control values after approximately 35—40 min. There were no changes in the diameters of the precapillary arterioles. The postcapillary venules dilated. Overall capillary flow appeared to be restricted, indicating an ischemic capillary bed. By the end of the experimental period, capillary sphincters began to open, and the initial ischemia appeared to be replaced by congestion. Apparently, halothane further increased vessel reactivity, which had been already elevated by the sublethal injury. These changes resulted in increased capillary flow, with the possibility of the development of increased capillary hydrostatic pressure favoring outward filtration of plasma. It appeared, however, that halo-thane maintained compensatory vascular patterns during sublethal trauma until late in the course of shock. Thus, while capillary blood flow may be impaired with deep halothane anesthesia, this does not necessarily occur with light levels of anesthesia. Furthermore, halothane does not reduce sensitivity to epinephrine, even in the presence of sublethal traumatic shock.

C. Myocardial Function

As mentioned in the introduction, any one of several variables have been proposed as a measurement of the state of myocardial inotropy. The effect of halothane on some of these variables will be described without further comment on the validity of the variables.

Early work by RAVENTOS (1956) showed a 50% inhibition of isotonic contrac-tion of the isolated tortoise atrium at a concentration of 39 mg-% halothane in Ringer's solution. Perfusion of the frog's heart with a fluid containing halothane 20 mg-% caused a moderate slowing and decrease in amplitude (KRANTZ et al., 1958). The isolated, spontaneously beating toad heart (NAYLER et al., 1959) also reacted to halothane by a decrease in rate and a weakening of the contractile force. ASHER and FREDERICKSON (1962) studied the effects of halothane on the isolated, perfused (LANGENDORF) rabbit heart. They noted a logarithmic dose-related de-pression of contraction.

GOLDBERG and ULLRICK (1967, 1968) studied the effects of halothane on iso-metric contractions of isolated trabeculae carneae of rats. Halothane concentra-tions in the perfusing solution were 0.10, 0.40, 1.65, and 2.35 vol-%. Peak de-veloped tension and maximum rate of tension development were decreased by as much as 53 and 57%, in direct proportion to the concentration of the anesthetic. Time to peak tension and total twitch duration were decreased by no more than 6.3%. Resting tension was affected only by the highest concentrations of halo-thane, which lowered it 6.8%. Relaxation time and muscle length were not altered. These experiments indicated a direct effect of halothane on isolated myocardium, apart from any circulatory, neurogenic, or hormonal influences. Because the decrease in peak tension was coupled to a parallel and proportional decrease in the rate of tension development, the authors concluded that the cardiac effects of halothane were primarily due to decreased active state intensity of the contractile elements of heart muscle.

GOLDBERG [1968 (1)] and GOLDBERG and PHEAR (1968) performed an extensive analysis of the changes in mechanical properties of isolated rat trabeculae carneae muscle produced by halothane. These later studies used different techniques than those outlined above. Instead of studying pure isometric contractions, they used a lever arrangement which allowed isometric contraction against a preload and isotonic contraction against a constant load (preload plus afterload). The cal-culated velocity of shortening at zero load (V_{max}) and the calculated maximal contraction at zero velocity (P_0) were both depressed by halothane in a dose-related fashion. Therefore, the force-velocity curve was shifted to the left and downward. Peak work, power, and developed tension were also depressed. From a theoretical viewpoint, the decrease in V_{max} could mean that both the maximum relative motion of thin and thick filaments and the rate of cyclic making and breaking of cross-bridges between filaments were depressed. However, the me-chanical equivalents of the rate of production of shortening energy per unit change in load and the amount of heat produced per unit of shortening (both estimated indirectly), were not reduced. Therefore, they concluded that the abnormality in cardiac muscle contraction in the presence of halothane was related to a defect in the utilization rather than in the liberation of energy. This implies that halothane affects the contractile elements by an indirect rather than a direct mechanism. Consistent with this hypothesis is the lack of alteration in both the extent of shortening of unloaded muscle and the instantaneous velocity of contractile element shortening at the time of the greatest decrease in development of tension. Possible indirect mechanisms could be related to excitation-contraction coupling, decreased availability of some essential substrate or ion such as a high energy phosphate compound or calcium, or decreased ability of cardiac myofibrils to hydrolyze ATP. Alterations of these variables could conceivably be the basis of the decrease in active state intensity coexisting with the absence of change in certain measurements of contractile element functions. BRODKIN et al. (1967) did observe that halothane decreased the ATPase activity of both myocardial and skeletal muscle myofibrillar preparations. These results support the last of the above hypotheses. GOLDBERG (1968) investigated the influence of external calcium concentration on the time required for an interpolated beat to achieve the same tension produced by the preceding normal beat (restitution curves) in the presence and absence of halothane. He found that the myocardial depression produced by halothane could be reversed by increasing the external calcium concentration. He suggested that this finding constituted indirect evidence that halothane might decrease the availability of intracellular calcium at a critical site in the vicinity of the contractile proteins.

BROWN and CROUT (unpublished data) have performed a study comparing inhalation anesthetic agents at equipotent levels. They determined MAC for ether, cyclopropane, methoxyflurane, halothane, and Ethrane in the cat and perfused isometrically contracting papillary muscles at these concentrations. All agents produced the same *qualitative* changes in isometric contraction: (1) depression of peak developed tension, (2) depression of dP/dt, (3) reduction in total time of contraction and time to peak tension, and (4) little change in the ratio of integrated force-time during contraction to total integrated force-time. *Quantitative* data, however, revealed considerable differences. When examined at equianalgesic concentrations, the five anesthetics depressed contraction unequally. In order of least to most depressant, the observed rank was ether, cyclopropane, methoxyflurane, halothane, Ethrane. Linear regression equations describing the log dose-response curves showed no differences in slope among those anesthetics. Responses to the anesthetics and log dose-response curves were not altered by the presence of 5.2×10^{-6} M of the *beta*-adrenergic blocking agent propranolol in the bath.

GOLDBERG and PHEAR (1969) studied the effects of halothane and paired electrical stimulation on isotonic contractions of isolated rat trabeculae carneae muscle. The two agents showed qualitatively opposite effects on extent of shortening and maximal rates of shortening and relaxation, essentially cancelling each other out. However, the decrease in diastolic compliance produced by halothane was not compensated for completely by paired stimulation. Decreased diastolic compliance means that smaller end-diastolic fiber length results at any given ventricular filling pressure, or a higher pressure at any given end-diastolic fiber length. This phenomenon could contribute to the depressed ventricular function curves seen with halothane.

CRAYTHORNE (1968) examined the effects of halothane on the relation between myocardial tension and frequency of contraction. When the interval between contractions is sufficiently long (300 sec), the strength of the subsequent heartbeat is not influenced by the previous beat. This "resting state contraction" was depressed by halothane. A very short interval between beats is associated with a decrease in tension: "negative inotropic effect of activation". As the interval between beats increases, there is an increase in tension: "positive inotropic effect of activation". Halothane lessened the positive inotropic effect but heightened the negative one. Tension decreased as rate of stimulation decreased from 150 to 30 impulses/min. If the tension at a given rate was plotted as a percentage of control at the same rate, the variance was less marked. The higher the concentration of anesthetic used, the smaller the variation of tension with rate.

AWALT and FREDERICKSON (1964) observed the expected decrease in peak developed tension in rabbit atria exposed to 1 and 1.5% halothane. However, amplitude and duration of the transmembrane action potential were not changed by halothane. They concluded that the effects of halothane on excitable tissue are not the result of primary alterations at the level of the cell membrane, and that halothane penetrates the membrane and exerts its depressant effect on contraction at some point within the cell.

PARADISE and GRIFFITH administered halothane for 2 h in sufficient quantity to produce and maintain a 50% decrease in the force of contraction of isolated rabbit atria (PARADISE and GRIFFITH, 1965). They could detect no resulting change in tissue concentration of potassium. In later studies (PARADISE and GRIFFITH, 1966), they showed a decrease in potassium and an increase in sodium content of rat ventricles perfused under the same conditions. Although anoxia and halothane produced similar changes in electrolyte concentrations, the authors felt that the two agents induced different biochemical changes in heart cells because: (1) force of contraction recovered more quickly and completely after exposure to halothane than after anoxia, (2) anoxia produced a gain in total water, and halothane did not, and (3) the coronary perfusion rate increased with anoxia but not with halothane.

FLACKE and ALPER (1962), using the canine heart-lung preparation, demonstrated the negative inotropic effect of halothane at concentrations greater than 1%. Their criteria were a rapid increase in atrial pressure and decrease in systemic output. Concentrations of 0.25 and 0.50% did not affect the heart. In a later investigation, ALPER and FLACKE (1963) compared the response of the halothane-anesthetized heart-lung preparation to augmentation in stroke work caused by an increased output (volume work) versus the augmentation caused by increased pressure (pressure work). Ventricular function curves were constructed. They concluded that the depression of contractility caused by halothane compromises the performance of the isolated heart more severely in the presence of increased arterial pressure. The heart is still able to increase its volume output, although at the expense of increased filling pressure. If this phenomenon applies to the intact circulation, the decrease in arterial pressure observed with halothane may be beneficial in that it may enable the heart to maintain an adequate cardiac output. Conversely, administration of a vasopressor, such as methoxamine or phenylephrine, which produces only an increase in total peripheral resistance could defeat the purpose by increasing arterial pressure to the detriment of flow to the tissues. In this same study, infusion of l-norepinephrine at a rate of 1—3 µg/min, enabled the heart under halothane to increase its output with normal filling pressures; it did not restore completely the ability of the heart to work against a high resistance.

MORROW et al. (1961) noted up to 70% decrease in myocardial contractile force in open-chest dogs prepared under chloralose anesthesia. THROWER et al. (1960) in open- or closed-chest dogs observed that halothane in concentrations of 0.5 to 1.0%, produced a minimal 15—20% depression in myocardial contractile force.

Li et al. (1968) in open-chest dogs anesthetized with pentobarbital, chloralose, or both, noted a decrease in myocardial contractile force from 180 to 112 g. There was also a decrease in the ascending slope of the myocardial contractile force recording.

Rushmer (1964) has observed a decrease in peak aortic flow in dogs previously anesthetized with pentobarbital.

The first data on true ventricular function curves were reported by Stirling et al. (1960). Their animals were premedicated with morphine and atropine and induced with thiopental. Thiopental was intermittently administered during the experiment. Venous return was controlled by pumping blood from a venous reservoir into the right atrium. In the presence of halothane, the relation between right ventricular work and right atrial pressure was depressed, that is, shifted to the right and actually flattened at higher atrial pressures.

Etsten and Shimosato (1966) and Shimosato et al. (1963) examined the effects of halothane in unpremedicated, nonoperated animals prepared under nitrous oxide and local anesthesia with procaine. To vary ventricular end-diastolic pressures, blood was infused or withdrawn in increments of 50—100 ml. The slope of the ventricular function curve (based on a ratio of stroke work to ventricular end-diastolic pressure) decreased in both ventricles linearly with increasing inspired concentrations of halothane. The correlation coefficients were — 0.94 on both the left and the right. The decrease in stroke work was accompanied by a parallel reduction in stroke power and mean ejection rate and was due primarily to a decrease in mean aortic pressure (Shimosato, 1964). When the heart was further stressed by increases in aortic pressure, accomplished by inflation of a balloon in the ascending aorta, there were no increases in stroke power or mean ejection rate (Etsten and Shimosato, 1964). It is known that in the *failing* heart, an increase in aortic pressure produces a negative inotropic effect (Ross et al., 1966). Since this change was not observed, the authors concluded that halothane evoked a metabolic depression, and that cardiac function was correlated with that state. It has been suggested that elevation of arterial pressure *per se* may increase the strength of the heart (Sarnoff and Mitchell, 1962). The fact that during halothane anesthesia the increase in aortic pressure was not associated with an increase in contractility may be related to a concomitant decreased level of myocardial tissue catecholamines (Laasberg et al., 1962; Li et al., in press).

Goldberg et al. [1962 (2)] studied the effects of digoxin on the myocardial depression produced by halothane in open-chest dogs. Pretreatment with digitalis significantly counteracted the negative inotropic effects of 1 and 2% halothane. The hypotensive effects of halothane were also reversed slightly. Shimosato and Etsten (1963) found analogous results in unpremedicated dogs: a depression of left and right ventricular function curves by halothane, and a partial restoration of these towards control by pretreatment with ouabain. They did not observe any protection against the hypotensive effects of halothane, however. The depression of cardiac output was reversed and thus also the increase in total peripheral resistance.

Spieckermann et al. (1968) studied the influence of barbiturates, halothane, and droperidol-fentanyl on the metabolism of high energy phosphates of the canine heart. During ischemia of the myocardium, there is a breakdown of high energy phosphates, especially of creatine phosphate (CP) and adenosinetriphosphate (ATP). The velocity of this breakdown is an index of the energy deficiency which builds up during anaerobic metabolism. As a measure of the velocity of breakdown of these high energy phosphates, two periods of ischemia were selected, corresponding to two exactly defined metabolic states: (1) "t-CP", corresponding to 3 μmol/g CP; and (2) "t-ATP", corresponding to 4 μmol/g ATP. At t-CP the heart can be safely resuscitated without danger of postischemic insufficiency. At t-ATP, resuscitation is just possible, although with a longer recovery time. During barbiturate anesthesia at 35 °C, t-CP = 3 min and t-ATP = 6 min. Compared with the conditions during barbiturate anesthesia, halothane anesthesia or droperidol-fentanyl analgesia produce no significant prolongation of t-CP, but a 3—4 fold prolongation of t-ATP. The cause, they felt, was a decrease in energy requirement, not an increase in the rate of energy production by glycolysis.

One of the earliest studies indicating that halothane causes myocardial depression was actually performed in man. SEVERINGHAUS and CULLEN (1958) administered 150 ml halothane vapor/minute to a series of premedicated patients in whom anesthesia had been induced with thiopental-succinylcholine. Ventilation was controlled, and the diluent mixture included 75% nitrous oxide. The patients were exposed to 15 min periods of halothane. The authors observed that administration of halothane in the presence of a sympathetic block produced by trimethaphan or high subarachnoid block with a spinal anesthetic, produced further decreases in cardiac output and arterial pressure and increases in total peripheral resistance and venous pressure. It was concluded that halothane depressed the myocardium directly. This conclusion was based on the correlation of left ventricular stroke work with right rather than left atrial pressure.

MORROW and MORROW (1961) studied the effects of halothane during thoracotomy in patients premedicated with meperidine, promethazine, and scopolamine. Anesthesia was induced with thiopental or cyclopropane and maintained with nitrous oxide-oxygen plus succinylcholine. Ventricular contractile force was measured by a Walton-Brodie strain gauge arch sutured onto the right ventricle. Administration of 2% halothane produced a decrease in myocardial contractile force in every patient, the average being 28% in 5 min. During a 10 min recovery period, arterial pressure increased, but myocardial contractile force decreased further. BLOODWELL et al. (1961) also observed depression of myocardial contractile force during thoracotomy in patients about to undergo open-heart surgery. Vaporizer concentrations of 0.5—1.3% halothane in oxygen produced decreases in myocardial contractile force of 4.4%, while 1.8—2.3% halothane lowered myocardial contractile force by 25.9%.

LUNDBORG et al. (1967) examined the effects of halothane in patients with heart disease undergoing cardiac catheterization. Stroke work, as well as the maximum rate of rise of left ventricular pressure (dP/dt) decreased at the same time that left ventricular end-diastolic pressure increased. These changes point to a decrease in myocardial function in man.

Evidence of myocardial depression was also seen by SMITH et al. [1968 (1)] in unpremedicated normal subjects. They measured the IJ complex of the ultralow frequency acceleration ballistocardiogram. This variable has shown a close relationship to ascending aortic acceleration, or Rushmer's initial ventricular impulse [WINTER et al., 1966, 1967; SMITH et al., 1968 (3)]. In fact, it may be an even more sensitive indicator of myocardial function than aortic acceleration. Although IJ amplitudes increased during the first 5 min of anesthesia, after that period any concentration of halothane of 0.8% or greater produced a dose-related decrease in amplitude. The maximum depression of the IJ amplitude was 60%.

LITTLE and GIVEN (1960) calculated indirectly some of the intervals of systole in man. Q-S_1 showed no significant decrease during 0.7—1.5% halothane. S_1-carotid pulse rise, Q-carotid pulse rise, and S_1-S_2 all increased. Heart rate decreased from 78 to 70. KADIS et al. (1969) demonstrated an increase in left ventricular ejection time (LVET, carotid pulse rise to incisura), left ventricular ejection time index (left ventricular ejection time corrected for changes in heart rate), pre-ejection period [(Q-S$_2$)-LVET], total duration of systole (Q-S$_2$), and duration of mechanical systole (S$_1$-S$_2$) during halothane anesthesia in concentrations ranging from 0.8 to 2.0% end tidal.

D. Arrhythmias

1. Incidence and Types

Early investigations of the incidence of arrhythmias during halothane anesthesia were hampered because continuous high-speed paper recording was too expensive and tape recorders were not available. Some arrhythmias, therefore, went undetected, rendering it impossible to correlate their incidence with other events occurring during anesthesia and surgery. Furthermore, only one lead could be monitored at a time. Recently, von der Groeben (1967, 1968) has recorded the three-orthogonal lead electrocardiogram and shown that arrhythmias appearing in one lead may be absent in the others.

Krantz et al. (1958) noted strongly inverted T-waves in dogs given halothane to the point of ventilatory arrest. Hall and Norris (1958) could detect no severe arrhythmias in dogs carried to ventilatory arrest with halothane.

Kuner et al. (1967) closely monitored 150 patients during anesthesia. With this careful attention, they noted arrhythmias in 61.7% of the patients. No difference between ostensibly normal patients and those with diagnosed cardiac disease was noted. Unfortunately, the patients were divided for analysis into many groups, but not by anesthetic agents. In a preliminary report on 2000 administrations of halothane (Ausherman and Adam, 1959), nodal rhythm, bradycardia, bigemini and extrasystoles were recorded, but no incidence was given. Illes and Defensor (1965) continuously monitored the electrocardiogram on 150 consecutive, unselected patients premedicated with meperidine, atropine, and occasionally promethazine or hydroxyzine. Arrhythmias of some type developed in 42% of the patients. The arrhythmias included ectopic beats, bigemini, and bradycardia at a rate of less than 25; again, the frequency of each type was not stated. Hyperventilation or increased depth of anesthesia with ether usually reversed the arrhythmias.

Dobkin (1958) recorded lead 2 of the electrocardiogram in 37 patients over 50 years of age, and in 11 younger patients with symptoms of cardiac disease. No patient received more than 0.5% halothane in 65% nitrous oxide. In none of the younger patients did a "major" disturbance of rhythm occur. Two of the older patients manifested runs of ventricular extra systoles and nodal rhythm. One patient developed S-T depression, which persisted until the anesthetic was discontinued. In another patient, extrasystoles seen preoperatively disappeared soon after induction of anesthesia. Hudon et al. [1957 (1)] recorded continuous electrocardiograms during halothane administration in 30 patients. They noted one episode each of nodal rhythm, bigemini, T-wave flattening, and ventricular extrasystoles. Sykes (1965) reported a case of heart block and cardiac arrest in a 3 year old girl being maintained with 0.5% halothane.

Murtagh (1960) produced deliberate hypotension with halothane in 30 patients undergoing thoracotomy. Direct mechanical stimulation of the heart and great vessels occurred in some of the patients. Systolic arterial pressure ranged between 60—80 torr. Continuous electrocardiographic monitoring revealed a change in rhythmic pattern in 7 out of 30 patients. Nodal rhythm was observed in 5 patients. Occasional premature atrial and ventricular extrasystoles were seen, but no runs of ventricular extrasystoles occurred. A wandering pacemaker (A-V dissociation), inverted P-waves, a high T-wave with an isoelectric take off, a small upward R and a prolonged downward S, a fall in voltage of QRS, and QRS electrical alternans with sinus rhythm were also noted. Seven normal, unpremedicated volunteer subjects (WYANT et al., 1958) experienced deliberate severe hypotension with halothane. Nodal rhythm was recorded in three subjects, ventricular extrasystoles in three, depressed ST segments in one, and no electrocardiographic change in two.

2. Hemodynamic Effect of Atrial Arrhythmias

Perhaps too much attention has been focused on ventricular arrhythmias, to the exclusion of atrial arrhythmias. Hemodynamic function is often well maintained during ventricular arrhythmias, unless the rate is very fast. Atrial arrhythmias, on the other hand, have been demonstrated to disturb hemodynamic function. LAVER and TURNDORF [1963 (1, 2)] produced A-V dissociation in man by using a combination of 1% halothane, d-tubocurarine, controlled ventilation, and some stimulation, such as a surgical incision. Arterial pressure invariably decreased and central venous pressure increased when A-V dissociation was present. SMITH et al. (unpublished data) observed A-V dissociation in six out of eleven normal unpremedicated subjects given halothane for circulatory studies. These arrhythmias were often produced by maneuvers which decreased arterial pressure and/or venous return, such as the Valsalva maneuver, increasing anesthetic concentration, or administering hexamethonium intravenously; and were often terminated by maneuvers which increased arterial pressure and/or venous return, such as lightening anesthesia, discontinuing the Valsalva maneuver, adding nitrous oxide to the inspired mixture, or placing a cold, wet pack on the subject's face during apnea (diving response). When normal rhythm changed to A-V dissociation, there was a definite decrease in mean arterial pressure, as well as stroke volume, cardiac output, and left ventricular work, as determined beat-to-beat by a ballistocardiograph-analog computer program. The greatest hemodynamic depression was observed when the P-wave began to emerge from the QRS and became a visible part of this complex. Thus it appears that during halothane anesthesia, not only is atrial contraction necessary for optimal ventricular performance, but improperly timed atrial contraction may actually interfere with ventricular performance.

3. Effect of CO_2

PURCHASE [1966 (2)] perfused 4 isolated cat hearts with halothane and 10% CO_2: 2 in 20% O_2, balance nitrogen, 2 in balance nitrogen. The latter two manifested ventricular extrasystoles. The author concluded that ventricular extrasystoles can occur independently of sympathetic activity, since they were seen in an isolated heart. It is known, however, that under similar circumstances (decreased pH), guinea pig atria can release norepinephrine in vitro [SMITH and CORBASCIO, 1966 (2)].

PURCHASE [1966 (1)] also studied cardiac arrhythmias during halothane anesthesia in cats. Factors influencing the onset of ventricular arrhythmias were the level of arterial pressure, Pa_{CO2} and arterial oxygen saturation. Cats whose mean arterial pressure was less than 60 torr during administration of 1—1.5% halothane seldom showed arrhythmias. Acutely-induced depressions in arterial pressure were able to abolish an existing arrhythmia. If Pa_{CO2} was elevated for 10 min by adding CO_2 to inspired gases when oxygen saturation was high, about 1/3 of the animals developed arrhythmias. Arrhythmias invariably occurred if Pa_{CO2} was greater than 55 torr and hemoglobin saturation was less than 90%. MUIR et al. (1959) investigated spontaneously ventilating cats anesthetized with 1.3%

halothane. Ventricular extrasystoles began in 14 out of the 16 cats within an hour. These arrhythmias were abolished with controlled hyperventilation at the same inspired concentration of anesthesia. The arrhythmias persisted if CO_2 was added to the mixture during hyperventilation. The disappearance of arrhythmias was thus identified with a decrease in Pa_{CO_2}, although no measurements were taken.

BLACK (1967, 1964) produced ventricular extrasystoles in each of eight children given atropine, thiopental, and 1.5% halothane, by adding carbon dioxide to the inspired gases. The first ventricular extrasystoles appeared when the Pa_{CO_2} values ranged from 104—150+. In the same study, in the presence of 1.5% methoxyflurane, similar levels of Pa_{CO_2} produced no change in rhythm. BLACK et al. (1959) also observed the effects of inhalation of CO_2 during anesthesia with 0.4—2.5% halothane inspired concentration in 15 unpremedicated patients. Coughing and gagging on the airway made these studies unsatisfactory when the P_{CO_2} was elevated during the administration of less than 1% halothane. These workers observed three kinds of arrhythmias in each patient: nodal rhythm (A-V dissociation), ventricular extrasystoles and multifocal ventricular tachycardia. Each subject showed a characteristic, and reproducible P_{CO_2} arrhythmia threshold, provided halothane concentration and rate of rise of Pa_{CO_2} were held constant. No consistent relationship was noted between the concentration of halothane and the Pa_{CO_2} threshold. Ventricular arrhythmias appeared at an average end-expiratory CO_2 level of 92 torr (range of 60—140 torr). Multifocal ventricular tachycardia occurred at an end-expiratory CO_2 level of 76 ($\pm$ 16) torr. Premature ventricular contractions always preceded multifocal ventricular tachycardia. No significant effects were noted when the Pa_{CO_2} was elevated 10—20 torr above the arrhythmic threshold. When the Pa_{CO_2} was reduced, the ventricular tachycardia gradually disappeared. On occasion, the return to normal rhythm was quite abrupt. Ventricular arrhythmias disappeared when the Pa_{CO_2} reached a level of 72 torr ($\pm$ 16). When the Pa_{CO_2} had been decreased to 60 torr, sinus rhythm was reestablished in 80% of the patients. During the reduction of Pa_{CO_2}, the arrhythmias did not appear to increase in severity. The arrhythmic threshold was significantly higher than that of cyclopropane, perhaps because of the lack of hypertension or a lesser release of catecholamines with CO_2 retention.

Adding carbon dioxide at a rate of 800—1000 ml/min produced arrhythmias in all 13 patients premedicated with pentobarbital, meperidine, and atropine, induced with thiopental-succinylcholine, and maintained with 1% halothane and nitrous oxide 70% (FUKUSHIMA et al., 1968). Ventricular arrhythmias appeared in 5—16 min at a Pa_{CO_2} of 72.0—98.2 torr (mean 86.1) and a pH of 6.88—7.20 (mean 7.10). Arterial pressure rose from 113/75 to 125/75. The arrhythmias consisted of unifocal premature ventricular contractions (3 patients), multifocal premature ventricular contractions (6 patients), ventricular bigemini (3 patients), and ventricular tachycardia (1 patient). Administration of propranolol, 3—5 mg intravenously, abolished all of these arrhythmias.

JOHNSTONE and NISBET (1961) examined the electrocardiographic response of patients to various maneuvers preformed under halothane anesthesia. Insertion of an endotracheal tube resulted in transient nodal rhythm in 3 out of 50 patients, and isolated ventricular extrasystoles in 8 patients, each of whom coughed after intubation. In deep (6—10% vaporizer concentration in 1—5 l/min oxygen) anesthesia, nodal rhythm was noted in 7 out of 50 patients, and occasional ventricular extrasystoles in one. In these same 50 patients, CO_2 retention was then allowed by rebreathing for 10—60 min. Ventricular extrasystoles appeared in 7 patients, bigemini in 10, and ventricular tachycardia in 1. In 10 patients, the rebreathing of CO_2 for 20 min followed by atropine, 0.5 mg intravenously, produced bigemini in 5, bifocal ventricular tachycardia in 2, multifocal ventricular tachycardia in 1, sinus tachycardia in 1, and no change in 1. During apneic diffusion oxygenation for 8—12 min, 8 out of 20 patients developed ventricular extrasystoles.

4. Administration of Epinephrine

In view of the dysrhythmic action of epinephrine and the ability of certain anesthetic agents such as cyclopropane and chloroform to "sensitize" the heart to epinephrine, the subject of epinephrine-halothane interaction has come under intensive study. Epinephrine can be introduced to the myocardium in two ways: either by endogenous release caused by excitement, surgical stimulation, or the anesthetic agent itself, or by exogenous administration by the anesthetist or surgeon. Sympathetic stimulation, of course, releases norepinephrine rather than epinephrine directly into the heart, but the arrhythmogenic properties of norepinephrine are just as potent as those of epinephrine.

SAITO et al. (1964) administered 1% vaporizer concentration halothane or 0.5% methoxyflurane to dogs for 30 min during controlled ventilation. Thereafter, epinephrine in doses of 10 and 100 µg/kg was injected. Although ventricular fibrillation occurred quite frequently with both concentrations of epinephrine during halothane anesthesia, it could not be elicited with the lower concentration during methoxyflurane anesthesia and occurred only once with the higher one.

DOBKIN and PURKIN (1959) provoked fatal (ventricular fibrillation) and serious (ventricular tachycardia) arrhythmias with intravenous epinephrine in 20 dogs. They observed that the incidence of arrhythmias was less with 1.0% halothane-ether azeotrope than with 0.5% halothane, although the two are not comparable in depth. They also noted that perphenazine was effective in preventing death during halothane and in reducing the duration and severity of arrhythmias during inhalation of either halothane or the azeotrope.

ROGOMAN et al. (1963) injected epinephrine subcutaneously, intramuscularly, or intravenously into twelve dogs each receiving thiopental or halothane on separate days. Five or 10 µg/kg epinephrine in a 1:200,000 solution, as well as 10 or 20 µg/kg in 1:100,000 solution, was injected subcutaneously or intramuscularly. The intravenous infusion rate of 1:200,000 epinephrine was increased until ventricular arrhythmias occurred. Subcutaneous and intramuscular injections of epinephrine produced more ventricular arrhythmias in dogs receiving thiopental 21 mg/kg than in those receiving 1 or 2% halothane. However, the amount of epinephrine required to produce ventricular tachycardia or ventricular fibrillation, when infused intravenously, was less with 1 or 2% halothane than with thiopental. The reason for the reversal in response to the two modes of injection is not apparent, although slower absorption of the injected epinephrine from subcutaneous tissue or muscle during halothane anesthesia may be one explanation. ISRAEL et al. (1962) administered 2% halothane, vaporizer concentration, to six dogs induced with thiopental-succinylcholine. Ventilation was controlled. Epinephrine was administered at a rate of 20 µg/kg/sec. Ventricular arrhythmias were seen in all animals. Neither high procaine spinal nor hyperventilation protected the animals against the arrhythmias. BOOKALLIL and LOMAZ (1962) reported that the subcutaneous infiltration of epinephrine into 37 children who were electrocardiographically monitored produced no arrhythmias. BRINDLE et al. (1957) reported that one out of 31 patients developed bizarre, prolonged ventricular arrhythmias during halothane 1—2% in N_2O-O_2, 50—50. Airway obstruction had occurred in this patient, and a total of 500 µg epinephrine was injected into the posterior cervical region. Later, the same authors (MILLAR et al., 1958) reported two cases of ventricular tachycardia, one occurring after

subcutaneous injection of epinephrine, the other "spontaneously". Serial determinations of catecholamine levels in peripheral venous plasma in the first patient
revealed levels of 0.02 μg/l of epinephrine 3 min before induction, 0.07 8 min
before injection of epinephrine and 57 min after induction, 1.78 13 min after
commencing injection, and 0.32 227 min after injection. VAREJES (1963) reported ventricular fibrillation after injection of 4 ml of 1:80,000 epinephrine
(20 μg) into the submucosa of the nasal septum. Halothane concentration was
1—2.5% and ventilation was spontaneous. Since meperidine 100 mg had been
given for premedication, Pa_{CO_2} and hence serum catecholamine levels were probably elevated. ROSEN and ROE (1963) reported cardiac arrest in two patients
anesthetized with halothane after injection of 50 ml of 1:100,000 epinephrine
and 30 ml of 1:200,000 epinephrine into the vaginal area. Interestingly enough,
opening of the chest revealed asystole, not ventricular fibrillation. MILLAR et al.
(1958) reported three cases of multifocal ventricular tachycardia during halothane
anesthesia, two of them after subcutaneous injection of 350—500 μg epinephrine.

JORDAN (1962) administered 3—45 ml (15—225 μg) topically applied 1:200,000
epinephrine in saline or 15—20 ml (75—100 μg) of the same concentration subcutaneously in 5.0% lidocaine. The total number of patients was 181 and the
total duration of surgery was 1—2 h. No arrhythmias were detected in 180 of
these patients. One patient developed persistent bigemini, which responded to a
decrease in halothane concentration. FORBES (1966) monitored the electrocardio-
graph lead three throughout halothane anesthesia and oral surgery in 100 patients
premedicated with atropine and meperidine and induced with thiopental and
succinylcholine. Halothane 2—3% was used for induction, 0.5—1% for maintenance. The first electrocardiogram was not taken until 5—8 min after induction.
One to 4 ml of 1% lidocaine with 1:200,000 epinephrine (5—20 μg) was injected
into the gums. Thirteen of the patients developed arrhythmias before injection
of this mixture: 7 with nodal rhythm, 3 with nodal rhythm plus ventricular extrasystoles, 2 with ventricular extrasystoles, and 1 with supraventricular extrasystoles. Another group of 11 patients developed arrhythmias 22 sec to 9 min
after injection: 1 with bigemini, 2 with bigemini and ventricular extrasystoles,
3 with ventricular extrasystoles, 2 with nodal rhythm plus ventricular extrasystoles, 2 with nodal rhythm, and 1 with atrial extrasystoles.

ANDERSEN and JOHANSEN (1963) administered infusions of epinephrine and
norepinephrine to 251 patients premedicated with atropine or scopolamine plus
meperidine or morphine and induced with thiopental-succinylcholine. The mean
vaporizer setting was 1.4% halothane. Ventilation was controlled. They demonstrated that increased ventricular excitability occurs just as readily with either
drug. The risk of evoking ventricular arrhythmias was marked if infusion rates
were greater than 10 μg/min, and if arteriosclerotic heart disease was present.

Since surgeons often find it necessary to inject a vasoconstrictor locally to
decrease bleeding, five alternatives present themselves: (1) use an anesthetic agent
or combination of agents known not to sensitize the heart; (2) use a vasoconstrictor
which does not produce ventricular arrhythmias; (3) use a *beta*-adrenergic blocking
agent intravenously either prophylactically or therapeutically; (4) use a combination of epinephrine plus a *beta*-blocking agent to infiltrate the desired region; or
(5) determine the safe amount of epinephrine to be used with a particular anesthetic agent. As far as the authors know, the fourth alternative has never been
tried. It would seem that if propranolol and epinephrine were absorbed into the
blood at equivalent rates, propranolol could block the arrhythmias produced by
epinephrine. At the same time, vasoconstriction would be enhanced and less epinephrine would be required, since propranolol blocks the vasodilating properties

of epinephrine, but not the vasoconstricting properties. Since propranolol is also a local anesthetic, it might be substituted for lidocaine under these circumstances. No one has determined the antiarrhythmic efficacy of the lidocaine which is usually injected with epinephrine. A potential disadvantage of the propranolol-epinephrine combination is that the action of propranolol may outlast that of epinephrine, with resulting myocardial depression.

The second, third and fifth alternatives listed above will be discussed in the next few paragraphs.

KATZ et al. (1962) have outlined the requirements for the safe injection of epinephrine during halothane anesthesia. These recommendations were based on careful studies of 100 patients receiving subcutaneous injection of 1:60,000 epinephrine, comparing these patients to controls receiving no injections. (One patient out of the 100 developed an arrhythmia severe enough — bigemini with increased arterial pressure — to warrant discontinuation of halothane.) Their recommendations include: (1) adequate ventilation of the patient, (2) epinephrine in a solution of 1:100,000 to 1:200,000, (3) the dose in adults not to exceed 10 ml of 1:100,000 in any given 10 min period, nor 30 ml/h. In comparison, the authors could not recommend the use of any epinephrine during cyclopropane anesthesia (MATTEO et al., 1963).

5. Injection of Other Cardiovascular-active Agents

TAKAORI and LOEHNING (1965) studied the effects of injections of isoproterenol, ephedrine and aminophylline separately or in combination during halothane anesthesia. Isoproterenol 10 µg/kg produced premature ventricular contractions in 5 out of 8 dogs and ventricular tachycardia in the others. Aminophylline 50 mg/kg produced premature ventricular contraction in 8 of 13 dogs. Ventricular arrhythmias persisted in three animals and reappeared in three other animals after subsequent injection of isoproterenol. One dog developed ventricular fibrillation immediately after isoproterenol. The one animal which had no change in rate or rhythm after aminophylline developed ventricular tachycardia after subsequent isoproterenol. Four out of 7 other dogs given 50 mg/kg aminophylline developed premature ventricular contractions. All four of these animals developed multifocal premature ventricular contractions after subsequent injection of 0.5 mg/kg ephedrine, three of these progressing to ventricular tachycardia and ventricular fibrillation. Two of the remaining three also showed ventricular tachycardia and ventricular fibrillation. After intravenous administration of 0.5 mg/kg ephedrine alone in 7 dogs, 4 dogs developed premature ventricular contractions and 2 developed secondary A-V block. Although these results are quite impressive, one would like to have seen comparable injections into conscious animals or animals anesthetized with pentobarbital.

KATZ and KATZ (1966) have suggested a non-arrhythmogenic alternative to epinephrine for use as a local vasoconstrictor. The polypeptide PLV-2 (2-phenyl-alinine-8-lysine vasopressin) can induce satisfactory local vasoconstriction without producing arrhythmias when injected into patients during halothane, cyclopropane, or trichlorethylene anesthesia. However, since the agent does produce coronary vasoconstriction (SMITH, 1967), the response of coronary circulation to combinations of anethetic agents plus PLV-2 should be examined.

LOEHNING and CZORNY (1960) administered phenylephrine, methoxamine, or mephentermine to dogs rapidly rendered severely hypotensive by halothane after induction with thiopental. Systolic arterial pressure was reduced to 20—40 mmHg within a 3—5 min period. Ventilation was controlled. A high incidence of ventricular cardiac irregularities was observed, including ventricular extrasystoles, multiple ventricular extrasystoles, paroxymal ventricular tachycardia, ventricular tachycardia, and ventricular fibrillation. Pretreatment with atropine did not prevent any of the irregularities except ventricular fibrillation.

McINTYRE (1965) administered phenylephrine to 50 patients anesthetized with thiopental-succinylcholine-nitrous oxide-halothane 1—3%. Dosage was 0.15 mg for the first 100—115 pounds, plus 0.025 mg for each additional 15 pounds. Runs of ventricular extrasystoles occurred in two patients for over 30 sec.

KATZ et al. (1967) compared the arrhythmic effects of dopamine and norepinephrine during pentobarbital, cyclopropane, or halothane anesthesia (1—2%) in open-chest cats. In pentobarbital-anesthetized cats, dopamine in doses of 1 to 100 µg/kg produced no ventricular arrhythmias. Doses of 25—100 µg/kg produced ventricular arrhythmias in cats anesthetized with cyclopropane or halothane. The arrhythmic threshold of dopamine was 25—100 times greater than that of norepinephrine. Pretreatment with 1-H56/28 consistently prevented dopamine arrhythmias at previous dose levels and increased the threshold four times. One encouraging factor was the appearance of the pressor effects of dopamine before any arrhythmic effects, suggesting the need for further careful studies in man.

6. Adrenergic Block

PETTER and SCHLAG (1965) anesthetized dogs with halothane or methoxyflurane and induced cardiac arrhythmias by administering small amounts of epinephrine intravenously. A Rauwolfia alkaloid, ajmaline, was effective in preventing and/or terminating epinephrine-induced atrial flutter and ventricular tachycardia. Pretreatment with ajmaline prevented epinephrine-induced arrhythmias at up to 1.5 times the previous challenging dose.

TE and CONN (1966) produced ventricular arrhythmias in 11 dogs by infusing 1:200,000 epinephrine "as rapidly as possible". The time of onset of arrhythmias averaged 40.8 sec. The infusion was discontinued, restarted, and 2 mg pronethalol, a *beta*-adrenergic blocking agent, was injected. Arrhythmias were reversed in 10 out of 11 dogs, even though previously, continuous administration of epinephrine had succeeded in maintaining the arrhythmias. Subsequently, epinephrine infusion was stopped and restarted simultaneously with the administration of 10 mg pronethalol. It is possible that the initial injection of pronethalol may still have been in effect.

IKEZONO et al. (1968) examined the effects of propranolol on epinephrine-induced arrhythmias in man and the cat. Thirty-five cats were maintained on 1% halothane. The threshold dose of epinephrine needed to produce at least ten premature ventricular contractions per minute was determined. In cats ventilated to normocapnia, the dose was 5.9 µg/kg. This increased to 21 µg/kg after administration of 50 µg/kg propranolol. In a second group of cats, after ventilation to an end-tidal CO_2 of 8%, one half the animals spontaneously developed premature ventricular contractions. In the remainder, the threshold dose of epinephrine was 0.68 µg/kg. This dose increased to 3.75 µg/kg after the injection of propranolol.

In patients, IKEZONO et al. (1968) assisted ventilation to maintain a normal P_{ACO_2}. Fifty-two patients were given propranolol 50 µg/kg before epinephrine was injected (0.15—4.6 µg/kg/h) or topically applied (35.7—1,254.8 µg/kg/h). In a second group of 62 patients, no propranolol was administered prophylactically. Epinephrine was also injected (0.54—10.7 µg/kg/h) or topically applied (15.0 to 279.0 µg/kg/h). The electrocardiogram was monitored continuously. No ventricular arrhythmias were observed in the first group. Thirteen patients developed ventricular arrhythmias in the second group. These arrhythmias were reverted after intravenous injection of 50 µg/kg propranolol.

McCLISH et al. (1968) believe that arrhythmias in patients with cardiovascular disease, particularly during surgery, are especially hazardous. They administered 1—2 mg propranolol intravenously to 115 patients to control 141 episodes of cardiac disturbance during light halothane anesthesia for cardiac surgery. Propranolol was successful in converting the arrhythmias to normal sinus rhythm in 94 of these episodes. Side effects encountered were sinus bradycardia (2 cases), atrio-ventricular block (1 case), hypotension (1 case), and bronchoconstriction (1 case).

HELLEWELL and POTTS (1966) noted ventricular extrasystoles in 11 out of 88 patients receiving halothane anesthesia. All of these disappeared approximately 1 min after injection of 1 mg propranolol. It would be interesting to compare the disappearance rate of arrhythmias in an equivalent group of patients, since spontaneous reversion is common.

WARNER (1968) reviewed the use of *beta*-adrenergic blocking agents to reverse arrhythmias during anesthesia. The present authors agree with his conclusion and with that of JOHNSTONE (1964, 1966) that the indications for the use of these agents is rare. As described above, ventricular arrhythmias during halothane are usually preventable or treatable by careful attention to several factors: avoidance of hypoventilation, with attendant increased Pa_{CO_2}, and hypertension, as well as careful — if any — injection of subcutaneous epinephrine. Arrhythmias which do not respond to increased ventilation, decreased depth of anesthesia, etc., particularly those produced by digitalis, may prove appropriate for treatment by beta-blockers. However, the dose of propranolol required to block digitalis-induced arrhythmias is several times that required to block *beta*-receptors. Thus, dangerously large amounts of propranolol may be required.

7. Mechanism of Arrhythmias

The mechanism of catecholamine-anesthetic agent arrhythmias is not yet fully understood [KATZ, 1967 (2)]. Some of the factors that may have a role include: (1) increased arterial pressure (MOE et al., 1948; DRESEL et al., 1960); (2) increased heart rate (DRESEL et al., 1960; VICK, 1966); and (3) release of potassium from the liver (O'BRIEN et al., 1954). Although the increase in arterial pressure is important in producing these arrhythmias, it is not absolutely essential, since isoproterenol, which decreases arterial pressure, can produce arrhythmias during anesthesia (KATZ, 1965). Similarly, the increase in heart rate and release of potassium in the liver, although important, are not essential [KATZ, 1967 (2)].

KOHLI et al. (1966) studied the influence of halothane and arterial pressure on the functional refractory period of A-V transmission in spinal vagotomized dogs. Halothane prolonged the functional refractory period, as did all anesthetics studied: ether, cyclopropane, thiopental and pentobarbital. Raising arterial pressure prolonged the functional refractory period both before and during administration of halothane.

GALINDO and SPROUSE (1962) studied ventricular excitability, refractoriness, and conduction in 22 open-chest dogs induced with 25 mg/kg thiopental. Halothane increased the absolute refractory period, both in absolute values and as a percentage of the total cardiac cycle. The relative refractory period decreased from 17.4 to 11.0 msec. Halothane increased the ventricular diastolic threshold by 50% in "deep" anesthesia; when anesthesia was deepened further, 90 min later, halothane decreased the ventricular diastolic threshold by about 40%.

MCLEOD and REYNOLDS (1964) have suggested that halothane may interfere with the stabilizing action of endogenous acetylcholine on the ventricle, thus producing a relative increase in ventricular automaticity.

Smith et al. (1962) based their studies on the assumption that any agent which slows conduction, shortens the refractory period, or lowers the threshold will favor the production and maintenance of ventricular fibrillation. They studied open-chest dogs induced with thiamylal. Halothane increased the drive stimulus-response (the interval between application of a drive impulse to the atria and the beginning of the QRS complex) from 123 to 155 msec. The latency, that is, the interval between the application of the test stimulus to the ventricle and the response by the ventricle, was used as an approximation of ventricular conduction time. Halothane increased that interval from 62.5 to 76.0 msec. Halothane also increased the absolute refractory period from 182 up to 208 msec, and displaced the strength-interval curve to the right. The mean diastolic threshold was increased by 0.7 mA at 280 msec following the R-wave, 9.8 mA at 180 msec and an insignificant amount (0.25 mA) at 160 msec.

E. Catecholamines

1. Plasma and Tissue Catecholamine Levels

Price et al. (1959), in an early study, could detect no change in arterial serum norepinephrine or epinephrine levels in 11 unpremedicated patients undergoing surgery. Inspired halothane concentrations varied from 0.5—3.0%. Hamelberg et al. (1960) examined venous plasma catecholamine levels in premedicated patients during halothane, noting no change after 1 h of light or deep surgical anesthesia. Elliott et al. (1968) induced ten normal subjects with thiopental-succinylcholine. Ventilation was spontaneous and the subjects were intubated. After 25 min of 1% halothane, vaporizer concentration, norepinephrine levels (trihydroxyindole method) went from 0.4 to 0.55, probably not a significant change.

Anton et al. (1964) measured urine, arterial plasma, and atrial tissue catecholamine levels in 25 patients undergoing thoracotomy and extracorporeal circulation. Serum epinephrine and norepinephrine levels increased during thoracotomy with ether or with halothane. During bypass, the levels continued to increase under ether, but failed to change significantly under halothane anesthesia. Atrial catecholamines did not change. Large increases in epinephrine and norepinephrine levels were found in urine samples obtained in the recovery room. Considerably higher excretion levels occurred in patients who had received ether anesthesia than in those previously under halothane anesthesia.

Etsten and Shimosato (1965) determined serum catecholamine levels at several intervals during halothane anesthesia in a patient with pheochromocytoma. Preanesthetic levels of norepinephrine and epinephrine were 1660 and 2540 µg/l. These were decreased by halothane to as low as 39 and 29 µg/l. Although these low levels were observed some time after considerable manipulation of the tumor, they indicate that halothane may have suppressed catecholamine release.

Li et al. (1964) measured catecholamine content in cardiovascular tissue in dogs. Halothane produced a significant decrease in epinephrine content in the right atrium and left atrium, but no significant change in right ventricular, left ventricular, aortic, and pulmonary artery tissues. Norepinephrine remained unchanged in all tissues examined.

2. Norepinephrine Release and Reuptake

Ngai et al. (1968) studied release of norepinephrine from myocardial sympathetic nerve endings in dogs by labelling myocardial norepinephrine stores with intra-arterial infusions of dl-^{3}H norepinephrine. Arterial and coronary sinus blood samples were obtained at intervals. In the four animals studied, no alteration in release of norepinephrine was observed during inhalation of halothane. NAITO and GILLIS (1968) examined the effect of halothane on norepinephrine reuptake, the major route for inactivation of the sympathetic neurotransmitter. They used sympathetically innervated atria prepared from cats induced with pentobarbital. Although halothane had pronounced negative inotropic actions, it did not affect the positive chronotropic response to sympathetic stimulation at frequencies from 0.5—8 Hz. Cocaine, at concentrations that are known to inhibit norepinephrine uptake, did potentiate this response, particularly to low frequency (0.5—2 Hz) stimulation. Halothane failed to influence the uptake and retention of ³HNE by slices of cat ventricle. Similar results were obtained with ether, cyclopropane, and methoxyflurane at equipotent concentrations (MAC) except for the fact that methoxyflurane significantly decreased retention of ³HNE with respect to the control. NAITO and GILLIS (1968) also examined the effects of 0.25 and 0.50% halothane in isolated cat atria. These concentrations decreased spontaneous contractile force 60—85% in 20—30 min. The spontaneous rate of contraction showed essentially no change. When exogenous norepinephrine was added to the media, atrial rate increased in proportion to the concentration used. No change in the slope of this line was produced by halothane. Thus halothane neither potentiated nor inhibited the effects of exogenous norepinephrine on atrial rate.They also noted that the spontaneous atrial rate between additions of norepinephrine was unaffected by halothane. Halothane did not significantly decrease retention of ³H-norepinephrine when compared with control. They concluded that halothane had little effect, if any, on the disposition of norepinephrine after its release from sympathetic nerve endings.

3. Response to Catecholamines

PRICE and PRICE (1962) tested the effect of six anesthetic agents on the response of isolated rabbit aortic strips to norepinephrine. Halothane was the only agent which depressed the response, and this depression was described as severe.

KADIS et al. [1969 (2)] attempted to explain the reported differences in the influence of halothane on the epinephrine response in isolated aortic strips (PRICE and PRICE, 1962), and in the rat mesoappendix preparation (MURRAY et al., 1963) (see page 84). During constant-flow perfusion with a Krebs-phosphate buffered solution, halothane depressed the epinephrine response in an isolated superior mesenteric artery segment of the rabbit. The addition of bovine albumin to the perfusing solution reversed the response from a depressant one to a pressor one. The authors concluded that differences in the perfusing fluid may explain the variation in results obtained in different experimental preparations.

FLACKE and ALPER (1962) studied the interaction between halothane and norepinephrine in the canine heart-lung preparation. The depressant effect of halothane on cardiac function was antagonized by norepinephrine, although complete reversal by norepinephrine was possible only with concentrations of halothane of 2% or less. The negative chronotropic action of halothane was undiminished during infusion of norepinephrine (1.2—3 µg/min), and the positive chronotropic effect of norepinephrine was not depressed in the presence of halothane (1.5% inspired concentration). High rates of infusion of norepinephrine (31 µg/min and above) in the presence of 1.5% halothane produced increases in heart rate significantly greater than those during the control period. They concluded that the depressant effects of halothane and the stimulating effects of norepinephrine on the heart are independent, and that the two drugs do not interact at the same receptor.

Andersen and Johansen (1963) infused epinephrine or norepinephrine into premedicated patients during halothane anesthesia. They found that if they were to avoid ventricular arrhythmias, the hypotensive action of halothane could be only partially corrected (up to 80% of control).

4. Adrenergic Blockade

Rein et al. (1963) examined the effect of guanethidine or reserpine pretreatment on the cardiac response to halothane in open-chest dogs. Atropine, 2 mg, was administered intravenously before measurements were made. The halothane-induced depression of myocardial contractile force (Walton-Brodie strain gauge) was not significantly changed by pretreatment with either agent, although inspired concentrations of 0.5 and 1.0% halothane did produce a significantly greater negative chronotropic and hypotensive effect. Comparable decrements were produced in these variables at 1.5 and 2.0% halothane anesthesia.

Morrow et al. (1961) noted no difference in the depressant response of heart rate, myocardial contractile force, and systolic arterial pressure to halothane in control dogs and in dogs previously subjected to total chronic cardiac denervation. The administration of atropine intravenously did not affect these results.

In open-chest dogs prepared under cyclopropane or halothane (Craythorne and Huffington, 1966), heart rate was the only variable to change when propranolol was injected during steady-state halothane anesthesia. Arterial pressure, cardiac output, stroke volume, myocardial contractile force, total peripheral resistance, and end-diastolic length did not change.

F. Blood Volume

Payne et al. (1959) measured blood volume in 12 patients, aged 32—61, premedicated with pentobarbital and atropine. Plasma volume was measured by the Evans blue dye method, and red blood cell volume estimated from a corrected hematocrit. Blood volume increased from 4.9 to 5.6 l, a statistically significant change. Since the hematocrit varies markedly from one region of the circulation to the other, this method is not as accurate as those tagging both plasma and red cells. Grable et al. (1962) measured blood volume in ten patients receiving pentobarbital and atropine for premedication. Ages ranged from 23—84 years. Red blood cells were tagged with 51 Cr and plasma protein with 125 I. After 30 min of "plane 2, stage 3" halothane, total blood volume had increased 10.1%, the increase being equally distributed between plasma and red blood cell volume. The change in red cell volume is difficult to interpret.

Morse et al. (1963), on the other hand, could detect no change in blood volume in ten normal unpremedicated volunteer subjects, aged 20—28 years, after 40, 60, and 100 min of a constant end-expired concentration of halothane. Red blood cell volume was determined by the 51 Cr method; total blood volume and plasma volume were calculated from the hematocrit. Differences in age of the subjects, methodology, premedication, and constancy of anesthetic depth could partially explain differences among these studies.

G. Blood Viscosity

Albert et al. (1964) studied the viscosity of blood withdrawn from ten patients during surgery plus anesthesia with halothane. Hematocrit decreased by 3.6%, total protein by 3.94%, blood viscosity by 2.97% and plasma viscosity by 2.77%.

The authors felt that the combined effect of hemodilution plus a change in plasma characteristics was responsible for the observed effect on viscosity.

In contrast, BEHAR and ALEXANDER (1966), and ARONSON et al. (1968) studied blood freshly drawn from unanesthetized humans. The anesthetic agent was then equilibrated with the blood *in vitro*. BEHAR and ALEXANDER noted that 1.2% halothane did not change whole blood viscosity. The instrument used was adequate for viscosity measurements only at shear rates of from 230—11.5 sec^{-1}. ARONSON et al. examined both halothane and methoxyflurane. The range of their three cone-plate viscometers totalled 1500—6.75 sec^{-1}. The Casson viscosity of blood and the apparent plasma viscosity were determined from the slope of the shear stress-shear rate relationship plotted on a square root scale. Yield stress was determined by extrapolation from the shear-stress intercept. Halothane, within concentrations equivalent to those used during clinical anesthesia, produced no discernible effect on either yield stress or apparent viscosity of blood or plasma. However, methoxyflurane resulted in a 6.5% decrease in plasma viscosity as measured by the capillary viscometric technique and 3% by the cone-plate viscometers.

ARONSON et al. (1967) studied the *in vitro* effects of halothane on surface tension and plasma electrophoretic mobility in human blood. Blood exposed to halothane in concentrations of 4—65 mg-% showed no change in surface tension of either blood or plasma, but a slight (+2.2%) albeit significant change in electrophoretic mobility of plasma albumin.

III. Methoxyflurane

A. Hemodynamics

1. Cardiac Output

SAITO et al. [1966 (2)] noted a dose-dependent depression of cardiac output in dogs during methoxyflurane anesthesia. In another study (SAITO et al., 1966) discontinuation of methoxyflurane was followed by protracted recovery of the depressed cardiac output, as might be expected from the high partition coefficients of this agent. BAGWELL and WOODS (1962) measured left ventricular output minus coronary flow with an electromagnetic flowmeter in 35 animals prepared the day before (closed-chest) or the day of (open-chest) the study. Animals were induced with either thiopental, halothane, or methoxyflurane. Ventilation was controlled. Cardiac output determinations performed during administration of methoxyflurane at vaporizer concentrations of 0.5, 0.7, and 1.0% were compared with those obtained at 0.25%. The decreases in cardiac output were about 27, 49, and 65%. DOBKIN and FEDORUK (1961) studied dogs premedicated with perphenazine and induced with thiopental. Cardiac output decreased from 2.98 to 2.06 l/min in animals breathing methoxyflurane spontaneously for 40—60 min, and from 3.45 to 2.60 in animals undergoing assisted ventilation.

HUDON et al. (1963) examined cardiac output in 20 patients premedicated with atropine plus a narcotic, and induced with either thiopental or methoxyflurane. Cardiac output decreased 19% in the first hour, 23% in the second hour, and 31.5% in the third hour of anesthesia and surgery. Since the amount of blood loss was not reported, it is impossible to ascertain whether these figures represent a true decompensation to methoxyflurane. WALKER et al. [1962 (1, 2)] studied five normal spontaneously ventilating subjects induced with thiopental-succinylcholine and stabilized with methoxyflurane at an unspecified concentration. The trachea was sprayed with 6% cocaine. Measurements taken after 35 min of steady-state anesthesia revealed a 9.8% decrease in cardiac index. Wyant et al. (1961) measured cardiac output in five normal unpremedicated spontaneously ventilating subjects induced with thiopental-succinylcholine. After 25—30 min of anesthesia, cardiac output changed very little from awake values, rising from 5.6—6.0 l/min. Ten minutes after a change to controlled ventilation (no blood gases measured), cardiac output fell to 4.3 l/min.

ALLARIA et al. (1967) noted that induction with 1% methoxyflurane in five patients decreased cardiac output and stroke volume, but that these variables returned to preinduction values after 10 min.

DEFARES (1965) has proposed the "circulatory index" as a more meaningful calculation than cardiac index. The standard calculation of cardiac index is:

$$CI = \frac{CO}{BSA}$$ where CI=cardiac index, CO = cardiac output, and BSA = body surface area.

The proposed calculation for circulatory index is:

$$CI = \frac{CO}{O_2 \text{ uptake}} - \frac{1}{(A-V) O_2},$$ where (A-V) O_2=arterial-venous oxygen difference. In other words, the circulatory index reflects the ability of the cardiac output to supply the body's oxygen needs. RESTALL et al. (1966) examined the cardiac index and circulatory index in six patients premedicated with pentobarbital, meperidine, and atropine and induced with thiopental and succinylcholine. Cardiac index during nitrous oxide (65%) oxygen-methoxyflurane (0.5% mean expired concentration) was 1.68—1.91 l/min/m². Values determined every 15 min showed no signs of the adaptation seen with halothane. However, measurements did not begin until 1 h after induction of anesthesia, and adaptation may have already occurred. Furthermore, measurements were taken during surgery. Infusion of 1 l lactated Ringer's solution into two of these patients was followed in 20 min by a slight increase in cardiac index, from 1.6 and 1.7 up to 1.8 and 2.1. The circulatory index for methoxyflurane was 0.22, compared to 0.22—0.25 seen by these investigators in awake subjects (DEFARES, 1965; REEVES, 1961).

2. Arterial Pressure

SAITO (1965) noted a profound concentration-dependent depression of mean arterial pressure with methoxyflurane in dogs. BAGWELL et al. (1962) reported a decrease in mean aortic pressure in 21 dogs which had undergone a thoracotomy 24 h previously. Pressure fell from 112 during the awake state down to 73, 59, 42, and 41 torr, at 0.50, 0.75, 1.00 and 1.25% inspired concentration. In 35 open- or closed-chest dogs induced with thiopental mean arterial pressure decreased 32, 51, and 60% at 0.5, 0.75, and 1.0% vaporizer concentration of methoxyflurane (BAGWELL and WOODS, 1962). Comparisons were made with 0.25% methoxyflurane as control. Arterial pressure was measured in 12 animals during the control period and after 30, 90, 150, and 210 min of methoxyflurane anesthesia. The corresponding values were 108.7, 81.3, 73,4, 76.3, and 67.5, indicating no adaptation unless adaptation had occurred prior to the 30-min measurement. DOBKIN and FEDORUK (1961) in dogs premedicated with perphenazine and induced with thiopental, observed a consistent decrease in systolic, diastolic, and mean arterial pressure after 90 min of methoxyflurane 1% inspired concentration. In spontaneously ventilating animals, these pressures fell from 145, 97, and 113 down to 119, 71, and 87. In dogs with assisted ventilation, they declined from 139, 102, and 109 to 94, 57, and 69. SHIMOSATO et al. (1968) studied open-chest dogs induced with chloralose or chloralose-urethane and paralyzed with gallamine. At blood concentrations of methoxyflurane averaging 17.0 mg- %, mean arterial pressure decreased 34.7%.

BRASSARD et al. (1963) studied arterial pressure in 30 unpremedicated dogs induced with methohexital. A thoracotomy was performed just before the study. Control measurements were taken when the animals began to struggle. Methoxyflurane was then introduced into the system at a vaporizer concentration of 0.5%. The concentration was increased every 15 min by 0.5% until a maximum of 2.0% was reached. The step changes in concentration were then reversed. Systolic and diastolic arterial pressures decreased about 12 and 14% for each step in methoxyflurane concentration. The changes in these variables lagged far behind the changes in concentration.

SPHIRE (1966) gathered retrospective data on 377 patients undergoing biliary surgery. The patients were induced with thiopental-succinylcholine. Neither premedication, concentration of methoxyflurane, nor type of ventilation was stated. A decrease in systolic arterial pressure of 25% or more was noted in 53.5% of the patients. In 26 patients, systolic pressure decreased more than 50% from the immediate preanesthetic level. The mean onset of hypotension was 24 min after induction of anesthesia. The mean duration was 15 min, with or without administration of a pressor agent.

McCAFFREY and MATE (1963) in a review of 1200 randomly premedicated and induced patients studied during surgery, noted an initial moderate drop in arterial pressure, which usually rose to and stabilized at a level slightly lower than the awake control. In his retrospective study, COPPOLINO (1963) observed no change in systolic, diastolic or mean arterial pressure during surgery and anesthesia with methoxyflurane.

NORTH and STEPHEN (1966) reported a stable arterial pressure (110—105 torr) in 209 patients during surgery (? premedication, ? induction), plus methoxyflurane. They commented on a sharp drop during induction but did not state its amount. ALLARIA (1967) in five patients anesthetized with 1% vaporizer concentration of methoxyflurane noted no change in arterial pressure. ROBERTS and CAM (1964) found a 30% decrease in mean arterial pressure in 50 patients induced with thiopental-succinylcholine and maintained with 0.5—1.0% vaporizer concentration methoxyflurane plus nitrous oxide. KNOX et al. (1962) reported a clinical evaluation of 75 patients induced with thiopental and maintained with methoxyflurane-nitrous oxide-oxygen. Decreases in arterial pressure were common, the degree of hypotension being dependent on the inspired concentration. The mean decrease in systolic arterial pressure was 15 torr.

Twenty-three patients were observed during surgery, after induction with thiopental or methoxyflurane plus nitrous oxide (HUDON et al., 1963). Ventilation was spontaneous or controlled. No change in mean arterial or pulse pressure was noted. BLACK and REA (1964) studied the circulatory effects of methoxyflurane during surgery. The children were premedicated with atropine, induced with thiopental, and maintained with nitrous oxide-oxygen-methoxyflurane, 0.5—1.5% vaporizer concentration. Mean arterial pressure did not change. The authors stated that they had observed the same lack of hypotension with halothane. GOETZINGER et al. (1962) described 31 patients induced with thiopental (5) or methoxyflurane-nitrous oxide (26). Ventilation was controlled or assisted. The decrease in arterial pressure was less than 20 torr in 26 patients, and greater than 20 torr in the other five. The relation between thiopental induction and hypotension was not stated.

MARUYAMA et al. (1966) studied methoxyflurane anesthesia in 120 infants and children premedicated with pentobarbital, meperidine, and scopolamine. Induction was performed with either methoxyflurane-nitrous oxide, halothane, cyclopropane, or thiopental. Ventilation was controlled. No change in arterial pressure was noted during induction with methoxyflurane (29 cases) which lasted 9 min. Induction with halothane (5 cases) decreased arterial pressure by a mean of 15%. During maintenance, arterial pressure increased from control in 8 of the 120 patients, did not change in 12, and decreased in 100. The mean change was 17.7 torr. LEWIS and SMITH (1965) studied 157 children induced with thiopental, cyclopropane, or methoxyflurane and maintained with methoxyflurane-nitrous oxide-oxygen. During the early period of methoxyflurane administration, systolic arterial pressure fell, usually by less than 20 torr. The authors had gathered the impression that those induced with cyclopropane seemed to be noticeably resistant to the hypotension produced by methoxyflurane.

WALKER et al. [1962 (1, 2)] noted a decrease in mean arterial pressure from 83.4 to 66.4 in five normal spontaneously ventilating patients induced with thiopental and succinylcholine. Measurements were taken after 35 min of steady-state anesthesia. ELLIOTT et al. (1968) induced ten normal subjects with thiopental-succinylcholine. Ventilation was spontaneous. After 25 min of 1% methoxyflurane, vaporizer concentration, mean arterial pressure had decreased from 82.1 to 70.4. WYANT et al. (1961) in a series of five unpremedicated volunteer subjects induced with thiopental and succinylcholine and maintained with methoxyflurane-oxygen, noted that mean arterial pressure decreased from 92 to 72 torr when ventilation was spontaneous. A further drop to 65 torr appeared when controlled ventilation was subsequently instituted. BLACK and McARDLE (1965) in 11 normal unpremedicated volunteer subjects induced with thiopental and maintained with methoxyflurane in 75% nitrous oxide, noted a statistically significant decrease in arterial pressure, measured by auscultation, from 89 to 82 torr.

a) Extra-Anesthetic Factors

MILLAR and MORRIS (1961) studied eight dogs anesthetized with thiopental. Two of these animals inhaled 0.61% methoxyflurane while breathing spontaneously. The systolic arterial pressure decreased from 140 down to 128 in 30 min, down to 116 in 60 min, and increased back to 142 by 120 min. Diastolic arterial pressure changed from 78 to 81, 66, and 78, respectively. However, Pa_{CO_2} rose from 24 to 135 torr and pH dropped from 7.54 down to 7.00 during the 120 min interval. In the other six dogs, ventilation was controlled. Systolic arterial pressure decreased from 155 down to 116, 107, and 97 torr, during the 30, 60, and 120 min intervals. Diastolic pressure decreased from 90 down to 71, 67, and 63 torr. Induced hypercarbia (Pa_{CO_2}=173—193, pH=6.86—6.83) resulted in a further drop in systolic arterial pressure to 88 and 91 and diastolic arterial pressure to 35 and 41. Hemorrhage of 20 ml/kg produced an arterial pressure of 44/24. A further hemorrhage of 10—14 ml/kg decreased arterial pressure to 37/16.

ANDREWS et al. (1966) withdrew approximately 50% of the blood volume in 45 min from dogs induced with thiamylal and maintained with 0.3—0.7% inspired concentrations of methoxyflurane or 0.6—1.2% of halothane. All dogs (7/9) which had survived hemorrhage during halothane survived a subsequent insult 1 week later under methoxyflurane. Six out of seven dogs survived the initial hemorrhage with methoxyflurane; only three survived the subsequent hemorrhage during halothane anesthesia.

MOSS and DOMER (1967) studied the response of arterial pressure to graded doses of histamine, acetylcholine, or epinephrine in nine dogs anesthetized with methoxyflurane, pentobarbital, or electronarcosis. The response to epinephrine was significantly greater during methoxyflurane anesthesia than during either of the other forms of anesthesia at both doses tested (0.5 and 1 μg/kg). Hemorrhage to a systemic arterial pressure of about 50% of control eliminated these differences. The response to acetylcholine was significantly greater during pentobarbital anesthesia than during methoxyflurane anesthesia at the two largest doses (4 and 8 μg/kg). No significant difference in responses was observed between methoxyflurane and electronarcosis. After hemorrhage, the response to acetylcholine was significantly greater during methoxyflurane anesthesia than during electronarcosis only at the lowest dose (0.5 μg/kg). In the control and in the animals undergoing hemorrhage, no differences in response to histamine were found between methoxyflurane anesthesia and electronarcosis or pentobarbital anesthesia.

3. Heart Rate

BAGWELL and WOODS (1962) could detect no significant change in heart rate during methoxyflurane anesthesia in dogs. DOBKIN and FEDORUK (1961) premedicated 18 dogs with perphenazine and induced them with thiopental. Administration of methoxyflurane decreased heart rate from 139 to 109 in spontaneously ventilating dogs and from 108 to 85 in dogs on assisted ventilation. SHIMOSATO et al. (1968) studied open-chest dogs induced with chloralose or chloralose-urethane and paralyzed with gallamine. At blood concentrations of methoxyflurane averaging 17.0%, heart rate decreased by 18.5%. The control heart rate was 141—202 in the presence of the cardiovagal block produced by gallamine. BRASSARD et al. (1963) studied heart rate in 30 unpremedicated dogs induced with methohexital. The chest was opened and closed just before the study. Control measurements were taken when the animal began to struggle. Methoxyflurane was then introduced into the system in steps of 0.5% as described under "Arterial Pressure". Heart rate decreased with each step until at 2% methoxyflurane it reached 80% of control level. No recovery of heart rate was seen as methoxyflurane concentration decreased, and a repeat run showed a trend towards a further decrease to about 70% of control.

CAMPBELL et al. (1962) monitored heart rate in 50 patients during anesthesia with methoxyflurane-nitrous oxide-oxygen. Premedication consisted of atropine plus a narcotic and/or barbiturate. Induction was accomplished in 41 patients with thiopental and in nine with methoxyflurane. No change in heart rate was observed, even at levels deep enough to produce hypotension. Heart rate did not change in 23 patients under controlled or spontaneous ventilation with methoxyflurane-nitrous oxide-oxygen (HUDON et al., 1963). Measurements were taken during surgery. McCAFFREY and MATE (1963) noted no significant change in heart rate in 1200 patients, unless anesthesia was judged to be too deep by clinical criteria. Again, measurements were taken during surgery. LEWIS and SMITH (1965) noted a slight, but significant decrease in heart rate during anesthesia and surgery with methoxyflurane in 157 children. In his retrospective study, COPPOLINO (1963) noted no change in heart rate in 200 patients during anesthesia and surgery.

BLACK and REA (1964) observed an increase in heart rate from 98 to 104 in ten children spontaneously breathing 0.5—1.5% methoxyflurane vaporizer concentration plus 75% nitrous oxide. The children were premedicated with atropine and induced with thiopental. MARUYAMA et al. (1966) observed a 4.7 beat/min decrease in heart rate in 120 infants and children during induction with methoxyflurane. The ultimate change in heart rate during maintenance with methoxyflurane-nitrous oxide was —12.6 beats/min. Twelve patients showed an increase, 24 no change, and 84 a decrease.

RESTALL et al. (1966) reported a gradual decrease in heart rate over a 2 h period in six patients during surgery for varicose veins. Measurements were not recorded until 1 h after induction.

WYANT et al. (1961) noted no change in heart rate in five normal unpremedicated subjects. ELLIOTT et al. (1968) induced ten normal subjects with thiopental-succinylcholine. Ventilation was spontaneous and the subjects were intubated. After 25 min of 1% methoxyflurane, vaporizer concentration, heart rate decreased from 86.3 to 74.0. Heart rate also decreased from 81 to 74 in 11 unpremedicated subjects induced with thiopental and maintained with 1.5% methoxyflurane in 75% N_2O (1965). WALKER et al. [1962 (1, 2)] in five normal volunteer patients induced with thiopental-succinylcholine observed an increase in heart rate from 74 up to 81 after 35 min of steady-state methoxyflurane anesthesia.

a) Extra-Anesthetic Factors

MILLAR and MORRIS (1961) could detect no change in heart rate in seven dogs given 0.7% methoxyflurane after induction with thiopental. Measurements were made for 2 h. Heart rate did not change when P_{CO_2} was increased to 173 to 193 torr nor when 20 ml/kg of blood was removed. However, heart rate did increase from 123 to 154 when a further 10—14 ml/kg was removed.

4. Stroke Volume

DOBKIN and FEDORUK (1961) saw no change in stroke volume in dogs premedicated with perphenazine, induced with thiopental, and maintained with methoxyflurane-oxygen in a non-rebreathing circuit. This was true during both spontaneous and assisted ventilation. BAGWELL and WOODS (1962) noted that stroke volume did change *pari passu* with cardiac output in open-chest dogs anesthetized with methoxyflurane-oxygen.

WYANT et al. (1961) in normal volunteer subjects noted changes in stroke volume usually parallel to those in cardiac output. Stroke volume fell from 78.3 ml during the awake period to 65 ml during spontaneous ventilation to 46.1 ml during subsequent controlled ventilation. WALKER et al. [1962 (1, 2)] observed a decrease in stroke index from 38 to 32 ml/m² in five normal volunteer subjects, unpremedicated but induced with thiopental-succinylcholine. Ventilation was spontaneous. The second determination was taken after 35 min of stable anesthesia.

5. Total Peripheral Resistance

CLARKE and CURRIE (1964) measured total peripheral resistance in ten dogs by excluding the heart from an extracorporeal circuit and measuring aortic and central venous pressures during a known rate of inflow from the pump-oxygenator. They noted a 38% decrease in total peripheral resistance when 0.5% methoxyflurane was administered to this system.

RESTALL et al. (1966) could detect no change in total peripheral resistance during 2 h of methoxyflurane anesthesia plus surgery. The values ranged from 1800—2000 dyne-sec-cm⁻⁵, somewhat higher than normal. The initial determinations were performed 1 h after induction of anethesia. HUDON et al. (1963) in 23 patients ranging from 18—83 years, noted a decrease in total peripheral resistance in seven patients, an increase in the other 16. By the end of 2 h of anesthesia, resistance had increased above awake control values in all 23 patients.

WYANT et al. (1961) noted a decrease in total peripheral resistance from about 1350 to about 1000 dyne-sec-cm⁻⁵ in volunteer subjects during methoxyflurane anesthesia and spontaneous ventilation. After controlled ventilation had been assumed, total peripheral resistance rose to about 1550 dyne-sec-cm^{-5}. The time factor may have played an important role, since controlled ventilation always followed spontaneous ventilation. WALKER et al. [1962 (1, 2)] noted a decrease in total peripheral resistance from 1356 to 1209 dyne/sec/cm^{-5} in normal volunteer subjects. However, the difference was not statistically significant.

6. Central Venous (Right Atrial) Pressure

DOBKIN and FEDORUK (1961) noted no change in mean central venous pressure when methoxyflurane anesthesia was administered to spontaneously ventilating dogs, and only a slight increase (4½ torr) in animals during assisted ventilation.

B. Regional Circulation

1. Pulmonary Circulation

WYANT et al. (1961) observed five normal unpremedicated subjects given methoxyflurane anesthesia after induction with methoxyflurane-nitrous oxide. Pulmonary arterial pressure did not change during either spontaneous or subsequent controlled ventilation. Calculated pulmonary resistance, on the other hand, increased from 260 to 400 dyne-sec-cm^{-5} when controlled ventilation was instituted. P_{CO_2} increased from 42 to 62 under spontaneous ventilation, but did not change when controlled ventilation was started. Thus, changes in blood gas tensions probably did not affect pulmonary resistance, but increased airway pressure may have.

2. Coronary Blood Flow

SAITO et al. (1965) observed a decrease in coronary blood flow upon administration of methoxyflurane to dogs. Statistically highly significant correlations were observed between left coronary blood flow and left ventricular work; less significant correlations occurred with mean arterial pressure and cardiac output. SAITO et al. (1966) also found that the ratio of coronary blood flow to cardiac output decreased as cardiac output decreased, while the ratio of coronary blood flow to mean aortic pressure remained relatively constant.

3. Renal Blood Flow

FABIAN (1966) studied five dogs in which electromagnetic flowmeters had been placed around renal arteries during thiamylal anesthesia. Methoxyflurane 0.5 to 0.7% was administered, producing a uniform increase in renal blood flow, ranging from 30—45%. BOBA (1965), in dogs prepared with pentobarbital, measured renal blood flow with the differential-pressure technique. Twenty-two animals were studied. Methoxyflurane administered in concentrations of 1.0—1.5% was sufficient to produce hypotension, apnea, and usually death. Under these circumstances, methoxyflurane decreased renal blood flow and increased renal vascular resistance. Methoxyflurane did not prevent the renal vascular response to trauma, nor did it modify the response once it had occurred.

4. Peripheral (Limb) Flow

MASSION and EMERSON (1968) studied the peripheral vascular effects of methoxyflurane in the canine isolated forelimb. The animals were induced with 30 mg/kg pentobarbital and ventilation was controlled. Two types of isolated-limb perfusion were employed: (1) a natural-flow preparation, in which the limb was perfused with blood from the intact brachial artery at the existing systemic pressure, and (2) a constant-flow preparation in which the limb was perfused by a Sigma Motor Pump at a steady rate and volume. Total limb vascular resistance decreased 29% in the five animals following inhalation of methoxyflurane at a 1.5% dial setting. The onset of the response was surprisingly rapid, occurring within 1 min. The fall in prevenous resistance paralleled total resistance closely, and venous resistance did not change significantly.

HAYASHI (1965) noted in normal volunteer subjects that either halothane or methoxyflurane increased both blood content of the toe and venous pressure of the ankle. These changes were accentuated by head-up tilt on a tilt table.

BLACK and McARDLE (1965) studied forearm blood flow as measured by a Whitney strain gauge in eleven normal unpremedicated patients induced with thiopental, maintained with 1.0—1.5% methoxyflurane in 75% N_2O, and studied before surgery. They observed no change in forearm blood flow or vascular resistance.

5. Microcirculation

ZAUDER et al. (1964), BAEZ et al. (1962), BAEZ and ORKIN [1964 (1, 2)] examined the effects of methoxyflurane on the rat mesoappendix preparation. In contrast to cyclopropane, diethyl ether, and halothane, methoxyflurane depressed spontaneous activity of the microcirculatory bed immediately. Both spontaneous vasomotion and sensitivity to epinephrine progressively declined as narcosis deepened. When anesthesia was discontinued and oxygen alone administered, venular dilation and sluggish venular blood flow persisted for 30—40 min, as might be anticipated from the physical properties of methoxyflurane.

ZAUDER et al. (1963, 1964) examined oxygen tensions in cerebral cortex, liver, renal cortex, and skeletal muscle of the dog during methoxyflurane anesthesia. The fall in skeletal muscle tension was slight until systemic hypotension ensued; at that time a decrease of 15—35% was noted. The decrease in renal oxygen tension, on the other hand, was considerably more marked. It occurred prior to any variations in arterial pressure. As anesthesia was deepened and systolic arterial pressure fell, there was a further concomitant drop in renal tension. Cerebral oxygen tension declined moderately in two out of four dogs studied. These decreases were independent of any variation in arterial pressure. With inspired concentrations of 0.25—1%, there occurred a moderate, but insignificant increase in hepatic oxygen tension.

C. Myocardial Function

CLARKE and CURRIE (1964) studied ten open-chest dogs premedicated with atropine and prepared under thiopental-pentobarbital anesthesia. Ventricular function curves were constructed by plotting left atrial pressure against left ventricular pressure work. When expressed as the area under the curve, ventricular function decreased by 36% during administration of 0.5% inspired methoxyflurane.

BRASSARD et al. (1963) measured myocardial contractile force with a Brodie-Walton strain gauge arch in 30 unpremedicated dogs induced with methohexital. A thoracotomy was performed immediately before the study. Control measurements were taken when the animal began to struggle. Methoxyflurane was then introduced into the system in steps of 0.5% every 15 min until a vaporizer concentration of 2.0% was reached. The step changes in concentration were then reversed. Myocardial contractile force decreased 12% for each 0.5% change in methoxyflurane concentration. There was a significant time lag between changes in inspired concentration of the anesthetic and changes in myocardial contractile force. BAGWELL et al. (1962) measured right ventricular contractile force in 21 dogs prepared 24 h previously. Anesthesia was induced in 12 animals with thiamylal and in nine with methoxyflurane. Myocardial contractile force during the control period averaged 89.3 g. During 0.5, 0.75, 1.0 and 1.25% inspired methoxyflurane inhalation, myocardial contractile force was 71.8, 59.3, 43.1, and 41.0 g, respectively. Since three of the animals anesthetized at 1.0% were not carried further to 1.25% because of extreme depression, the last value is somewhat misleading. BAGWELL and WOODS (1962) studied 16 open-chest dogs, six induced with thiopental and ten with methoxyflurane. Ten additional animals were prepared 24 h previously. Values obtained at 0.25% were used as control values. Right ventricular contractile force was depressed about 24% at 0.5% inspired concentration of methoxyflurane, 36% at 0.75%, and 40% at 1.0%. Again, only five out of 20 animals studied in this group breathed the highest concentration. In six animals, left ventricular contractile force was measured. This variable decreased by 25% at 0.5% methoxyflurane, and 55% at 0.75%. Stroke work in these animals decreased by 57 and 65% at the two concentrations.

ETSTEN and SHIMOSATO (1964) suggested that the action of methoxyflurane upon the inotropic state of the *in situ* canine heart was different from that of halothane, even though the hemodynamic effects of the two agents were similar, that is, they both decreased cardiac output, arterial pressure, and total peripheral resistance as well as ventricular stroke work and power at any given end-diastolic ventricular pressure. During methoxyflurane anesthesia, the mean ejection rate (stroke velocity) was not altered at any given ventricular end-diastolic pressure or end-diastolic volume. The afterload (mean aortic pressure) was reduced. The decreased afterload in the presence of unaltered velocity of shortening is perhaps correlated with a shift of the force-velocity curve to the left, predominantly on the force side. Ventricular stroke power was also decreased during methoxyflurane anesthesia. A further decrease in ventricular stroke work and mean ejection rate occurred during an intentional increase in mean aortic pressure up to control level. This change in afterload evoked a negative inotropic effect, as shown by a further shift of the estimated force-velocity curve to the left. The concomitant reductions of shortening velocity and stroke work and power are consistent with a decrease in myocardial contractility. The authors believed that methoxyflurane anesthesia exerts a negative inotropic effect upon the contractile machinery of the heart, and that this negative inotropism may be enhanced by an increase in aortic pressure.

In a later investigation, SHIMOSATO et al. (1968) studied the effects of methoxyflurane on myocardial mechanics in eight open-chest dogs anesthetized with chloralose or chloralose-urethane. Left ventricular volumes were determined by the thermodilution technique. Any change in volume can affect myocardial force (tension) which, according to LaPlace's Law is dependent on ventricular radius as well as pressure. Force-velocity curves were determined from a pure isovolumic contraction produced by rapid application of an aortic tourniquet. In all computations, it was assumed that the left ventricle may be represented as a homogeneous thin-walled sphere, and that all portions of the ventricle contract simultaneously and equally. Ventricular end-diastolic volume varied only 2% during inhalation of methoxyflurane, producing arterial blood concentrations of 17.0 mg-%. Maximum dP/dt of the left ventricular pressure decreased 51.1%. Estimated maximal force at zero velocity (P_0) decreased 45.1%, while maximum velocity of the contractile element (V_{max}) decreased only 2.6%. Sympathetic stimulation during the pre-methoxyflurane period increased both V_{max} and P_0. However, when the sympathetic stimulus was repeated during anesthesia, there was an increase only in P_0. The authors concluded that methoxyflurane exerted a direct negative inotropic effect upon the intrinsic contractile state of the myocardium.

SUGAI et al. (1968), from the same laboratories, studied the effects of methoxyflurane on myocardial mechanics in isolated cat papillary muscle preparations. Recordings were taken at 22 °C. The maximal force and the rate of force development during isometric contraction of the isolated heart muscle showed a dose-dependent decrease. The time between the stimulation and peak force of contraction and the time between the start and peak force of contraction both exhibited a dose-dependent reduction. However, the time between stimulation and start of muscle contraction was prolonged with increasing concentrations of methoxyflurane. The force-velocity curve shifted to the left during methoxyflurane anesthesia. The decrease in P_0 on the force-velocity curve was more pronounced than the decrease in V_{max}. Net shortening, power, and work of an isotonic contraction also showed a dose-dependent decrease during methoxyflurane anesthesia. Dynamic stiffness was unaltered. They concluded that the duration of the active state, as well as its intensity, decreased under methoxyflurane anesthesia. The shift of the force-velocity curve to the left under methoxyflurane, with a more pronounced decrease on its force-axis than on its velocity axis, can be explained by a shortening duration of the active state.

WAKAI et al. (1965) noted a depression of contractile force in isolated frog heart preparations, both with methoxyflurane 18.8 mg-% and with halothane (unspecified concentration). Halothane perfused after methoxyflurane had a transient restorative effect on the heart, after causing a short period of A-V dissociation or bigemini. This transient restoration was not observed when methoxyflurane was perfused after halothane. Methoxyflurane perfused after epinephrine sensitization of the heart consistently caused A-V block and sudden ventricular arrest.

CRAYTHORNE (1968) exposed isolated atrial strips to methoxyflurane at vaporizer concentrations of 0.25, 0.74, 1.18, 1.49, 1.74 and 2.1%. Methoxyflurane decreased the positive inotropic effect of activation (see page 187) *and* negative inotropic effect of activation. Tension decreased as rate of stimulation decreased from 150 to 30 impulses/min. If the tension at a given rate was presented as a percentage of the contraction at the same rate, the variance was less marked. The higher the anesthetic concentration, the smaller was the variation of tension with rate.

CRAYTHORNE and GORMAN (1968) investigated the depression of myofibrillar ATPase by methoxyflurane. The authors found no depression of enzyme activity after incubation for 8 min with 5 mM/l methoxyflurane. They observed a 4% depression from control with 10 mM/l, 8% with 15, 16% with 20, and 35% with 40. After incubation for 2 min with 40 mM/l methoxyflurane, a 17% depression from control occurred; 26% after 4 min, 31% after 6, and 35% after 8. The concentrations of methoxyflurane were high in this study, but the tension to which the myofibrils were actually exposed is comparable to that seen during clinical anesthesia.

PARADISE and GRIFFITH (1965) noted in isolated rat atria that a concentration of halothane or methoxyflurane required to produce a 50% depression in peak force of contraction did not change the potassium or water content.

D. Arrhythmias

All of the anesthetic ethers appear to have a property in common: they are said not to increase ventricular irritability over that seen in the awake state. Thus, one gains the impression that the heart is more stable during methoxyflurane anesthesia than during halothane anesthesia. We have mentioned in the introduction to this chapter, however, that this point is difficult to prove.

1. Incidence and Types

BRASSARD et al. (1963) studied 30 unpremedicated dogs induced with methohexital. The chest was opened and closed just prior to the study. Methoxyflurane was increased and then decreased in steps of 0.5%. Four of the dogs manifested disturbances in cardiac rhythm. Bigeminal rhythm occurred during inhalation of 0.5% methoxyflurane in one animal; another developed ventricular extra systoles at this concentration. Both arrhythmias cleared spontaneously as depth increased. One episode of isorhythmic dissociation occurred at high concentrations. A fourth animal developed idioventricular rhythm, which progressed to ventricular fibrillation.

HUDON (1961), in a survey of 939 patients, stated that cardiac rhythm "remained stable" during anesthesia with methoxyflurane-nitrous oxide. Ventilation was controlled or assisted. The patients were premedicated with atropine or meperidine and induced with thiopental-decamethonium, thiopental-succinylcholine, or nitrous oxide-oxygen-azeotrope. The authors stated that the drug could be used with epinephrine, although no dosage was mentioned. ANDERSEN and ANDERSEN (1961) monitored the electrocardiogram in 21 patients premedicated with atropine plus a narcotic, induced with methoxyflurane, and maintained with 0.5—1.0% (vaporizer concentration) methoxyflurane. Ventilation was spontaneous or assisted. No electrocardiographic abnormalities were noted.

RICHARDS and BACHMAN (1964) observed no arrhythmias in 120 infants and children premedicated with atropine or scopolamine plus occasional pentobarbital and morphine sulfate, induced with cyclopropane or methoxyflurane, and maintained with methoxyflurane-nitrous oxide. They used an ECG and stethoscope for monitoring. Administration of intravenous atropine was not associated with arrhythmias. LEWIS and SMITH (1965) monitored lead 2 of the ECG in 11 children during methoxyflurane-nitrous oxide anesthesia after induction with cyclopropane or thiopental. Ventilation was spontaneous. No "significant" changes in the electrocardiogram were observed. ARTUSIO et al. (1960) described 100 patients premedicated with a belladonna derivative plus a barbiturate and induced with methoxyflurane. Ventilation was spontaneous. The anesthetic systems used included open-drop, semi-closed and closed-circle, and nonrebreathing. The only type of arrhythmia noted was a "wandering pacemaker". CAMPBELL et al. (1962) carefully examined the electrocardiogram in 26 patients premedicated with a belladonna plus a narcotic and/or barbiturate, induced with methoxyflurane or thiopental, and maintained with methoxyflurane-nitrous oxide. Ventilation was spontaneous. The most frequent electrocardiographic abnormality observed was A-V and isorhythmic dissociation, which occurred in 5 out of the 26 cases. Two patients developed occasional ventricular extrasystoles. Other findings included one patient with cyclic inversion of the P-wave, and one whose T-waves became tall and spiked. KNOX et al. (1962) noted four cases of A-V dissociation in 20 patients continuously monitored with an electrocardiogram. Induction was with methoxyflurane or thiopental. Ventilation was assisted or controlled. WYANT et al. (1961) in studies on five normal volunteer subjects, could detect no electrocardiographic changes.

2. Effect of Increased CO_2

MILLAR and MORRIS (1961) added CO_2 to the inspired mixture in four dogs receiving methoxyflurane-oxygen anesthesia. Arterial CO_2 tension and pH were

14*

173 mmHg and 6.86 after 30 min and 193 and 6.83 after 60 min. No cardiac arrhythmias were observed.

BLACK (1964) premedicated ten children with atropine and induced them with thiopental. The only electrocardiographic changes noted during spontaneous ventilation, as Pa_{CO_2} rose from 40 torr (control) to 45 torr (methoxyflurane) were minor alterations in the configurations of the P- and T-waves. In two of these children, Pa_{CO_2} was deliberately elevated to 87 and 90 torr; no arrhythmias occurred. In two children receiving halothane, ventricular arrhythmias occurred at 65 and 71 torr Pa_{CO_2}. BLACK (1967) also administered exogenous CO_2 to eight children receiving 1.5% vaporizer concentration of methoxyflurane. The rate of rise of Pa_{CO_2} was 6—8 torr/min. Maximum values of Pa_{CO_2}, determined from finger-stick blood, ranged from 96—150+ torr. Again, no arrhythmias were noted.

3. Administration of Epinephrine and Other Agents

ISRAEL et al. (1962) injected epinephrine into 12 dogs induced with thiopental-succinylcholine and anesthetized with 1% methoxyflurane for 25 min. The rate of infusion was 20 μg/sec, and the total dose was 20 μg/kg. Ventricular fibrillation occurred in one animal, superventricular tachycardia in 3, nodal rhythm in 11, ventricular extrasystoles in 11, ventricular tachycardia in 8, bigemini in 5, and multifocal ventricular extrasystoles in 5. In an extension of this study, ISRAEL et al. (1962) injected epinephrine at the same rate into ten additional dogs. Ventricular arrhythmias were seen in all animals. Neither high procaine spinal anesthesia nor hyperventilation protected the animals against the arrhythmias. In fact, the one animal which suffered ventricular fibrillation had received spinal anesthesia. The incidence of ventricular fibrillation was definitely less in the animals receiving methoxyflurane than in those receiving halothane (see page 193).

Moss (1967) observed that the arrhythmic response to epinephrine was greater in dogs anesthetized with methoxyflurane than in those anesthetized with pentobarbital or electronarcosis.

BAMFORTH et al. (1961) anesthetized 20 dogs with cyclopropane or methoxyflurane on separate days. Epinephrine was administered intravenously over a 5-sec interval. During anesthesia with cyclopropane, 10 μg/kg epinephrine produced ventricular tachycardia in 16 out of 20 dogs. The other four animals required a dose of 20 μg/kg. During anesthesia with methoxyflurane and administration of 10 μg/kg epinephrine, ventricular tachycardia occurred in only three animals. The most common arrhythmia, seen in 9 out of 20 animals, was complete A-V block. Atrio-ventricular nodal rhythm occurred five times, and S-A tachycardia twice. Fifteen animals were then given 20 μg/kg. Ventricular tachycardia was produced in two animals and ventricular fibrillation in one of these. Seven animals developed complete A-V block; three sinoatrial tachycardia, and one A-V nodal rhythm. In ten of the animals, 50 μg/kg epinephrine was then administered. There were three instances of A-V block and three of S-A tachycardia. Marked electrocardiographic changes occurred in several of these animals, suggesting coronary insufficiency following these large doses of epinephrine.

SAITO et al. (1964) administered 0.5% methoxyflurane in oxygen to dogs for 30 min under intermittent positive pressure ventilation. Thereafter, epinephrine in doses of 10 and 100 μg/kg was injected intravenously. Ventricular fibrillation could not be elicited from 10 μg/kg of epinephrine, while one out of ten animals injected with 100 μg/kg of epinephrine experienced ventricular fibrillation. This is in contrast to those animals anesthetized with 1% halothane; ventricular fibrillation occurred quite frequently with both doses of epinephrine.

ROBERTS and CAM (1964) used epinephrine infiltrations "without incidence" in eight spontaneously ventilating patients induced with thiopental-succinylcholine and maintained with 0.5—1.0% vaporizer concentration methoxyflurane plus nitrous oxide. The dose of epinephrine was not stated.

NORTH and STEPHEN (1966) described the local injection and topical administration of 1:1,000—1:300,000 epinephrine in 741 patients receiving methoxyflurane anesthesia. The higher concentration was administered by accident. Electrocardiographic and careful pulse monitoring did not reveal "serious" irregularities or tachycardias. Premature ventricular contractions were not considered serious. JACQUES and HUDON (1963) monitored 150 patients premedicated with atropine and meperidine, induced with thiopental or methoxyflurane, and maintained with methoxyflurane-nitrous oxide-oxygen. Ventilation was controlled. Subcutaneous injection or topical application of epinephrine in lidocaine, hexylcaine, or cocaine was performed, even though the latter can potentiate epinephrine. In one patient, 1 ml of 1:1,000 epinephrine (1000 µg!) was inadvertently injected. No ventricular arrhythmias were observed. Only a transient nodal rhythm with the cocaine-epinephrine mixture was seen. ARENS (1968) monitored the ECG in 100 patients age 1—80 years during anesthesia with 0.25—0.50% methoxyflurane vaporizer concentration. Ventilation was assisted. Ninety patients received 10 ml or more of 1:200,000 epinephrine in 2% lidocaine. Ten patients received "three drops" of 1:1,000 epinephrine applied topically to the eye. In no case were ventricular arrhythmias detected. Eight patients developed nodal rhythm prior to injection of epinephrine. Three of these arrhythmias reverted to normal spontaneously, the other five reverted within 2—3 min after injection of epinephrine. In five other patients, nodal rhythm developed after injection of epinephrine and reverted to normal sinus rhythm within 10 min.

SPHIRE (1966) administered ephedrine (59 patients), methamphetamine (8), methoxamine (3), or phenylephrine (1), to patients receiving methoxyflurane-nitrous oxide. No arrhythmias were noted after administration of these agents. However, the author used an R-wave monitor, which will detect only the grossest of arrhythmias.

E. Catecholamines

1. Plasma Levels

ELLIOTT et al. (1968) induced anesthesia in ten normal subjects with thiopental-succinylcholine. Ventilation was spontaneous and the subjects were intubated. After 25 min of 1% methoxyflurane, vaporizer concentration, norepinephrine levels (trihydroxyindole method) showed essentially no change: 0.496 µg/ml before methoxyflurane to 0.538 during methoxyflurane. MILLAR and MORRIS (1961) determined arterial plasma levels of catecholamines in dogs given 0.6% vaporizer concentration of methoxyflurane under controlled ventilation. Epinephrine levels during the control period were 0.08 µg/l. After 30, 60 and 120 min of methoxyflurane, they were 0.14, 0.28, and 0.08. Norepinephrine levels remained relatively constant: 0.19 during control period and 0.22—0.26 during methoxyflurane. When hypercarbia was induced by adding exogenous CO_2, Pa_{CO_2} increased from about 30 up to 173—193. Plasma epinephrine levels increased to 0.74—1.4 and norepinephrine to 0.58—0.93 µg/l. After hemorrhage of 20 ml/kg, epinephrine levels were 0.50 and norepinephrine levels were 0.15 µg/l. After hemorrhage of a further 10—14 ml/kg, epinephrine levels rose to 2.2 and norepinephrine levels to 0.5 µg/l.

LI et al. (1968), using a modified trihydroxyindole method, determined arterial and adrenal venous plasma levels of norepinephrine and epinephrine in ten dogs induced with chloralose, pentobarbital, and gallamine. Methoxyflurane administered at 0.5% inspired concentration for 30 min produced no change in arterial plasma norepinephrine or epinephrine levels, a finding confirming the results described above. However, adrenal venous plasma concentrations decreased markedly during methoxyflurane, and rebounded during emergence from methoxyflurane. Epinephrine levels (µg/l) were 103.1 during the control period; 46.1 with 16 to 20 mg-% of methoxyflurane in arterial blood; 35.7 with 21—25 mg-% methoxyflurane in arterial blood; 185.9 with 5—10 mg-% methoxyflurane in arterial blood (recovery), and 101.0 with 1—4 mg-% methoxyflurane in arterial blood (recovery). Corresponding norepinephrine levels were 39.9, 18.0, 13.0, 98.7 and 41.3 µg/l. These results confirm that arterial plasma catecholamine concentrations do not necessarily reflect the release of catecholamines. As discussed in the introduction, these levels are influenced by many other factors, such as dilution, breakdown, uptake, and release from sympathetic nerve endings.

2. Response to Norepinephrine; Disposition of Norepinephrine

BLACK and McARDLE (1965) reported that the intra-arterial infusion of norepinephrine at a rate of 2 µg/min for 2 min into three subjects decreased calf blood flow to zero. Methoxyflurane was said not to affect this response. However, since the control response was maximal, it is difficult to say whether methoxyflurane actually did exert any influence.

NAITO and GILLIS (1968) studied the effects of 0.1 and 0.23% methoxyflurane in isolated cat atria. These concentrations decreased spontaneous contractile force 60—85% in 20—30 min. Spontaneous rate showed essentially no change. When exogenous norepinephrine was added to the perfusing medium, atrial rate increased in proportion to the concentration used. No change in the slope of this response was produced by either concentration of methoxyflurane. Thus, methoxyflurane neither potentiated nor inhibited the effects of exogenous norepinephrine on atrial rate. These investigators also noted that methoxyflurane did not affect the atrial rate as measured between additions of norepinephrine. They concluded that in clinical concentrations, neither methoxyflurane nor halothane exerted an effect either on uptake of norepinephrine by nerve endings or on catechol-O-methyl transferase metabolism. The uptake of tritiated norepinephrine by atrial slices from the perfusion medium, gave an atrial/perfusing medium ratio of 3.14 during the control period and 2.64 during 0.25% methoxyflurane, a significant difference. Thus methoxyflurane significantly decreased retention of ^{3}H-norepinephrine when compared to the control, the only agent of those tested (ether, cyclopropane, halothane) to do so.

3. Response to Adrenergic Blockade

ELLIOTT et al. (1968) induced ten normal subjects with thiopental-succinylcholine. Ventilation was spontaneous and the subjects were intubated. Administration of propranolol, 1 mg intravenously, to these subjects after 25 min of 2% methoxyflurane vaporizer concentration, resulted in a decrease in arterial pressure from 77.6 to 68.9, with no change in heart rate. No change in arterial pressure was seen in ten subjects given ether. Since pH was normal in these subjects and became depressed in the presumably hypercarbic subjects receiving methoxyflurane, the authors concluded that the pH level was more important than the norepinephrine level in determining the effects of propranolol.

F. Miscellaneous Effects

ARONSON et al. (1967) studied the *in vitro* effects of methoxyflurane on surface tension and plasma electrophoretic mobility in human blood. In blood exposed to methoxyflurane in concentrations of 8—143 mg-%, no change was observed in surface tension of blood or plasma, nor in electrophoretic mobility of plasma albumin.

IV. Fluroxene

Since the number of investigations on the remaining anesthetic agents is small, only the four major circulatory groups will be discussed: hemodynamics, myocardial function, regional flow, and arrhythmias.

A. Hemodynamics

BAGWELL et al. (1964, 1966) studied 14 animals, 7 induced with fluroxene, 7 with thiopental. A thoracotomy had been performed 48 h prior to the study.

Table 3. *Cardiovascular dynamics and blood levels of fluroxene during increasing concentrations in the inspired gas*
(Values= mean ± S.E.)

Arterial blood levels (mg/100 ml)	Change from control (%)				increase
	decrease				
	MAP	TAF	HR	SV	PR
32.4 ± 1.5	13 ± 6.9	23 ± 5.6	11 ± 4.0	20 ± 5.9	24.9 ± 12.4
41.3 ± 2.4	32 ± 2.9	34 ± 2.4	11 ± 3.6	27 ± 3.6	1.3 ± 6.5
51.2 ± 3.5	48 ± 4.2	54 ± 5.0	20 ± 3.6	36 ± 4.3	27.8 ± 17.9
64.1 ± 4.7	66 ± 2.8	68 ± 7.7	25 ± 7.2	55 ± 10.6	35.0 ± 4.1

MAP= Mean aortic pressure
TAF = Total aortic flow
HR = Heart rate
SV = Calculated stroke volume (aortic flow/heart rate).
PR = Calculated peripheral resistance (mean pressure/aortic flow).
From: BAGWELL, E. E., GADSDEN, R. H., RISINGER, K. B. H., WOODS, E. F.: Blood levels and cardiovascular dynamics during fluroxene anaesthesia in dogs. Canad. Anaesth. Soc. J. 13, 378—389 (1966).
By permission.

Table 3 shows the arterial blood levels of fluroxene and the corresponding changes in several hemodynamic variables. The values of all variables except heart rate and total peripheral resistance were concentration dependent. In the animals induced with thiopental, a reasonably constant arterial concentration of fluroxene (23.3—27.2 mg-%) was maintained for 2 h. Total aortic flow and stroke volume changed very little during that period, while mean arterial pressure decreased from 88.4% of control down to 81.9% of control, heart rate decreased from 90.4 to 82.9% and total peripheral resistance from 123.7 to 112.4%.

MILLAR et al. (1962) summarized the administration of fluroxene to 131 patients of all ages undergoing surgery on the heart or great vessels. They stated that during anesthesia, arterial pressure remained at or near normal levels in every case. GAINZA et al. (1956) commented on changes in arterial pressure during anesthesia and surgery in 100 patients of all ages, induced with thiopental or fluroxene. Sudden hypotension of undefined levels occurred in several patients. The hypotension appeared before the usual signs of deep anesthesia were noted, before any change in the electroencephalogram, and occasionally while the patient was still moving. However, anesthetic concentrations were unpredictable, since the patients were anesthetized with open-drop or closed-circle techniques.

Zeedick et al. (1966) described changes in arterial pressure and heart rate during anesthesia and surgery in an unstated number of patients premedicated with a variety of narcotics and induced with a barbiturate or fluroxene. Ventilation was spontaneous. Mean arterial pressure on admission ranged from 120/74—131/80, and heart rate from 86—90. Immediately after induction, arterial pressure was 114/86—125/74, and heart rate 82—87. The maximum arterial pressure during surgery was 120/68—148/88, heart rate 89—98; the minimum values were 108/64 to 111/67 and 78—85. Although no statistics were available, it appeared that arterial pressure in patients receiving narcotics for premedication was consistently higher than in those receiving no premedication.

Fluroxene in 40 patients of all ages produced an increase in heart rate of 10—20 beats/min (Orth and Dornette, 1955). If "marked depth" of anesthesia was produced, systolic arterial pressure decreased from 120 down to 80—90. Sadove et al. (1965), in 37 patients induced with thiopental and anesthetized with fluroxene, noted a "tachycardia" in 6 patients, "bradycardia" in 3 patients, and no change in heart rate in 28 patients.

Concentrations of fluroxene in the blood or clinical estimates of depth were correlated with arterial pressure during anesthesia induced and maintained with fluroxene in 17 patients (Dundee et al., 1957). Premedication was variable, and most values were measured during surgery. Nevertheless, the absolute changes in arterial pressure showed a surprisingly linear relationship with the other two variables. At blood levels of about 5 mg-%, mean arterial pressure was 18 to 20 mmHg above awake control. At 40—50 mg-%, the mean arterial pressure had dropped 20—30 mmHg below control.

Virtue et al. (1962) studied the effects of fluroxene in ten normal spontaneously ventilating subjects premedicated with intravenously administered atropine or scopolamine. Values before and during anesthesia were cardiac output (dye-dilution), 4.94 and 5.42 l/min; heart rate, 65 and 79; systolic arterial pressure 119 and 108 torr; central venous pressure, 7.7 and 9.4 torr; and total peripheral resistance, 1440 and 1160 dyne-cm-sec^{-5}. None of these changes were statistically significant. However, the administration of halothane to the same subjects induced statistically significant changes only in arterial pressure.

B. Regional Circulation

Zauder et al. (1964) measured tissue oxygen tension in four regions in dogs induced with 25 mg/kg pentobarbital. Ventilation was controlled to maintain a constant end-tidal PCO_2. During light planes of fluroxene anesthesia, no significant changes in the oxygen tension of the brain, kidney, liver, or muscle were seen. As anesthesia was deepened and arterial pressure depressed, there was a moderate drop of about 40% in both muscle and renal oxygen tension. The decline in hepatic tension was more marked. Cerebral oxygen tension was not significantly affected.

C. Myocardial Function

Bagwell et al. (1966) studied right ventricular myocardial contractile force in 14 dogs induced with thiopental or fluroxene. The animals had undergone a thoracotomy 48 h prior to the study. During maintenance with fluroxene for 2 h after thiopental induction, essentially no changes were seen in ventricular contractile force. After induction with fluroxene, the changes in myocardial contractile force were qualitatively proportional to the concentration of fluroxene in the arterial blood: 32.4 mg-%, —15%; 41.3 mg-%, —34%; 51.2 mg-%, —46%; 64.1 mg-%, —57%.

D. Arrhythmias

DORNETTE et al. (1962) noted only an occasional nodal rhythm in 256 spontaneously ventilating patients maintained with fluroxene after variable premedications and inductions. The number of patients continuously monitored was not mentioned. GAINZA et al. (1956) monitored the ECG in 100 patients induced with thiopental or fluroxene and maintained with fluroxene by an open-drop or closed-circle system. Ventilation was spontaneous. The only electrocardiographic abnormality observed was a wandering pacemaker. Again, the incidence was not stated. SADOVE et al. (1965) monitored the electrocardiogram in 37 patients receiving fluroxene. Neither concentration, premedication, nor induction was described. Extrasystoles were noted in three patients, pulsus alternans in one. DUNDEE et al. (1957) performed continuous three limb-lead electrocardiographic studies on eleven spontaneously ventilating patients induced and maintained with fluroxene (? premedication). Periods of monitoring ranged from 125—185 min and depth of anesthesia from electroencephalographic levels 2—7. A normal tracing was found in four patients and sinus tachycardia in three during deep anesthesia. Atrio-ventricular dissociation, occasionally in the form of isorhythmic dissociation, occurred during light anesthesia, but reverted to normal when anesthesia was deepened. The only "marked" abnormality observed was temporary inversion of the T-wave in lead 2, occurring in one patient during very deep anesthesia.

ISRAEL et al. (1962) injected epinephrine at the rate of 20 µg/kg/sec into 12 dogs receiving 4% and 12 receiving 4.8% vaporizer concentration of fluroxene after induction with thiopental-succinylcholine. Ventilation was controlled. One animal in the first group manifested ventricular fibrillation. The other 11 developed supraventricular tachycardia (1), nodal rhythm or A-V dissociation (10), premature ventricular contractions (10), ventricular tachycardia (6), bigemini (4), idioventricular rhythm (9), and multifocal premature ventricular contractions (2). In the second group receiving the higher concentration, the incidence was essentially the same: supraventricular tachycardia (1), nodal rhythm or A-V dissociation (10), premature ventricular contractions (11), ventricular tachycardia (7), bigemini (3), idioventricular rhythm (9), multifocal premature ventricular contractions (5), but no ventricular fibrillation. GAINZA et al. (1956) administered 10 µg/kg/sec epinephrine for 10 sec to four animals during the awake state and 15 min after equilibration with fluroxene. Fewer premature ventricular contractions occurred during fluroxene than before.

DORNETTE et al. (1962) administered 1 µg/kg epinephrine over a period of 15 sec to five patients receiving fluroxene anesthesia at moderate concentrations. The electrocardiogram was observed for 15 min after injection of the epinephrine. Three patients developed frequent premature ventricular contractions, one developed depressed S-T segments, and one showed no change. The authors concluded from these data that the use of epinephrine with fluroxene was safe.

V. Teflurane

A. Hemodynamics

WARNER et al. (1967) studied the effects of teflurane in eight unpremedicated dogs induced and maintained with teflurane. Arterial pressure remained stable when the concentration in the rebreathing bag was 10—25%. Higher concentrations produced a progressive decline in arterial pressure. Arterial pressure was virtually abolished at concentrations of approximately 35%.

van Poznak (1964) in a clinical assessment of teflurane found that arterial pressure progressively declined with increasing depth of anesthesia. Artusio et al. (1967) studied teflurane in 150 patients premedicated with pentobarbital and atropine and induced with either teflurane, thiopental, nitrous oxide, or cyclopropane. Measurements were taken during surgery. Ventilation was controlled if tidal volume fell below 275 ml. Teflurane produced a mean drop in arterial pressure of 10% from control values when administered in a closed system, and 2% in a semi-closed system. Heart rate decreased by 5%.

Levin and Corssen (1968) administered teflurane to 45 patients, age 3 to 83 years. Preanesthetic medication included pentobarbital plus a belladonna derivative or droperidol. Anesthesia was induced and maintained with teflurane-nitrous oxide-oxygen. Heart rate did not change significantly. A transient decrease in arterial pressure (? magnitude) was noted in four patients. In the five patients in whom cardiac output was measured by the dye-dilution method, cardiac output decreased by 18.3% from awake control values. It is probable, therefore, that stroke volume decreased and total peripheral resistance increased.

B. Arrhythmias

van Poznak (1964) stated that in dogs anesthetized with teflurane, cardiac rhythm remained regular and rapid. Injection of epinephrine (? amount) produced no arrhythmias. Warner et al. (1967) in 18 dogs induced and maintained with teflurane, observed cardiac arrhythmias infrequently at flowmeter concentrations of 10—25% teflurane. Occasional nodal rhythm, premature ventricular contractions, and S-T depression were the only electrocardiographic findings. Of 12 dogs receiving intravenous epinephrine, none developed ventricular tachycardia with a dose of 10 μg/kg. Two developed ventricular tachycardia with 15 μg/kg, and 20 μg/kg produced ventricular fibrillation in three animals. Multiple premature ventricular contractions, bigeminal rhythm, and A-V dissociation were observed in most dogs given 15 μg/kg.

On the other hand, humans are apparently much more prone to arrhythmias during teflurane. In a study by Artusio (1967), 48 out of 150 patients developed arrhythmias, including ventricular fibrillation in one patient. Supra-ventricular arrhythmias were present in 14 patients (9.3%), and ventricular arrhythmias in 34 (22.7%). In patients not receiving propranolol (136), supra-ventricular arrhythmias occurred in 13 patients (9.6%), and ventricular arrhythmias in 32 (23.5%). When propranolol 2—4 mg was administered intravenously to 14 patients before induction, supra-ventricular arrhythmias developed in one patient (7%), and ventricular arrhythmias in two (14%). Most arrhythmias were transient. Those associated with depth of anesthesia were easily reversed by decreasing concentration of the anesthetic agent in the inspired mixture.

Levin and Corssen (1968) noted arrhythmias in 33 out of 45 patients anesthetized with teflurane. Most of the arrhythmias occurred during induction and orotracheal intubation. When 10% teflurane was used at the end of induction just before the endotracheal tube was inserted, cardiac arrhythmias occurred in 58% of the patients. Decrease of concentration to 5% was followed by cessation of arrhythmias in 17 of these patients. Droperidol 1—2 ml given before induction in five patients did not seem to influence the incidence of arrhythmias. Propranolol 1—2 mg administered intravenously 1 min before induction in seven patients was rewarded by arrhythmias in four of these patients during anesthesia The side effects of propranolol plus teflurane were quite alarming — severe bradycardia in three patients and asystole of 6 sec in one.

VI. Halopropane

A. Hemodynamics

FABIAN et al. (1962) studied the effects of halopropane in 56 unpremedicated dogs induced with thiamylal. Ventilation was usually spontaneous. A 20% increase in heart rate was seen during induction. During maintenance, heart rate returned to control values. Arterial pressure remained within control values at a moderate anesthetic depth. However, when ventilation was controlled and inspired concentration of halopropane exceeded 1.5%, hypotension of about 25% did occur. At inspired concentrations of greater than 3.0%, the mean decrease in arterial pressure was about 50%.

MERKEL and EGER (1963) studied six unpremedicated dogs induced with thiopental on each of four separate days: halothane and halopropane were administered during spontaneous as well as controlled ventilation. This is one of the few studies in which a reasonable attempt has been made to compare anesthetic agents at equipotent levels, although no control measurements were taken. Various cardiovascular variables were compared at MAC (the minimum alveolar concentration required to prevent response to a standard stimulus) and at multiples of MAC. Tables 4 and 5 show the values of circulatory variables at different alveolar concentrations of halothane and halopropane. Table 4 represents values during spontaneous ventilation and Table 5 during controlled ventilation. During spontaneous ventilation, cardiac output was greater and arterial pressure lower with halopropane than with halothane. Thus total peripheral resistance was lower with halopropane at comparable levels of anesthesia. Mean central venous pressure with either agent showed a linear and parallel increase with increasing alveolar concentrations, with no significant differences between agents. As indicated in the last column of each table, no tendency for recovery was shown with either agent. During controlled ventilation with both agents, total peripheral resistance increased at MAC 1.5 or 2 before falling. With halothane, resistance did not fall as much during spontaneous ventilation. Total peripheral resistance was always greater with halothane. At MAC 1, cardiac output was greater with halopropane, but the difference between the two agents disappeared at higher concentrations. Mean arterial pressure was always higher at equivalent MAC concentrations with halothane than with halopropane. Central venous pressure rose linearly with increasing concentration under all conditions. Heart rate generally showed a progressive slowing with increasing alveolar anesthetic concentrations of either agent, but with halopropane during spontaneous ventilation, heart rate began to increase at higher concentrations, presumably due to CO_2 retention. At MAC 1.0, heart rate was greater with halopropane than with halothane.

In 396 patients receiving a variety of premedications and inductions, FABIAN et al. (1962) observed a change in heart rate only during induction with halopropane-oxygen. Arterial pressure remained constant at all times. STEPHEN and NORTH (1964) evaluated halopropane during anesthesia and surgery in 82 patients after variable premedications and inductions. Decreases in systolic arterial pressure greater than 20 torr occurred in 44% of the patients. In 14%, the arterial pressure decreased more than 40 torr. Hypotension, when it occurred, was usually noted during induction and before the surgical incision was made.

Table 4. *The means and standard deviations of various physiologic variables at different alveolar concentration of halothane (H) and halopropane (HP) during spontaneous ventilation*

		MAC 1.0	MAC 1.5	MAC 2.0	MAC 2.5
Number of dogs	H	6	6	6	6
represented by data	HP	6	6	6	2
Mean arterial pressure	H	119 ± 10	96 ± 14	76 ± 10	64 ± 12
(torr)	HP	98 ± 12	78 + 18	62 ± 17	62
Mean venous pressure	H	−0.6 ± 2.3	−0.5 + 2.1	+1.8 ± 3.2	+4.8 ± 4.0
(cm H_2O)	HP	−1.3 ± 3.0	+2.1 ± 3.4	+4.9 ± 3.1	4.5
Cardiac output	H	1.99 ± 0.52	1.75 ± 0.41	1.66 ± 0.40	1.49 ± 0.48
(l/min)	HP	2.43 ± 0.42	2.05 ± 0.55	1.89 ± 0.49	2.63
Total peripheral					
resistance	H	5,100 ± 1,320	4,680 ± 1,140	3,780 ± 730	3,540 ± 1,100
(dynes sec/cm⁵)	HP	3,290 ± 330	3,060 ± 500	2,570 ± 700	1,840
Cardiac rate	H	127 ± 27	124 ± 23	117 ± 22	114 ± 18
	HP	130 ± 29	120 ± 9	110 ± 9	124
Arterial P_{CO_2}	H	41.3 ± 3.2	46.7 ± 2.9	54.5 ± 4.8	69.3 ± 9.5
(torr)	HP	45.6 ± 6.9	47.2 ± 8.9	74 ± 9.5	108.5
Arterial pH	H	7.349 ± 0.103	7.289 ± 0.066	7.228 ± 0.082	7.127 ± 0.071
	HP	7.318 ± 0.078	7.310 ± 0.062	7.132 ± 0.041	6.972

		MAC 3.0	MAC 3.5	MAC 4.0	R-1.0
Number of dogs	H	5	4	1	6
represented by data	HP	0	0	0	6
Mean arterial pressure	H	67 ± 8	75 ± 16	64	121 ± 3
(torr)	HP	—	—	—	101 ± 9
Mean venous pressure	H	+5.4 ± 2.5	+11.8 ± 4.5	+9.5	+0.7 ± 3.2
(cm H_2O)	HP	—	—	—	+0.3 ± 2.2
Cardiac output	H	1.67 ± 0.24	1.06 ± 0.33	1.63	2.20 ± 0.47
(l/min)	HP	—	—	—	2.36 ± 0.46
Total peripheral					
resistance	H	3,100 ± 520	3,750 ± 1,000	2,800	4,580 ± 960
(dynes sec/cm⁵)	HP	—	—	—	3,560 ± 680
Cardiac rate	H	124 ± 11	132 ± 20	110	122 ± 13
	HP	—	—	—	126 ± 18
Arterial P_{CO_2}	H	82.4 ± 12.7	115 ± 31	88	44.5 ± 5.6
(torr)	HP	—	—	—	46.8 ± 6.8
Arterial pH	H	7.070 ± 0.075	6.950 ± 0.117	7.050	7.281 ± 0.037
	HP	—	—	—	7.280 ± 0.070

R-1.0 indicates recovery values at MAC 1.0.
From: Merkel, G., and Eger, E. I.: A comparative study of halothane and halopropane anesthesia. Anesthesiology **24**, 346 (1963).
By permission

Virtue et al. (1963) anesthetized eight normal volunteer male subjects premedicated with scopolamine and induced with halopropane. Ventilation was at first spontaneous, and then controlled. Anesthesia was carried to a depth of minimal electroencephalographic burst suppression. Mean cardiac output values during awake and spontaneous and controlled ventilation periods under anesthesia were 5.91, 6.74, and 5.91 l/min. Comparative values for systolic arterial pressure were 118, 92, and 84 torr, the latter two being significantly different from control. Venous pressure values were 6.9, 8.9, and 7.7 torr. Heart rate was 73, 93, and 96, a significant increase. Dye appearance time was 9.90, 6.20 and 6.69 sec, a significant decrease. Total peripheral resistance dropped from 1,100 to 704 and 773 dyne-sec-cm⁻⁵, again a significant decrease.

Table 5. *The means and standard deviations of various physiologic variables at different alveolar concentrations of halothane (H) and halopropane (HP) during controlled ventilation*

		MAC 1.0	MAC 1.5	MAC 2.0	MAC 2.5
Number of dogs	H	6	6	6	6
represented by data	HP	6	6	6	4
Mean arterial pressure	H	111 ± 22	108 ± 22	91 ± 21	65 ± 26
(torr)	HP	100 ± 21	86 ± 19	58 ± 19	36 ± 10
Mean venous pressure	H	$+1.1 \pm 0.6$	$+2.3 \pm 2.4$	$+4.3 \pm 1.6$	$+6.0 \pm 0.9$
(cm H_2O)	HP	$+0.2 \pm 2.4$	$+2.2 \pm 2.7$	$+5.4 \pm 3.3$	$+8.4 \pm 2.2$
Cardiac output	H	1.82 ± 0.49	1.45 ± 0.37	1.11 ± 0.32	0.87 ± 0.32
(l/min)	HP	2.36 ± 0.54	1.90 ± 0.47	1.20 ± 0.55	0.87 ± 0.48
Total peripheral					
resistance	H	$5,490 \pm 2,440$	$6,230 \pm 2,100$	$6,870 \pm 1,600$	$5,800 \pm 2,210$
(dynes sec/cm^5)	HP	$3,340 \pm 810$	$3,640 \pm 1,100$	$3,380 \pm 1,000$	$2,360 \pm 570$
Heart rate	H	118 ± 27	106 ± 15	109 ± 15	106 ± 9
	HP	130 ± 16	122 ± 12	120 ± 20	93 ± 27
Arterial P_{CO_2}	H	33.2 ± 3.4	32.2 ± 3.6	33.5 ± 4.2	33.4 ± 1.6
(torr)	HP	32.8 ± 3.6	33.5 ± 3.7	31.7 ± 3.7	29.8 ± 2.8
Arterial pH	H	7.426 ± 0.035	7.451 ± 0.037	7.446 ± 0.070	7.446 ± 0.046
	HP	7.374 ± 0.030	7.395 ± 0.030	7.399 ± 0.031	7.449 ± 0.069

		MAC 3.0	MAC 3.5	MAC 4.0	R-1.0
Number of dogs	H	5	3	2	6
represented by data	HP	2	1	0	6
Mean arterial pressure	H	59 ± 24	65	56	118 ± 10
(torr)	HP	25	22	—	99 ± 15
Mean venous pressure	H	$+7.1 \pm 0.6$	$+7.7$	$+10.5$	$+3.7 \pm 1.1$
(cm H_2O)	HP	$+7.8$	$+9.0$	—	$+1.6 \pm 2.1$
Cardiac output	H	0.75 ± 0.24	0.69	0.53	1.65 ± 0.56
(l/min)	HP	0.58	0.40	—	2.22 ± 0.46
Total peripheral					
resistance	H	$5,050 \pm 2,300$	7,070	7,330	$6.003 \pm 2,000$
(dynes sec/cm^5)	HP	2,770	3,050	—	$3,720 \pm 1,000$
Heart rate	H	106 ± 9	120	114	105 ± 14
	HP	107	103	—	130 ± 22
Arterial P_{CO_2}	H	33.9 ± 3.3	36.3	32.5	35.8 ± 7.3
(torr)	HP	31.0	28.0	—	35.3 ± 3.0
Arterial pH	H	7.430 ± 0.041	7.413	7.413	7.415 ± 0.059
	HP	7.465	7.475	—	7.363 ± 0.090

R-1.0 indicates recovery values at MAC 1.0.
From: MERKEL, G., and EGER, E. I.: A comparative study of halothane and halopropane anesthesia. Anesthesiology 24, 346 (1963).
By permission

B. Arrhythmias

FABIAN et al. (1962) noted a 24% incidence of arrhythmias in dogs. Nodal rhythm was the most common arrhythmia, although bigemini occurred in 5% of the animals. In six dogs anesthetized with halopropane (MERKEL and EGER, 1963), premature ventricular contractions appeared in one animal, but only after apnea occurred. Another developed nodal rhythm during spontaneous ventilation.

STEPHEN and NORTH (1964) administered an epinephrine challenge to 17 dogs at light halopropane and five dogs at deep halopropane anesthesia. All animals developed ventricular fibrillation. As seen in Table 6, an equivalent challenge during inhalation of other anesthetic agents produced a lower incidence of ventricular fibrillation.

The high incidence of arrhythmias with halopropane in man was the main factor leading to the discontinuation of its investigation as a clinical agent. Fabian et al. (1962) noted cardiac arrhythmias in about 20% of 396 patients. These occurred mainly during induction and consisted of wandering pacemaker, premature ventricular contractions, and bigemini. The ventricular abnormalities could usually be abolished by controlling ventilation. Virtue et al. (1963) monitored the electrocardiogram in 30 patients anesthetized with halopropane during surgery. They too noted that premature ventricular contractions and episodes of bigemini were frequent during spontaneous ventilation and that these disappeared when controlled ventilation was assumed. Stephen and North (1964), on the basis of their investigations in 82 patients, felt that the high incidence of arrhythmias contraindicated the clinical use of halopropane. Ventilation was usually controlled. Arrhythmias were observed in 56% of the patients, significant arrhythmias

Table 6. *Ventricular fibrillation in dogs*

Anesthetic	Dogs	Challenging dose epinephrine µg/kg				Total dogs fibrillating
		5	10	20	50	
Ethyl ether (deep)	7	0	0		0	0/7
Methoxyflurane (light)	10	0	0		1	1/10
Methoxyflurane (deep)	11	0	2		4	6/11
Cyclopropane (light)	5	0	1	0	0	1/5
Cyclopropane (deep)	5	3	1	0	1	5/5
Halothane (light)	5	0	0	1	0	1/5
Halothane (deep)	5	3	1	1		5/5
Halopropane (light)	17	12	2			17/17
Halopropane (deep)	5	2	2	0		5/5
Chloroform	5	4	1			5/5

Response to epinephrine challenge during light or deep anesthesia with ethyl ether, methoxyflurane, cyclopropane, halothane, halopropane, and chloroform.
From: Stephen, C. R., North, W. C.: Halopropane — a clinical evaluation. Anesthesiology **25**, 600 (1964).
By permission.

in 39%. Significant arrhythmias included atrial and premature ventricular contractions, runs of ventricular tachycardia, and multifocal premature ventricular contractions. Ventricular arrhythmias usually began as bigemini.

Katz (1964, 1966) and Lord et al. (1968) have performed elegant studies on halopropane-induced arrhythmias. The first series analyzed the genesis of the arrhythmias; the second described the use of halopropane as a tool to investigate antiarrhythmic agents.

In cats with an arterial pH of 7.32 Katz (1966) observed arrhythmias with 1—2% halopropane in oxygen in 45 of 73 animals. The rhythm disturbance consisted primarily of frequent supraventricular and ventricular premature contractions. The frequency of ectopic beats was usually 50% or greater. In 72 out of 73 cats, inhalation of 1% halopropane, 10% CO_2, and 89% O_2 resulted in arrhythmias which persisted as long as the inhalation continued. The latter arrhythmias could not be distinguished electrocardiographically from those produced by halopropane-oxygen alone. Of the 28 animals in which normal sinus rhythm was maintained during halopropane-oxygen, injection of a small amount of epinephrine (1 µg/kg) produced arrhythmias in 26. Halopropane-oxygen arrhythmias were abolished by decerebration, spinal cord transsection, Hydergine (mixed hydrogenated ergot alkaloids) (1—20 µg/kg), or pretreatment with reserpine (0.1 mg/kg intraperitoneally for 1 day); but not by vagotomy, atropine (2 mg/kg) or ethylbenztropine (0.1—0.2 mg/kg). The halopropane-carbon dioxide arrhythmias were abolished by spinal cord transsection, by prolonged reserpine pretreatment (7 days), but not by vagotomy, atropine, decerebration, Hydergine, acute bilateral adrenalectomy, or reserpine pretreatment (1 day). The halopropane-epinephrine arrhythmias were not abolished by vagotomy, atropine, decerebration, spinal cord transsection, or reserpine (7 days). The author concluded that the presence of suprapontine structures was necessary for the halopropane arrhythmias, while halopropane-CO_2 arrhythmias required an intact pons and medulla. The halopropane-epinephrine arrhythmias did not require the presence of any of these structures. Although cholinergic blocking drugs and vagotomy did not affect the three types of arrhythmias, the sympathetic nervous system and/or catecholamines played an important role in their genesis.

To analyze the antiarrhythmic properties of stereoisomers of a *beta*-adrenergic blocking agent (H 56/28), LORD et al. (1968) produced arrhythmias in cats by inhalation of 1% halopropane plus 10% carbon dioxide, or by injection of epinephrine during inhalation of 1% halopropane in oxygen. Dextro-H 56/28, which has local anesthetic properties but only 1/40 the *beta*-receptor blocking activity of the levo form, manifested a weak and transient antiarrhythmic effect on the halopropane-carbon dioxide arrhythmias and did not significantly increase the threshold dose of epinephrine required to produce an arrhythmia during halopropane administration. However, levo H 56/28, when tested against the halopropane-CO_2 and halopropane-epinephrine arrhythmias, exhibited a marked, prolonged antiarrhythmic effect, which was attributed to its *beta*-adrenergic blocking action.

C. Catecholamines

FABIAN et al. (1962) determined arterial plasma catecholamine levels in 14 patients before, during, and 1 h after halopropane anesthesia. A fluorometric method was used. Control levels of epinephrine and norepinephrine were 0.116 and 1.61 µg/l. During anesthesia and surgery, the levels were 0.070 and 1.11. One hour after anesthesia, the levels were 0.257 and 1.12.

D. Miscellaneous Effects

VIRTUE et al. (1963) determined blood volume and hematocrit in 12 patients before and after 1 h of steady-state halopropane anesthesia. The patients were premedicated with meperidine and scopolamine and induced with thiopental-succinylcholine. Neither variable changed.

VII. Nitrous Oxide

For years nitrous oxide has been considered as a pleasantly inert substance, useful primarily for diluting oxygen and for maintaining a slight amount of basal anesthesia. Only PRICE and HELRICH (1955) had suggested that it possessed myocardial depressant properties in the canine heart-lung preparation. Recent investigations have shown nitrous oxide to be a complex, interesting agent, perhaps most nearly analogous to a weak cyclopropane. Of necessity, most investigators have studied nitrous oxide in combination with other agents, since nitrous oxide by itself does not provide sufficient anesthesia, and since the stage-two excitement often seen with maximum allowable amounts of nitrous oxide in oxygen can mask any of its primary cardiovascular effects.

A. Hemodynamics

CRAYTHORNE and DARBY (1965) studied the cardiovascular effects of nitrous oxide in 12 dogs premedicated with atropine. Ventilation was controlled. During steady-state maintenance of halothane anesthesia, no change in heart rate, arterial pressure, central venous pressure, or cardiac output was produced by adding nitrous oxide (50 or 75%). Sympathetic blockade produced by 20 ml af 0.5% lidocaine injected into the epidural space did not alter this lack of change. However, in 6 out of 13 animals receiving 75% nitrous oxide and 3 out of 9 animals receiving 50% nitrous oxide, the authors noted a sympathetic "burst" shortly after onset of administration of nitrous oxide. These bursts were characterized by an increase in arterial pressure and heart rate and rarely lasted more than 20 sec.

SMITH and CORBASCIO [1966 (1)] studied the effects of nitrous oxide in dogs induced with thiopental and maintained with oxygen or with halothane-oxygen plus succinylcholine. Ventilation was controlled. Nitrous oxide ranging in concentration from 20—80% in oxygen produced no significant changes in cardiac output, stroke volume, heart rate, left or right ventricular pressures, left ventricular minute work or mean aortic pressure. However, there was a 10% increase in mean aortic pressure at higher concentrations, and a statistically significant 16% increase in total peripheral resistance. Nitrous oxide administered with halothane did not change the depression in most variables produced by halothane alone. The depression in mean aortic pressure was lessened, although not significantly. The decrease in total peripheral resistance noted with halothane-oxygen was abolished by nitrous oxide.

LUNDBORG et al. (1966) alternated between halothane 1% in nitrogen-oxygen and halothane-nitrous oxide-oxygen 43 times in eight dogs. Anesthesia was induced with halothane, and succinylcholine was infused at 150 mg/h. The presence of nitrous oxide did not significantly change cardiac output ($+3.3\%$) but did change stroke volume (-11.2%), heart rate ($+14.2\%$), left ventricular stroke work (-5.9%), left ventricular pressure (4.6%), total peripheral resistance ($+5.3\%$), and arterial pressure ($+8.8\%$).

COOPERMAN et al. (1968) studied the circulation in six unpremedicated normal volunteer subjects. There were no significant changes in cardiac output, heart rate, and total peripheral resistance when nitrous oxide-oxygen-d-tubocurarine anesthesia was maintained for 45 min after induction with thiopental. WYANT et al. (1962) studied five normal unpremedicated subjects under thiopental-nitrous oxide-d-tubocurarine (45 mg) anesthesia. Cardiac output fell from 5.4 to 4.8 l/min and stroke volume from 66 to 52 ml. Arterial pressure dropped slightly, while total systemic resistance rose slightly, neither significantly.

In ten young spontaneously ventilating male volunteers (HORNBEIN et al., 1969), adding 70% nitrous oxide to halothane anesthesia resulted in stimulation of the circulation at 0.8% end-tidal halothane concentration, depression of circulation at 1.5% halothane, and depression of responsiveness of circulatory variables to increased Pa_{CO_2} at both halothane concentrations. The effect of N_2O at lower halothane concentrations appeared to be associated with stimulation of the sympathetic nervous system. This effect was not observed at higher halothane and CO_2 concentrations, presumably because of depressant actions of the combination of all three agents. At equipotent concentrations (MAC), 0.3% halothane —

70% N_2O depressed circulation less than 0.8% halothane-oxygen. SMITH et al. (1968, 1969) reported observations in eleven unpremedicated normal volunteer subjects induced and maintained with halothane-oxygen. Ventilation was controlled. During a steady state of halothane anesthesia as determined by measurements of alveolar concentration and selected cardiovascular variables, halothane-oxygen was changed either to halothane-nitrous oxide-oxygen or to halothane-nitrogen-oxygen. Circulatory measurements were taken immediately before and 15 min after the change in mixture. In eight subjects, hexamethonium 100 mg was administered slowly intravenously and the changes in inspired gas mixture repeated. Only heart rate changed ($+ 4.5\%$) when nitrogen was added. Table 7 shows the results of adding nitrous oxide. It can be seen that nitrous oxide produced a stimulation of the peripheral vascular system. The authors also noted that the response to nitrous oxide was more prominent at deep levels of halothane anesthesia than at light levels, in contrast to the results reported by HORNBEIN et al. (1969). Pretreatment with hexamethonium changed the response to addition of nitrous oxide from a predominantly vascular one to a predominantly cardiac one. The response to nitrous oxide was undoubtedly influenced by the presence of halothane. To confirm these results, further studies need to be performed with nitrous oxide-oxygen alone.

The investigations described above, conducted under controlled conditions in animals and in man, contradict clinical observations. Several British observers have reported that the addition of nitrous oxide to halothane-oxygen can decrease arterial pressure to markedly low levels (YOUNG and LODGE, 1959; JOHNSTONE, 1959, 1961; APIVAR, 1959; BLOCH, 1963) while discontinuation of nitrous oxide is followed by an increase in arterial pressure (BLOCH, 1963). An explanation for this phenomenon is difficult. It is possible that enough vasoconstriction accompanies nitrous oxide to give a falsely low indirect blood pressure reading in patients with decreased body temperature. BLOCH (1963) described shivering and increased muscle tension in many of his patients. JOHNSTONE noted a considerable diminution of the digital pulse wave in his subjects. Accidental hypothermia does occur during halothane anesthesia, particularly in air-conditioned operating rooms (SMITH, 1962). We have observed that during hypothermia of 30—32 °C, withdrawal of halothane and substitution of nitrous oxide produced a disappearance of Korotkov sounds as estimated aurally and a marked decrease as measured by microphone, a profound decrease of the digital plethysmographic pulse, but an increase in blood pressure as recorded through an intraarterial needle (unpublished data). Withdrawal of nitrous oxide and addition of halothane reversed these changes. Without a direct pressure measurement, this phenomenon would have been interpreted as cardiovascular collapse.

JOHNSTONE (1959, 1961) proposed another explanation. He ascribed the phenomenon to the effects of acute hypoxia under conditions in which the sympathoadrenal system is less able to respond to the stimulus of acute hypoxia — that is, during halothane anesthesia. The rapid onset and reversal of the hypotension favor this interpretation. Also, the original case reports (YOUNG and LODGE, 1959; APIVAR, 1959) described closed anesthetic systems in which hypoxia with nitrous oxide easily occurs. However, a later report by JOHNSTONE (1961) involved a partial rebreathing system, using total gas flows of 8 l/min. When nitrous oxide-oxygen 4/1 l is administered to normal human subjects after breathing room air, arterial P_{O_2} actually increases during the first 5 min. An excessively low arterial P_{O_2} need not occur when 70% nitrous oxide is added to halothane-oxygen anesthesia in man (EGER, et al., unpublished data). Adequate ventilation must, of course, be maintained.

As discussed above, $PaCO_2$ rises when N_2O is added to halothane in spontaneously ventilating subjects (Hornbein et al., 1969). The combination of N_2O, CO_2, and halothane may accentuate circulatory depression at deeper levels of anesthesia. The cases reported by Johnstone (1959, 1961) were carried at deep levels of halothane. In fact, Johnstone (personal communication) states that the phenomenon is more likely to occur in debilitated patients with marked halothane-induced hypotension.

Another possible explanation is the second gas effect (Epstein et al., 1964). The addition of a low solubility gas in high concentrations in the presence of a second gas or vapor in low concentrations increases the uptake of that second gas. We have noted that the addition of nitrous oxide to steady-state halothane anesthesia will increase the alveolar concentration of halothane briefly. Unless compensation is made for this increase by lowering the inspired concentration of halothane, it is difficult to evaluate the effects of addition of nitrous oxide.

B. Regional Circulation

Miller et al. (1966) studied unpremedicated patients during surgery. Although it was not mentioned by the authors, an inspection of their table, which listed mean values only, revealed the possibility of a higher systolic and diastolic arterial pressure and renal plasma flow, but a lower glomerular filtration rate and urine flow, with halothane-nitrous oxide-oxygen than with halothane-oxygen.

Cooperman et al. (1968) studied the splanchnic circulation in unpremedicated normal volunteer subjects during nitrous oxide-oxygen-tubocurarine anesthesia after induction with thiopental. Hyperventilation with normocarbia and with hypocarbia was instituted during anesthesia. Splanchnic blood flow decreased from 2.06 down to 1.12 and up to 1.40 during the control, anesthesia-normocarbia, and anesthesia-hypocarbia periods. Splanchnic vascular resistance changed from 44 to 96 to 77. Oxygen concentration did not change from the first to the second periods, but did increase in the third (hypocarbia) period.

Zauder et al. (1963, 1964) measured tissue oxygen tension in the brain, kidney, liver, and muscle in dogs anesthetized with pentobarbital. When air was changed to nitrous oxide-oxygen, no change in any tissue oxygen tension was noted. Galindo (1965) could detect no change in hepatic artery vascular resistance in four dogs given 75% nitrous oxide in oxygen.

C. Catecholamines

Hamelberg et al. (1960) measured plasma concentrations of epinephrine and norepinephrine in patients premedicated with meperidine plus atropine or scopolamine. After 1 h of anesthesia with thiopental-nitrous oxide, no changes in plasma concentrations were observed. Smith et al. (1968) noted a statistically significant increase in plasma norepinephrine concentrations from 0.86 to 1.19 µg/l 15 min after nitrous oxide was added to halothane-oxygen anesthesia in unpremedicated volunteer subjects. No changes in epinephrine levels were detected. Addition of air instead of nitrous oxide produced no changes in catecholamine levels. After pre-treatment with hexamethonium, no change in catecholamine levels occurred when nitrous oxide was added (Smith et al., 1969).

D. Myocardial Contractility

Craythorne and Darby noted a depression of myocardial contractile force in dogs when nitrous oxide was added to halothane-oxygen anesthesia. Myocardial

contractile force increased during the sympathetic bursts described above, sometimes to values greater than those seen during the control period.

LUNDBORG et al. (1966) substituted nitrous oxide for nitrogen or vice versa
42 times in eight unpremedicated dogs anesthetized with halothane. When nitrous
oxide was compared to nitrogen, left ventricular end-diastolic pressure increased
2.6 torr, right atrial pressure increased 0.9 torr and dP/dt decreased 9.7%, all
significant changes. These changes reflect a decrease in myocardial function.

SMITH, et al. (1970) (Table 7) found no change in the ultra-low frequency
acceleration ballistocardiogram (Bcg) upon addition of 70% nitrous oxide to
halothane-oxygen in man. After administration of hexamethonium, however,
addition of nitrous oxide increased the Bcg by 34.7%. The Bcg is an excellent
indicator of myocardial contractility in man.

Table 7. *Response to addition of 70% nitrous oxide to steady-state halothane-oxygen anesthesia*

Variable	% change (± S.D.)	
	Before hexamethonium	After hexamethonium
Ultra-low frequency acceleration		
ballistocardiogram	0.6 ± 17.1	34.2 ± 22.9
Cardiac output	− 2.9 ± 17.9	23.9 ± 19.8
Stroke volume	− 5.5 ± 15.5	10.9 ± 16.8
Heart rate	1.6 ± 6.0	12.2 ± 11.0
Total peripheral resistance	14.8 ± 19.6	6.4 ± 21.1
Mean arterial pressure	11.5 ± 16.8	31.7 ± 23.1
Right atrial pressure (torr)	2.2 ± 1.0	0.66 ± 1.3
Peripheral venous pressure	35.3 ± 109.3	14.8 ± 41.1
Forearm blood flow	−18.3 ± 26.0	−6.0 ± 27.5
Forearm venous compliance	−16.1 ± 35.1	0.2 ± 47.9

From: SMITH, N. TY, EGER, E. I., II, STOELTING, R. K., WHAYNE, T. F., CULLEN, D. and
Kadis, L. B.: The cardiovascular and sympathomimetic responses to the addition of nitrous
oxide to halothane in man. Anesthesiology 32, 410 (1970). By permission.

VIII. Miscellaneous Agents

VIRTUE et al. (1966) investigated the effects of difluoromethyl 1,1,2-trifluoro-
2-chloroethyl ether (compound 347, Ethrane) in dogs, volunteer subjects, and
patients. In 3 out of 16 dogs given epinephrine during anesthesia with Ethrane
(amount unstated) ventricular fibrillation developed immediately after injection.
Ventilation was spontaneous, but $PaCO_2$ levels were not recorded. Cardiac output
in eight normal volunteer subjects premedicated with atropine was 6.60 l/min.
After induction with Ethrane and during anesthesia with Ethrane-oxygen, cardiac
output was 5.31 l/min; during anesthesia with Ethrane-air, it rose to 6.22 l/min.
The differences from the control value were not significant. Corresponding values
for systolic arterial pressure were 120, 80, and 79 torr. The changes from control were significant. Values for central venous pressure were 8, 7 and 8 torr.
Heart rate went from 76 to 86 and 89, a significant change. Arterial carbon
dioxide tension went from 35.9 to 44.4 and 47.0 torr. The last value represented
a significant increase from control. Eleven patients, premedicated with meperidine
and scopolamine, were induced with thiopental or Ethrane. The mean decrease in
systolic arterial pressure in these patients was 25 torr.

15*

Dobkin et al. (1968) evaluated Ēthrane in 100 patients given atropine and secobarbital or diazepam for premedication. They were induced with thiopental-gallamine. Anesthesia was maintained with a vaporizer concentration of 0.5 to 3.0% Ēthrane in 60% nitrous oxide. Arterial pressure fell from 147/90 to 123/81 20 min after induction. Heart rate did not change. In eleven patients studied in more detail, cardiac index decreased about 13% after induction with thiopental-gallamine. Addition of Ēthrane induced a further lowering (9%). The corresponding decreases in stroke index were 10 and 20%. Total peripheral resistance increased 7% after induction, and rose 24% above control during administration of Ēthrane. Left ventricular minute work decreased 20% during induction and a further 7% during maintenance. The authors detected no pulse or electrocardiographic irregularities, although the extent of monitoring was not stated. Serum norepinephrine and epinephrine concentrations were 0.94 and 0.68 μg/l before anesthesia and 1.27 and 0.49 μg/l 30 min after anesthesia.

In 1959, Burn et al. (1959) studied the effect of 1,1,2-trifluro-1,2-dichloro-ethane. This compound produced a decrease in cardiac output in the canine heart-lung preparation. The authors felt that this compound has 1/3 the cardiovascular depressant action of halothane, but less than 1/3 the potency. Arrhythmias occurred in the heart-lung preparation and in intact cats during administration of this agent.

Acknowledgements

The authors wish to thank Drs. Aldo N. Corbascio and E. I. Eger, II, for their invaluable criticisms and suggestions. They also acknowledge the important assistance of Miss Helen Busch in preparing the manuscript.

The survey of the literature for this chapter was concluded in January, 1969.

References

Abbott, B. C., Mommaerts, W. F. H. M.: Study of inotropic mechanisms in papillary muscle preparation. J. Gen. Physiol. **42**, 533 (1959).

Ahlgren, I., Aronsen, K. F., Ericsson, B., Fajgelj, A.: Hepatic blood flow during different depths of halothane anaesthesia in the dog. Acta Anaesth. Scand. Suppl. **25**, 285 (1966).

— — Hepatic blood flow during different depths of halothane anaesthesia in the dog. Acta Anaesth. Scand. **11**, 91 (1967).

Akester, J. M., Brody, M. J.: Effects of halothane on vascular resistance and responses to sympathetic nerve stimulation in mucsle and skin. Clin. Research. **15**, 404 (1967).

Albert, S. N., Jain, S. C., Shadid, J. N.: Studies on blood viscosity and its significance in anesthesia. Med. Ann. Dist Columbia **33**, 372 (1964).

Alexander, S. C., Wollman, H., Cohen, P. J., Chase, P. E., Behar, M.: Cerebrovascular response to PaCO$_2$ during halothane anesthesia in man. J. Appl. Physiol. **19**, 561 (1964).

Allaria, B., Galligari, G., Bottani, G., Castelli, S.: A study of cardiac output employing the Wetzler-Boger sphygmographic method during anesthesia with fluothane, penthrane and neuroleptanalgesia. Anesthesiology Anes. E. Rianimaz **8**, 29 (1967).

Alper, M. H., Flacke, W.: Halothane and cardiac work. Anesthesiology **24**, 121 (1963).

— Gillis, R. A., Flacke, W.: Actions of halothane and ether on coronary flow in the dog. Pharmacologist **9**, 186 (1967).

Andersen, N., Andersen, E. W.: Methoxyflurane: a new volatile anaesthetic agent. Acta Anaesth. Scand. **5**, 179 (1961).

— Johansen, S.: Incidence of catecholamine-induced arrhythimas during halothane anesthesia. Anesthesiology **24**, 51 (1963).

Andrews, I. C., Zauder, H. L., Orkin, L. R.: Methoxyflurane and halothane anesthesia during controlled bleeding in dogs. Anesthesiology **27**, 207 (1966).

Anton, A. H., Gravenstein, J. S., Wheat, M. W., Jr.: Extracorporeal circulation and endogenous epinephrine and norepinephrine in plasma, atrium, and urine in man. Anesthesiology **25**, 262 (1964).

Apivar, D.: Collapse after halothane. Anaesthesia **14**, 296 (1959).

Arens, J. F.: Methoxyflurane and epinephrine administered simultaneously. Anesthesia & Analgesia **47**, 391 (1968).

ARONSON, H. B., LAASBERG, L. H., CHARM, S., ETSTEN, B. E.: Influence of anesthetic agents upon plasma electrophoretic mobility and surface tension as related to blood viscosity, Anesthesia & Analgesia 46, 642 (1967).
— LEVESQUE, P. R., CHARM, S., ETSTEN, B. E.: Influence of anaesthetics on rheology of human blood, Canad. Anaesth. Soc. J. 15, 244 (1968).
ARTUSIO, J. F., JR., VAN POZNAK, A., HUNT, R. E., TIERS, F. M., ALEXANDER, M.: A clinical evaluation of methoxyflurane in man. Anesthesiology 21, 512 (1960).
— — WEINGRAM, J., SOHN, Y. J.: Teflurane, a nonexplosive gas for clinical anesthesia. Anesthesia & Analgesia 46, 657 (1967).
ASHER, M., FREDERICKSON, E. L.: Halothane versus chloroform. Anesthesia & Analgesia 41, 429 (1962).
AUSHERMAN, H. M., ADAM, A.: Fluothane: a new nonexplosive volatile anesthetic agent. Southern. Med. J. 52, 46 (1959).
AWALT, C. H., FREDERICKSON, E. L.: The contractile and cell membrane effects of halothane. Anesthesiology 25, 90 (1964).
BABAD, A. A.: Effect of hyperthyroidism and hypothyroidism on halothane and oxygen requirements in dogs. Anesthesiology 29, 172 (1968).
BACHMAN, L.: The antidiuretic effects of anesthetic agents. Anesthesiology 16, 939 (1955).
BAEZ, S., ORKIN, L. R.: (1) Microcirculatory effects of anesthesia on shock. Intern. Anesth. Clin. 2, 365 (1964).
— — (2) Anesthetics and the microcirculation. Effects of the anesthetics on the circulation, p. 182. (by PRICE, H. L., Ed.). Springfield, Illinois (USA): Charles C. Thomas 1964.
— ZAUDER, H. L., ORKIN, L. R.: Effects of various anesthetic agents on the reaction of the microcirculation. Federation Proc. 21, 120 (1962).
BAGWELL, E. E.: Effects of halothane on coronary flow and myocardial metabolism in dogs, Pharmacologist 7, 177 (1965).
— GADSDEN, R. H., RISINGER, K. B. H., WOODS, E. F.: Blood levels and cardiovascular dynamics during fluroxene anaesthesia in dogs. Canad. Anaesth. Soc. J. 13, 378 (1966).
— WOODS, E. F.: Cardiovascular effects of methoxyflurane. Anesthesiology 23, 51 (1962).
— — Blood levels and cardiovascular dynamics during Fluomar anesthesia in dogs. Federation Proc. 23, 179 (1964).
— — GADSDEN, R. H.: Blood levels and cardiovascular dynamics during methoxyflurane inhalation in dogs. Anesthesiology 23, 243 (1962).
BAMFORTH, B. J., SIEBECKER, K. L., KRAEMER, R., ORTH, O. S.: Effect of epinephrine on the dog heart during methoxyflurane anesthesia. Anesthesiology 22, 169 (1961).
— — STEINHAUS, J. E., ORTH, S. O.: A clinical comparison of chloroform and halothane by a blind study technique. Anesthesiology 21, 273 (1960).
BARRY, K. G., MAZZE, R. I., SCHWARTZ, F. D.: Prevention of surgical oliguria and renal-hemodynamic suppression by sustained hydration, New Engl. J. Med. 270, 1371 (1964).
BEHAR, M. G., ALEXANDER, S. C.: In vitro effects of inhalational anesthetics on viscosity of human blood. Anesthesiology 27, 567 (1966).
BENDIXEN, H. H., HEDLEY-WHYTE, J., LAVER, M. B.: Impaired oxygenation in surgical patients during general anesthesia with controlled ventilation; a concept of atelectasis. New Engl. J. Med. 269, 991 (1963).
BERNE, R. M., LEVY, M. N.: Effects of acute reduction of cardiac output on the renal circulation of the dog. J. Clin. Invest. 29, 444 (1950).
— — Effect of acute reduction in cardiac output on the denervated kidney. Am. J. Physiol. 171, 558 (1952).
BISCOE, T. J., MILLAR, R. A.: (1) The effect of cyclopropane, halothane, and ether on sympathetic ganglionic transmission. Brit. J. Anaesthesia 38, 3 (1966).
— — (2) Effects of cyclopropane, halothane, and ether on central baroreceptor pathways. J. Physiol. (London) 184, 535 (1966).
— — Effects of inhalation anaesthetics on carotid body chemoreceptor activity. Brit. J. Anaesthesia 40, 2 (1968).
BLACK, G. W.: A review of the pharmacology of halothane. Brit. J. Anaesthesia 37, 688 (1965).
— Comparison of cardiac rhythm during halothane and methoxyflurane anesthesia at normal and elevated levels of PaCO$_2$, Acta Anaesth. Scand. 11, 103 (1967).
— LINDE, H. W., DRIPPS, R. D., PRICE, H. L.: Circulatory changes accompanying respiratory acidosis during halothane (Fluothane) anaesthesia in man. Brit. J. Anaesthesia 31, 238 (1959).
— MCARDLE, L.: The effects of halothane on the peripheral circulation in man. Brit. J. Anaesthesia 34, 2 (1962).
— — The effects if methoxyflurane (Penthrane) on the peripheral circulation in man. Brit. J. Anaesthesia 37, 947 (1965).

Black, G. W., Rea, J. L.: Effects of methoxyflurane (Penthrane) anaesthesia in children. Brit. J. Anaesthesia **36**, 26 (1964).

Blackmore, W. P., Erwin, K. W., Wiegand, O. F., Lipsey, R.: Renal and cardiovascular effects of halothane. Anesthesiology **21**, 489 (1960).

Blinks, J. R.: On the measurement of myocardial contractility. Anesthesiology **28**, 800 (1967).

Bloch, M.: Some systemic effects of nitrous oxide. Brit. J. Anaesthesia **35**, 631 (1963).

Bloodwell, R. D., Brown, R. C., Christenson, G. R., Goldberg, L. I., Morrow, A. G.: The effect of fluothane on myocardial contractile force in man. Anesthesia & Analgesia **40**, 352 (1961).

Boba, A.: The effects of methoxyflurane on the renal blood flow of the dog. Anesthesiology **26**, 240 (1965) (Work-in-Progress).

Boettner, R. B., Ankeney, J. L., Middleton, H.: Effect of halothane on splanchnic and peripheral flow in dogs. Anesthesia & Analgesia **44**, 214 (1965).

Bookallil, M., Lomaz, J. G.: Some observations on the use of halothane ("Fluothane") in paediatric anaesthesia. Med. J. Australia **49**, 666 (1962).

Bosomworth, P. P., Nikolowski, Z., Tetirick, J. E., Edwards, C. B., Hamelberg, W.: Halothane versus cyclopropane in shock. Anesthesiology **24**, 125 (1963).

Bourgeois-Gavardin, M., Lawrence, J. H. A., Fabian, L. W., Dent, S. J., Stephen, C. R.: Fluothane: incidence and significance of hypotension. Southern Med. J. **52**, 53 (1959).

Brady, A. J.: Time and displacement dependence of cardiac contractility: Problems in defining active state and force-velocity relations. Federation Proc. **24**, 1410 (1965).

— Active state in cardiac muscle. Physiol. Rev. **48**, 570 (1968).

Brassard, R., Johnson, C. A., Buckley, J. J., Matthews, J. H.: Methoxyflurane: effects upon cardiac contractility, rhythmicity, and blood pressure in dogs. Canad. Anaesth. Soc. J. **10**, 264 (1963).

Braunwald, E.: The control of ventricular function in man. Brit. Heart J. **27**, 1 (1965).

— Ross, J., Jr., Sonnenblick, E. H.: Mechanisms of contraction of the normal and failing heart. Med. Progr. Rep. New Engl. J. Med. Boston, Mass. (USA): Little, Brown and Co. 1967.

Breakstone, G. E.: Zone metering of halothane anesthesia for pediatric dental procedures. Oral Surg. **15**, 548 (1962).

Brewster, W. R., Jr., Isaacs, J. P., Wainø-Andersen, T.: Depressant effect of ether on myocardium of the dog and its modification by reflex release of epinephrine and norepinephrine. Am. J. Physiol. **175**, 399 (1953).

Bridges, B. E., Jr., Eger, E. I. II.: Effect of hypocapnia on level of halothane anesthesia in man. Anesthesiology **27**, 634 (1966).

Brindle, G. F., Gilbert, R. G. B., Millar, R. A.: Use of fluothane in anaesthesia for neurosurgery: a preliminary report, Canad. Anaesth. Soc. J. **4**, 265 (1957).

Brodkin, W. E., Goldberg, A. H., Kayne, H. L.: Depression of myofibrillar ATPase activity by halothane. Acta Anaesth. Scand. **11**, 97—101 (1967).

Bryce-Smith, R., O'Brien, H. D.: Fluothane: a non-explosive volatile anaesthetic agent. Brit. Med. J. **1956 II**, 969.

Burn, J. H., Epstein, H. G.: Hypotension due to halothane. Brit. J. Anaesthesia **31**, 199 (1959).

— Feigan, G. A., Paton, W. D. M.: Some pharmacological actions of Fluothane. Brit. Med. J. **1957 II**, 479.

— Goodford, P. J.: The properties of the anaesthetic substance 1:1:2-trifluoro-1:2-dichloroethane. Brit. J. Anaesthesia **31**, 518 (1959).

Burns, T. H. S., Mushin, W. W., Organe, G. S. W., Robertson, J. D.: Clinical investigations of fluothane. Brit. Med. J. **1957 II**, 483.

Caffrey, J. A., Eckstein, J. W., Hamilton, W. K., Abboud, F. M.: Forearm venous and arterial responses to halothane and cyclopropane. Anesthesiology **26**, 786 (1965).

Campbell, M. W., Hvolboll, A. P., Brechner, V. L.: Penthrane: a clinical evaluation in 50 cases. Anesthesia & Analgesia **41**, 134 (1962).

Carson, J. S., Harkness, T. T., Hampton, L. J., Chase, H. F.: Clinical experiences with Fluothane, a new nonexplosive anesthetic. Ann. Surg. **149**, 100 (1959).

Chatas, G. J., Gottlieb, J. D., Sweet, R. B.: Cardiovascular effects of d-tubocurarine during Fluothane anesthesia. Anesthesia & Analgesia **42**, 65 (1963).

Christensen, M. S., Høedt-Rasmussen, K., Lassen, N. A.: Cerebral vasodilation by halothane anesthesia in man and its potentiation by hypotension and hypercapnia. Brit. J. Anaesthesia **39**, 927 (1967).

Clarke, C. P., Currie, T. T.: The cardiac and peripheral vascular effects of methoxyflurane. Anaesthesia **19**, 514 (1964).

COHN, J. M.: Comparative cardiovascular effects of tyramine, ephedrine and norepinephrine in man. Circulation Research **16**, 174 (1965).

COOPERMAN, L. H., WARDEN, J. C., PRICE, H. L.: Splanchnic circulation during nitrous oxide anesthesia and hypocarbia in normal man. Anesthesiology **29**, 254 (1968).

COPPOLINO, C. A.: Penthrane, cardiovascular stability and postoperative analgesia. J. Intern. Coll. Surgeons **40**, 131 (1963).

COVELL, J. W., ROSS, J., JR., SONNENBLICK, E. H., BRAUNWALD, E.: Comparison of force-velocity relation and ventricular function curve as measures of contractile state of intact heart. Circulation Research **19**, 364 (1966).

CRAYTHORNE, N. W. B.: The influence of anesthetics on the variability of myocardial contraction with heart rate. Anesthesiology **29**, 182 (1968).

— DARBY, T. D.: Cardiovascular effects of nitrous oxide in the dog. Brit. J. Anaesthesia **37**, 560 (1965).

— GORMAN, H. M.: Depression of myofibrillar ATPase by methoxyflurane. Proc. 4th World Congress of Anaesthesiologists, London, England 1968.

— HUFFINGTON, P. E.: Effects of propranolol on the cardiovascular response to cyclopropane and halothane. Anesthesiology **27**, 580 (1966).

CRISTOFORO, M. F., BRODY, M. J.: Non-adrenergic vasoconstriction produced by halothane and cyclopropane anesthesia. Anesthesiology **28**, 242 (1967) (Abstract).

— — (1) The effects of halothane and cyclopropane on skeletal muscle vessels and baro-receptor reflexes. Anesthesiology **29**, 36 (1968).

— — (2) Non-adrenergic vasoconstriction produced by halothane and cyclopropane anesthesia. Anesthesiology **29**, 44 (1968).

DECHÊNE, J. P., HÉBERT, C., McCLISH, A.: Halothane-ether in cardiac surgery. Canad. Anaesth. Soc. J. **9**, 61 (1962).

DEFARES, J. G.: A critique of the cardiac index and the introduction of a more rational index of cardiac performance. Am. Heart J. **69**, 571 (1965).

DÉRY, R., PELLETIER, J., JACQUES, A.: Comparison of cardiovascular, respiratory, and metabolic effects of halothane-ether azeotropic mixture with those of methoxyflurane anaesthesia in man. Canad. Anaesth. Soc. J. **11**, 394 (1964).

DEUTSCH, S., GOLDBERG, M., STEPHEN, G. W., WU, W. H.: Effects of halothane anesthesia on renal function in normal man. Anesthesiology **27**, 793 (1966).

— LINDE, H. W., DRIPPS, R. D., PRICE, H. L.: Circulatory and respiratory actions of halothane in normal man. Anesthesiology **23**, 631 (1962).

DOBKIN, A. B.: Circulatory dynamics during light halothane anaesthesia. Brit. J. Anaesthesia **30**, 568 (1958).

— FEDORUK, S.: Comparison of the cardiovascular, respiratory, and metabolic effects of methoxyflurane and halothane in dogs. Anesthesiology **22**, 355 (1961).

— HARLAND, J. H., FEDORUK, S.: Trichlorethylene and halothane in a precision system. Anesthesiology **23**, 58 (1962).

— HEINRICH, R. G., ISRAEL, J. S., LEVY, A. A., NEVILLE, J. F., JR., OUNKASEM, K.: Clinical and laboratory evaluation of a new inhalation agent: Compound 347. Anesthesiology **29**, 275 (1968).

— PURKIN, N.: The effect of perphenazine on epinephrine-induced cardiac arrhaythmis in dogs. I. Anaesthesia with Fluothane and Fluothane-ether azeotrope. Canad. Anaesth. Soc. J. **6**, 243 (1959).

DORNETTE, W. H. L., MILLER, G. L., SHEFFIELD, W. E., CAVALLARO, R. J., POE, M. F.: Cardiovascular system. Anesthesia & Analgesia **41**, 612 (1962).

DRESEL, P. E., MACCANNELL, K. L., NICKERSON, M.: Cardiac arrhythmias induced by minimal doses of epinephrine in cyclopropane-anesthetized dogs. Circulation Research **8**, 948 (1960).

DUNDEE, J. W.: Clinical pharmacology of general anesthetics. Clin. Pharm. Therap. **8**, 91 (1966).

— LINDE, H. W., DRIPPS, R. D.: Observations on trifluoroethylvinyl ether. Anesthesiology **18**, 66 (1957).

EBERLY, V. E., GILLESPIE, J. R., TYLER, W. S., FOWLERS, M. E.: Cardiovascular values in the horse during halothane anesthesia. Am. J. Vet. Research **29**, 305 (1968).

EGER, E. I., II, SMITH, N. T., STOELTING, R. K., WHITCHER, C. E.: The cardiovascular effects of various alveolar halothane concentrations in man. Anesthesiology **29**, 185 (1968).

EGER, W., HÜGIN, W.: Ballistocardiographic measurements during halothane anesthesia. Anaesthetist **10**, 38 (1961).

EISELE, J. H., TRENCHARD, D., STUBBS, J., GUZ, A.: The immediate cardiac depression by anaesthetics in conscious dogs. Brit. J. Anaesthesia **41**, 86 (1969).

ELLIOTT, J., BLACK, G. W., McCULLOUGH, H.: Catecholamine and acid-base changes during anaesthesia and their influence upon the action of propranolol. Brit. J. Anaesthesia **40**, 615 (1968).

Emerson, T. E., Massion, W. H.: Direct and indirect vascular effects of cyclopropane and halothane in the dog forelimb. J. Appl. Physiol. 22, 217 (1967).
Epstein, R. M.: Splanchnic circulatory responses during anaesthesia. Acta Anaesth. Scand. Suppl. 25, 290 (1966).
— Deutsch, S., Cooperman, L. H., Clement, A. J., Price, H. L.: Splanchnic circulation during halothane anesthesia and hypercapnia in normal man. Anesthesiology 27, 654 (1966).
— Rackow, H., Silanitre, E., Wolf, G. L.: Influence of the concentration effect on the uptake of anesthetic mixtures: The second gas effect. Anesthesiology 25, 364 (1964).
Etsten, B., Li, T. H.: Effects of anesthetics on the heart. Am. J. Cardiol. 6, 706 (1960).
— Shimosato, S.: Myocardial contractility: performance of the heart during anesthesia. Clin. Anesth. 3, 55 (1964).
— — Halothane anesthesia and catecholamine levels in a patient with pheochromocytoma. Anesthesiology 26, 688 (1965).
— — Influence of stress upon the performance of the heart during halothane and ether anesthesia, Suppl. 23. Proc. Second European Congress Anaesth. 1966.
Fabian, L. W.: Effects of methoxyflurane on renal function and circulation: Symposium on methoxyflurane, April 1966, Pittsburgh and New York.
— Gee, H. L., Dowdy, E. G., Dunn, R. E., Carnes, M. A.: Laboratory and clinical investigation of a new fluorinated anesthetic compound halopropane ($CHF_2CF_2CH_2Br$). Anesthesia & Analgesia 41, 707 (1962).
— Smith, D. P., Carnes, M. A.: Tolerance of acute hypovolemia during cyclopropane and halothane anesthesia. II. Anesthesia & Analgesia 41, 272 (1962).
Farman, J. V.: Circulatory effects of atropine during halothane anaesthesia. Brit. J. Anaesthesia 39, 226 (1967).
Farmati, O., Freeman, A., Moya, F.: Changes in retinal arterial blood pressure during cyclopropane and halothane anesthesia in children. Canad. Anaesth. Soc. J. 14, 26 (1967).
Flacke, W., Alper, M. H.: Actions of halothane and norepinephrine in the isolated mammalian heart. Anesthesiology 23, 793 (1962).
— — Seifen, E.: The action of volatile anesthetic agents on cardiac work, on coronary flow, and on myocardial oxygen consumption in the dog. Biochem. Pharmacol. 12, 121 (1963).
Forbes, A. M.: Halothane, adrenaline, and cardiac arrest. Anaesthesia 21, 22 (1966).
Frederickson, E. L.: Electrophysiological changes in cardiac muscle incident to anesthetics. In: Toxicity of anesthetics, p. 142 (Fink, B. R., Ed.). Baltimore (Maryland): William and Wilkins Comp. 1968.
Freeman, J.: Survival of bled dogs after halothane and ether anaesthesia. Brit. J. Anaesthesia 34, 235 (1962).
Fry, D. L.: Discussion. Federation Proc. 21, 991 (1962).
Fukushima, K., Fujita, T., Fujiwara, T., Ooshima, H., Sato, T.: Effect of propranolol on the ventricular arrhythmias induced by hypercarbia during halothane anaesthesia in man. Brit. J. Anaesthesia 40, 53 (1968).
Gainza, E., Heaton, C. E., Willcox, M., Virtue, R. W.: Physiological measurements during anaesthesia with Fluoromar. Brit. J. Anaesthesia 28, 411 (1956).
Galindo, A. H.: Hepatic circulation and hepatic function during anesthesia and surgery. II. Effect of various anesthetic agents. Canad. Anaesth. Soc. J. 12, 337 (1965).
— Baldwin, M.: Intracranial pressure and internal carotid blood flow during halothane anesthesia in the dog. Anesthesiology 24, 318 (1963).
— Sprouse, J. H.: The effect of anesthesia on cardiac excitability produced by single pulse electrical stimulation. Anesthesia & Analgesia 41, 659 (1962).
Garfield, J. M., Alper, M. H., Gillis, R. A., Flacke, W.: A pharmacological analysis of ganglionic actions of some general anesthetics. Anesthesiology 29, 79 (1968).
Gleason, W. L., Braunwald, E.: Studies on the first derivative of the ventricular pressure pulse in man. J. Clin. Invest. 41, 80 (1962).
Goetzinger, B. R., Welt, P. J. L., Massion, W. H.: Preliminary observations on methoxyflurane anesthesia. J. Oklahoma State Med. Assoc. 55, 202 (1962).
— Goldberg, A. H.: (1) Effects of halothane on force-velocity, length-tension, and stress-strain curves of isolated heart muscle. Anesthesiology 29, 192 (1968).
— (2) Cardiovascular function and halothane. In: Clinical anesthesia, Chapter 3, p. 23. Philadelphia (Pennsylvania): Davis Company 1968.
— Maling, H. M., Gaffney, T. E.: (1) Protection by digitalization against the negative inotropic effect of halothane in dogs. Anesthesiology 23, 150 (1962).
— — — (2) The value of prophylactic digitalization in halothane anesthesia. Anesthesiology 23, 207 (1962).
— Phear, W. P. C.: Alterations in mechanical properties of heart muscle produced by halothane. J. Pharmacol. Exptl Therap. 162, 101 (1968).

GOETZINGER, B. R., PHEAR, W. P. C.: Effects of halothane and paired electrical stimulation on isotonic contractions of isolated heart muscle. Anesthesiology 38, 341 (1969).
— ULLRICK, W. C.: Effects of halothane on isometric contractions of isolated heart muscle. Anesthesiology 28, 838 (1967).
GORLIN, R., SONNENBLICK, E. H.: Regulation of performance of the heart. Am. J. Cardiol. 22, 16 (1968).
GRABLE, E., FINCK, A. J., ABRAMS, A. L., WILLIAMS, J. A.: The effect of cyclopropane and halothane on the blood volume in man. Anesthesiology 23, 828 (1962).
GREIFENSTEIN, F. E.: Excess lactate during halothane-oxygen and halothane-nitrous oxide-oxygen anesthesia. Anesthesia & Analgesia 45, 362 (1966).
VON DER GROEBEN, J.: Decision rules in electrocardiography and vectorcardiography. Circulation 36, 136 (1967).
— WHITCHER, C. E., FITZGERALD, J., OMODT, L.: Computer analysis and monitoring of cardiac arrhythmias in surgical patients. Presented at Association of University Anesthetists' Annual Meeting, Los Angeles, Calif., March 1968.
GUYTON, A. C.: Regulation of cardiac output. Anesthesiology 29, 314 (1968).
HALL, K. D., NORRIS, F. H., JR.: Respiratory and cardiovascular effects of Fluothane in dogs. Anesthesiology 19, 339 (1958).
HALL, L. W.: Bromochlorotrifluoroethane (Fluothane): a new volatile anesthetic agent. Vet. Record 69, 615 (1957).
— LITTLEWORT, M. C. G.: Cardiac irregularities in cats under halothane aneasthesia. Brit. J. Anaesthesia 31, 488 (1959).
HAMELBERG, W., SPROUSE, J. H., MAHAFFEY, J. E., RICHARDSON, J. A.: Catecholamine levels during light and deep anesthesia. Anesthesiology 21, 297 (1960).
HAMILTON, W. K., LARSON, C. P., BRISTOW, J. D., RAPAPORT, E.: Effect of cyclopropane and halothane on ventricular mechanics; a change in ventricular diastolic pressure-volume relations. J. Pharmacol. Exptl Therap. 154, 566 (1966).
HANSEN, J. M., DAVIES, J. I., HARDY, H. M.: Fluothane; Clinical appraisal and report of its use in 1,000 cases. J. Kansas Med. Soc. 60, 126 (1959).
HAUSWIRTH, O., SCHAER, H.: Effects of halothane on the sino-atrial node. J. Pharmacol. Exptl Therap. 158, 36 (1967).
HAYASHI, K.: Clinical studies on the effect of various anesthetics on the vascular volume of the human toe, evaluated by a photoconductive plethysmograph. Med. J. Hiroshima Univ. 13, 235 (1965).
HELLEWELL, J., POTTS, M. W.: Propranolol during controlled hypotension. Brit. J. Anaesthesia 38, 794 (1966).
HILL, A. V.: Heat of shortening and dynamic constants of muscle. Proc. Roy. Soc. London B 126, 136 (1938).
— Abrupt transition from rest to activity in muscle. Proc. Roy. Soc. London B 136, 399 (1949).
HORNBEIN, T. F., MARTIN, W. E., BONICA, J. J., FREUND, F. G., PARMENTIER, P.: The nitrous oxide effects on the circulatory and ventilatory responses to halothane. Anesthesiology 31, (1969).
HUCKABEE, W. E.: Relationships of pyruvate and lactate during aneraobic metabolism: I. Effects of infusion of pyruvate or glucose and of hyperventilation; II. Exercise and formation of O_2 debt; III. Effect of breathing low-oxygen gases. J. Clin. Invest. 37, 244 (1958).
HUDON, F.: Methoxyflurane. Canad. Anaesth. Soc. J. 8, 544 (1961).
— JACQUES, A., BOIVIN, P.-A.: Fluothane-ether: an azeotropic mixture. Canad. Anaesth. Soc. J. 5, 403 (1958).
— — CLAVET, M., HOUDE, J.: Clinical observations on Fluothane anaesthesia. Canad. Anaesth. Soc. J. 4, 221 (1957).
— — DÉRY, R., ROUX, J., MENARD, J.: Respiratory and haemodynamic effects of methoxyflurane anaesthesia. Canad. Anaesth. Soc. J. 10, 442 (1963).
HUTCHIN, P., McLAUGHLIN, J. S., HAYES, M. A.: Renal response to acidosis during anesthesia and operation (I—IV). Ann. Surg. 154, 9 (1961).
IKEZONO, E., YASUDA, K., HATTRORI, Y.: Effects of propranolol on epinephrine-induced arrhythmias during halothane anesthesia in man and cats. Anesthesiology 29, 199 (1968).
ILLES, I. A., DEFENSOR, N. C.: Incidence and detection of cardiac arrhythmias during halothane anesthesia. Anesthesia & Analgesia 44, 529 (1965).
ISRAEL, J. S., CRISWICK, V. G., DOBKIN, A. B.: Effect of epinephrine on cardiac rhythm during anesthesia with methoxyflurane (Penthrane) and trifluoroethyl vinyl ether (Fluoromar). Acta Anaesth. Scand. 6, 7 (1962).

Israel, J. S., Dobkin, A. B., Robidoux, H. J., Jr.: The effect of sympathetic blockade or hyperventilation on epinephrine-induced cardiac arrhythmias during anaesthesia with halothane and methoxyflurane. Canad. Anaesth. Soc. J. 9, 125 (1962).

Jacques, A., Hudon, F.: Effect of epinephrine on the human heart during methoxyflurane anaesthesia. Canad. Anaesth. Soc. J. 10, 53 (1963).

Jewell, B. R., Blinks, J. R.: Drugs and the mechanical properties of heart muscle. Ann. Rev. Pharm. 8, 113 (1968).

— Wilkie, D. R.: Mechanical properties of relaxing muscle. J. Physiol. (London) 152, 30 (1960).

Johnstone, M.: The human cardiovascular response to Fluothane anaesthesia. Brit. J. Anaesthesia 28, 392 (1956).

— Collapse after halothane. Anaesthesia 14, 410 (1959).

— Halothane-oxygen: a universal anesthetic. Brit. J. Anaesthesia 33, 29 (1961).

— Beta-adrenergic blockade with pronethalol during anaesthesia. Brit. J. Anaesthesia 36, 224 (1964).

— Propranolol in anesthesia. Am. J. Cardiol. 18, 479 (1966).

— Evans, V., Murphy, P. V.: The halothane-ether azeotrope: an illogical mixture. Canad. Anaesth. Soc. J. 8, 53 (1961).

— Nisbet, H. I. A.: Ventricular arrhythmia during halothane anaesthesia. Brit. J. Anaesthesia 33, 9 (1961).

Jordan, W. S.: Effect of epinephrine during halothane anesthesia in man. Anesthesiology 23, 152 (1962).

Kadis, L. B., Baez, S., Orkin, L. R.: (2) Effect of anesthetic agents on the response of isolated small arteries to epinephrine. Circulation Research 1969 (in press).

— Smith, N. Ty., Eger, II, E. I., Whitcher, C. E., Cullen, D.: (1) Indirect methods for monitoring the performance of the heart during anesthesia: the time interval of electrical and mechanical systole. Anesthesiology 30, 343 (1969) (Abstract).

Katz, R. L.: Cardiac arrhythmias with halopropane and cyclopropane in the cat. Federation Proc. 23, 180 (1964).

— The effect of alpha and beta-adrenergic blocking agents on cyclopropane-catecholamine cardiac arrhythmias. Anesthesiology 26, 289 (1965).

— Neural factors affecting cardiac arrhythmias induced by halopropane. J. Pharmacol. Exptl Therap. 152, 88 (1966).

— Clinical experience with neurogenic cardiac arrhythmias. Bull. N.Y. Acad. Med. 43, 1106 (1967).

— Katz, G. J.: Surgical infiltration of pressor drugs and their interaction with volatile anaesthetics. Brit. J. Anaesthesia 38, 712 (1966).

— Lord, C. O., Eakins, K. E.: Anesthetic-dopamine cardiac arrhythmias and their prevention by beta adrenergic blockade. J. Pharmacol. Exptl Therap. 158, 40 (1967).

— Matteo, R. S., Papper, E. M.: The injection of epinephrine during general anesthesia with halogenated hydrocarbons and cyclopropane in man. Anesthesiology 23, 597 (1962).

Kohli, J. D., Tuttle, R. R., Dresel, P. E., Innes, I. R.: Influence of anesthetics and arterial blood pressure on functional refractory period of atrioventricular conduction. J. Pharmacol. Exptl Therap. 153, 505 (1966).

Knox, P. R., North, W. C., Stephen, C. R.: Methoxyflurane — a clinical evaluation. Anesthesiology 23, 238 (1962).

Krantz, J. C., Jr., Park, C. S., Truitt, E. B., Jr., Ling, A. S. C.: Anesthesia LVII. A further study of the anesthetic properties of 1,1,1, trifluoro-2,2-bromochlorethane (Fluothane). Anesthesiology 19, 38 (1958).

Kubota, Y., Vandam, L. D.: Circulatory effects of halothane in patients with heart disease. Clin. Pharmacol. Therap. 3, 153 (1962).

Kudo, Y.: Electrocardiographic studies on the oculocardiac reflex. Japan. J. Anesthesia 14, 851 (1965).

Kuner, J., Enescu, V., Utsu, F., Boszormenyi, E., Bernstein, H., Corday, E.: Cardiac arrhythmias during anesthesia. Diseases of Chest 52, 580 (1967).

Laasberg, L. H., Li, T. H., Etsten, B. E.: Effect of halothane on myocardial catecholamines. Federation Proc. 21, 329 (1962).

Laver, M. B., Turndorf, H.: (1) Atrial activity and systemic blood pressure during anesthesia in man. Circulation Research 28, 63 (1963).

— — (2) Atrial activity during halothane anesthesia in man. Anesthesiology 24, 133 (1963).

Levin, K., Corssen, G.: Teflurane: a new halogenated gaseous anesthetic — first clinical experience. Mich. Med. 67, 466 (1968).

Lewis, A. A., Smith, R. M.: The use of methoxyflurane in children. Anesthesia & Analgesia 44, 347 (1965).

LI, T. H., GAMBLE, C., ETSTEN, B.: Stellate ganglionic transmission and myocardial contractile force during halothane anesthesia. Anesthesiology 29, 444 (1968).
— LAASBERG, L. H., ETSTEN, B. E.: Effects of anesthetics on myocardial catecholamines. Anesthesiology 25, 641 (1964).
— SHAUL, M. S., ETSTEN, B. E.: Decreased adrenal venous catecholamine concentrations during methoxyflurane anesthesia. Anesthesiology 29, 1145 (1968).
LINDGREN, P., WESTERMARK, L., WÅHLIN, Å.: Blood circulation in skeletal muscles under halothane anaesthesia in the cat. Acta Anaesth. Scand. 9, 83 (1964).
— — — Blood circulation in the skin of the cat under halothane anaesthesia. Acta Anaesth. Scand. 9, 191 (1965).
LITTLE, D. M., JR., GIVEN, J. B.: Measurement of electrical and mechanical events of the cardiac cycle during halothane anesthesia. Anesthesiology 21, 106 (1960).
LLAURADO, J. G.: Aldosterone excretion following hypophysectomy in man: relation to urinary Na/K ratio. Metabolism 6, 556 (1957).
LOEHNING, R. W., CZORNY, V. P.: Halothane-induced hypotension and the effect of vasopressors. Canad. Anaesth. Soc. J. 7, 304 (1960).
LONG, J. P., PITTINGER, C. B.: Laboratory observations on the cardiovascular and respiratory effects of Fluothane. Anesthesiology 19, 106 (1958).
LORD, C. O., KATZ, R. L., EAKINS, K. E.: Antiarrhythmic properties of stereoisomers of a beta-adrenergic blocking agent (H 56/28). Anesthesiology 29, 288 (1968).
LUNDBORG, R. O., MILDE, J. H., THEYE, R. A.: Effect of nitrous oxide on myocardial contractility of dogs. Canad. Anaesth. Soc. J. 13, 361 (1966).
— RAHIMTOOLA, S. H., SWAN, H. J. C.: Halothane administration and left ventricular function in man. Anesthesia & Analgesia 46, 377 (1967).
LYNN, R. B., SHACKMAN, R.: The peripheral circulation during general anesthesia and surgery. Brit. Med. J. 1951 II, 333.
MACLEOD, D. P., REYNOLDS, A. L.: Effects of acetylcholine on adrenaline-induced sub-atrial rhythms in the sensitized cat heart. Canad. J. Physiol. 42, 431 (1964).
MAHAFFEY, J. E., ALDINGER, E. E., SPROUSE, J. H., DARBY, T. D., THROWER, W. B.: The cardiovascular effects of halothane. Anesthesiology 22, 982 (1961).
MARUYAMA, F. S., SCOTT, E. B., SANKAWA, H., LEIGH, M. D.: Anesthesia with methoxyflurane in children. Amesthesia & Analgesia 45, 396 (1966).
MASSION, W. H., EMERSON, T. E.: Peripheral vascular effects of diethyl ether and methoxyflurane in the isolated forelimb. Anesthesia & Analgesia 47, 515 (1968).
MATTEO, R. S., KATZ, R. L., PAPPER, E. M.: The injection of epinephrine during general anesthesia with halogenated hydrocarbons and cyclopropane in man. Anesthesiology 24, 327 (1963).
MAZUZAN, J. E., HANNA, C., ABAJIAN, J., JR.: Effect of halothane on the heart. Anesthesiology 23, 156 (1962).
MAZZE, R. I., SCHWARTZ, F. D., SLOCUM, H. C., BARRY, K. G.: Renal function during anesthesia and surgery. I. The effects of halothane anesthesia. Anesthesiology 24, 279 (1963).
MCCAFFREY, F. W., MATE, M. J.: Methoxyflurane (Penthrane): a report of 1200 cases. Canad. Anaesth. Soc. J. 10, 103 (1963).
MCCLISH, A., ANDREW, D., MOISAN, A., MORIN, Y.: Intravenous propranolol for cardiac disturbances in relation to halothane anesthesia for cardiovascular surgery. Can. Med. Assoc. J. 99, 388 (1968).
MCDOWALL, D. G.: The effects of clinical concentrations of halothane on the blood flow and oxygen uptake of the cerebral cortex. Brit. J. Anaesthesia 39, 186 (1967).
— HARPER, A. M., JACOBSON, I.: Cerebral blood flow during halothane anaesthesia. Brit. J. Anaesthesia 35, 5 (1966).
MCGREGOR, M., DAVENPORT, H. T., JEGIER, W., SEKELJ, P., GIBBONS, J. E., DEMERS, P. P.: The cardiovascular effects of halothane in normal children. Brit. J. Anaesthesia 30, 398 (1958).
MCHENRY, L. C., JR., SLOCUM, H. C., BIVENS, H. E., MAYES, H. A., HAYES, G. J.: Hyperventilation in awake and anesthetized man. Arch. Neurol. Psychiat. 12, 270 (1965).
MCINTYRE, J. W. R.: Effects of phenylephrine during halothane anesthesia in man. Canad. Anaesth. Soc. J. 12, 634 (1965).
MERIN, R. G.: Myocardial metabolism and hemodynamics in the halothane-depressed canine heart. Anesthesiology 30, 346 (1969).
— ROSENBLUM, I.: The effect of halothane on certain aspects of myocardial substrate utilization and hemodynamics in the intact dog. Federation Proc. 26, 503 (1967).
MERKEL, G., EGER, E. I., II: A comparative study of halothane and halopropane anesthesia. Anesthesiology 24, 346 (1963).

MIDDLETON, M. D., ROTH, G. J., SMUCKLER, E. A., NYHUS, L. M.: The effect of high concentration of halothane on the isolated perfused bovine liver. Surg. Gynecol. Obstet. **122**, 817 (1966).

MILLAR, R. A., BISCOE, T. J.: Effect of halothane on baroreceptors. Lancet **1963** II, 765.

— — Postganglionic sympathetic discharge and the effect of inhalation anaesthetics. Brit. J. Anaesthesia **38**, 92 (1966).

— GILBERT, R. G. B., BRINDLE, G. F.: Ventricular tachycardia during halothane anaesthesia. Anaesthesia **13**, 164 (1958).

— MORRIS, M. E.: A study of methoxyflurane anaesthesia. Canad. Anaesth. Soc. J. **8**, 210 (1961).

MILLER, G. L., DORNETTE, W. H. L., CAVALLARO, R. J.: Fluoromar as the anesthetic agent of choice for cardiac operations. Anesthesia & Analgesia **41**, 128 (1962).

MILLER, J. R., STOELTING, V. K., RHAMY, R. K.: A comparison of the effects on renal tubular function of halothane-oxygen and halothane-nitrous oxide-oxygen anesthesia. Anesthesia & Analgesia **45**, 41 (1966).

— TOWNLEY, N., STOELTING, V. K., RHAMY, R. K.: Effect of halothane anesthesia on renal tubular function in man. Anesthesia & Analgesia **44**, 236 (1965).

MOE, G. K., MALTON, S. D., RENNICK, B. R., FREYBURGER, W. A.: The role of arterial pressure in the induction of idioventricular rhythms under cyclopropane anesthesia. J. Pharmacol. Exptl Therap. **94**, 319 (1948).

MORRIS, L. E., FELDMAN, S. A.: Influence of hypercarbia and hypotension upon liver damage following halothane anaesthesia. Anaesthesia **18**, 32 (1963).

MORROW, D. H., GAFFNEY, T. E., HOLMAN, J. E.: The chronotropic and inotropic effects of halothane. Anesthesiology **22**, 915 (1961).

— MORROW, A. G.: The effects of halothane on myocardial contractile force and vascular resistance. Anesthesiology **22**, 537 (1961).

— PIERCE, G. E.: Effect of halothane on systemic venous reactivity. J. Sci. Research **8**, 115 (1968).

MORSE, H. T., LINDE, H. W., MISHALOVE, R. D., PRICE, H. L.: Relation of blood volume and hemodynamic changes during halothane anesthesia in man. Anesthesiology **24**, 790 (1963).

MOSS, C. M.: Electroanesthesia: comparison of its cardiovascular effects to those of pentobarbital and methoxyflurane. Bull. Tulane Univ. Med. Fac. **26**, 226 (1967).

— DOMER, F. R.: Comparisons of selected cardiovascular responses in dogs anesthetized with electricity, pentobarbital or methoxyflurane. Anesthesia & Analgesia **46**, 287 (1967).

MOYERS, J., PITTINGER, C. B.: Changes in blood pressure and pulse rate during Fluothane anesthesia: a comparative clinical study. Anesthesiology **20**, 605 (1959).

MUIR, B. J., HALL, L. W., LITTLEWORT, M. C. G.: Cardiac irregularities in cats under halothane anaesthesia. Brit. J. Anaesthesia **31**, 488 (1959).

MUNCHOW, O. B., DENSON, J. S.: Modification by light cyclopropane and halothane anesthesia of the chronotropic effect of atropine in man. Anesthesia & Analgesia **44**, 782 (1965).

MURRAY, J. F., GOLD, P., JOHNSON, B. L., JR.: Circulatory effects of hematocrit variations in normovolemic and hypervolemic dogs. J. Clin. Invest. **42**, 1150 (1963).

MURTAGH, G. P.: Controlled hypotension with halothane. Anaesthesia **15**, 235 (1960).

NAITO, H., GILLIS, C. N.: Anesthetics and response of atria to sympathetic nerve stimulation. Anesthesiology **29**, 259 (1968).

NAYLER, W. G.: The action of Fluothane, chloroform and hypothermia on the heart. Australian J. Exptl Biol. Med. Sci. **37**, 279 (1959).

NEILL, R. S., NIXON, B. A.: Halothane and tubocurarine. A study of changes in blood pressure. Anaesthesia **20**, 250 (1965).

NELSON, R. M., HENRY, J. W., LYMAN, J. H.: Influence of l-norepinephrine on renal blood flow, renal vascular resistance, and urine flow in hemorrhagic shock. Surgery **50**, 115 (1961).

NGAI, S. H., BOLME, P.: (1) Effects of anesthetics on circulatory regulatory mechanisms in the dog. J. Pharmacol. Exptl Therap. **153**, 495 (1966).

— — (2) Effects of anesthetics on cardiovascular responses to hypothalamic and mesencephalic stimulation in dogs. Anesthesiology **27**, 223 (1966).

— OZERNITSKY, S., DIAZ, P. M.: The effects of anesthetics on the release of norepinephrine from sympathetic nerves. Anesthesiology **29**, 207 (1968).

NOBLE, M. I., TRENCHARD, D., GUZ, A.: Left ventricular ejection in conscious dogs. I. Measurement and significance of the maximum acceleration of blood from the left ventricle. Circulation Research **19**, 139 (1966).

NORTH, W. C., STEPHEN, C. R.: Methoxyflurane — a second look at 4 years of experience. Anesthesia & Analgesia **45**, 117 (1966).

O'BRIEN, G. S., EID, C. H., MURPHY, Q. R., JR., MEEK, W. J.: Effects of elimination of hepatic circulation on cyclopropane-epinephrine ventricular tachycardia and arterial serum potassium in dogs. J. Pharmacol. Exptl Therap. **112**, 374 (1954).

ORTH, O. S., DORNETTE, W. H. L.: Fluoromar as an anesthetic agent. Federation Proc. 14, 376 (1955) (Abstract).
OZORIO, H. P. L.: Control of abnormal hypertensive responses by halothane. Anesthesiology 24, 885 (1963).
PAPPER, E. M., NGAI, S. H.: Kidney function during anesthesia. Ann. Rev. Med. 7, 213 (1956).
PARADISE, R. R., GRIFFITH, L. K.: Influence of halothane, chloroform and methoxyflurane on potassium content of rat atria. Anesthesiology 26, 195 (1965).
— — Electrolyte content of perfused rat ventricles exposed to halothane or anoxia. J. Pharmacol. Exptl Therap. 54, 281 (1966).
PATTERSON, S. W., STARLING, E. H.: On mechanical factors which determine output of ventricles. J. Physiol. (London) 48, 357 (1914).
PAUCA, A., SYKES, M. K.: Upper limb blood flow during thiopentone-halothane anaesthesia. Brit. J. Anaesthesia 39, 758 (1967).
PAYNE, J. P., GARDINER, D., VERNER, I. R.: Cardiac output during halothane anaesthesia. Brit. J. Anaesthesia 31, 87 (1959).
PETTER, A., SCHLAG, G.: Treatment of epinephrine induced cardiac arrhythmias during anesthesia with halogenated inhalation anesthetics. Anaesthetist 14, 68 (1965).
PHILIPPART, C.: Fluothane et débit coronaire. Acta Anaesth. Belgica 14, 219 (1963).
PODOLSKY, R. J.: Mechanism of muscular contraction. Am. J. Med. 30, 708 (1961).
PRICE, H. L.: General anesthesia and circulatory homeostasis. Physiol. Revs 40, 187 (1960).
— Circulation during anesthesia and operation. Springfield (Illinois): Charles C. Thomas 1967.
— COHEN, P. J.: Effects of anesthetics on the circulation. Springfield (Illinois): Charles C. Thomas 1964.
— HELRICH, M.: The effects of cyclopropane, diethyl ether, nitrous oxide, thiopental, and hydrogen ion concentration on the myocardial function of the dog heart-lung preparation. J. Pharmacol. Exptl Therap. 115, 206 (1955).
— DEUTSCH, S., DAVIDSON, I. A., CLEMENT, A. J., BEHAR, M. G., EPSTEIN, R. M.: Can general anesthetics produce splanchnic visceral hypoxia by reducing regional blood flow? Anesthesiology 27, 24 (1966).
— LINDE, H. W., JONES, R. E., BLACK, G. W., PRICE, M. L.: Sympatho-adrenal responses to general anesthesia in man and their relation to hemodynamics. Anesthesiology 20, 563 (1959).
— — MORSE, H. T.: Central nervous actions of halothane affecting the systemic circulation. Anesthesiology 24, 770 (1963).
— PRICE, M. L.: Has halothane a predominant circulatory action? Anesthesiology 27, 764 (1966).
— — Relative ganglion-blocking potencies of cyclopropane, halothane, and nitrous oxide, and the interaction of nitrous oxide with halothane. Anesthesiology 28, 349 (1967).
— — MORSE, H. T.: Effects of cyclopropane, halothane, and procaine on the vasomotor "center" of the dog. Anesthesiology 26, 55 (1965).
PRICE, M. L., PRICE, H. L.: Effects of general anesthetics on contractile responses of rabbit aortic strips. Anesthesiology 23, 16 (1962).
PRYS-ROBERTS, C., KELMAN, G. R., KAIN, M. L., GREENBAUM, R., BAY, J.: Cardiac output and blood carbon dioxide levels in man. Brit. J. Anaesthesia 39, 687 (1967).
PURCHASE, I. F. H.: The effect of halothane on the sympathetic nerve supply to the myocardium. Brit. J. Anaesthesia 37, 915 (1965).
— (1) Cardiac arrhythmias occurring during halothane anaesthesia in cats. Brit. J. Anaesthesia 38, 13 (1966).
— (2) The effect of halothane on the isolated cat heart. Brit. J. Anaesthesia 38, 80 (1966).
RAVENTOS, J.: The action of Fluothane — a new volatile anaesthetic. Brit. J. Pharmacol. 11, 394 (1956).
— DEE, J.: The action of the halothane-diethyl ether azeotropic mixture on experimental animals. Brit. J. Anaesthesia 31, 46 (1959).
REEVES, J. T., GROVER, R. F., FILLEY, G. F., BLOUNT, S. G., JR.: Cardiac output in normal resting man. J. Appl. Physiol. 16, 276 (1961).
REIN, J., AUSTEN, W. G., MORROW, D. H.: Effects of guanethidine and reserpine on the cardiac responses to halothane. Anesthesiology 24, 672 (1963).
RESTALL, C. J., MILDE, J. H., THEYE, R. A.: Circulatory indices of methoxyflurane, halothane and ether anesthesia. Anesthesia & Analgesia 45, 330 (1966).
RICHARDS, C. C., BACHMAN, L.: Methoxyflurane anesthesia for pediatric neurosurgical operations: clinical evaluation of 120 cases. Anesthesia & Analgesia 43, 144 (1964).
ROBERTS, R. B., CAM, J. F.: Methoxyflurane: a clinical study of fifty selected cases. Brit. J. Anaesthesia 36, 494 (1964).
ROGOMAN, E. P., JOHNSTON, A. E., CONN, A. W.: The use of epinephrine during halothane anaesthesia with respect to ventricular irritabliity in dogs. Anesthesiology 42, 109 (1963).

Rosen, M., Roe, R. B.: Adrenaline infiltration during halothane anaesthesia: a report of two cases of cardiac arrest. Brit. J. Anaesthesia **35**, 51 (1963).

Ross, J., Jr., Covell, J. W., Sonnenblick, E. H., Braunwald, E.: Contractile state of the heart characterized by force-velocity relations in variably afterloaded and isovolumic beats. Circulation Research **18**, 149 (1966).

Rushmer, R. F.: Cardiovascular dynamics, 2nd ed., Chapter 2. Philadelphia (Pennsylvania): W. B. Saunders 1961.

— Effects of nerve stimulation and hormones on heart: role of heart in general circulatory regulation. In: Handbook of physiology, Vol. 1, Sect. 2, p. 533. Washington, D.C.: American Physiol. Soc. 1962.

— Initial ventricular impulse: a potential key to cardiac evaluation. Circulation **29**, 268 (1964).

Sadove, M. S., Balagot, R. C., Linde, H. W.: The effects of Fluoromar on certain organ functions. Anesthesia & Analgesia **36**, 758 (1965).

Saito, T.: Epinephrine induced cardiac arrhythmias during methoxyflurane and halothane anesthesia in dogs. Japan. J. Anesth. **13**, 347 (1964).

— Coronary circulation during inhalation anesthesia in dogs. Japan. J. Anesth. **14**, 815 (1965).

— Wakisaka, K., Okazaki, K.: (1) Hemodynamic effects of halothane in relation to oxygen supply and halothane uptake of the myocardium and whole body in dogs. Tokushima J. Exp. Med. **13**, 149 (1966).

— — Yudate, T., Okazaki, K., Hirano, T., Maoka, N.: (2) Coronary and systemic circulation during (inhalation) anesthesia in dogs. Far East J. Anaesth. **5**, 105 (1966).

Sarnoff, S. J., Mitchell, J. H.: Control of function of heart. In: Handbook of physiology, Vol. 1, Sect. 2, p. 489. Washington, D.C.: American Physiol. Soc. 1962.

Schmahl, F. W.: Effects of anesthetics on regional cerebral blood flow and the regional content of some metabolites of the brain cortex of the cat. Acta Neurol. Scand. **41** (Suppl. 14), 156 (1965).

Segar, W. E., Riley, P. A., Jr., Barila, T. G.: Urinary composition during hypothermia. Am. J. Physiol. **185**, 528 (1956).

Sessler, A. D., Theye, R. A.: Metabolic and circulatory aspects of halothane anesthesia. Anesthesiology **27**, 226 (1966).

Severinghaus, J. W., Cullen, S. C.: Depression of myocardium and body oxygen consumption with Fluothane in man. Anesthesiology **19**, 165 (1958).

Shimosato, S.: Discussion: effects of anesthetics on the circulation, p. 135 (Price, H. L., Cohen, P. J., Ed.). Springfield (Illinois): Charles C. Thomas Comp. 1964.

— Etsten, B. E.: Performance of digitalized heart during halothane anesthesia. Anesthesiology **24**, 41 (1963).

— Li, T. H., Etsten, B.: Ventricular function during halothane anesthesia in closed-chest dogs. Circulation Research **12**, 63 (1963).

— Shanks, C., Etsten, B. E.: The effects of methoxyflurane and sympathetic nerve stimulation on myocardial mechanics. Anesthesiology **29**, 538 (1968).

Shinozaki, T., Mazuzan, J. E., Abajian, J., Jr.: Halothane and the heart. Brit. J. Anaesthesia **39**, 79 (1968).

Shipley, R. E., Study, R. S.: Factors regulating renal blood flow and urine flow following acute changes in renal artery perfusion pressure. Am. J. Physiol. **163**, 750 (1950).

— — Changes in renal blood flow, extraction of inulin, glomerular filtration rate, tissue pressure and urine flow with acute alterations of renal arterial blood pressure. Am. J. Physiol. **167**, 676 (1951).

Smith, N. Ty.: Subcutaneous, muscle, and body temperatures in anesthetized man. J. Appl. Physiol. **17**, 306 (1962).

— Pressor agents. Calif. Med. **107**, 33 (1967).

— van Citters, R. L., Verdouw, P. D.: (3) Relation between the pneumocardiogram and aortic flow in the baboon. Ballistocardiography and Circulatory Performance. Bibliotheca Cardiologica **24**: 34 Basel: Karger (1969).

— — — The relation between the ultra-low frequency ballistocardiogram, the acceleration pneumocardiogram, and ascending aortic flow acceleration in the baboon. Proc. 2nd World Congress on Ballistocardiography and Cardiovascular Dynamics, Oporto 1969.

— Corbascio, A. N.: (1) The cardiovascular effects of nitrous oxide during halothane anesthesia in the dog. Anesthesiology **27**, 560 (1966).

— — (2) Myocardial resistance to metabolic acidosis. Arch. Surg. **92**, 892 (1966).

— Eger, E. I., II, Kadis, L. B.: Use of an analog computer to study cardiovascular effects of anaesthetic and ancillary agents. Progress in Anesthesiology Proc. Fourth World Congress of Anaesthesiologists, London, 597 (1969).

SMITH N. TY., EGER, E. I., II, STOELTING, R. K., WHITCHER, C. E.: (1) Cardiovascular effects of halothane in man. Studies during induction and sudden changes in concentration. J. Am. Med. Assoc. **206**, 1495 (1968).

— — WHITCHER, C. E., STOELTING, R. K., CULLEN, D., KADIS, L. B.: The cardiovascular and sympathomimetic responses to the addition of nitrous oxide to halothane in man. Anesthesiology **32**, 410 (1970).

— — — — WHAYNE, T. F.: (2) The circulatory effects of the addition of nitrous oxide to halothane anesthesia in man. Anesthesiology **29**, 212 (1968).

— WHITCHER, C. E.: Hemodynamic effects of gallamine and d-tubocurarine administered during halothane anesthesia. J. Amer. Med. Assoc. **199**, 704 (1967).

SMITH, S. L., WEBB, W. R., FABIAN, L. W., HAGAMAN, V. D.: Cardiac excitability in ether, cyclopropane and halothane anesthesia. Anesthesiology **23**, 766 (1962).

SONNENBLICK, E. H.: Determinants of active state in heart muscle: force, velocity, instantaneous muscle length, time. Federation Proc. **24**, 1396 (1965).

— BRAUNWALD, E., MORROW, A. G.: Contractile properties of human heart muscle: studies on myocardial mechanics of surgically excised papillary muscle. J. Clin. Invest. **44**, 966 (1965).

— — WILLIAMS, J. F., JR., GLICK, G.: Effects of exercise on myocardial force-velocity relations in intact unanesthetized man: relative roles of changes in heart rate, sympathetic activity, and ventricular dimension. J. Clin. Invest. **44**, 2051 (1965).

— MORROW, A. G., WILLIAMS, J. F., JR.: Effects of heart rate on dynamics of force development in intact human ventricle. Circulation **33**, 945 (1966).

— ROSS, J., JR., COVELL, J. W., BRAUNWALD, E.: Alterations in resting length-tension relations of cardiac muscle induced by changes in contractile force. Circulation Research **19**, 980 (1966).

SPHIRE, R. D.: Hypotension and other problems associated with methoxyflurane administration. Anesthesia & Analgesia **45**, 737 (1966).

SPIECKERMANN, P. G., BRÜCKNER, J., EBERLEIN, H. J., GREBE, D., KÜBLER, W., LOHR, B., BRETSCHNEIDER, H. J.: The influence of barbiturates, halothane, and droperidolfentanyl on the metabolism of high energy phosphates of the dog heart. Proc. Fourth World Congress of Anaesthesiologists, London 1968.

STARR, I., HORWITZ, O., MAYOCK, R. L., KRUMBHAAR, E. B.: Standardization of the ballistocardiogram by simulation of the heart's function at necropsy, with a clinical method for the estimation of cardiac strength and normal standards for it. Circulation **1**, 1073 (1950).

— MAYOCK, R. L., HORWITZ, O., KRUMBHAAR, E. B.: On the initial force of cardiac contraction, standardization of ballistocardiogram by physiological experiments performed at necropsy. Trans. Assoc. Am. Physicians **62**, 154 (1949).

— OGAWA, S.: Incoordination of the cardiac contraction in clinical conditions; as judged by the ballistocardiogram and the pulse derivative. Am. J. Med. Sci. **224**, 663 (1962).

STEPHEN, C. R., GROSSKREUTZ, D. C., LAWRENCE, J. H. A., FABIAN, L. W., BOURGEOIS-GAVADIN, M., COUGHLIN, J.: Evaluation of Fluothane for clinical anaesthesia. Canad. Anaesth. Soc. J. **4**, 246 (1957).

— NORTH, W. C.: Halopropane — a clinical evaluation. Anesthesiology **25**, 600 (1964).

STIRLING, G. R., MORRIS, K. N., ORTON, R. H., BOAKE, W. C., RACE, D. R., KINROSS, F., THOMSON, J. W., CROSBY, W.: Halothane and circulatory occlusion: some experimental and clinical observations. Brit. J. Anaesthesia **32**, 262 (1960).

SUGAI, N., SHIMOSATO, S., ETSTEN, B. E.: Effect of methoxyflurane upon myocardial mechanics. Anesthesiology **29**, 215 (1968).

SUMMERS, F. W., KOONS, R. A., DENSON, J. S.: The effects of d-tubocurarine on blood pressure during Fluothane anesthesia in man. Anesthesia & Analgesia **41**, 17 (1962).

SUTHERLAND, A., HASELBY, K., ABEL, F. L.: Comparative measurements of ventricular contractility. Federation Proc. **28**, 327 (1969).

SYKES, M. K.: Repeated cardiac arrest with halothane. A case report. Brit. J. Anaesthesia **37**, 208 (1965).

TAKAORI, M., LOEHNING, R. W.: Ventricular arrhythmias during halothane anaesthesia: effect of isoproterenol, aminophylline, and ephedrine. Canad. Anaesth. Soc. J. **12**, 275 (1965).

TAYLOR, J. S., DENSON, J. S.: Comparison of the effects of some inhalation anesthetic agents on forearm blood flow. Anesthesiology **28**, 271 (1967).

TE, L. T., CONN, A. W.: Effect of adrenergic beta-receptor blocker on epinephrine-induced cardiac arrhythmias during halothane anesthesia. Canad. Anaesth. Soc. J. **13**, 242 (1966).

THEYE, R. A.: Myocardial and total oxygen consumption with halothane. Anesthesiology **28**, 1042 (1967).

— MILDE, J. H., MICHENFELDER, J. D.: Effect of hypocapnia on cardiac output during anesthesia. Anesthesiology **27**, 778 (1966).

THEYE, R. A., SESSLER, A. D.: Effect of halothane anesthesia on rate of canine oxygen consumption. Anesthesiology 28, 661 (1967).

THOMPSON, D. D., PITTS, R. F.: Effects of alteration of renal arterial pressure on sodium and water excretion. Am. J. Physiol. 168, 490 (1952).

THROWER, W. B., DARBY, T. D., ALDINGER, E. E., SPROUSE, J. H.: Effects of halothane (Fluothane) anesthesia on ventricular contractile force in the human and dog. Federation Proc. 19, 274 (1960).

TOMLIN, P. J.: Methoxyflurane. Brit. J. Anaesthesia 37, 706 (1965).

— SCHLOBOHM, R. M., CARSON, S. A. A., MORRIS, L. E.: The effects of hypothermia, hypercapnia and pH upon cardiac output in the halothane anaesthetized dog. Brit. J. Anaesthesia 38, 660 (1966).

TUOHY, G. F., THEYE, R. A.: Comparative haemodynamics during operation, unreplaced blood loss, and anaesthesia with ether or halothane in nitrous oxide and oxygen. Brit. J. Anaesthesia 36, 212 (1964).

VAN POZNAK, A.: Laboratory and clinical investigations of teflurane. J. Am. Assoc. Nurse Anesthetists 19, 38 (1964).

VAREJES, L.: The use of solutions containing adrenaline during halothane anaesthesia. Anaesthesia 18, 507 (1963).

VICK, R. L.: Effects of altered heart rate on chloroform-epinephrine cardiac arrhythmia. Circulation Research 18, 316 (1966).

VIRTUE, R. W., LUND, L. O., PHELPS, M., VOGEL, J. H. K., BECKWITT, H., HERON, M.: Difluoromethyl 1,1,2-Trifluoro-2-Chloroethyl ether as an anaesthetic agent: results with dogs, and a preliminary note on observations with man. Canad. Anaesth. Soc. J. 13, 233 (1966).

— VOGEL, J. H. K., PRESS, P., GROVER, R. F.: Respiratory and hemodynamic measurements during anesthesia. J. Am. Med. Assoc. 179, 224 (1962).

— YOUNG, R. V., LUND, L. O., VOGEL, J. H. K., GROVER, R. F.: Halopropane anesthesia in man. Laboratory and clinical studies. Anesthesiology 24, 217 (1963).

WAKAI, I., MIYAKE, S., TASHIRO, M., ODA, M.: A study of the direct effects of Fluothane and Penthrane on the isolated heart preparation. Japan. J. Anaesth. 14, 472 (1965).

WALKER, J. A., EGGERS, G. W. N., ALLEN, C. R.: (1) Cardiovascular effects of methoxyflurane anesthesia. Anesthesiology 23, 164 (1962) (Abstract).

— — — (2) Cardiovascular effects of methoxyflurane in man. Anesthesiology 23, 639 (1962).

WALLACE, A. G., SKINNER, N. S., JR., MITCHELL, J. H.: Hemodynamic determinants of the maximal rate of rise of left ventricular pressure. Am. J. Physiol. 205, 30 (1963).

WALTHER, W. W., SLACK, W. K., CHEW, H. E. R.: The cardiac output under halothane anaesthesia with induced hypotension. Lancet 1964 II, 1266.

WALTON, R. P., HAUCK, A. L.: Direct recording of heart force with the strain gage arch. Dept. of Pharmacology, Medical College of South Carolina, Charleston, S.C. (1966).

WARD, R. J., ALLEN, G. D., DEVENY, L. J., GREEN, H. D.: Halothane and the cardiovascular response to endotracheal intubation. Anesthesia & Analgesia 44, 248 (1965).

WARNER, W. A.: Beta-adrenergic blocking agents and anaesthesia: a review. Canad. Anaesth. Soc. J. 15, 42 (1968).

— ORTH, O. S., WEBER, D. L., LAYTON, J. M.: Laboratory investigation of teflurane. Anesthesia & Analgesia 46, 32 (1967).

WENTHE, F. M., PATRICK, R. T., WOOD, E. H.: Effects of anesthesia with halothane on the human circulation. Anesthesia & Analgesia 41, 381 (1962).

WIGGERS, C. J.: Pressure pulses in the cardiovascular system. Aberdeen (Scotland): University Press 1927.

WILKIE, D. R.: Facts and theories about muscle. Progr. in Biophys. and Biophys. Chem. 4, 288 (1954).

— Mechanical properties of muscle. Brit. Med. Bull. 12, 177 (1956).

WINTER, P. J., DEUCHAR, D. C., NOBLE, M. I. M., GUZ, A.: The ballistocardiogram and left ventricular ejection in the dog. Proc. 1st World Congress on Ballistocardiography and Cardiovascular Dynamics, Basel. Ballistocardiography and Cardiovascular Dynamics (Basel) (1966), p. 248.

— — — TRENCHARD, D., GUZ, A.: Relationship between the ballistocardiogram and the movement of blood from the left ventricle in the dog. Cardiovasc. Res. 1, 194 (1967).

WOLLMAN, H., ALEXANDER, S. C., COHEN, P. J., CHASE, P. E., MELMAN, E., BEHAR, M. G.: Cerebral circulation of man during halothane anesthesia. Anesthesiology 25, 180 (1964).

WYANT, G. M., CHANG, C. A., MERRIMAN, J. E.: The effect of anesthesia upon pulmonary circulation. Anesthesia & Analgesia 41, 338 (1962).

— — RAPICAVOLI, E.: Methoxyflurane (Penthrane): a laboratory and clinical study. Canad. Anaesth. Soc. J. 8, 477 (1961).

WYANT, G. M., COCKINGS, E. C., MUIR, J. M.: Halothane and diethyl ether. Anesthesia & Analgesia **42**, 188 (1963).
— MERRIMAN, J. E., HARLAND, J. H., DONALDSON, H. V.: The cardiovascular effects of azeotropic halothane-ether. Canad. Anaesth. Soc. J. **7**, 91 (1960).
— — KILDUFF, C. J., THOMAS, E. T.: The cardiovascular effects of halothane. Canad. Anaesth. Soc. J. **5**, 384 (1958).
YOSHIDA, T., OSHIKA, M., NISHIDA, A.: Study on hemodynamics during Fluothane anesthesia. Japan. J. Anaesth. **14**, 575 (1965).
YOUNG, T. M., LODGE, A. B.: Collapse after halothane. Case reports. Anaesthesia **14**, 156 (1959).
ZAUDER, H. L., BAEZ, S., ORKIN, L. R.: Tissue perfusion during anesthesia. Clin. Anesthesia **3**, 79 (1964).
— MASSA, L. S., ORKIN, L. R.: Effects of general anesthetics on tissue oxygen "tensions". Anesthesiology **24**, 142 (1963).
ZEEDICK, J. F., THOMAS, G. J., OLIVO, N., JEROSKI, E.: Clinical experience with fluroxene-nitrous oxide-oxygen anesthesia as a non-flammable anesthetic. Anesthesia & Analgesia **45**, 790 (1966).

Liver. C. Trey (see p. 502)

4.5. General Anesthesia and the Kidney

RICHARD I. MAZZE and JOHN P. BUNKER

In 1905, PRINGLE, MAUNSELL and PRINGLE reported the effects of ether anesthesia on water and non-protein nitrogen excretion in eight patients undergoing a variety of minor and major surgical procedures. Urine was collected in seven periods: prior to, during, and after surgery. Urine flow averaged 50 ml/h on the day prior to surgery, increased during the induction of anesthesia, fell progressively to 1.2 ml/h during the operation, and returned toward normal postoperatively. The average urine output in the 24 h following surgery was 17 ml/h or about 400 ml for the day. Changes in non-protein nitrogen excretion paralleled those in urine flow but were less marked. PRINGLE noted that those patients who had the smallest urine output postoperatively had vomited the most and had received the smallest quantities of fluids on the day of surgery.

Since PRINGLE's report, many investigators have measured renal function during anesthesia and surgery (BURNETT et al., 1949; HABIF et al., 1951; MILES et al., 1952; MAZZE et al., 1963; DEUTSCH et al., 1966; GORMAN and CRAYTHORNE, 1966; and DEUTSCH et al., 1967). The pattern of response has been one of depression of all measured function: urine flow, glomerular filtration rate (GFR), renal blood flow (RBF), and electrolyte excretion. This consistent and generalized depression of renal function can be attributed to many factors, including the type and duration of the surgical procedure (HAYES and GOLDENBERG, 1963); the physical status of the patient, expecially that of the cardiovascular and renal systems (BARRY et al., 1964; SEITZMAN et al., 1963); preoperative and intraoperative blood volume, fluid, and electrolyte balance (BOBA and LANDMESSER, 1961; HUTCHIN et al., 1961; and MAZZE and BARRY, 1967); and to a lesser degree, the choice of anesthetic agent (GORMAN and CRAYTHORNE, 1966). Fortunately, the changes in renal function associated with anesthesia and surgery are almost always reversible.

Indirect Circulatory Effects

Profound disturbances in the circulation may accompany anesthesia and surgery and can be expected to result in equally profound disturbances in renal function. The quantitative effects of circulatory depression on renal function can be anticipated from the following considerations:

In the 70 kg male, the kidneys weigh approximately 300 g or 0.4% of the total body weight. They receive about 20—25% of the cardiac output: 90% of this going to the cortex, 8—10% to the medulla, and 1—2% to the papilla. The average renal arterial-venous oxygen difference is 1.7 ml/ 100 ml of blood and is independent of blood flow. This contrasts with the relatively constant oxygen consumption and the inverse relationship of arterial-venous oxygen difference and blood flow of other organs. DEETJEN and KRAMER (1960) and THURAU (1961) have explained the anomalous behaviour of the kidney by showing that the significant variable is GFR rather than RBF. A reduction in blood flow is accompanied by a decrease in GFR. Since $^3/_4$ to $^5/_6$ of the energy turnover of the kidney is concerned with sodium reabsorption, less glomerular filtration means less filtered sodium, less sodium reabsorption, and smaller oxygen requirements. In dogs, when blood pressure is dropped to levels at which GFR ceases, oxygen consumption drops from 4—6 µmoles/gm/min to 1.0—1.5 µmoles/gm/min.

During general anesthesia, renal blood flow may be depressed as a consequence of hypotension, renal vasoconstriction, or a combination of both. All anesthetic agents are myocardial depressants. Whether or not hypotension occurs depends on the depth of anesthesia and whether compensatory peripheral vasoconstriction occurs. The administration of either cyclopropane or diethyl ether is accompanied by increased blood levels of catecholamines (PRICE et al., 1959) and peripheral vasoconstriction which tend to support blood pressure but at the price of a marked increase in renal vascular resistance (DEUTSCH et al., 1967), decreased renal blood flow, and a marked depression of renal function. Halothane and thiopental, though not provoking a catecholamine response, are associated with a moderate increase in renal vascular resistance (DEUTSCH et al., 1966) as blood is shunted away from the kidneys to compensate for hypotension induced by myocardial depression and peripheral vasodilation. As a consequence, renal function falls, but the depression in renal function with halothane and thiopental is considerably less than with the catecholamine releasers. In a third category are central nervous system depressant drugs with alpha adrenergic blocking activity (JANSSEN et al., 1963) such as de-hydrobenzperidol, a butyrophenone derivative, which is used in combination with the short-acting narcotic, fentanyl, in the anesthetic technique called "neurolept analgesia". The administration of an alpha adrenergic blocking agent will, of course, lead to peripheral, including renal, vasodilation. GORMAN and CRAYTHORNE (1966) report no change in renal function and only a slight decrease in blood pressure where this technique is used for general anesthesia. Thus, if blood pressure can be maintained, an agent which prevents renal vasoconstriction and has only minimal myocardial depressant effects should produce the least depression of renal function. Neurolept analgesia, with its alpha blocking property and only slight cardiac depressant effect appears to come closest to this ideal.

Sympathetic Nervous System

The effects of the sympathetic nervous system on renal circulation and function during anesthesia are clearly of critical importance and merit detailed examination.

The blood vessels of the kidney are richly supplied with sympathetic constrictor fibers derived from the T_4-L_1 spinal cord segments via the coeliac and renal plexuses. There is no sympathetic dilator or parasympathetic innervation of the kidney. Under a wide variety of physiologic conditions, normal and abnormal, RBF is regulated to maintain stability of GFR. In the unanesthetized patient in the supine position, completely at rest, and in an environment of neutral temperature, there is very little, if any, tonic sympathetic control (SMITH, 1939). Were the individual to sit up or stand, situations which represent mild stress, RBF falls slightly but GFR is maintained. As the stress increases, RBF decreases significantly. filtration fraction increases, and GFR remains constant, suggesting efferent renal arteriolar constriction. Finally, during severe stress, GFR decreases. Judged by their depressant effects on RBF and GFR, general anesthesia, along with syncope, pain, severe exercise and hemorrhage represents severe stress. It is assumed that the major renal effects of each is mediated via sympathetic nervous system stimulation.

Perhaps the best evidence for the role of the sympathetic nervous system in the renal effect of anesthesia is provided by BERNE's (1952) experiments in dogs with one normal and one denervated kidney. Prior to induction of pentobarbital or chloralose anesthesia, the RBF and GFR of a denervated and normally innervated kidney are the same. However, following induction of anesthesia, RBF and GFR on the normally innervated side decreases while no changes are seen on the denervated side. These changes must be due to an anesthetic induced increase in vasoconstrictor tone of the innervated kidney.

16*

Apart from the marked influence which sympathetic nervous system activity clearly plays, a considerable degree of autoregulation may occur during anesthesia with a least some anesthetic agents. In the absence of anesthesia, RBF and GFR of the denervated, isolated, perfused kidney can be shown to be relatively independent of arterial pressure. Similarly, in animals anesthetized with intravenous pentobarbital or chloralose but with normally innervated and perfused kidneys, RBF and GFR vary only slightly over an arterial pressure range of 80—180 mmHg. (Shipley and Study, 1951; and Ochwadt, 1961). In contrast, evidence of autoregulation does not accompany anesthesia with the inhalation agents. Decreases in RBF and GFR of 50% or more are seen with ether and cyclopropane (Habif et al., 1951) and halothane (Mazze et al., 1963) in patients with stable blood pressures above 80 mmHg.

The effects of sympathetic innervation are probably limited to the circulation, and have no effect on tubular reabsorptive or secretory function. Denervation natriuresis is described but this is usually accompanied by increases in RBF and GFR. Excretion of a relatively fixed proportion of the increased filtered load is a more likely explanation of this phenomenon than withdrawal of impulses stimulating tubular reabsorption (Kamm and Levinsky, 1965).

Endocrine System

Endocrine effects on renal function during anesthesia are of equal importance and closely tied to the circulatory effects discussed above. Most important in regulating urine volume is the anti-diuretic hormone (ADH). Renin-angiotensin, aldosterone, epinephrine, and norepinephrine also play important roles in electrolyte excretion and regulation of renal blood flow.

1. ADH. Anti-diuretic hormone, an octapeptide, is formed in cells of the supraoptic and paraventricular nuclei of the hypothalmus. The hormone is transported to the posterior lobe of the pituitary by the axons which make up the supraopticohypophyseal tracts. Release of ADH is controlled by osmoreceptors in the carotid body and the pituitary which are sensitive to osmolality changes of approximately 2%.

Whether or not narcotics, such as morphine, and general anesthetics stimulate secretion of ADH is still unresolved. Evidence in the affirmative comes principally from two sources. Duke et al. (1951) injected 4—32 µg of morphine into the supraoptic nuclei of dogs after water diuresis had been established. The rate of urine flow fell rapidly with the degree and duration of inhibition roughly in proportion to the dose of morphine. Control injection of the same volume of saline into the supraoptic nuclei produced only a fleeting change in the rate of urine flow, and injection of morphine into the hypothalmus produced little or no change in systemic blood pressure, RBF or GFR. From this it was concluded that the inhibitory action of morphine on urine flow in their experiment was due to the liberation of ADH. The same investigators injected morphine, 0.25—5.0 mg/kg into dogs undergoing water diuresis both before and after section of the supraoptic tracts. Before operation, morphine invariably caused an inhibition of the rate of urine flow — whereas there were no changes in urine volume when morphine was administered after operation.

It is generally assumed that general anesthetic agents, as well as morphine, may initiate an ADH response and its attendant renal effects. Perhaps the best case for an anesthetic induced ADH response is offered by Aprahamian and his associates (1959). They point out that inhalation agents of low molecular weight and medium or low potency, such as diethyl ether and nitrous oxide, represent in anesthetic concentrations a sufficient osmolal stimulus for the release of ADH by the posterior pituitary. Their report of a marked increase in urinary solute concentration accompanying a marked fall in urine volume during the induction of diethyl ether anesthesia is typical of, and therefore additional presumptive evidence of an ADH effect. In contrast, anesthetic concentrations of cyclopropane do not represent a significant osmolal increase; and although cyclopropane causes an intense antidiuresis, the reciprocal changes in urinary solute concentration and urine volume, typical of an ADH response, and seen with ether, were conspicuously absent.

The principal evidence against morphine or general anesthesia induced ADH response comes from the studies of BACHMAN (1955). He observed that morphine, 2.5 mg/kg, ether, and cyclopropane caused the expected antidiuretic effect in normal dogs undergoing a water diuresis. When these animals were then subjected to high pituitary stalk and hypothalamic tract section, in order to produce diabetes insipidus, morphine, ether, and cyclopropane still produced the same degree of antidiuresis. The intensity of this effect appeared to be related to the depth of anesthesia produced by the inhalation agents. Though RBF was not measured, BACHMAN expressed the opinion that the changes observed in his experiments were due to the renal hemodynamic depressant effects of these agents.

During water diuresis in man, PAPPER et al. (1957) reported that 5—10 mg of morphine produced a decrease in urine flow in 17 of 22 experiments. However, in 8 of these, the diminution of urine flow was not accompanied by a significant rise in urine osmolality as one would expect with an ADH response. In 16 of the 17, there was a decrease in GFR and in solute excretion, changes that alone or together are sufficient to account for a decrease in the rate of urine flow.

To establish beyond doubt an ADH effect following the administration of anesthetics, it would be necessary to demonstrate a decrease in urine flow, a reciprocal increase in urinary solutes and no change in renal hemodynamics, together with an increase in circulating ADH. Because of the multiple systemic effects of anesthetics and the difficulty involved in ADH assay, these conditions have not yet been met. In the absence of such evidence, it seems reasonable to assume that ADH and altered renal hemodynamics are together responsible for the decrease in urine flow associated with the administration of narcotics and general anesthetic agents.

2. Epinephrine and Norepinephrine. The catecholamines, epinephrine and norepinephrine, are the neurohumoral transmitter substances of the sympathetic nervous system. In man, about ten times more epinephrine than norepinephrine is found in the adrenal glands while norepinephrine is the predominant sympathomimetic substance in the sympathetic nerves and is the adrenergic mediator liberated by their stimulation (EULER, 1954).

Both epinenephrine and norepinenephrine produce marked renal vasoconstriction, especially of the efferent arterioles, with a decrease in RBF and, to a lesser degree, GFR (JACOBSON et al., 1951). Sodium, chloride, and potassium excretion are depressed, probably due to the decreased filtered load or to increased reabsorption from the tubules. Antidiuresis occurs following administration of epinephrine and norepinephrine, and ERANKO et al. (1953) suggest that ADH may be responsible.

Anesthesia with ether and cyclopropane produces an increase in circulating catecholamines (PRICE et al., 1959) as discussed above. It is difficult to determine how much of the renal effect of these anesthetic agents is due to the increase in catecholamines and how much to their other systemic effects.

3. Renin-Angiotensin. An additional hormonal pathway capable of affecting renal function is the renin-angiotensin system. Renin is a proteolytic enzyme produced by the juxtaglomerular cells of the afferent arterioles. Renin reacts with an alpha-2 globulin of plasma to form

angiotensin-I. This substance is ultimately converted into the strongly pressor and renal vascular constricting substance, angiotensin II. The latter substance is one of the main factors involved in aldosterone release.

Control of renin release is complex (Vander, 1967) and is influenced by several factors which are in turn affected by administration of anesthesia. Sodium content of tubular fluid, catecholamine levels, sympathetic nerve impulses, and intra-luminal pressure of afferent arterioles are probably all involved.

Deutsch et al. (1967) have reported increased renin activity in two non-operated subjects anesthetized with cyclopropane and two with halothane. In contrast, three of four subjects anesthetized with morphine, thiopental, nitrous oxide and muscle relaxants showed a decrease in renin activity and one showed an increase. The authors suggest that a fall in renin activity might explain the relatively greater reduction in GFR than in RBF observed with this technique in comparison with cyclopropane or halothane. However, the number of patients is too small and the data too fragmentary for conclusions to be drawn at this time.

4. Aldosterone. Aldosterone, the hormone responsible for moment to moment control of sodium excretion, is formed in the zona glomerulosa of the adrenal cortex. Its release is primarily dependent on volume depletion as mediated by baroreceptors in the carotid sinus. Impulses originating there are carried by the vagus nerve to an integrative center in the dorsal medulla.

Anesthetic agents are known to sensitize the carotid baroreceptors. Trichlor-ethylene, chloroform, and ether cause large increases in discharge frequency following carotid sinus pressure (Robertson et al., 1956). Cyclopropane causes lesser changes (Price and Widdicombe, 1962). It has been suggested that anesthetics may change the circulatory pressures which activate the baroceptors, may act on the central nervous pathways for the baroreceptor reflexes, or on the afferent or efferent limb of the reflex arc, thereby causing aldosterone secretion. It is also possible that anesthetic agents cause aldosterone release indirectly by affecting circulating angiotensin level; by causing ADH release, which in turn stimulates secretion of ACTH, which then stimulates the zona glomerolusa to liberate aldo-sterone (Hilton, 1960); or by stimulating the sympathetic nervous system, thereby causing renal vasoconstriction, leading to renin and angiotensin formation, which in turn stimulates aldosterone formation (Davis, 1961); or by causing peripheral vasodilatation, the expanded vascular compartment stimulating baroreceptors in the same manner as a decrease in blood volume.

Despite anesthesia induced aldosterone release and the sodium retention it produces, it is well known that serum sodium falls following general anesthesia and surgery. This change has been ascribed to dominance of ADH effect, liberation of endogenous sodium-free water from oxidation of fat, and overadministration of sodium-free fluids. Indeed, the postoperative patient has been thought to be intolerant to sodium administration and the practice of infusing small volumes of sodium-free fluid has developed.

Hayes et al. (1957, 1959) demonstrated that both the antidiuresis and sodium retention described above could be reduced in patients having major surgery by infusing a liter or more of Ringer's lactate solution 8—12 h preoperatively and continuing the administration of sodium-containing fluids throughout the post-operative period. It was their opinion that postoperative sodium intolerance was due at least in part to preoperative and intraoperative sodium restriction.

Shires et al. (1961, 1969) supported Hayes' conclusions and presented evidence that postoperative sodium intolerance was due to an acute contraction of the functional extracellular fluid volume. Using ^{125}I-tagged serum albumin, ^{51}Cr-tagged red blood cells and ^{35}S-tagged sodium sulfate to measure simultaneously the plasma volume, red cell mass, and extracellular space they found reductions of up to 28% in the latter compartment which they correlated with the degree of surgical trauma. They postulated the loss of large volumes of isotonic fluid into a third space, not in ready communication with the more mobile, and functionally significant, interstitial fluid volume. SHIRES (1964) recommended infusion of large volumes of RINGER's lactate solution, 500—1000 ml/h during operation, up to a total of 4 l, to prevent contraction of the functional extracellular volume which in turn supports the intravascular volume. Using this regimen, he noted a marked reduction in sodium retention which he attributed to decreased aldosterone secretion.

SHIRES' position has not gone unchallenged. VIRTUE et al. (1966), CLELAND et al. (1966), and most recently ROTH et al. (1969) used similar isotopic techniques and were not able to demonstrate significant deficits in extracellular fluid volume. ROTH et al. (1969) noted a deficit in extracellular fluid of only 5.7% in animals subjected to $1^1/_2$ h of profound hemorrhagic shock, whereas in similar experiments, SHIRES et al. (1964) had reported as much as a 43% deficit in extracellular fluid. ROTH attributes the discrepancy in results primarily to errors inherent in the single-sample radiosulfate dilution method and to other methodologic considerations. In rebuttal, MIDDLETON, MATHEWS, and SHIRES (1969) have reproduced their earlier studies using a multiple-sample ^{35}S-tagged radiosulfate dilution technique. The matter is far from settled.

Direct Effects of Anesthetics on Renal Function

Any direct effects of anesthetic agents on renal function are obscured by the marked indirect hemodynamic and endocrine effects considered above. However, recent reports of the effects of anesthetic agents on active sodium transport in a variety of experimental preparations (toad bladder, frog skin, squid giant axon) strongly suggest that such effects should occur in the renal tubule. In the isolated toad bladder, cyclopropane and nitrous oxide have been shown to give rise to a dose dependent stimulation and halothane to a dose dependent inhibition of active sodium transport (ANDERSEN, 1966). Ether produces a biphasic response: initial stimulation followed by inhibition of ion transport both in the toad bladder (ANDERSEN, 1966) and in the squid giant axon (SCHWARTZ, 1968).

In an effort to elucidate the mechanism of the above responses, and because epinephrine has been found to stimulate sodium transport in frog skin, ANDERSEN (1967) performed additional experiments in bladders from toads previously treated with reserpine, alpha and beta adrenergic blocking agents and with epinephrine. Cyclopropane was used as the test gas. In untreated bladders, cyclopropane produced a dose dependent stimulation of sodium transport, while in reserpinized bladders and those treated with the alpha blockers, phenoxybenzamine and phentolamine, cyclopropane produced dose dependent inhibition of sodium transport. The beta blockers had no effect upon the bladder response to cyclopropane. ANDERSEN also observed that the stimulation of sodium transport after the simultaneous administration of epinephrine and cyclopropane far exceeded the stimated additive effect of the two drugs. He concluded that the synergism of cyclopropane and epinephrine on sodium transport in toad bladder is transmitted through an alpha receptor. He further concluded that the enhancement of sodium transport brought about by ether and nitrous oxide may possibly occur through a similar interaction with epinephrine, while inhibition of sodium transport by anesthetic agents may be a direct effect.

It can be assumed that such marked effects of anesthetic agents on sodium transport must play a role in the alterations of renal function which accompany anesthesia. No direct studies of renal tubular function during anesthesia are available, however, and one can only speculate what these effects might be from indirect evidence. Total urinary excretion of sodium is known to decrease markedly with all anesthetic agents. A decrease in total sodium excretion would, of course, be consistent with a cyclopropane-induced stimulation of tubular rearbsorption, but could not be distinguished from the effect of a decreased filtered load. More difficult to rationalize, however, is the decrease in total urinary sodium excretion which accompanies anesthetic agents such as halothane, which appear to depress active sodium transport. If sodium reabsorption falls, urinary sodium excretion should rise. To explain this paradox, it would be necessary to assume a fall in glomerular filtration of sodium which is quantitatively larger than the fall in tubular reabsorption. The validity of such speculations can, of course, only be established by direct studies of the effects of anesthetics on renal tubular function.

Summary of Anesthetic Effects on Renal Function

Table 1 summarizes published reports of changes in renal function observed during general anesthesia in man. Only the broadest comparisons of anesthetic agents can be made from this data. In general, decreases in RBF were greater than those in GFR with a resultant increase in filtration fraction. Urine volume and sodium excretion were always decreased while changes in potassium excretion were variable. Anesthetic depression was dose dependent in those studies where depth of anesthesia was noted.

Nephrotoxicity

Surgical Renal Failure. The changes in renal function which ordinarily accompany general anesthesia spontaneously revert toward normal when anesthesia is discontinued. Renal blood flow and GFR usually return to normal within a few hours after the termination of surgery, although the ability to excrete a water load may be impaired for several days (Hayes and Goldenberg, 1963). The persistence of abnormalities in renal function, such that the kidneys are not able to vary urine volume and content appropriately in response to homeostatic needs, occasionally occurs. This condition can vary from one of mild impairment to anuric renal shutdown. Renal failure is probably never due to the choice of anesthetic agent alone; rather, it is more likely due to a combination of factors, of which the anesthetic agent is a minor one. The nature and duration of the surgical procedure, the prior existence of renal and/or cardiovascular disease and the preoperative, intraoperative, and postoperative management of fluid and electrolyte balance are the major factors involved in surgical renal failure.

In the healthy patient undergoing a relatively minor operation, any well administered anesthetic and virtually any fluid regimen, from no fluids on the day of surgery to several liters of dextrose in water or salt solution, will be tolerated. Renal function will be depressed on the day of surgery, but 24 hrs later RBF, GFR, urine flow, and the ability to excrete a water load will have returned to normal.

In other patients, anesthesia and surgery may carry markedly increased risks of postoperative renal failure. Patients undergoing surgery of the aorta, those having procedures in which large volumes of blood may be transfused, older patients having lengthy or extensive surgical procedures, patients with pre-existing cardiac or renal disease, patients with obstetric complications such as abruptio placentae, and patients who have suffered major trauma all face an increased

Table 1. Results of renal function studies during general anesthesia

Author	Agent	Depth	Premedication	% of control						Remarks
				RBF	GFR	Filt. fract.	Urine Vol.	Na excret.	K excret.	
BURNETT (1949)	Ether	1st—2nd Pl.	None	62	78	131	55	—	—	No fluid information
HABIF (1951)	Ether	2nd Plane	Atropine, meperidine	48	61	132	42	37	48	250 ml/h of 5% dextrose normal saline
MILES (1952)	Ether	Light / Deep	Atropine / Atropine	65 / 42	78 / 57	124 / 142	—	—	—	No fluid information
BURNETT (1949)	Cyclopropane	1st—2nd Pl.	None	46	69	148	56	—	—	No fluid information
HABIF (1951)	Cyclopropane	2nd Plane	Meperidine, atropine	31	45	156	32	16	32	250 ml/h of 5% dextrose normal saline
MILES (1952)	Cyclopropane	Light / Deep	Atropine / Atropine	72 / 34	74 / 45	109 / 150	—	—	—	No fluid information
DEUTSCH (1967)	Cyclopropane	2nd Plane	None	58	61	114	35	33	122	Hydrated with 1 l of 4% fructose
MAZZE (1963)	Halothane	0.5—1.0%	Morphine, scopolamine	39	52	134	43	43	117	No fluids during surgery
	Halothane	1.2—3.0%	Morphine, scopolamine	31	42	126	36	36	108	
BARRY (1964)	Halothane	0.5—1.0%	Morphine, scopolamine	88	92	104	—	—	—	Hydrated during and before surgery with 15 ml/h of 1/3 normal saline
	Halothane	1.2—3.0%	Morphine, scopolamine	53	60	110	—	—	—	
DEUTSCH (1966)	Halothane	2nd Plane	None	62	81	139	37	36	—	Hydrated with 1 l of 4% fructose
HABIF (1951)	Thiopental	2nd Plane	Meperidine, atropine	70	68	97	48	30	57	250 ml/h of 5% dextrose normal saline
DEUTSCH (1968)	Thiopental, nitrous oxide	Light	Morphine, atropine	89	77	86	—	—	—	Hydrated with 1 l of 4% fructose
GORMAN (1966)	Neurolept-analgesia	2nd Plane	None	97	97	100	58	66	80	No fluids during surgery

likelihood of such renal injury (Teschan et al., 1955; Franklin and Merrill, 1960). To minimize this danger, these patients must be carefully prepared with special attention to the renal and cardiovascular systems. Preoperative, intra-operative, and postoperative fluid, acid-base, and electrolyte balance must be monitored and corrections made when necessary. It is particularly important to adjust fluid balance throughout the operation itself, and to do this it is necessary to introduce an indwelling urethral catheter prior to surgery to measure urine flow rate and to replace measured fluid volume and estimated insensible losses with a physiologic salt solution. The use of an osmotic diuretic, such as mannitol, may be necessary to maintain urine flow rate at 60—100 ml/h during and after surgery if hydration alone is not adequate for this purpose (Mazze and Barry, 1967). Finally, an anesthetic method and agent should be chosen with minimal depression of renal function.

Methoxyflurane Induced Renal Insufficiency. The possibility of a specific anesthetic induced nephrotoxicity has recently been reported by Crandell et al. (1966). They reported that in 13 of 41 patients who received methoxyflurane for abdominal surgery, renal failure with high urine volumes occurred. Urine volumes were 2.5—4.0 l per day with a negative fluid balance, elevation of serum sodium, serum osmolality, and blood urea nitrogen, and a relatively fixed urine osmolality close to that of serum. These patients were unable to concentrate urine despite fluid deprivation and Pitressin administration, suggesting that the difficulty was of renal origin and not due to ADH deficiency. Impairment lasted from 10—20 days in most patients, but in three, abnormalities persisted for longer than one year. Pezzi et al. (1966) had previously noted a similar syndrome in 16% of 123 patients undergoing abdominal surgery with methoxyflurane. However, all of their patients suffered major medical or surgical complications which they acknowledge might have significantly contributed to the observed renal difficulties. (Their report appeared as a letter to the editor with a definitive study still unpublished.)

Earlier, in a study of hepatic and renal function, North and Stephen (1965) had noted an elevation in blood urea nitrogen with methoxyflurane anesthesia, but other elements of high output renal failure were not present. Paddock et al. (1964) observed the development of renal failure in three of their patients anesthetized with methoxyflurane. Pathological examination of the kidney in the two patients who died with this syndrome showed moderate arterial and arteriolar nephrosclerosis, with the tubules containing calcium oxalate crystals. Additional study by these authors of kidney sections from 200 autopsies and of renal function in 40 healthy males who received methoxyflurane anesthesia failed to confirm an association of this anesthetic agent with renal injury in healthy patients.

In the four years since the publication of Crandell et al. (1966) and Pezzi et al. (1966) only a few case reports of high output renal insufficiency associated with methoxyflurane administration have appeared in the literature. However, a controlled, randomized, prospective, clinical evaluation had not been done until the study recently reported by Mazze et al. (1971). Administration of methoxyflurane differed somewhat from the usual clinical circumstance in that premedication was omitted, a barbiturate was not used for induction and nitrous oxide was not included in the maintenance anesthetic gas mixture. Findings in this study agreed with those of Crandell et al. (1966) and went even further: abnormalities were found in every patient. Mazze et al. (1971) noted polyuria unresponsive to ADH administration, marked weight loss, delayed return to preoperative concentrating ability, hypernatremia, serum hyperosmolality, elevated BUN and serum creatinine, increased serum uric acid and a decrease in uric acid clearance. None of the halothane (control) patients responded in this fashion. Polyuria and dehydration following operation added difficulty to the postoperative management in six of the twelve patients studied. One patient had a combined urinary output (6 l) and nasogastric drainage (2 l) of 8 l per day for several days. All of the patients receiving methoxyflurane had increases in serum uric acid greater than the largest increase in any control patient. Nephrotoxicity was not permanent in any of the patients in this series though abnormalities persisted for as long as 68 days in one patient. As administered in the study by MAZZE et al. (1971), methoxyflurane produced definite evidence of tubular dysfunction. Its continued use in clinical anesthesia should be reconsidered in light of this and future studies of the agent's renal effects.

Inappropriate ADH Secretion. An additional type of renal failure secondary to anesthesia and surgery has been reported by DEUTSCH et al. (1966). They noted a sustained and inappropriate secretion of ADH in elderly patients having major surgery receiving hypotonic fluids intra and postoperatively. The patients exhibited hyponatremia with low serum osmolality in the face of a persistent excretion of a hypertonic urine. Clinically, the patients developed a variety of diffuse neurological symptoms ranging from restlessness and disorientation to profound stupor. Improvement followed restriction of fluids.

Summary

The depressant effects of general anesthetics agents on renal function appear to be largely secondary to their effects on the cardiovascular, sympathetic, and endocrine systems. Renal function is also markedly affected by the type and duration of the surgical procedure, the physical status of the patient, especially the cardiovascular and renal systems, and preoperative and intraoperative fluid, acid-base, and electrolyte balance. With the apparent exception of the newly introduced neurolept analgesia, all anesthetics depress renal function with decreases in urine volume, sodium excretion, RBF, and GFR being noted. Renal blood flow and function are most markedly depressed by anesthetic agents which initiate the reflex release of catecholamines (diethyl ether, cyclopropane) and are least affected by anesthetic agents which minimize or prevent sympathetic nervous system responses.

A direct effect of anesthetics on renal tubular function can be assumed. It has been shown that cyclopropane and nitrous oxide enhance sodium transport in the isolated toad bladder, while halothane causes depression and ether a biphasic response. Enhancement of sodium transport seems to be mediated by alpha adrenergic receptors while depression appears to be a direct effect.

Finally, the changes in renal functions associated with anesthesia and surgery appear to be self limiting, returning toward normal at the end of anesthesia and surgery. However, in those patients whose renal function is barely adequate to maintain homeostasis, a major surgical procedure, a period of hypotension or hypovolemia, or similar stress may be sufficient to cause renal decompensation or oliguric renal failure.

References

ANDERSEN, N. B.: Effect of general anesthetics on sodium transport in the isolated toad bladder. Anesthesiology **27**, 304 (1966).
— Synergistic effect of cyclopropane and epinephrine on sodium transport in toad bladder. Anesthesiology **28**, 438 (1967).
APRAHAMIAN, H. A., VANDERVEEN, J. L., BUNKER, J. P., MURPHY, A. J., CRAWFORD, J. D.: The influence of general anesthetics on water and solute excretion in man. Ann. Surg. **150**, 122 (1959).

Bachman, L.: The antidiuretic effects of anesthetic agents. Anesthesiology 16, 939 (1955).

Barry, K. G., Mazze, R. I., Schwartz, F. D.: Prevention of surgical oliguria and renal-hemodynamic suppression by sustained hydration. New Engl. J. Med. 270, 1371 (1964).

Berne, R. M.: Hemodynamics and sodium excretion of denervated kidney in anesthetized and unanesthetized dog. Am. J. Physiol. 171, 148 (1952).

Boba, A., Landmesser, C. M.: Renal complications after anesthesia and operation. Anesthesiology 22, 781 (1961).

Burnett, C. H., Bloomberg, E. L., Shortz, G., Compton, D. W., Beecher, H. K.: A comparison of the effects of ether and cyclopropane anesthesia on the renal function of man. J. Pharmacol. Expt Therap. 96, 380 (1949).

Cleland, J., Pluth, J. R., Tauxe, W. N., Kirklin, J. W.: Blood volume and body fluid compartment changes soon after closed and open intracardiac surgery. J. Thoracic Cardiovascular Surg. 52, 689 (1966).

Crandell, W. B., Pappas, S. G., Macdonald, A.: Nephrotoxicity associated with methoxy-flurane anesthesia. Anesthesiology 27, 591 (1966).

Davis, J. O.: A critical evaluation of the role of receptors in the control of aldosterone secretion and sodium excretion. Prog. Cardiovasc. Dis. 4, 27 (1961).

Deetjen, P., Kramer, K.: Original Na-Rückresorption und O_2-Verbrauch der Niere. Klin. Wschr. 38, 680 (1960).

Deutsch, S., Goldberg, M., Dripps, R. D.: Postoperative hyponatremia with the inappropriate release of antidiuretic hormone. Anesthesiology 27, 250 (1966).

— — Stephen, G. W., Wu, W.: Effects of halothane anesthesia on renal function in normal man. Anesthesiology 27, 793 (1966).

— Pierce, E. C., Jr., Vandam, L. D.: Cyclopropane effects of renal function in normal man. Anesthesiology 28, 547 (1967).

— — — Effects of anesthesia with thiopental, nitrous oxide and neuromuscular blockers on renal function in normal man. Anesthesiology 29, 184 (1968).

Duke, H. N., Pickford, M., Watt, J. A.: The antidiuretic action of morphine: its site and mode of action in the hypothalamus of the dog. Quart. J. Exptl Physiol. 36, 149 (1951).

Eranko, O., Karvonen, M. J., Laamanen, A., Pitkanen, M. E.: The antidiuretic action of adrenaline and noradrenaline in the water-loaded dog. Acta Pharmacol. Toxicol. 9, 345 (1953).

Euler, U. S.: III. Epinephrine and norepinephrine. Adrenaline and noradrenaline distribution and action. Pharmacol. Revs 6, 15 (1954).

Franklin, S. S., Merrill, J. P.: Acute renal failure. New Engl. J. Med. 262, 761 (1960).

Gorman, H. M., Craythorne, N. W. B.: The effects of a new neuroleptanalgesic agent (Innovar) on renal function in man. Acta Anaest, Scand. Suppl. 24, 111 (1966).

Habif, D. V., Papper, E. M., Fitzpatrick, H. F., Lowrance, P., McC. Smythe, C., Bradley, S. E.: The renal and hepatic blood flow, glomerular filtration rate, and urinary output of electrolytes during cyclopropane, ether, and thiopental anesthesia, operation, and the immediate postoperative period. Surgery 30, 241 (1951).

Hayes, M. A., Byrnes, W. P., Goldenberg, I. S., Greene, N. M., Tuthill, E.: Water and electrolyte exchanges during operation and convalescence. Surgery 46, 123 (1959).

— Goldenberg, I. S.: Renal effects of anesthesia and operation mediated by endocrines. Anesthesiology 24, 487 (1963).

— Williamson, R. J., Heidenreich, W. F.: Endocrine mechanisms involved in water and sodium metabolism during operation and convalescence. Surgery 41, 353 (1957).

Hilton, J. G.: Adrenocorticotropic action of antidiuretic hormone. Circulation 21, 1038 (1960).

Hutchin, P., McLaughlin, J. S., Hayes, M. A.: Renal response to acidosis during anesthesia and operation: I. The effect of acute dilutional hyponatremia on hydrogen ion and free water excretion during metabolic acidosis in anesthetized dogs. Ann. Surg. 154, 9 (1961).

— — — Renal response to acidosis during anesthesia and operation: II. The effect of operative trauma on hydrogen ion and free water excretion during metabolic acidosis. Ann. Surg. 154, 145 (1961).

— — — Renal response to acidosis during anesthesia and operation: III. Maintenance of homeostasis in acute respiratory acidosis during intravenous infusion of Ringer's lactate and 5% glucose in water. Ann. Surg. 154, 161 (1961).

Jacobson, W. E., Hammarsten, J. F., Heller, B. I.: The effects of adrenaline upon renal function and electrolyte excretion. J. Clin. Invest. 30, 1503 (1951).

Janssen, P. A. J., Niemegeers, J. E., Schellekens, K. H. L., Verbruggen, F. J., van Nueten, J. M.: The pharmacology of dehydrobenzperidol, a new potent and short acting neuroleptic agent chemically related to haloperidol. Arzneimittel-Forsch. 13, 205 (1963).

Kamm, D. E., Levinsky, N. G.: The mechanism of denervation natriuresis. J. Clin. Invest. 44, 93 (1965).

MAZZE, R. I., BARRY, K. G.: Prevention of functional renal failure during anesthesia and surgery by sustained hydration and mannitol infusion. Anesthesia & Analgesia **46**, 61 (1967).
— SCHWARTZ, F. D., SLOCUM, H. C., BARRY, K. G.: Renal function during anesthesia and surgery. I. The effects of halothane anesthesia. Anesthesiology **24**, 279—284 (1963).
— SHUE, G. L., JACKSON, S. H.: Methoxyflurane nephrotoxicity a randomized prospective clinical evaluation. J. Am. Med. Assoc. (1971) (in press).
MIDDLETON, E. S., MATHEWS, R., SHIRES, T.: Radiosulphate as a measure of the extracellular fluid in acute hemorrhagic shock. Ann. Surg. **170**, 174 (1969).
MILES, B. E., DE WARDENER, H. E., CHURCHILL-DAVIDSON, H. C., WYLIE, W. D.: The effect on the renal circulation of pentamethonium bromide during anesthesia. Clin. Sci. **11**, 73 (1952).
NORTH, W. C., STEPHEN, C. R.: Hepatic and renal effects of methoxyflurane in surgical patients. Anesthesiology **26**, 257 (1965).
OCHWADT, B.: Relation of renal blood supply to diuresis. Prog. Cardiovasc. Dis. **III**, 501 (1961).
PADDOCK, R. B., PARKER, J. W., GUADAGNI, N. P.: The effects of methoxyflurane on renal function. Anesthesiology **25**, 707 (1964).
PAPPER, S., SAXON, L., BURG, M. B., SEIFER, H. W., ROSENBAUM, J. D.: The effect of morphine sulfate upon the renal excretion of water and solute in man. J. Lab. Clin. Med. **50**, 692 (1957).
PEZZI, P. J., FROBESE, A. S., GREENBERG, S. R.: Methoxyflurane and renal toxicity. Lancet **1966 I**, 823.
PRICE, H. L., LINDE, H. W., JONES, R. E., BLACK, G. W., PRICE, M. L.: Sympathoadrenal responses to general anesthesia in man and their relation to hemodynamics. Anesthesiology **20**, 563 (1959).
— WIDDICOMBE, J.: Actions of cyclopropane on carotid sinus baroreceptors and carotid body chemoreceptors. J. Pharmacol. Exptl Therap. **135**, 233 (1962).
PRINGLE, H., MAUNSELL, R. C. B., PRINGLE, S.: Clinical effects of ether anaesthesia on renal activity. Brit. Med. J. **2**, 542 (1905).
ROBERTSON, J. D., SWAN, A. A. B., WHITTERIDGE, D.: Effect of anaesthetics on systemic baroreceptors. J. Physiol. London **131**, 463 (1956).
ROTH, E., LAX, L., MALONEY, J. V., Jr.: Ringer's lactate solution and extracellular fluid volume in the surgical patient: a critical analysis. Ann. Surg. **169**, 149 (1969).
SCHWARTZ, E. A.: Effect of diethylether on sodium efflux from squid axons. Current Trends in Mod. Biol. **2**, 1 (1968).
SEITZMAN, D. M., MAZZE, R. I., SCHWARTZ, F. D., BARRY, K. G.: Mannitol diuresis: A method of renal protection during surgery. J. Urol. **90**, 139 (1963).
SHIPLEY, R. E., STUDY, R. S.: Changes in renal blood flow, extraction of inulin, glomerular filtration rate, tissue pressure and urine flow with acute alterations of renal artery blood pressure. Am. J. Physiol. **167**, 676 (1951).
SHIRES, T.: Shock and metabolism. Surg. Gynecol. Obstet. **124**, 284 (1964).
— COLN, D., CARRICO, J., LIGHTFOOT, S.: Fluid therapy in hemorrhagic shock. Arch. Surg. **88**, 688 (1964).
— WILLIAMS, J., BROWN, F.: Acute change in extracellular fluids associated with major surgical procedures. Ann. Surg. **154**, 803 (1961).
SMITH, H. W.: Physiology of the renal circulation. Harvey Lectures **35**, 166 (1939—40).
TESCHAN, P. E., POST, R. S., SMITH, L. H., ABERNATHY, R. S., DAVIS, J. H., GRAY, D. M., HOWARD, J. N., JOHNSON, K. E., KLOPP, E., MUNDY, R. L., O'MEARA, M. P., RUSH, B. F.: Post-traumatic renal insufficiency in military casualties. Am. J. Med. **18**, 172 (1955).
THURAU, K.: Renal Na-reabsorption and O_2 uptake in dogs during hypoxia and hydrochlorothiazide infusion. Proc. Soc. Exptl. Biol. Med. **106**, 714 (1961).
VANDER, A. J.: Control of renin release. Physiol. Rev. **47**, 359 (1967).
VIRTUE, R. W., LE VINE, D. S., AIKAWA, J. K.: Fluid shifts during the surgical period: RISA and S^{35} determinations following glucose, saline or lactate infusion. Ann. Surg. **163**, 523 (1966).

4.6. Respiratory System

Edwin S. Munson

With 10 Figures

All anesthetic drugs are capable of producing ventilatory depression if administered in sufficient amounts. However, used clinically, anesthetics produce varying degrees of functional impairment. The rational management of ventilation during anesthesia and surgery requires an understanding of the relative effects of drug actions as well as the physiologic changes that occur during the anesthetized state.

Clinicians for generations have evaluated ventilatory adequacy by means of visual and tactile assessment of the rate and excursion of the reservoir bag and chest wall. These methods do not permit quantitative evaluation of ventilatory function. The relationship between the rate and volume of ventilatory exchange has been stressed by SEVERINGHAUS and LARSON (1965) as a concept necessary for critical appraisal of drug action. Oxygenation of arterial blood and removal of metabolically produced CO_2 depends on gas exchange at the alveolar level. Endogenous CO_2 is transported from the lung to ambient air usually at a rate of about 200 ml/min. This quantity of excreted CO_2 represents about 5 % of the total volume removed from the alveoli each minute. This relationship defines alveolar ventilation:

$$\text{Alveolar ventilation} = \frac{CO_2 \text{ Output/min}}{\text{Alveolar } CO_2 \text{ Concentration}}$$

Any reduction in alveolar ventilation at constant CO_2 output results in an increased alveolar (arterial) PCO_2. Therefore, any increase in arterial PCO_2 above normal is diagnostic of alveolar hypoventilation. However, hypoventilation may exist at a normal or low PCO_2 in certain circumstances following prolonged hyperventilation (see below).

I. Physiologic Changes During Anesthesia

Alveolar ventilation normally represents the major portion (70%) of the total expired ventilatory volume. The difference is accounted for by that portion of the ventilatory exchange that does not participate in alveolar gas exchange, i.e., the physiologic dead space. An estimate of the uniformity of distribution of pulmonary blood flow within the lung can be obtained from measurement of physiologic dead space which more recently has been termed wasted ventilation. Increase in wasted ventilation occurs when the normal relationship between alveolar ventilation and perfusion is altered, producing areas of the lung that are hypoperfused relative to ventilation. This inequality between ventilation and circulation produces an arterial to alveolar PCO_2 difference. The development of this CO_2 gradient appears to be related to the duration of anesthesia rather than to any specific anesthetic agent. Because both ventilation and perfusion are distributed in a non-uniform fashion, the ratio of ventilation to perfusion that prevails in the lung as a whole will be found in only very few of the respiratory elements (WEST, 1962). Where ventilation is too high in respect to perfusion, the system can be visualized as one in which part of the inspired gas is adequately matched to the gas flow, while the remainder is in excess. Similarly, gas exchange in overperfused alveoli can be analyzed in terms of an ideal component of perfusion, which matches ventilation, and an "excess perfusion". Since it is impossible to measure either "excess ventilation" or "excess perfusion", the relationship is usually expressed in terms of the contribution to wasted ventilation and venous admixture.

ASKROG et al. (1964) found a mean increase in wasted ventilation of 26% in patients mechanically ventilated and anesthetized with halothane, cyclopropane, or nitrous oxide. Their data suggest a progressive increase in the proportion of poorly perfused areas of the lung. In a subsequent report, ASKROG et al. (1966) showed that during halothane anesthesia the magnitude of the arterial to alveolar PCO_2 difference correlated with changes in pulmonary artery pressure. Indeed, the authors demonstrated that restoration of pulmonary artery pressure (and presumably flow) following the rapid infusion of isotonic saline or head-down tilt, diminished the difference between arterial and alveolar PCO_2. This suggests that elevation of pulmonary artery pressure improves circulation to the non-dependent portions of the lung. In contrast, it has been pointed out that patients anesthetized with halothane and who are allowed to ventilate spontaneously do not develop changes in wasted ventilation (MARSHALL, 1966). This indicates that other factors may have influence on the pulmonary circulation. Intubation of the trachea may have advantage in promoting adequate ventilation by reducing the proportion of wasted ventilation. The effects of a given "excess ventilation" or "excess perfusion" will be influenced by the gas considered (SAIDMAN and EGER, 1967). Specifically, for soluble gases such as diethyl ether or methoxyflurane, blood represents a relatively good reservoir with the result that excess ventilation will be quite effective in producing an increase in the rate of rise of the alveolar concentrations of these agents. Consequently, the extent to which hyperventilated elements contribute to the dead space will be minor. On the other hand, the volume of a relatively insoluble gas such as nitrous oxide or cyclopropane that can be taken up by blood is more limited, and excess ventilation will be rather inefficient in changing the alveolar concentration. In a similar manner, it is possible to show that when excess perfusion is present, its effects on soluble gases will be much more pronounced than the effects of gases of low solubility.

Non-uniformity of ventilation and perfusion may account for the observed right-to-left shunting that occurs during general anesthesia. Even with a high inspired O_2 concentration the alveolar to arterial PO_2 difference may be as great as 200 mmHg. NUNN (1964) has recommended that inspired gases during anesthesia contain an O_2 concentration of at least 35% to insure adequate oxygenation. Progressive atelectasis during constant-volume ventilation has been assumed to be the basis for the increased right-to-left shunt and resultant arterial hypoxemia. Although COLGAN and WHANG (1968) reported no significant changes in shunting, lung compliance, and functional residual capacity during anesthesia with spontaneous breathing, periodic hyperinflation of the lungs has been suggested as a useful preventive measure. Arterial hypoxemia can also occur during air breathing following nitrous oxide anesthesia and after prolonged hyperventilation (see below).

Anesthetics also may influence gas exchange and lung mechanics by direct effects on conducting airways. The effects of halothane and cyclopropane on total pulmonary resistance have been compared in dogs before and during airway constriction produced by histamine or vagal nerve stimulation (HICKEY et al., 1969).

Over a wide range of anesthetic concentrations, mean resistance change in the unstimulated airways of animals anesthetized with halothane was half the mean value obtained in similar animals anesthetized with cyclopropane. Although both anesthetics prevented severe bronchospasm of vagal nerve stimulation in small and large airways, comparison at equivalent levels of anesthesia showed that halothane was a more potent bronchodilator than cyclopropane.

In the search for a mechanism responsible for postoperative lung complications and altered function, the effects of anesthetics on pulmonary surfactant have been investigated. Although halothane (1.2%) and chloroform (2.4%) have been shown to alter surfactant function during ventilation in freshly excised dogs' lungs (WOO et al., 1969), studies in rats and dogs following halothane and diethyl ether anesthesia demonstrated no measurable effect on the surface tension characteristics of surfactant (ZELKOWITZ et al., 1968). The results of this later study are

Table 1. *Human MAC and lipid solubility values*
(37 °C)
(SAIDMAN et al., 1967)

Agent	MAC (Vol-%)	Oil/Gas partition coefficient
Methoxyflurane	0.16	970
Halothane	0.77	224
Diethyl ether	1.92	65
Fluroxene	3.4	47.7
Cyclopropane	9.2	11.8
Nitrous oxide	101[a]	1.4

[a] Calculated value.
Note the relationship MAC X O/G= K.

supported by studies of surface activity of the alveolar lining substance in lung extracts prepared from sequential lung biopsies of anesthetized patients (MILLER and THOMAS, 1967). These observations have not explained the method of production of atelectasis following general anesthesia and suggest that other pathophysiologic mechanisms are involved.

II. Depth of Anesthesia

The magnitude of the effect that inhalation anesthetics have on ventilation is dependent in part on the level of anesthesia. In the past, anesthetic depth was estimated by evaluation of reflex responses, electroencephalographic activity or by degree of depression of various physiologic systems. With the advent of the concept of minimum (alveolar) anesthetic concentration (MAC), definition of a standard of anesthetic potency is possible (EGER et al., 1965). MAC is defined as that alveolar concentration of an inhalation anesthetic which just prevents movement in response to a standard stimulus (usually the surgical incision) in 50% of patients. MAC values for the various agents in man (SAIDMAN et al., 1967) are shown in Table 1. Using this concept, the alveolar concentration (partial pressure) of one anesthetic may be expressed in equivalent analgesia potency to MAC of other anesthetics. For example, an alveolar concentration of methoxyflurane of

0.16% is equivalent in analgesic potency to an alveolar halothane concentration of 0.77%. In order to correlate anesthetic effect with anesthetic depth (dosage), levels of anesthesia greater than MAC may be expressed empirically as multiples of MAC. A value of 2 MAC halothane indicates an alveolar concentration of halothane 2 times MAC or 1.54% halothane and is therefore numerically equivalent to an alveolar concentration of methoxyflurane of 0.32%. This method permits the comparison of drug effects at equivalent depths of anesthesia.

III. Resting Ventilation

Induction of anesthesia with most inhalation agents characteristically produces changes in both ventilatory performance and function. The response in non-

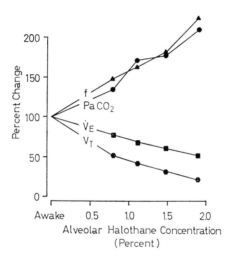

Fig. 1. Graphic representation of per cent changes in respiratory frequency (f), arterial PCO_2, expiratory volume (V_E), and tidal volume (V_T) in 12 non-medicated subjects awake and at various alveolar halothane concentrations. Data plotted from MUNSON et al. (1966)

medicated, non-stimulated subjects is an increase in the frequency of breathing and a decrease in tidal volume. This combination usually produces a decrease in effective ventilatory exchange with a resultant proportional rise in the arterial PCO_2. Changes observed during halothane anesthesia are illustrated in Fig. 1. The frequency of breathing increases with increasing depth of anesthesia. The magnitude of this response during halothane anesthesia is surpassed only by that of fluroxene (MUNSON et al., 1966) and trichlorethylene (TALCOTT et al., 1965). Increase in respiratory frequency may be valuable in the assessment of relative depth of anesthesia (Fig. 2). Although respiratory frequency increases with all agents, the magnitude of changes over a wide range of cyclopropane and methoxy-flurane concentrations is small, making rate changes a less useful clinical sign of anesthetic depth with these agents than with halothane, fluroxene or diethyl ether. Tidal volume decreases with most agents with increasing depth of anesthesia, thus providing another useful response for the assessment of relative anesthetic

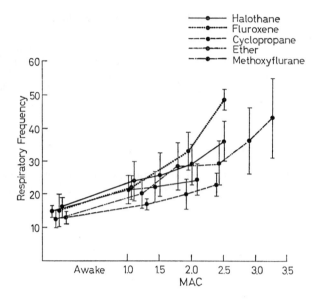

Fig. 2. Comparison of mean (± S.D.) changes in respiratory frequency (breaths per minute) for subjects awake and at various levels (MAC) of anesthesia for 5 agents. Rectilinear regression slopes showed significant differences between fluroxene and diethyl ether and between fluroxene and methoxyflurane. From LARSON et al. (1969)

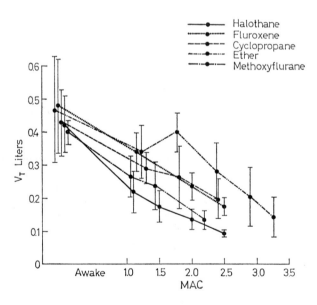

Fig. 3. Comparison of mean (± S.D.) change in tidal volume (V_T) in subjects awake and at various levels (MAC) of anesthesia for 5 agents. Reduction in tidal volume was greatest with halothane. Differences between halothane and ether were significant at each level of anesthesia. From LARSON et al. (1969)

depth (Fig. 3). The addition of other depressant drugs and the presence of metabolic acidosis and surgical stimulation may alter these responses during clinical
anesthesia. During CO_2 challenge subjects anesthetized with fluroxene, cyclopropane or diethyl ether show relatively greater increases in respiratory frequency
than with either halothane or methoxyflurane. Interestingly, ANDREWS and ORKIN
(1968) found that severely hemorrhaged dogs anesthetized with halothane were
able to respond with greater increases in respiratory frequency, and therefore
minute ventilation, than methoxyflurane hemorrhaged animals. The role of cate-
cholemines in this regard remains, as yet, undefined.

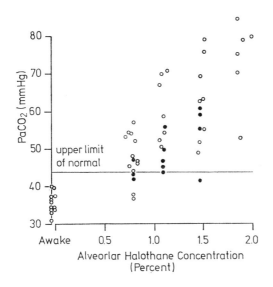

Fig. 4. The relationship of arterial PCO_2 to alveolar halothane concentration in 12 non-
medicated, intubated patients is shown. Open circles represent values obtained prior to
surgical stimulation, whereas closed circles represent values during surgery. In both non-
stimulated and stimulated groups, mean PCO_2 values were increased above normal limits.
Note that arterial PCO_2 increases rectilinearly with increasing anesthetic depth. From
MUNSON and LARSON (1968)

Studies in both dog and man have shown that alveolar ventilation decreases
with increasing depth of halothane anesthesia. MERKEL and EGER (1963) demonstrated a rectilinear rise in arterial PCO_2 in dogs above an alveolar halothane
concentration of 0.7%. Studies in man at known halothane alveolar concentrations
show similar findings. In non-medicated, intubated patients in the absence of
surgical stimulation, mean arterial PCO_2 values at light levels of anesthesia are
significantly increased above awake control values (Fig. 4). Above an alveolar
halothane concentration of 0.8%, arterial PCO_2 increased markedly with increasing
anesthetic depth. Patients with relatively low awake arterial PCO_2 values tend to
maintain lower arterial PCO_2 values with increasing depth of anesthesia. Likewise,
patients with higher awake alveolar PCO_2 values show higher arterial PCO_2
values. This was not observed in similar studies with methoxyflurane (LARSON
et al., 1969).

A comparison of mean resting arterial PCO_2 values for five anesthetics at equivalent levels of anesthesia is shown in Fig. 5. At light levels of anesthesia (1.1 MAC) halothane, fluroxene, cyclopropane and methoxyflurane produce significant elevation of arterial PCO_2 when compared to awake values. At each level of anesthesia studied, halothane and methoxyflurane show the greatest depression of alveolar ventilation during spontaneous ventilation. Fluroxene and cyclopropane show relatively less depression. Only with diethyl ether does the increase in the frequency of breathing offset the decrease in tidal ventilation sufficiently to maintain alveolar ventilation, and hence PCO_2 within the normal range. Comparison

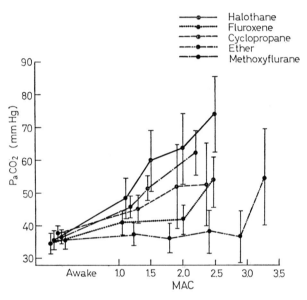

Fig. 5. Mean (± S.D.) arterial PCO_2 values during resting, spontaneous ventilation in 43 subjects awake and during various levels of anesthesia. Note that halothane and methoxyflurane produce the greatest rise in arterial PCO_2 values at any anesthetic level while diethyl ether has little effect even at relatively profound levels of anesthesia. From Larson et al. (1969)

of the relationship between total ventilation and arterial PCO_2 for diethyl ether and halothane illustrates this point (Fig. 6). Even at relatively deep levels of ether anesthesia PCO_2 is maintained at or *below* normal values. Relative increase in ventilation above awake values at normal levels of PCO_2 indirectly reflects a disproportionate increase in wasted ventilation. In contrast to these findings Marshall and Grange (1966) found no change in wasted ventilation in patients anesthetized with diethyl ether in air and allowed to breathe spontaneously. The mechanism by which diethyl ether maintains PCO_2 normal is unknown. Muallem et al. (1969) have shown in dogs that the stimulant effect of diethyl ether probably originates within the central nervous system. The halothane-ether azeotrope has also been shown to produce mild ventilatory depression in pre-medicated patients (Dery et al., 1964).

The acidemia that accompanies ventilatory depression is due to an increased arterial PCO_2 since standard bicarbonate remains essentially normal. This is substantiated by reports of a lack of an appreciable metabolic acidosis in both anesthetized infants (BLACK and McKANE, 1965) and adults (HOLMDAHL and PAYNE, 1960). However, MILLAR and MARSHALL (1965) reported small reductions in standard bicarbonate (less than 2.2 mM/l) following several hours of hyperventilation in patients anesthetized with halothane during induced mild hypothermia. This non-respiratory acidosis is believed not to represent a true metabolic acidosis since the change was rapidly reversed on return to normocarbia. The effect is not associated with the development of metabolically produced acids but is apparently related to the migration of bicarbonate ions from blood to less well-buffered tissues.

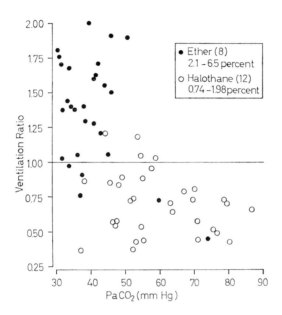

Fig. 6. The ventilation ratio [ventilation (V_E) anesthetized divided by ventilation awake] is plotted as a function of arterial PCO_2 for 20 subjects maintained at constant depth ether and halothane anesthesia. Figures in parentheses indicate the number of subjects studied. The range of alveolar anesthetic concentrations are also noted. Even at relatively deep levels of ether anesthesia PCO_2 is maintained at near normal levels. The corresponding ventilatory ratio increase during ether anesthesia indicates a disproportionate increase in wasted ventilation. Data taken from LARSON et al. (1969) and MUNSON et al. (1966)

If adequate ventilation and near-normal arterial PCO_2 values are desired during surgery, ventilation must be at least assisted with most agents at anything more than the lightest level of anesthesia. Augmenting ventilation, while permitting the patient to initiate ventilatory effort, can lower arterial PCO_2 5—10 mmHg, depending on the depth of anesthesia (SEVERINGHAUS and LARSON, 1965). In order for assisted ventilation to be effective in lowering arterial PCO_2 during anesthesia, alveolar ventilation must be increased and maintained greater than that resulting from spontaneous breathing. Intermittent assistance by occasional augmentation of tidal ventilation has no appreciable effect on lowering arterial PCO_2. At deep levels of anesthesia further elevation of the apneic threshold occurs so that assisted ventilation alone is unable to produce adequate alveolar ventilation. Controlled ventilation is therefore required if further rise in arterial PCO_2 is to be prevented.

The concept of adequate ventilation proposed by Morris (1963) using the apneic threshold during nitrous oxide anesthesia combined with subapneic amounts of d-tubocurarine represents a special technic. Intermittently controlled ventilation may allow the central respiratory centers to maintain resting ventilation at a near normal value. However, any alteration in ventilatory threshold or sensitivity by the addition of drugs, such as halothane or opiates, will result in respiratory acidosis.

The use of controlled ventilation may produce other responses during anesthesia. The loss of respiratory rate and depth may impair the clinical assessment of the depth of anesthesia. Hyperventilation also increases the rate of rise of the alveolar anesthetic concentration, and therefore anesthetic depth, particularly with the agents that are most soluble in blood (Eger, 1964). In addition, the resultant respiratory alkalosis shifts the hemoglobin dissociation curve to the left and may alter regional blood flows, such as in the brain and fetus. If an increase in mean intrathoracic pressure occurs during controlled ventilation venous return to the heart may be compromised with resultant circulatory depression.

Apnea may occur in the anesthetized patient following prolonged periods of hyperventilation. If arterial PCO_2 is reduced below the apneic threshold, the resumption of spontaneous ventilation is dependent on the rate of CO_2 production and subsequent rise in PCO_2 and the absolute position of the apneic threshold on the ventilatory response curve. Eger and Severinghaus (1961) showed that during apnea following hyperventilation the arterial PCO_2 rises primarily as a function of metabolism. After equilibration of the alveolar PCO_2 with mixed venous blood, PCO_2 rises at a rate of 2—4 mmHg/min.

Arterial PCO_2 need not rise, however, to the point that was required to initiate ventilation prior to hyperventilation. Edelist and Osorio (1969) demonstrated that the apneic threshold is shifted to the left an average of 7 mmHg following prolonged periods of controlled ventilation to arterial PCO_2 levels of 20 mmHg. These findings are consistent with a decrease in cerebrospinal fluid (CSF) bicarbonate concentration which restores CSF pH to normal in the presence of a reduced PCO_2. As a result, the same arterial PCO_2 in the posthyperventilation period may initiate a greater than normal ventilatory response. However, loss of CO_2 stores during prolonged hyperventilation may produce a state termed "posthyperventilation hypoxia" (Salvatore et al., 1969). This syndrome is characterized by reduced "functional" CO_2 excretion, a normal arterial PCO_2, and a reduced arterial PO_2. This paradox shows alveolar ventilation to be adequate for CO_2 clearance but inadequate in terms of oxygen uptake. Ivanov and Nunn (1969) studied various methods in anesthetized patients for elevating end-expiratory PCO_2 at the end of prolonged hyperventilation. They found that the addition of 5% CO_2 to the inspired gases was more rapid and reliable than methods which utilized either the removal of soda lime from the anesthetic apparatus or a step reduction in minute ventilation.

Central nervous system stimulants have been used to increase ventilation in depressed patients. However, most analeptics have brief duration of action and may be hazardous in the treatment of drug induced ventilatory depression. One double blind study compared the effectiveness of doxapram, ethamivan, and methylphenidate in a large postoperative series (Wolfson et al., 1965). Doxapram appeared to be most potent with reference to respiratory stimulation while cardiovascular effects were most marked with methylphenidate. No indication for the routine use of these drugs was provided by this study, but neither was there shown any contraindication to this considered application. The use of such a therapy should also consider resultant increases in cerebral and cardiac O_2 consumption and the abilities of the circulatory, as well as the respiratory system, to supply increased metabolic needs.

IV. Ventilatory Response

The level of resting arterial PCO_2 during anesthesia does not always indicate the degree of ventilatory depression. Decreased responsiveness of respiratory control mechanisms may be more accurately assessed by changes in the slope and position of the ventilatory response to arterial CO_2 and the response to hypoxia at constant PCO_2. CO_2 response can be rapidly determined with a rebreathing technique using a 4-l bag prefilled with 8% CO_2 in O_2 (READ, 1967), or by the slower but more interpretable steady state (> 5 min) breathing of 2—4 levels of increased CO_2. The slope represents a change in ventilation per change in PCO_2 and is expressed in units of liters per minute per mmHg PCO_2. Within the range studied (40—60 mmHg) this response is usually a linear function (see Figs. 7 and 9). Normal slopes vary from 0.5—3.0 l/min/m², while normal arterial PCO_2 is much less variable (37—42 mmHg in men, 34—40 mmHg in women). Although BRAND-STATER et al. (1965) showed that at constant depth anesthesia in dogs for a period up to 8 h does not produce changes in the ventilatory response to inhaled CO_2, confirmation in other species is lacking. Since ventilatory response may be depressed at relatively deep levels of anesthesia PCO_2 levels above 70 mmHg might be required to demonstrate significant increases in ventilation at deeper levels of anesthesia.

It is interesting that relatively wide fluctuations in ventilation do not alter anesthetic requirement. EISELE et al. (1967) demonstrated that arterial PCO_2 levels ranging from 15—90 mmHg had no influence on halothane MAC in dogs. Similar findings have been found during hyperventilation in man (BRIDGES and EGER, 1966). Increase in arterial PCO_2 above this level may provide further increase in the relative depth of narcosis producing progressing depression of ventilation, and eventually, apnea. Changes in responsiveness may represent depression of central or peripheral chemoreceptors or depression of other areas. MITCHELL et al. (1963) produced mild respiratory depression to apnea in cats by perfusing chemosensitive areas on the ventrolateral surfaces of the medulla with dilute solutions of procaine. KATZ and NGAI (1962) and NGAI et al. (1965) studied the effects of diethyl ether, trichlorethylene, halothane and methoxyflurane in cats. Their findings indicate that these agents are primarily respiratory depressants through their actions on the central regulatory and integratory mechanisms. It is possible that central chemosensitive areas in man might also be depressed by the inhalation anesthetic agents.

The effect of halothane on ventilatory response has been quantitated in dogs (Fig. 7) by BRANDSTATER et al. (1965). At a constant alveolar halothane partial pressure, ventilatory response to CO_2 was reproducible for periods up to 8 h. With increasing alveolar halothane concentration a progressive rectilinear depression of ventilatory response was observed. The response to CO_2 diminished when arterial PCO_2 levels approached 100 mmHg. Further increase in PCO_2 results in a further depression of ventilation, i.e., a negative slope. These authors also found that cyclopropane, when compared to halothane, caused little change in ventilatory response until relatively deep levels of anesthesia were obtained.

Similar depression of ventilatory response during anesthesia has been reported in unmedicated human subjects (LARSON et al., 1969). Data for 43 subjects anesthetized with five agents at various levels of anesthesia are shown in Fig. 8.

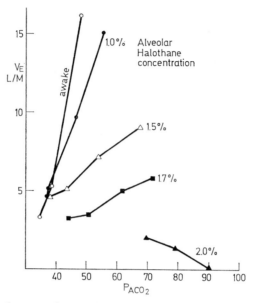

Fig. 7. Effect of halothane on the ventilatory response to CO_2. A family of curves in a dog shows a progressive decrease in ventilatory responsiveness with increasing depth of halothane anesthesia. At deep levels (2 % halothane) a negative slope is observed as ventilation approaches apnea. From BRANDSTATER et al. (1965)

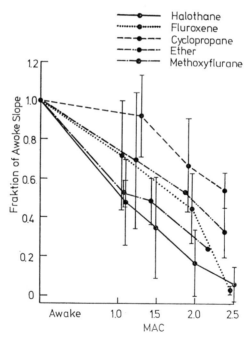

Fig. 8. Mean (± S.D.) slopes of ventilatory response to CO_2 for 43 subjects are shown at various levels (MAC) of anesthesia. Values on the ordinate are expressed as fractions of the awake values. Halothane and methoxyflurane show the greatest depression of ventilatory response of all the agents studied. From LARSON et al. (1969)

Halothane shows the greatest depression of CO_2 responsiveness when compared to the other agents at equivalent levels of anesthesia. Ventilatory response to CO_2 during light levels of anesthesia is equally depressed by halothane, fluroxene, methoxyflurane, and diethyl ether. In another study, DUNBAR et al. (1967) also showed that methoxyflurane produced profound respiratory depression at deep levels of anesthesia. One possible explanation for the relative lack of ventilatory response depression during cyclopropane anesthesia may be related to circulating catecholamines. Cyclopropane has been shown to increase plasma catecholamine levels in man (particularly norepinephrine) in proportion to both cyclopropane concentration and PCO_2 (PRICE et al., 1959, 1960).

The occurrence of hypothermia during anesthesia may mask the usual ventilatory warning of the development of hypercapnia. REGAN and EGER (1966) studied ventilatory response to hypercapnia and hypoxia during moderate hypothermia (32—28 °C) in dogs. At constant depth halothane anesthesia ventilatory depression progressively decreased with falling body temperatures.

Due to the relative lack of potency of nitrous oxide, evaluations of the ventilatory effects of this agent usually have been made in combination with other drugs. Often these other agents have been respiratory depressants. Under these conditions nitrous oxide has been shown to have either a mild stimulant (ECKENHOFF and HELRICH, 1958) or ventilatory sparing effect (HORNBEIN et al., 1969). This later study showed that at approximately equivalent levels of anesthesia (MAC) the combination of 0.3% halothane and 70% nitrous oxide depressed both resting ventilation and the response to CO_2 less than the degree of depression observed when 0.8% halothane was administered without nitrous oxide. However, at deeper levels of anesthesia the addition of nitrous oxide to both 0.8 and 1.5% halothane elevated resting arterial PCO_2 only slightly, but had little effect on CO_2 responsiveness. These findings suggest that nitrous oxide, in combination with halothane, stimulates the sympathetic nervous system. This hypothesis is consistent with studies of CUNNINGHAM et al. (1963) who demonstrated that intravenously infused norepinephrine (8—15 µg/min) increased the slope of the CO_2 response curve by 30%. This is of interest in regard to the finding of mean cyclopropane slopes 30—50% greater at 1.9 and 2.4 MAC than those for halothane at comparable levels of anesthesia (Fig. 8). The results of LUNDHOLM and SVEDMYR (1966) show that the respiratory stimulation mechanism of norepinephrine (0.2 µg/kg/min) seems at least in part to be related to possible influence on O_2 sensitive receptors. Epinephrine (0.1 µg/kg/min) also stimulates ventilation, but in contrast to norepinephrine the stimulation is thought to result from increases in CO_2 production and plasma PCO_2 levels.

V. Other Drugs

Patients often receive supplemental drugs in the form of belladonna agents, barbiturates, and opiates. These drugs, either alone or in combination with the inhalation agents, may modify resting ventilation and ventilatory response to CO_2. Atropine and other belladonna drugs may effect a small increase in arterial PCO_2 by dilating conducting airways, thereby increasing the proportion of wasted ventilation (SEVERINGHAUS and STUPFEL, 1955). Secobarbital in usual premedicant doses (100 mg intravenously) in adult patients produces no appreciable effect on the slope of the CO_2 response curve (STEPHEN et al., 1969). However, induction of anesthesia with large doses of thiopental may depress ventilatory response to CO_2 for several hours (MERKEL and EGER, 1963). Relatively small dosages of pentobarbital (100 mg) have been shown to produce serious central nervous system depression and increased respiratory failure in bronchitic patients with severe airway obstruction (GOLD et al., 1969).

All opiates may elevate PCO_2 and alter the CO_2 response curve, displacing it to the right and/or flattening the slope. At equal analgesic doses, morphine is less depressant to respiration than any other narcotic. At the other extreme, fentanyl may produce apnea without loss of consciousness, and in this state, no respiratory response to CO_2 occurs, but respiration can be maintained voluntarily by reminding the subject to breathe. Opiates are often used in an attempt to slow respiratory rate and thereby reduce the minute dead space ventilation during anesthesia.

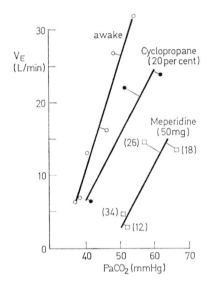

Fig. 9. Ventilatory response curves in a subject awake and at constant depth cyclopropane anesthesia. The addition of 50 mg meperidine to cyclopropane elevated the resting arterial PCO_2 10 mmHg and produced a parallel shift of the response curve to the right. Numbers in parentheses indicate the time course (min) following meperidine injection

Although opiates may contribute significant analgesia and thus reduce MAC (SAIDMAN and EGER, 1964; MUNSON et al., 1965), there is no evidence that the addition of opiate produces a more efficient ventilation (i.e., a lower arterial PCO_2) at equivalent levels of anesthesia. In fact, LARSON (unpublished data) has shown that arterial PCO_2 rises when doses of an opiate sufficient to slow respiratory rate are administered during halothane anesthesia, even if alveolar halothane concentration is reduced. Tachypnea probably acts as a compensatory mechanism to maintain a more normal arterial PCO_2. Opiates reduce respiratory rate, but do not increase tidal volume by a corresponding amount; hence, arterial PCO_2 rises. The interaction of meperidine and cyclopropane is shown in Fig. 9. Twelve minutes following the intravenous injection of 50 mg of meperidine during constant depth cyclopropane anesthesia, arterial PCO_2 increased 10 mmHg. Following CO_2 challenge (with no appreciable change in slope) resting arterial PCO_2 after 34 min remained elevated.

Ventilatory response to CO_2 has also been measured during Innovar-nitrous oxide anesthesia in man (DUNBAR et al., 1967). In 7 patients, anesthesia induced by the injection of a single dose of Innovar (fentanyl 0.25 mg and dehydrobenzperidol 12.5 mg), and maintained with nitrous oxide (67%), markedly depressed the slope of the CO_2 response curve for periods greater than 60 min. This shows that this form of neuroleptanalgesia profoundly depresses ventilation with a maximal effect quantitatively equal to that seen at 2—2.5 MAC for fluroxene or halothane.

VI. Surgical Stimulation

Surgical stimulation produces a small but appreciable effect on reducing resting arterial PCO_2 toward normal during light levels of halothane anesthesia (Fig. 1,

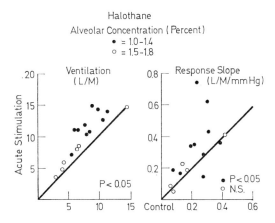

Fig. 10. Changes in expired ventilation and ventilatory response following acute tail clamp stimulation are shown for 9 dogs at 2 levels of halothane anesthesia. Points above the identity line indicate relative increases from control values. Changes for both responses were significant at alveolar halothane concentrations less than 1.4%. Data plotted from REGAN, EGER, and MUNSON (unpublished data)

closed circles). In 10 patients at alveolar concentrations of halothane between 0.8 and 1.5%, mean arterial PCO_2 values were decreased 6 mmHg during the stimulation of surgery. This effect of noxious somatic afferent stimulation on ventilation has also been observed in dogs. REGAN, EGER, and MUNSON in an unpublished study showed that during acute noxious stimulation minute ventilation and CO_2 responsiveness was increased at alveolar halothane concentrations of 1.4% or less but was unchanged at deeper levels (Fig. 10). Prolonged continuous stimulation (tail clamping) did not alter CO_2 responsiveness during light or deep levels of anesthesia. These data together with those shown in Fig. 1 show that the noxious stimulation of surgery has a small but appreciable effect which tends to oppose the ventilatory depressant effects of halothane. The effect of acute sensory stimulation is presumably related to the development of an alerting or arousal reaction transmitted to medullary centers via neural pathways in the midbrain reticular formation. These observations suggest that chronic surgical stimulation, if of unvarying intensity, probably cannot be depended upon to maintain normal ventilation.

VII. Recovery

Fink (1955) directed attention to the phenomenon of diffusion anoxia which occurs at the termination of nitrous oxide anesthesia when the patient breathes room air. The resultant hypoxemia is related to the differential solubility between nitrous oxide and nitrogen, the former being 34 times more soluble in blood than the latter. As a result, the excretion of nitrous oxide into the alveoli is greater (several liters in the first few minutes following air breathing) than the uptake of nitrogen from the alveoli into the blood. The dilution of alveolar O_2 and CO_2 by excreted nitrous oxide may reduce arterial O_2 saturation.

This "excretion-ventilation" or "dilution effect" has received critical reappraisal by Frumin and Edelist (1969). Using electrode technics for accurate and reproducible arterial PO_2 and PCO_2 determinations, these investigators concluded that the entity of diffusion anoxia does not exist as a clinically significant phenomenon providing patients are free of cardiopulmonary disease and capable of maintaining normal ventilation. However, hypoxemia may occur in the immediate postanesthetic period following respiratory obstruction or the development of ventilatory-perfusion changes. In such instances the administration of oxygen will eliminate or reduce considerably any hypoxemia resulting from such causes.

Summary

Ventilatory performance and function may be influenced directly by the effects of drugs on central regulatory and integratory mechanisms, and indirectly by other effects. These include altered PO_2, body temperature, acid-base balance, sympatho-adrenal stimulation, blood pressure, cardiac output, cerebral blood flow, dead space, airway resistance, muscle function, and postural and mechanical chest limitation. In addition, prolonged hyperventilation tends to be self perpetuating by lowering CSF bicarbonate concentration.

References

Andrews, I. C., Orkin, L. R.: Methoxyflurane and halothane anesthesia during controlled bleeding in dogs: Effect on respiration. Anesthesiology 29, 171—173 (1968),
Askrog, V. F.: Changes in (a-A) CO_2 difference and pulmonary artery pressure in anesthetized man. J. Appl. Physiol. 21, 1299—1305 (1966).
— Pender, J. W., Smith, T. C., Eckenhoff, J. E.: Changes in respiratory dead space during halothane, cyclopropane, and nitrous oxide anesthesia. Anesthesiology 25, 342—352 (1964).
Black, G. W., McKane, R. V.: Respiratory and metabolic changes during methoxyflurane and halothane anaesthesia. Brit. J. Anaesthesia 37, 409—413 (1965).
Brandstater, B., Eger, E. I., II, Edelist, G.: Constant-depth halothane anesthesia in respiratory studies. J. Appl. Physiol. 20, 171—174 (1965).
Bridges, B. E., Jr., Eger, E. I., II: The effect of hypocapnia on the level of halothane anesthesia in man. Anesthesiology 27, 634—637 (1966).
Colgan, F. J., Whang, T. B.: Anesthesia and atelectasis. Anesthesiology 29, 917—922 (1968).
Cunningham, D. J. C., Hey, E. N., Patrick, J. M., Lloyd, B. B.: The effect of noradrenaline on the relation between pulmonary ventilation and the alveolar PO_2 and PCO_2 in man. Ann. N.Y. Acad. Sci. 109, 756—771 (1963).
Dery, R., Pelletier, J., Jacques, A.: Comparison of cardiovascular, respiratory, and metabolic effects of halothane-ether azeotropic mixture with those of methoxyflurane anaesthesia in man. Can. Anaesth. Soc. J. 11, 394—409 (1964).
Dunbar, B. S., Ovassapian, A., Smith, T. C.: The effects of methoxyflurane on ventilation in man. Anesthesiology 28, 1020—1028 (1967).
Eckenhoff, J. E., Helrich, M.: Effect of narcotics, thiopental and nitrous oxide upon respiration and respiratory response to hypercapnia. Anesthesiology 19, 240—253 (1958).

EDELIST, G., OSORIO, A.: Postanesthetic initiation of spontaneous ventilation after passive hyperventilation. Anesthesiology 31, 222—227 (1969).

EGER, E. I., II: Respiratory and circulatory factors in uptake and distribution of volatile anaesthetic agents. Brit. J. Anaesthesia 36, 155—171 (1964).

— SAIDMAN, L. J., BRANDSTATER, B.: Minimum alveolar anesthetic concentration: A standard of anesthetic potency. Anesthesiology 26, 756—763 (1965).

— SEVERINGHAUS, J. W.: The rate of rise of $PaCO_2$ in the apneic anesthetized patient. Anesthesiology 22, 419—425 (1961).

EISELE, J. H., EGER, E. I., II, MUALLEM, M.: Narcotic properties of carbon dioxide in the dog. Anesthesiology 28, 856—865 (1967).

FINK, B. R.: Diffusion anoxia. Anesthesiology 16, 511—519 (1955).

FRUMIN, M. J., EDELIST, G.: Diffusion anoxia: A critical reappraisal. Anesthesiology 31, 243 to 249 (1969).

GOLD, M. I., REICHENBERG, S., FREEMAN, E.: Respiratory depression in the sedated bronchitic patient. Anesthesiology 30, 492—499 (1969).

HICKEY, R. G., GRAF, P. D., NADEL, J. A., LARSON, C. P., Jr.: The effects of halothane and cyclopropane on total pulmonary resistance in the dog. Anesthesiology 31, 334—343 (1969).

HOLMDAHL, M. H., PAYNE, J. P.: Acid-base changes under halothane, nitrous oxide and oxygen anesthesia during spontaneous respiration. Acta Anaesthesiol. Scand. 4, 173—180 (1960).

HORNBEIN, T. F., MARTIN, W. E., BONICA, J. J., FREUND, F. G., PARMENTIER, P.: Nitrous oxide effects on the circulatory and ventilatory responses to halothane. Anesthesiology 31, 250—260 (1969).

IVANOV, S. D., NUNN, J. F.: Methods of elevation of PCO_2 for restoration of spontaneous breathing after artificial ventilation of anaesthetized patients. Brit. J. Anaesthesia 41, 28—37 (1969).

KATZ, R. L., NGAI, S. H.: Respiratory effects of diethyl ether in the cat. J. Pharmacol. Exptl Therap. 138, 329—336 (1962).

LARSON, C. P., Jr., EGER, E. I., II, MUALLEM, M., BUECHEL, D. R., MUNSON, E. S., EISELE, J. H.: The effects of diethyl ether and methoxyflurane on ventilation: II. A comparative study in man. Anesthesiology 30, 174—184 (1969).

LUNDHOLM, L., SVEDMYR, N.: Studies on the stimulating effects of adrenaline and noradrenaline on respiration in man. Acta Physiol. Scand. 67, 65—75 (1966).

MARSHALL, B. E.: Physiological shunting and deadspace during spontaneous respiration with halothane-oxygen anaesthesia and the influence of intubation on the physiological deadspace. Brit. J. Anaesthesia 38, 912—922 (1966).

— GRANGE, R. A.: Changes in respiratory physiology during ether/air anaesthesia. Brit. J. Anaesthesia 38, 329—338 (1966).

MERKEL, G., EGER, E. I., II: A comparative study of halothane and halopropane anesthesia. Including method for determining equipotency. Anesthesiology 24, 346—357 (1963).

MILLAR, R. A., MARSHALL, B. E.: Acid-base changes in arterial blood associated with spontaneous and controlled ventilation during anaesthesia. Brit. J. Anaesthesia 37, 492—504 (1965).

MILLER, R. N., THOMAS, P. A.: Pulmonary surfactant: Determinations from lung extracts of patients receiving diethyl ether or halothane. Anesthesiology 28, 1089—1093 (1967).

MITCHELL, R. A., LOESCHCKE, H. H., MASSION, W. H., SEVERINGHAUS, J. W.: Respiratory responses mediated through superficial chemosensitive areas on the medulla. J. Appl. Physiol. 18, 523—533 (1963).

MORRIS, L. E.: Concept of adequate ventilation using the apnoeic threshold during curare and nitrous oxide anaesthesia. Brit. J. Anaesthesia 35, 35—42 (1963).

MUALLEM, M., LARSON, C. P., JR., EGER, E. I., II: The effects of diethyl ether on $PaCO_2$ in dogs with and without vagal, somatic and sympathetic block. Anesthesiology 30, 185—191 (1969).

MUNSON, E. S., LARSON, C. P., JR.: Halothane and pulmonary ventilation. Clin. Anesth. 1, 139—151 (1968).

— — BABAD, A. A., REGAN, M. J., BUECHEL, D. R., EGER, E. I.: The effects of halothane, fluroxene and cyclopropane on ventilation: A comparative study in man. Anesthesiology 27, 716—728 (1966).

— SAIDMAN, L. J., EGER, E. I.: Effect of nitrous oxide and morphine on the minimum anesthetic concentration of fluroxene. Anesthesiology 26, 134—139 (1965).

NGAI, S. H., KATZ, R. L., FARHIE, S. E.: Respiratory effects of trichlorethylene, halothane and methoxyflurane in the cat. J. Pharmacol. Exptl Therap. 148, 123—130 (1965).

NUNN, J. F.: Factors influencing the arterial oxygen tension during halothane anaesthesia with spontaneous respiration. Brit. J. Anaesthesia 36, 327—341 (1964).

Price, H. L., Linde, H. W., Jones, R. E., Black, G. W., Price, M. L.: Sympatho-adrenal responses to general anesthesia in man and their relationship to hemodynamics. Anesthesiology 20, 563—575 (1959).
— Lurie, A. A., Black, G. W., Sechzer, P. H., Linde, H. W., Price, M. L.: Modification by general anesthetics (cyclopropane and halothane) of circulatory and sympathoadrenal responses to respiratory acidosis. Ann. Surg. 152, 1071—1077 (1960).
Read, D. J. C.: A clinical method for assessing the ventilatory response to carbon dioxide. Australasian Ann. Med. 16, 20—32 (1967).
Regan, M. J., Eger, E. I., II: Ventilatory responses to hypercapnia and hypoxia at normothermia and moderate hypothermia during constant-depth halothane anesthesia. Anesthesiology 27, 624—633 (1966).
Saidman, L. J., Eger, E. I., II: Effect of nitrous oxide and of narcotic premedication on the alveolar concentration of halothane required for anesthesia. Anesthesiology 25, 302—306 (1964).
— — The influence of ventilation/perfusion abnormalities upon the uptake of inhalation anesthetics. In: Clinical anesthesia, pp. 80—87. (Duncan, A., Holaday, M. D., Eds.). Philadelphia: F. A. Davis Co. 1967.
— — Munson, E. S., Babad, A. A., Muallem, M.: Minimum alveolar concentrations of methoxyflurane, halothane, ether and cyclopropane in man: Correlation with theories of anesthesia. Anesthesiology 28, 994—1002 (1967).
Salvatore, A. J., Sullivan, S. F., Papper, E. M.: Postoperative hypoventilation and hypoxemia in man after hyperventilation. New Engl. J. Med. 280, 467—470 (1969).
Severinghaus, J. W., Larson, C. P., Jr.: Respiration in anesthesia. In: Handbook of Physiology-Respiration, Vol. II, pp. 1219—1264 (Fenn, W. O., Rahn, H., Eds.). Washington, D.C.: American Physiological Society 1965.
— Stupfel, M.: Respiratory dead space increase following atropine in man, and atropine, vagal or ganglionic blockade and hypothermia in dogs. J. Appl. Physiol. 8, 81—87 (1955).
Stephen, G. W., Banner, M. P., Wollman, H., Smith, T. C.: Respiratory pharmacology of mixtures of scopolamine with secobarbital and with fentanyl. Anesthesiology 31, 237—242 (1969).
Talcott, D. A., Larson, C. P., Jr., Buechel, D. R.: Respiratory effects of trichlorethylene in man. Anesthesiology 26, 262—263 (1965).
West, J. B.: Regional differences in gas exchange in the lung of erect man. J. Appl. Physiol. 17, 873—878 (1962).
Wolfson, B., Siker, E. S., Ciccarelli, H. E.: A double blind comparison of doxapram, ethamivan and methylphenidate. Am. J. Med. Sci. 249, 391—398 (1965).
Woo, S. W., Berlin, D., Hedley-Whyte, J.: Surfactant function and anesthetic agents. J. Appl. Physiol. 26, 571—577 (1969).
Zelkowitz, P. S., Modell, J. H., Giammona, S. T.: Effects of ether and halothane inhalation on pulmonary surfactant. Am. Rev. Resp. Dis. 97, 795—800 (1968).

4.7. Metabolic Effects of Anesthetics

Nicholas M. Greene

The metabolic responses to general anesthesia are the result of many simultaneous and interrelated biochemical reactions. Some are caused by the anesthetic acting directly on cell metabolism. Others are secondary to anesthetically induced changes in, for example, blood gas tensions, organ blood flows, and neuro-endocrine function. Clear differentiation between direct and indirect effects is often difficult. The metabolic alterations concerned, be they direct or indirect, are manifestations of abnormal function and as such they are basic to a full understanding of the anesthetic state. Unfortunately, our present understanding of the metabolic effects of anesthesia is incomplete. In part this is due to limitations inherent in the present state of the art and science of human biochemistry. In part it is due to limitations resulting from the fact that until very recently few modern biochemical research technics have been applied to the field of anesthesia. Enough information is, however, available on the metabolic effects of anesthetics to warrant review at this time. Since all compounds capable of depressing neuronal function do not have metabolic effects in common, the present review is restricted to the effects of inhalation anesthetics, old and new, with the separate field of the metabolic effects of nonvolatile "anesthetics" omitted. Emphasis is placed on data which have become available since the subject was reviewed in 1963 (Greene, 1963). Since the question of whether the metabolic effects of anesthetics represent a cause of anesthesia or a result of anesthesia is considered in another chapter (Chapter 6.3), the effects of anesthetics upon body metabolism as a whole will be emphasized rather than their effects upon cerebral metabolism.

The subject divides itself into three parts: direct effects of anesthetics upon cell metabolism; indirect effects; and the sum of direct and indirect effects, i.e. effects *in vitro*.

I. Direct Effects

Direct effects of anesthetics upon cell metabolism are best evaluated by *in vitro* technics which allow control or elimination of the variables introduced by the indirect effects found in *in vivo* experiments. *In vitro* experiments are particularly appropriate for measurement of the effect of inhalation anesthetics upon enzyme activity, and it is surprising that so few data are available on the direct effects of anesthetics upon enzyme systems. Greene and Spencer studied the effect of diethyl ether upon lactate dehydrogenase activity *in vitro* and found that in clinically effective concentrations ether produces inhibition averaging 12.6%. The reason for this inhibition is not clear but may represent a nonspecific binding of ether to enzyme protein. This inhibition of lactate dehydrogenase corresponds to comparable inhibition of carbonic anhydrase observed *in vivo* in man during ether anesthesia (Christian and Greene). However, Galla (1967) found in a preliminary report an increase in erythrocyte transketolase activity in dogs during halothane anesthesia. This not only indicates that the pentose phosphate pathway of glucose metabolism is unaffected by halothane anesthesia, but also that the inhibition of enzyme activity associated with ether is not representative of a general tendency for interactions to take place between inhalation anesthetics and enzymes.

Although the effect of ether on lactate dehydrogenase and carbonic anhydrase activity is significant from a statistical point of view, it is doubtful if 12% inhibition is significant from a metabolic point of view. The specific activities of most enzyme systems are such that 80—90% inhibition is required before the biochemical reactions an enzyme catalyzes are significantly impaired. The relationship between lactate and pyruvate is normally dependent in part upon lactate dehydrogenase activity, but it is also dependent upon the availability of reduced and oxidized nicotinamide-adenine-dinucleotide (NADH and NAD). It is more likely that the disturbance of the normal lactate: pyruvate ratio observed *in vivo* during ether anesthesia is a result of abnormal concentrations of NAD and NADH than the result of impaired lactate dehydrogenase activity. The same can be said of the carbonic anhydrase inhibition noted during ether anesthesia. Its magnitude is not great enough to have any significant effect on either the rate of formation of H_2CO_3 from CO_2 and water, or on the rate of formation of CO_2 from H_2CO_3, and carbon dioxide homeostasis is but little affected due to this cause during ether anesthesia.

The transport of sodium ions across most biologic membranes is an active process the energy for which is derived in large part from adenosine triphosphate (ATP) through the action of the enzyme adenosine triphosphatase (ATPase). Although there are hazards of overinterpretation and oversimplification when the effects of anesthetics on sodium transport are interpreted in terms of their effect on ATPase activity, it is nonetheless interesting to note that halothane in concentrations of 2, 5 and 8% was found by ANDERSEN (1966) to be associated with a dose-dependent depression of active sodium transport in the toad bladder, while ether produced a biphasic response consisting of an initial stimulation followed by inhibition at all three concentrations studied (5, 15, and 25%). Cyclopropane (10, 30, and 60%) and nitrous oxide (30 and 80%), on the other hand, produced a dose-related stimulation of active sodium transport. The effect of nitrous oxide in ANDERSEN's experiments may have been related to the partial pressure of nitrous oxide employed. GOTTLIEB and SAVRAN showed that nitrous oxide produced a dose-related inhibition of sodium transport in frog skin which paralleled the depressant action of nitrous oxide on nerve excitability; this effect was only observed, however, at partial pressures of 6.8 atmospheres and above. ANDERSEN has also shown (1967) that active sodium transport was inhibited by cyclopropane when toads were pretreated with reserpine to deplete their tissues of catecholamines, indicating that the stimulatory effect of cyclopropane on active sodium transport is related to the action of epinephrine and norepinephrine. As ANDERSEN has noted, anesthetically induced inhibition of sodium transport could be due to inhibition of ATPase, inhibition of aerobic metabolism necessary for sodium transport, or stabilization of cell membranes. The possibility that anesthetics may affect ATPase is supported by the observations of UEDA (1965) on the inhibitory effect of ether on firefly bioluminescence. The light of firefly lanterns is produced by the action of the enzyme, luciferase, acting on the luminescent substrate, luciferin. ATP, magnesium and oxygen are also required for the reaction. When excess luciferin and luciferase are present, the intensity of the light produced is a function of the amount of ATP available. UEDA found that when ATP concentration is plotted against light produced the normal curve is shifted to the right in the presence of 6% ether, suggesting that inhibition of bioluminescence may be the result of inhibition of ATP utilization rather than ATP synthesis. One of the factors involved in ATP utilization *in vivo* is, of course, ATPase activity. However, UEDA and MIETANI have also shown that in clinically effective concentrations halothane produces no significant inhibition *in vitro* of the ouabain-sensitive $Na^+K^+ATPase$ of rabbit brain microsomes. Inhibition was noted only in the presence of concentrations which are lethal *in vivo*. Whether the differences between these two studies on ATPase are the result of differences in pharmacologic properties of ether and halothane, or whether they represent differences in the types of ATPase studied is undetermined.

HOECH et al. used rat tissue slices to evaluate the *in vitro* effect of halothane upon tissue oxygen consumption. They found that 1% halothane was associated with a significant depression of consumption of oxygen by unstimulated as well as cation-stimulated brain slices. Liver and heart slices were, however, less sensitive to the effects of halothane. Oxygen consumption of liver and heart slices was unaffected by 1% halothane, and it was only upon exposure to concentrations of 2% halothane that significant degrees of inhibition of oxygen sconumption were noted. The experiments of HOECH et al. are an illustration of the fact that the metabolic response to anesthetics is not the same for all tissues. These same investigators also found that anaerobic glycolysis in rat brain homogenates was unaffected by concentrations of halothane which significantly depressed oxygen consumption. This suggests that at least in the rat brain the decrease in oxygen consumption during halothane anesthesia is not the result of unavailability of substrates entering into the tricarboxylic acid cycle but that instead the decrease in oxygen consumption is associated with alterations of tricarboxylic acid cycle metabolism or electron transport systems.

A technic for measuring the direct effect of anesthetics upon cell metabolism based upon the use of cell cultures has recently been introduced by FINK and KENNY. Employing monolayer mouse heteroploid or mouse sarcoma I cultures, these investigators studied the effects on multiplication rates of therapeutic concentrations of chloroform, diethyl, ether fluroxene, halothane, methoxyflurane, trichlorethylene, and nitrous oxide. All anesthetics decreased the rate of multiplication of cells. In an attempt to determine why anesthetics decreased multiplications rates, FINK and KENNY investigated in detail the metabolic effects of 0.4, 0.8, and 1.6% halothane. They found that halothane was associated with a dose-related increase in glucose uptake. For example, in the presence of 0.8% halothane glucose uptake rose from control values of 3.5—$13.6 \, \mu M/cell \times 10^6$. This was associated with a simultaneous decrease in oxygen uptake from 1.00 in the control state to 0.53 during exposure to 0.8% halothane. Output of lactic acid also rose, from control levels of 0.7 to levels of $23.7 \, \mu M/cell \times 10^6$ with halothane. The increase in glycolysis and decrease in oxygen uptake were accompanied by an increase in the amount of glucose which was calculated as undergoing metabolism by being reduced (from 0—$12.1 \, \mu M/cell \times 10^6$) and a decrease in the calculated amount of glucose being oxidized (from 3.5—$1.5 \, \mu M/cell \times 10^6$). These changes in anaerobic and aerobic metabolism resulted in significant alterations in the amount of ATP produced during exposure to halothane and in the metabolic sources of the ATP which was produced. The amount of ATP produced by oxidative metabolism was $133 \, \mu M/cell \times 10^6$ in the absence of halothane, but only $57 \, \mu M/cell \times 10^6$ in the presence of 0.8% halothane. This decrease corresponded to an increase in the amount of ATP synthesized by glycolytic means, from 9—$24.2 \, \mu M/cell \times 10^6$. The authors hypothesized that the accelerated glycolysis and the inhibition of oxidative metabolism associated with exposure to halothane were the result of changes in permeability of mitochondrial membranes produced by a direct action of the anesthetic. Decreased permeability of mitochondrial membranes to pyruvate, to tricarboxylic acid metabolites such as oxaloacetate and malate, or to compounds such as α-glycerophosphate and dihydroxyacetone phosphate would significantly impair normal oxidative phosphorylative processes occuring within mitochondria. Alteration in mitochondrial membrane permeability to compounds such as α-glycerophosphate would also influence extramitochondrial concentration of NAD because of the relationship of such compounds to shuttle systems responsible for transport of NADH across mitochondrial membranes. Resultant changes in cytoplasmic NAD concentrations could impair extramito-chondrial metabolic processes such as lactate metabolism.

The *in vitro* findings of FINK and KENNY are supported by the *in vivo* data obtained by SCHWEIZER and her associates. These investigators studied 50 patients during ether anesthesia and 50 patients during halothane anesthesia. They found blood levels of lactate and pyruvate were consistently higher following ether than following halothane anesthesia, the lactate:pyruvate ratio also being higher with ether. On the other hand, blood levels of acetyl coenzyme A, citrate, malate, and α-ketoglutarate were unaffected by either anesthetic. They suggested that the increased blood levels of glycolytic metabolites in the presence of normal levels of tricarboxylic acid cycle metabolites could be ascribed to a depressant effect produced by ether on mitochondrial membrane shuttle systems, or to a direct depressant effect of ether on intramitochondrial electron transport mechanisms. That they found evidence of interference with mitochondrial membrane permeability during ether but not during halothane anesthesia even though FINK and KENNY found that halothane impaired membrane permeability may be in part due to the fact that blood levels of metabolites are at best very indirect indices of events transpiring within or immediately adjacent to mitochondria. Perhaps longer duration of halothane anesthesia in the patients of SCHWEIZER et al. would have resulted in changes analogous to those observed by FINK and KENNY. And perhaps if FINK and KENNY had studied the response of cell cultures to exposure to ether they might also have found changes similar to those they observed following exposure to halothane.

The *in vitro* observations of FINK and KENNY are also confirmed by the findings of COHEN and MARSHALL. Using an *in vitro* rat liver mitochondrial preparation, COHEN and MARSHALL studied the effect of halothane on the rate of uptake of oxygen in the presence of exogenously added adenosine diphosphate (ADP). They found that clinically effective concentrations of halothane produced a dose-related, reversible depression of mitochondrial uptake of oxygen which consisted of two parts: depression of the respiratory chain within mitochondria, and loss of mitochondria respiratory control. The decreases in mitochondrial function which were observed by COHEN and MARSHALL could in part be due to an anesthetically induced decrease in permeability of mitochondrial membranes to substrates required for normal oxygen consumption as hypothesized by FINK and KENNY and by SCHWEITZER et al. The significance of the *in vitro* findings of SNODGRASS and PIRAS that halothane is an uncoupler of oxidative phosphorylation producing a loss of respiratory control which precedes depression of phosphorylation is difficult to interpret inasmuch as the concentrations of halothane which produced this effect were considerably in excess of those used in clinical practice.

The above evidence strongly suggests that anesthetics may affect cell metabolism by altering the permeability of the membranes investing mitochondria. Since the majority of enzymes involved in oxidative phosphorylation, in oxygen consumption and in energy production are located within mitochondria, changes in membrane permeability would be expected to have profound metabolic consequences. But there are also data suggesting that anesthetics may affect metabolism by altering the rate at which substrates cross cell membranes. These include data on the effects of anesthetics upon the rate of entry of monosaccharides into red cells. Red cells are a convenient model for such studies because they are living, readily available human cells. In addition, transport mechanisms for monosaccharides in human erythrocytes are not dependent upon insulin, a circumstance which permits experimental study of the effect of anesthetics upon sugar metabolism in a system devoid of the possibility that anesthetics may affect sugar metabolism by affecting insulin activity. The mechanism by which sugars cross human erythrocyte membranes is not one of simple physical diffusion. Neither is it an active transfer process in which metabolic energy is expended to move sugar molecules against a concentration gradient. Instead, transport is achieved by a process of altered or facilitated diffusion. By this is meant that monosaccharides which are normally excluded from cell membranes react with and form complexes with intramembranous carriers at the external surface of the cell membrane. The sugar-carrier complex so formed moves toward the inner part of the membrane by a process of thermal agitation (diffusion) with dissociation of the complex back into free carrier and free sugar at the inner surface of the membrane, the free sugar then diffusing into the cytoplasm. Since entry does not require the expenditure of metabolic energy, it is unaffected by changes in oxygen tension [GREENE, 1965 (1)] or by ouabain (GREENE and CERVENKO). The rate of entry of monosaccharides into human red cells is, however, significantly accelerated for unknown reasons by carbon dioxide (GREENE and CERVENKO). Inhalation anesthetics inhibit this transport mechanism in human red cells in a complex manner best explained by hypothesizing that the anesthetics act as competitive inhibitors of the intramembranous carriers [GREENE, 1965 (2)]. The inhibition by anesthetics cannot be due solely to a nonspecific stabilization of the membrane because of the fact that while high concentrations of anesthetics decrease the rate of entry of monosaccharides into red cells, lower concentrations accelerate entry [GREENE, 1965 (2)]. This unusual phenomenon can readily be explained on the basis that anesthetics act as competitive inhibitors of a carrier system in which countertransport mechanisms also exist, as they do in red cells [GREENE, 1965 (2)]. In the presence of countertransport systems, competitive inhibitors act to increase rate of transport when present in low concentrations but decrease rate of entry when present in high concentrations.

In vitro data suggesting that anesthetics affect membrane transport of monosaccharides receive confirmatory support from *in vivo* experiments. For example, while DRUCKER et al. (1959) found that ether anesthesia does not alter the normal response to intravenous fructose tolerance tests, intravenous glucose tolerance tests indicate decreased tissue utilization of glucose during ether anesthesia (HENNEMAN and BUNKER, 1961). Since glucose and fructose share the same glycolytic pathways after they are converted to fructose-6-phosphate (GREENE, 1963), it is likely that glycolysis is unaffected by ether but that instead transport of glucose or glucose-6-phosphate into cells is impaired. The fact that intravenous pyruvate tolerance tests are abnormal during ether anesthesia (DRUCKER et al., 1957) supports the possibility that while glycolysis is unaffected by ether anesthesia, oxidative phosphorylation is affected, perhaps by ether-induced alterations in mitochondrial membrane permeability. Whether ether affects glucose uptake in all tissues or only in some is unknown, but the latter is suggested by the observation of GALLA et al. (1962) that glucose utilization by canine myocardium is uninfluenced by ether anesthesia at a time when total body glucose uptake is depressed.

Data comparable to the above have also been reported with other anesthetics. Halothane does not affect the normal response to intravenous fructose tolerance tests (in dogs) but decreases the rate of uptake of glucose following intravenous glucose tolerance tests (GALLA and WILSON). Decreases in glucose utilization have also been observed in man during cyclopropane anesthesia (CERVENKO and GREENE).

II. Indirect Effects

Indirectly mediated metabolic effects of anesthetics fall into two categories: those resulting from physiologic alterations produced by anesthesia, such as changes in organ blood flow, changes in arterial gas tensions, or changes in neuro-endocrine function; and those resulting from iatrogenically introduced factors, such as operative trauma, blood loss, and drugs and fluids used during anesthesia and surgery.

Increased Sympathetic Activity. Certain inhalation anesthetics, notably cyclopropane and ether, are associated with increased activity of the sympathetic nervous system (PRICE et al., 1959; DEUTSCH et al., 1962). Stimulation of the sympathetic nervous system is also associated with altered metabolism (HAVEL). It has therefore been suggested that the metabolic effects of anesthetics are in part or in whole due to their effect on the sympathetic nervous system. The classic observation of BREWSTER et al. that total sympathetic block produced by injection of local anesthetic agent into the peridural space prevents much of the normal metabolic response of dogs to ether emphasizes the importance of such a relationship. However, the magnitude of sympathetic responses and the associated metabolic changes seen during ether and cyclopropane anesthesia vary with different species (BUNKER et al., 1951; PRICE et al., 1959; DEUTSCH et al., 1962), with age (BUNKER et al., 1952), and with the use of drugs for premedication or induction of anesthesia (BASS et al., 1953; STEPHEN et al., 1957; HUNTER, 1959). The metabolic changes in peripheral blood observed during clinical ether anesthesia in adult man are no greater than the changes found in the course of normal daily human activity (BEECHER et al.).

Although a reflex increase in sympathetic activity may contribute to the metabolic changes associated with certain anesthetics, *all* the metabolic changes of *all* inhalation anesthetics cannot be related to the ability of the anesthetic to produce an increased activity of the sympathetic nervous system. Anesthetics such as halothane and methoxyflurane do not produce reflex stimulation of the sympathetic nervous system, yet they may be associated with metabolic changes, including hyperglycemia, which, in the case of ether or cyclopropane, are attributed to changes in autonomic tone. When sympathetic nervous system stimulation does occur, it affects metabolism in 2 ways. First, tissue metabolism is directly affected. Stimulation of the splanchnic nerves innervating the liver, for example, results in increased hepatic glycogenolysis. Second, the direct effects of sympathetic stimulation on tissue metabolism are accentuated if the sympathetic stimulation is widespread enough to result in increased blood levels of catecholamines, particularly epinephrine. The catecholamines so released further increase hepatic glycogenolysis after being delivered to the liver by the vascular system. The role of circulating catecholamines in determining the metabolic response to sympathetic stimulation is illustrated by studies in which hematogenous delivery of epinephrine to the liver has been prevented by previous bilateral adrenalectomy. As early as 1933, for example, BANERJI and REID observed that bilateral adrenalectomy decreased but did not eliminate the hyperglycemia produced by ether anesthesia in rabbits, although subsequently JOHNSON reported that in such a preparation ether hyperglycemia was completely absent. Unfortunately, these early experiments do not take into account the metabolic effects which adrenalectomy might have due to elimination of ether-induced elevations of blood corticosteroid levels and they have not been subsequently repeated in de-medullated animals. It is therefore impossible to quantitate today the relative roles played by direct and indirect responses to sympathetic stimulation in explaining anesthetically induced hyperglycemia, but obviously both direct and indirect factors are important. They are important not only in explaining hyperglycemia but also in explaining the elevated blood levels of acids such as lactate and pyruvate which are seen during certain types of anesthesia. For example, total sympathetic blockade eliminates the increase in blood lactate and pyruvate observed during ether anesthesia in the dog (BREWSTER et al.). But total sympathetic blockade does two things: it denervates the liver, and it prevents the release of epinephrine from the adrenal medullae. The importance of the latter is demonstrated by the fact that the intravenous infusion of epinephrine in the absence of anesthesia produces changes in lactate and pyruvate [GREENE, 1961 (2)] analogous to those observed during ether anesthesia.

Hormonal Effects. Inhalation anesthetics are associated with elevation of plasma levels of adrenal cortical hormones (VIRTUE et al.; HAMMOND et al.; NISHIOKA et al.). These increases are not due to decreased rates of hormone utilization during anesthesia, but rather to increased production of hormones by the adrenal cortex secondary to elevated output of adrenocorticotropic hormone (ACTH) by the pituitary (OYAMA et al.). The increased output of ACTH is in part produced by the anesthetic agent itself, but it is accentuated by afferent impulses arising from the operative site (HAMMOND et al.). Metabolically the adrenal cortical hormones have profound effects. HENNEMAN and BUNKER in 1957 first called attention to the fact that the metabolic changes observed during anesthesia closely resemble those seen in a patient with Cushing's syndrome and emphasized that part of the changes in carbohydrate metabolism during anesthesia are due to this cause.

Metabolic responses associated with anesthesia and surgery may also be contributed to by alteration of circulating levels of thyroid hormone. GREENE and GOLDENBERG were unable to detect an effect of ether or spinal anesthesia on thyroid activity as determined by blood protein-bound iodine (PBI) levels, but a rise in blood PBI levels was observed associated with the start of operation.

The effects of anesthetics on insulin activity, while of basic importance in evaluating the metabolic response to anesthesia, have not been studied adequately enough to date to draw conclusions. GALLA and WILSON found that the response to insulin in dogs was unaffected by halothane anesthesia. On the other hand, HENNEMAN and VANDAM (1960) felt that insulin activity in man was inhibited by ether anesthesia, a conclusion which in turn has been questioned (GREENE, 1963).

Operation. As indicated above, metabolic responses to anesthesia and surgery include changes due to operative trauma which are in addition to those resulting from anesthesia alone. Metabolic responses to afferent stimuli arising from the site of surgery include changes in endocrine homeostasis but other metabolic effects of surgery have been but little studied. It is essential that they be borne in mind, however, for failure to dissociate the metabolic effects of anesthesia from the effects of anesthesia plus surgery has led in the past and continues to lead to erroneous concepts of the role anesthesia itself plays.

Hemorrhage during anesthesia and surgery is accompanied by metabolic changes which may significantly add to the metabolic changes induced by anesthesia itself. Metabolic effects of hemorrhage may be the result of decreased blood volume, the use of cold ACD blood transfusions, or both (BUNKER, 1966; SCHWEIZER et al.). The metabolic response to hemorrhage may also be modified by anesthesia, although how and why remains controversial. On the one hand, it has been reported by DRUCKER et al. (1965) that cyclopropane is associated with a greater accentuation of anaerobic metabolism during experimental hemorrhagic shock than is an anesthetic such as halothane which causes peripheral vasodilation. On the other hand, DOBKIN and his associates (1966) found that all the inhalation anesthetic agents (halothane, ether, trichlorethylene, methoxyflurane, fluroxene, and chloroform) except cyclopropane were associated with accentuation of the metabolic acidosis and anaerobiosis associated with graded hemorrhagic shock.

Pulmonary Changes. Metabolic responses to anesthesia are accentuated if accompanied by changes in pulmonary function great enough to affect arterial oxygen and carbon dioxide levels. The most pronounced metabolic changes are those due to hypoxia. In the unanesthetized state when hypoxia is associated with arterial oxygen tension levels of 30—40 mmHg in normal subjects or to 50—60 mmHg in patients with heart disease (GREENE, 1964) significant changes in blood lactate and pyruvate levels occur. Similar changes also occur if hypoxia occurs during general anesthesia and may be additive to the changes due to the anesthetic agent itself. While the majority of the metabolic changes occurring during hypoxia are due to decreased availability of molecular oxygen at the tissue level, hypoxia is also a potent stimulant of the sympathetic nervous system, and in the intact animal approximately one third of the metabolic effects of hypoxia are due to the reflex increase in activity of the sympathetic nervous system produced by the hypoxia itself (GREENE and PHILLIPS).

The metabolic effects of high oxygen tensions are of no significance during clinical anesthesia. The effects of changes in carbon dioxide tension are mediated principally through secondary alterations in organ blood flow.

Changes in Organ Blood Flow. Anesthesia may cause decreases in organ blood flow by decreasing cardiac output, by lowering arterial perfusing pressure, or by increasing vascular resistance consequent to anesthetically induced increases in sympathetic tone. Depending upon the magnitude of the changes in organ blood flow, as well as upon their etiology, tissue oxygen tensions may decrease to the point where metabolic evidence of hypoxia become evident (GREENE and WILLENKIN; WILLENKIN and GREENE).

Changes in hepatic blood flow are of particular interest during anesthesia because of the prominent metabolic role played by the liver, and thus while inhalation anesthetics have been recognized for some time as being associated with decreases in hepatic blood flow (HABIF et al.; LEVY et al.), in recent years the subject has been the object of renewed interest in an attempt to define the magnitude and significance of the observed changes. PRICE et al. (1965), for example, found in ten normal nonoperative subjects that during cyclopropane anesthesia splanchnic vascular resistance increased, as did arterial perfusing pressure. The latter, however, did not increase as much as the former, with the result that splanchnic blood flow diminished. All these alterations could be reversed by blockade of sympathetic ganglia, indicating that the changes were secondary to reflex increases in sympathetic vasoconstrictor tone produced by the anesthetic agent. EPSTEIN and his associates (1966) found that halothane anesthesia in nine normal nonoperative subjects was also accompanied by significant decreases in hepatic blood flow. Control hepatic blood values before anesthesia averaged 1,881 ml/min, while during anesthesia they averaged 1,321 ml/min. This decrease was not due to a decrease in splanchnic vascular resistance but instead was due to a fall in mean arterial pressure from 91.3—63.3 mmHg. These results during cyclopropane and halothane anesthesia differ somewhat from the findings of COOPERMAN et al. These investigators found that when arterial carbon dioxide tension remained normal during nitrous oxide-oxygen-muscle relaxant anesthesia splanchnic vascular resistance doubled and blood flow diminished correspondingly. However, when hyperventilation reduced arterial carbon dioxide tension to 18 mmHg, even though splanchnic vascular resistance remained high there was a slight increase in blood flow. During normocarbia oxygen consumption was unaffected by anesthesia. During respiratory alkalosis, however, a pronounced increase in oxygen demand occurred (59 ml/min when pCO_2 was normal, 88 ml/min when pCO_2 was 18 mmHg). The increase in oxygen consumption during respiratory alkalosis was considerably in excess of the modest increase in hepatic blood flow, and the question can be raised whether respiratory alkalosis during anesthesia is associated with development of splanchnic hypoxia or splanchnic oxygen debt.

Respiratory acidosis is accompanied by an increase in splanchnic vascular resistance, but hepatic blood flow shows no consistent change, either increasing, decreasing, or remaining unchanged depending upon changes in blood pressure (EPSTEIN et al., 1961).

PRICE and his associates in 1966 examined in considerable detail whether general anesthetics can produce splanchnic hypoxia and changes in splanchnic metabolism by reducing regional blood flow. They measured splanchnic oxygen consumption, splanchnic blood flow, splanchnic vascular resistance, and arterial and hepatic vein lactate and pyruvate levels in 35 normal subjects during halothane and cyclopropane anesthesia. They found significant decreases in splanchnic blood flow with each anesthetic, the decrease with cyclopropane being associated with an increase in vascular resistance while with halothane splanchnic resistance remained unaltered. At the time splanchnic blood flow was diminished during anesthesia there was no consistent change in splanchnic oxygen consumption with either anesthetic. The decreases in flow during anesthesia in the presence of unchanged oxygen consumption were associated with metabolic evidence of hypoxia during cyclopropane as evidenced by the appearance of excess lactate production, but despite the fact that blood flow was equally diminished during halothane anesthesia excess lactate was not present during halothane. However, restoration of blood flow to normal values during halothane and during cyclopropane anesthesia gave no evidence that an oxygen debt had been incurred during the periods of reduced flow. Furthermore, excess lactate production during cyclopropane anesthesia was eliminated by the administration of a beta-adrenergic blocking agent. The authors concluded that splanchnic blood flow produced by anesthesia was unassociated with tissue hypoxia, and that the excess lactate during cyclopropane anesthesia resulted from metabolic changes produced by an increase in sympathetic activity rather than from lack of adequate amounts of oxygen.

Changes in organ blood flow during anesthesia may also affect the cerebral circulation. They are most frequently the result of changes in arterial carbon dioxide tension and if severe enough have been described as being accompanied by changes in carbohydrate metabolism. ALEXANDER et al. found that when arterial carbon dioxide tension is decreased below 20 mmHg by hyperventilation during nitrous oxide anesthesia, there is a decrease in cerebral aerobic metabolism and an increase in anaerobic glucose utilization.

Renal blood flow is almost invariably decreased during inhalation anesthesia as a result of increased renal vascular resistance (HABIF et al.; APRAHAMIAN et al.; DEUTSCH et al., 1967). Metabolic responses to changes in renal blood flow include apparent elevations of renal excretory thresholds. The rate at which glucose is excreted in the urine during hyperglycemia, for example, is diminished by a decrease in renal blood flow, and the hyperglycemia of ether anesthesia may be accentuated by the changes in renal blood flow induced by the ether.

III. In Vivo Changes

In vivo changes during anesthesia are the result of both the direct as well as the indirect effects of anesthesia on metabolism. The *in vivo* changes have been particularly studied in relation to changes in oxygen consumption, to changes in blood glucose levels, and to changes in blood levels of fixed acids.

Oxygen Consumption. Oxygen consumption is always decreased by general anesthesia below levels observed during normal activity because the state of general anesthesia is a more basal state. Beyond that, however, it is not always clear what effect general anesthetics, particularly inhalation anesthetics, have on total body oxygen consumption. Part of the problem lies in accurate determination of oxygen consumption in the presence of an anesthetic agent which may not only interfere with methods for measurement of oxygen but which may also continue to be taken up by the body for long periods and so prevent establishment of the physiologic steady state required for oxygen consumption measurements (THEYE and MESSICK, 1968). Part of the problem also lies in differentiating between effects of the inhalation anesthetic itself and effects of other drugs which may be administered during anesthesia. It has only been in recent years that these methodologic and experimental problems have been successfully solved, at least in the case of halothane. Particularly noteworthy has been the work of THEYE and his associates. While others had previously demonstrated a decrease in oxygen consumption during clinical anesthesia in man (SEVERINGHAUS and CULLEN; NUNN and MATTHEWS; BERGMAN), it was THEYE and TUOHY who accurately quantitated the importance of premedication and thiopental in determining changes in oxygen consumption during halothane anesthesia. In 9 patients who received barbiturate and narcotic premedication and in whom anesthesia was induced with thiopental, oxygen consumption was 84% of predicted basal levels during halothane anesthesia. In 10 patients who received the same premedication but no thiopental, oxygen consumption during equal levels of halothane anesthesia was 88% of predicted. And in 10 patients in whom neither premedication nor thiopental induction were employed, oxygen consumption was 100% of predicted basal levels.

The means by which pulmonary ventilation is achieved during anesthesia also affects oxygen consumption. During spontaneous ventilation a portion of the oxygen consumption is due to the work of respiration, a source of oxygen consumption not present during controlled ventilation (NUNN and MATTHEWS). In seven subjects studied by THEYE and TUOHY during controlled respiration oxygen consumption was found to average 84% of predicted basal levels, while under identical anesthetic conditions but with spontaneous respirations oxygen consumption was 100% of predicted.

During anesthesia cardiac output and cardiac work also change and may produce changes in oxygen consumption. THEYE also studied this aspect of oxygen consumption during halothane in the most controlled and thorough investigation to date of the effect of any inhalation anesthetic upon total body oxygen consumption. THEYE minimized changes in cardiac output and blood pressure by employing spinal anesthesia and an extracorporeal pump to bypass the right side of the heart. He was thereby able to measure separately both total body oxygen consumption and myocardial oxygen consumption. He found that at a time when halothane anesthesia was associated with an 8% reduction in total body oxygen consumption, the decrease in oxygen consumption in tissues other than the heart averaged 7%. He further found that when changes in myocardial oxygen consumption occurred they were directly related to decreases in myocardial work produced by halothane. He concluded that while halothane had a slight depressant effect on noncardiac oxygen consumption, it had no direct effect on myocardial oxygen consumption, only an indirect effect mediated though changes in myocardial work. THEYE calculated on the basis of these and other data (THEYE and SESSLER) that when oxygen consumption in the dog is decreased 23 ml/m²/min by halothane anesthesia, 12 ml of the decrease is due to decreased myocardial work and 11 ml of the decrease is due to direct depression of oxygen consumption in the remainder of body tissues.

The anatomic sites in which extramyocardial decreases in oxygen consumption occur during halothane anesthesia have not been fully defined. There is a tendency for cerebral oxygen consumption to decrease (McDOWALL et al.; WOLLMAN et al.; COHEN et al., 1964), but the changes observed have not proven to be consistent enough or of great enough magnitude to be of statistical significance in man. Oxygen consumption in the liver has also been shown to be slightly but insignificantly decreased during halothane anesthesia in man (PRICE et al., 1966). It is most likely that halothane causes a decrease in oxygen consumption by interference with mitochondrial function in many tissues, as discussed above, but that these changes which are measurable *in vitro* exceed the accuracy of methods available for measurement of changes in oxygen consumption *in vivo*.

The effect of inhalation anesthetics other than halothane on total body oxygen consumption must be regarded as unproven in the absence of studies as controlled and as accurate as those employed by THEYE for halothane. It is not unlikely that inhalation anesthetics such as ether and cyclopropane which are associated with pronounced neuroendocrine responses may be associated with increases in oxygen consumption above basal levels (ALBERS et al.) even in the presence of controlled ventilation.

Blood Glucose levels are well recognized as being increased during ether anesthesia (GREENE, 1963). The usual explanation for this phenomenon is that ether causes an increase in sympathetic activity which in turn causes an increase in hepatic glycogenolysis. Liver glycogen levels have been reported decreased at a time when blood levels of glucose are increased during ether anesthesia in man (ANNAMUNTHODO et al.), but it is unlikely that this is the sole etiology of ether hyperglycemia, or even its most major cause. If it were the most important factor, equal or more pronounced hyperglycemia would be expected during anesthesia with an agent such as cyclopropane since it is associated with a more consistent and more pronounced stimulation of the sympathetic nervous system in man than ether is. Cyclopropane anesthesia, however, is accompanied by slight or even no elevation of blood glucose (CERVENKO and GREENE). Similarly, an anesthetic such as halothane which does not cause an increase in sympathetic activity would not be expected to be associated with increased blood levels of glucose, yet modest elevations of blood sugar have been reported (BURNAP et al.; COHEN et al., 1964; KEATING et al.; SCHWEIZER et al.; VIRTUE et al.). Indeed, the decrease in hepatic glycogen levels during halothane anesthesia in man (KEATING et al.) is comparable to that observed during ether anesthesia. The hyperglycemia of ether is best explained as the result of a balance between an increased rate of input of glucose into the blood stream and a decreased rate of removal of glucose from blood. Factors involved include proven or possible decreases in membrane transport of glucose, decreased glucose utilization, impaired insulin activity, stimulation of the sympathetic nervous system, decreased renal excretion, and increased circulating levels of adrenal cortical hormones.

The same complexities which determine blood glucose levels during ether anesthesia also occur in varying degrees with other inhalation anesthetics. They have been best studied during cyclopropane and during halothane. During cyclopropane anesthesia there is a decrease in tissue utilization of glucose (CERVENKO and GREENE). The decrease in glucose uptake occurs at a time when blood levels of glucose are unchanged or declining, thereby suggesting that there is a simultaneous decrease in glucose production during cyclopropane anesthesia. The most likely place for this to occur is within the liver, and PRICE et al. (1966) have shown in the two subjects in whom hepatic glucose production was measured that such does occur. In one subject hepatic glucose production decreased from control levels of 300 mg/min before anesthesia to 165 mg/min during cyclopropane anesthesia, and in the other a decrease from 120—0 mg/min occurred. The explanation for these findings at a time when an increase in lactate and pyruvate production occurred, which the authors (PRICE et al., 1966) ascribed to increased sympathetic activity rather than to anaerobic carbohydrate metabolism, remains unclear. Similarly, halothane is associated with simultaneous changes in both glucose production as well as glucose utilization (GALLA, 1967; GALLA and WILSON, 1964).

Fixed Acids which are of greatest interest in anesthesia are lactic acid and pyruvic acid. The relationship between the two

$$\text{Lactate} + \text{NAD}^+ \rightleftharpoons \text{Pyruvate} + \text{NADH}$$

consists of a reversible reaction catalyzed by lactate dehydrogenase which is also dependent upon tissue concentrations of oxidized and reduced NAD. While pyruvate enters into a series of reactions including conversion to glucose or lactate, as well as entry into fat, protein or tricarboxylic acid cycle metabolism, lactate represents a metabolic "dead end". It undergoes no reactions without being first metabolized to pyruvate. Pyruvic acid levels may increase for a variety of reasons, including increased glycolysis, with a resulting increase in lactate. Lactate levels may also increase without parallel increases in pyruvate, most frequently because of an imbalance between concentrations of NAD and NADH. The ratio between NAD and NADH is in part a function of availability of normal amounts of molecular oxygen. The lactate:pyruvate ratio and "excess" lactate, or the amount of lactate present beyond that due to concurrent increases in pyruvate, have been employed as metabolic indices of the adequacy of tissue oxygenation. The ratio between NAD and NADH is also, however, dependent upon mitochondrial metabolic shuttle systems which maintain normal extramitochondrial concentrations of NAD and NADH. Alterations in lactate:pyruvate ratios and "excess" lactate levels have been ascribed to changes in mitochondrial membrane permeability (SCHWEIZER et al.; FINK and KENNY).

Certain inhalation anesthetics are associated with increased lactate:pyruvate ratios in blood and with the appearance of "excess" lactate. This is particularly frequent with ether (GREENE, 1961; SCHWEITZER et al.). It also occurs, though less consistently, with cyclopropane anesthesia (GREENE, 1961; PRICE et al., 1966). Although increased lactate:pyruvate ratios during cyclopropane may be related to the presence or absence of respiratory acidosis, during halothane anesthesia arterial carbon dioxide tensions do not affect blood levels of these metabolites (COHEN et al., 1964), and whether or not "excess" lactate occurs during halothane anesthesia appears to depend upon other factors, including operative trauma (LOWENSTEIN et al.; GREIFENSTEIN; PRICE et al., 1966). What is not fully defined is the etiology and significance of increased lactate:pyruvate ratios and "excess" lactate when they occur during uneventful and uncomplicated inhalation anesthesia. Certainly they could reflect tissue hypoxia even in the presence of normal arterial oxygenation, and anesthetics such as ether and cyclopropane have been shown to be associated in man with decreased tissue oxygen tension in at least one organ, skin (GREENE et al., 1959), but whether decreases in organ blood flow occur during anethesia in metabolically more active organs to the extent that anaerobic carbohydrate metabolism occurs has been a matter of debate. The most definitive study of this problem is that by PRICE and his associates (1966). As discussed above, these investigators compared the effects of an anesthetic, cyclopropane, which is known to increase sympathetic activity, with the effects of an agent, halothane, which decreases peripheral vascular resistance in order to determine whether anesthetics can produce splanchnic visceral hypoxia by reducing regional blood flow. Estimated hepatic blood flow was decreased by approximately the same percentage by both anesthetics, the decrease in hepatic blood flow with halothane being the result of decreased arterial perfusing pressure, while the decrease in hepatic flow with cyclopropane was due to hepatic vasoconstriction. During the period of decreased hepatic blood flow, "excess" lactate was produced during cyclopropane but not during halothane anesthesia. This suggested that it was not the decrease in blood flow but rather the increased sympathetic activity associated with cyclopropane which caused the "excess" lactate during cyclopropane anesthesia. This was further suggested by the observation that restoration of blood flow to control levels during cyclopropane as well as during halothane anesthesia gave no evidence that an oxygen debt had developed during the period of decreased flow. Ganglionic and alpha-adrenergic blocking agents administered during cyclopropane anesthesia did not affect "excess" lactate production even though they did restore blood flow to normal. This indicated further that the "excess" lactate was due to an effect of the cyclopropane other than the ability of cyclopropane to alter blood flow, a possibility confirmed by the fact that a beta-adrenergic blocking agent abolished the production of "excess" lactate. The authors concluded that neither anesthetic causes anaerobic metabolism by producing splanchnic ischemia but that cyclopropane produces "excess" lactate by a mechanism which is reversible by beta-adrenergic blockade. Their data also led PRICE and his co-workers to the conclusion that the increase in "excess" lactate was related more to a cyclopropane-induced increase in pyruvate consumption than to an increase in lactate production. There is, however, a puzzling aspect of these studies, namely, that if beta-adrenergic stimulation associated with cyclopropane were the entire explanation of the findings, then not only would lactate and pyruvate levels change in the manner observed but also glycogenolysis and glucose production should increase. In the two subjects in whom it was measured, hepatic glucose production decreased rather than increased during cyclopropane anesthesia.

Final interpretation of the significance of blood lactate and pyruvate levels during anesthesia is not yet possible. Blood levels of these substances may represent two phenomena which vary in relative importance with the anesthetic agent employed and with the circumstances under which anesthesia is administered. In some situations, abnormalities of lactate and pyruvate levels may reflect impairment of mitochondrial membrane shuttle systems produced by the anesthetic itself. In other situations, altered lactate and pyruvate levels may indicate that the rate of consumption of oxygen by mitochondria exceeds the rate at which oxygen is delivered to mitochondria to the extent that mitochondrial or perimitochondrial hypoxia develops. In either case, increased lactate:pyruvate ratios or "excess" lactate represent abnormal cellular metabolism.

Summary

The most important development in studies of the metabolic effects of anesthetics has been the recent demonstration that anesthetics may alter the rate of transport of metabolites across biologic membranes. The membranes affected include cell membranes as well as mitochondrial membranes. Inhalation anesthetics generally have little effect on glycolysis but may significantly alter oxidative phosphorylation and mitochondrial oxygen consumption. The direct effects of anesthetics on cell metabolism may be overshadowed *in vitro* by secondary effects anesthetics exert on endocrine balance, organ blood flow, and changes in oxygen and carbon dioxide tensions.

References

Albers, C., Brendel, W., Usinger, W.: Kreislauf respiratorischer Stoffwechsel und Atmung in Äthernarkose. Arch. exp. Pathol. Pharmakol., Naunyn-Schmiedeberg's **226**, 278 (1955).

Alexander, S. C., Cohen, P. J., Wollman, H., Smith, T. C., Reivich, M., Molen, R. A. U.: Cerebral carbohydrate metabolism during hypocarbia in man. Studies during nitrous oxide anesthesia. Anesthesiology **26**, 624 (1965).

Andersen, N. B.: Effect of general anesthetics on sodium transport in the isolated toad bladder. Anesthesiology **27**, 304 (1966).

— Synergistic effect of cyclopropane and epinephrine on sodium transport in toad bladder. Anesthesiology **28**, 438 (1967).

Annamunthodo, H., Keating, V., Patrick, S. J.: Liver glycogen alteration in anaesthesia and surgery. Anaesthesia **13**, 429 (1958).

Aprahamian, H. A., Vanderveen, J. L., Bunker, J. P., Murphy, A. J., Crawford, J. D.: The influence of general anesthetics on water and solute excretion in man. Ann. Surg. **150**, 122 (1959).

Banerji, H., Reid, C.: The adrenals and anesthetic hyperglycemia. J. Physiol. (London) **78**, 370 (1933).

Bass, W. P., Watts, D. T., Chase, H. F.: Ether hyperglycemia as influenced by premedication and Pentothal induction. Anesthesiology **14**, 18 (1953).

Beecher, H. K., Francis, L., Anfinsen, C. B.: Metabolic effects of anesthesia in man. I. Acid-base balance during ether anesthesia. J. Pharmacol. exptl Therap. **98**, 38 (1950).

Bergman, N. A.: Components of the alveolar-arterial oxygen tension difference in anesthetized man. Anesthesiology **28**, 517 (1967).

Brewster, W. R., Jr., Bunker, J. P., Beecher, H. K.: Metabolic effects of anesthesia: mechanism of metabolic acidosis and hyperglycemia during ether anesthesia in the dog. Amer. J. Physiol. **171**, 37 (1952).

Bunker, J. P.: Metabolic effects of blood transfusion. Anesthesiology **27**, 446 (1966).

— Beecher, H. K., Briggs, B. D., Brewster, W. R., Jr., Barnes, B. A.: Metabolic effects of anesthesia. II. A comparison of the acid-base equilibrium in man and dogs during ether and cyclopropane anesthesia. J. Pharmacol. Exptl Therap. **102**, 62 (1951).

— Brewster, W. R., Jr., Smith, R. M., Beecher, H. K.: Metabolic effects of anesthesia in man: acid-base balance in infants and children during anesthesia. J. Appl. Physiol. **5**, 233 (1952).

Burnap, T. K., Galla, S. J., Vandam, L. D.: Anesthetic, circulatory and respiratory effects of Fluothane. Anesthesiology **19**, 307 (1958).

Cervenko, F. W., Greene, N. M.: Effect of cyclopropane anesthesia on glucose assimilation coefficient in man. Anesthesiology **28**, 914 (1967).

Christian, G., Greene, N. M.: Blood carbonic anhydrase activity in anesthetized man. Anesthesiology **23**, 179 (1962).

Cohen, P. J., Marshall, B. E.: Effects of halothane on respiratory control and oxygen consumption of rat liver mitochondria. In: Toxicity of anesthetics (Fink, B. R., Ed.). Baltimore: The Williams & Wilkins Co. 1968.

— Wollman, H., Alexander, S. C., Chase, P. E., Behar, M. G.: Cerebral carbohydrate metabolism in man during halothane anesthesia: Effects of $PaCO_2$ on some aspects of carbohydrate utilization. Anesthesiology **25**, 185 (1964).

Cooperman, L. H., Warden, J. C., Price, H. L.: Splanchnic circulation during nitrous oxide anesthesia and hypocarbia in normal man. Anesthesiology **29**, 254 (1968).

Deutsch, S., Linde, H. W., Price, H. L.: Circulatory and sympathoadrenal responses to cyclopropane in the dog. J. Pharmacol. Exptl Therap. **135**, 354 (1962).

DEUTSCH, S., PIERCE, E. C., JR., VANDAM, L. D.: Cyclopropane effects on renal function in normal man. Anesthesiology **28**, 547 (1967).
DOBKIN, A. B.: Effect of Fluothane on acid-base balance. Anesthesiology **20**, 10 (1959).
— BYLES, P. H., NEVILLE, J. F., JR.: Neuroendocrine and metabolic effects of general anaesthesia and graded haemorrhage. Canad. Anaesth. Soc. J. **13**, 453 (1966).
— FEDORUK, S.: A comparison of the cardiovascular, respiratory and metabolic effects of methoxyflurane and halothane in dogs. Anesthesiology **22**, 355 (1961).
— HARLAND, J. H., FEDORUK, S.: Trichlorethylene and halothane in a precision system: Comparison of cardiorespiratory and metabolic effects in dogs. Anesthesiology **23**, 58 (1962).
DRUCKER, W. R., COSTLEY, C., STULTS, R., HOLDEN, W. D., CRAIG, J., MILLER, M., HOFFMAN, N., WOODWARD, H.: Studies of carbohydrate metabolism during ether anesthesia: effect of ether on glucose and fructose metabolism. Metabolism **8**, 828 (1959).
— — — MILLER, M., CRAIG, J. W., WOODWARD, H.: The effect of ether anesthesia on pyruvate metabolism. Surg. Forum **7**, 185 (1957).
— DAVIS, H. S., BURGET, D., POWERS, A. L., SIEVERDING, E.: Effect of halothane and cyclopropane anesthesia on energy metabolism in hypovolemic animals. J. Trauma **5**, 503 (1965).
EPSTEIN, R. M., DEUTSCH, S., COOPERMAN, L. H., CLEMENT, A. J., PRICE, H. L.: Splanchnic circulation during halothane anesthesia and hypercapnia in man. Anesthesiology **27**, 654 (1966).
— WHEELER, H. D., FRUMIN, M. J., HABIF, D. V., PAPPER, E. M., BRADLEY, S. E.: The effect of hypercapnia on estimated hepatic sulfobromophthalein clearance during general anesthesia in man. J. Clin. Invest. **40**, 592 (1961).
FINK, B. R., KENNY, G. E.: Metabolic effects of volatile anesthetics in cell culture. Anesthesiology **29**, 505 (1968).
GALLA, S. J.: Glucose pool size, turnover rate and $C^{14}O_2$ production during halothane anesthesia in dogs. Anesthesiology **28**, 251 (1967).
— HENNEMAN, D. H., SCHWEIZER, H. J., VANDAM, L. D.: Effects of ether anesthesia on myocardial metabolism in dogs. Am. J. Physiol. **202**, 241 (1962).
— WILSON, E. P.: Hexose metabolism during halothane anesthesia in dogs. Anesthesiology **25**, 96 (1964).
GOTTLIEB, S. F., SAVRAN, S. U.: Nitrous oxide inhibition of sodium transport. Anesthesiology **28**, 324 (1967).
GREENE, N. M.: (1) Lactate, pyruvate, and excess lactate production in anesthetized man. Anesthesiology **22**, 404 (1961).
— (2) Effect of epinephrine on lactate, pyruvate, and excess lactate production in normal human subjects. J. Lab. Clin. Med. **58**, 682 (1961).
— Inhalation anesthetics and carbohydrate metabolism. Baltimore: Williams and Wilkins Co. 1963.
— (1) Glucose permeability of human erythrocytes and the effects of inhalation anesthetics, oxygen, and carbon dioxide. Yale J. Biol. and Med. **37**, 319 (1965).
— (2) Inhalation anesthetics and permeability of human erythrocytes to monosaccharides. Anesthesiology **26**, 731 (1965).
— CERVENKO, F. W.: Inhalation anesthetics, carbon dioxide, and glucose transport across red cell membranes. Acta Anaesth. Scand. Suppl. **28**, (1967).
— DAVIS, M. T., BELL, J. K. S.: Effects of general anesthetics on tissue oxygen tension in man: skin. Anesthesiology **20**, 830 (1959).
— GOLDENBERG, I. S.: The effect of anesthesia on thyroid activity in humans. Anesthesiology **20**, 125 (1959).
— PHILLIPS, A. D'E.: Metabolic response of dogs to hypoxia in the absence of circulating epinephrine and norepinephrine. Am. J. Physiol. **189**, 475 (1957).
— SPENCER, E. L., JR.: Diethyl ether and lactate dehydrogenase activity in vitro. Anesthesiology **24**, 23 (1963).
— TALNER, N. S.: Blood lactate, pyruvate and lactate-pyruvate ratios in congenital heart disease. New Engl. J. Med. **270**, 1331 (1964).
— WILLENKIN, R. L.: Skeletal muscle oxygen tension and metabolism during hemorrhagic hypotension and subsequent vasopressor administration. Yale J. Biol. and Med. **35**, 429 (1963).
GREIFENSTEIN, F. E.: Excess lactate during halothane-oxygen and halothane-nitrous oxide-oxygen anesthesia. Anesthesia & Analgesia **45**, 362 (1966).
HABIF, D. V., PAPPER, E. M., FITZPATRICK, H. F., LOWRANCE, P., SMYTHE, C. McC., BRADLEY, S. E.: The renal and hepatic blood flow, glomerular filtration rate, and urinary output of electrolytes during cyclopropane, ether, and thiopental anesthesia, operation, and the immediate postoperative period. Surgery **30**, 241 (1951).

Hammond, W. G., Vandam, L. D., Davis, J. M., Carter, R. D., Ball, M. R., Moore, F. D.:
Studies in surgical endocrinology: IV. Anesthetic agents as stimuli to change in corticosteroids and metabolism. Ann. Surg. 148, 199 (1958).

Havel, R. J.: The autonomic nervous system and intermediary carbohydrate and fat metabolism. Anesthesiology 29, 702 (1968).

Haworth, J., Duff, A.: A note on trichlorethylene anaesthesia. Brit. Med. J. 1943 I, 381.

Henneman, D. H., Bunker, J. P.: Pattern of intermediary carbohydrate metabolism in
Cushing's syndrome. Am. J. Med. 23, 34 (1957).

— — Effects of general anesthesia on peripheral blood levels of carbohydrate and fat metabolites and serum inorganic phosphorus. J. Pharmacol. Exptl Therap. 133, 253 (1961).

— Vandam, L. D.: Effect of epinephrine, insulin, and tolbutamide on carbohydrate metabolism during ether anesthesia. Clin. Pharmacol. Ther. 1, 694 (1960).

Hewer, C. L., Hadfield, C. F.: Trichlorethylene as an inhalation anaesthetic. Brit. Med. J.
1941 I. 924.

Hoech, G. P., Jr., Matteo, R. S., Fink, B. R.: Effect of halothane on oxygen consumption
of rat brain, liver and heart and anaerobic glycolysis of rat brain. Anesthesiology 27, 770
(1966).

Hunter, A. R.: Halothane and blood sugar. Brit. J. Anaesthesia 31, 490 (1959).

Johnson, S. R.: Mechanisms of hyperglycamia during anesthesia: Experimental study.
Anesthesiology 10, 379 (1949).

Keating, V., Patrick, S. J., Annamunthodo, H.: Halothane and carbohydrate metabolism.
Anaesthesia 14, 268 (1959).

Levy, M. L., Palazzi, H. M., Nardi, G. L., Bunker, J. P.: Hepatic blood flow variations
during surgical anesthesia in man measured by radioactive colloid. Surg. Gynecol. Obstet.
112, 289 (1961).

Lowenstein, E., Clark, J. D., Villareal, Y.: Excess lactate production during halothane
anesthesia in man. J. Am. Med. Assoc. 190, 1110 (1964).

McDowall, D. G., Harper, A. M., Jacobson, I.: Cerebral blood flow during halothane
anaesthesia. Brit. J. Anaesthesia 35, 394 (1963).

Nishioka, K., Levy, A. A., Dobkin, A. B.: Effect of halothane and methoxyflurane anaesthesia on plasma cortisol concentration in relation to major surgery. Canad. Anaesth. Soc. J.
15, 441 (1968).

Nowill, W. K., Stephen, C. R., Searles, P. W.: Evaluation of trichloroethylene as an
anesthetic and analgesic agent. Arch. Surg. 66, 35 (1953).

Nunn, J. F., Matthews, R. L.: Gaseous exchange during halothane anaesthesia: The steady
respiratory state. Brit. J. Anaesthesia 31, 330 (1959).

Oyama, T., Saito, T., Isomatsu, T., Samejima, N., Uemura, T., Arimura, A.: Plasma levels
of ACTH and cortisol in man during diethyl ether anesthesia and surgery. Anesthesiology
29, 559 (1968).

Price, H. L., Deutsch, S., Cooperman, L. H., Clement, A. J., Epstein, R. M.: Splanchnic
circulation during cyclopropane anesthesia in normal man. Anesthesiology 26, 312 (1965).

— — Davidson, I. A., Clement, A. J., Behar, M. G., Epstein, R. M.: Can general anesthetics produce splnachnic visceral hypoxia by reducing regional blood flow? Anesthesiology 27, 24 (1966).

— Linde, H. W., Jones, R. E., Black, G. W., Price, M. L.: Sympathoadrenal responses to
general anesthesia in man and their relation to hemodynamics. Anesthesiology 20, 563
(1959).

Schweizer, O., Howland, W. S., Sullivan, C., Vertes, E.: The effect of ether and halothane
on blood levels of glucose, pyruvate, lactate and metabolites of the tricarboxylic acid cycle
in normotensive patients during operation. Anesthesiology 28, 814 (1967).

Severinghaus, J. W., Cullen, S. C.: Depression of myocardium and body oxygen consumption with Fluothane. Anesthesiology 19, 165 (1958).

Snodgrass, P. J., Piras, M. M.: Effects of halothane on rat liver mitochondria. Biochemistry
5, 1140 (1966).

Stephen, C. R., Grosskreutz, D. C., Lawrence, J. H., Fabian, L. W., Bourgeois-Gavardin, M., Coughlin, J.: Evaluation of Fluothane for clinical anaesthesia. Canad. Anaesth.
Soc. J. 4, 246 (1957).

Theye, R. A.: Myocardial and total oxygen consumption with halothane. Anesthesiology 28,
1042 (1967).

— Messick, J. M., Jr.: Measurement of oxygen consumption by spirometry during halothane anesthesia. Anesthesiology 29, 361 (1968).

— Sessler, A. D.: Effect of halothane anesthesia on rate of canine oxygen consumption.
Anesthesiology 28, 661 (1967).

— Tuohy, G. F.: Oxygen uptake during light halothane anesthesia in man. Anesthesiology
25, 627 (1964).

UEDA, I.: Effects of diethyl ether and halothane on firefly luciferin bioluminescence. Anesthesiology 26, 603 (1965).
— MIETANI, W.: Microsomal ATPase of rabbit brain and effects of general anesthetics. Biochem. Pharmacol. 16, 1370 (1967).
VIRTUE, R. W., HELMREICH, M. L., GAINZA, E.: The adrenal cortical response to surgery. I. The effect of anesthesia on plasma 17-hydroxycorticosteroid levels. Surgery 41, 549 (1957).
— PAYNE, K. W., CARANNA, L. J., GORDON, G. S., REMBER, R. R.: Observations during experimental and clinical use of Fluothane. Anesthesiology 19, 478 (1958).
WILLENKIN, R. L., GREENE, N. M.: Skeletal muscle oxygen tension and metabolism during induced hypotension and during vasopressor administration. Anesthesiology 24, 168 (1963).
WOLLMAN, H., ALEXANDER, S. C., COHEN, P. J., CHASE, P. E., MELMAN, E., BEHAR, M. G.: Cerebral circulation of man during halothane anesthesia: Effects of hypocarbia and of d-tubocurarine. Anesthesiology 25, 180 (1964).

4.8. Endocrine System

Leroy D. Vandam

In keeping with developments in other fields of medicine, current knowledge of the endocrine system has completely altered the original concept of several unrelated ductless glands each secreting a hormone in turn acting on its own target tissue. The body in its wisdom, to paraphrase W. B. Cannon, has evolved a neuro-endocrine arrangement whereby, with few exceptions, hormonal secretion is regulated by the central nervous system, with a system of checks and balances and a degree of interaction among the hormones hitherto unsuspected. In conformity with integrative action, it is probable that each hormone exerts its effect at the cellular level through a final common pathway, cyclic AMP (adenosine 3', 5' monophosphate), Butcher (1968). New humoral substances are found from time to time, secreted by organs not in the ductless category such as lung, kidney, liver, even neoplasms. Elaborate combinations of hormones act in consort to regulate such physiological functions as maintenance of the blood volume or the renal compensation for alterations in body water and electrolytes. Furthermore, we are just beginning to recognize the variety of humoral substances that act as transmitters in the central nervous system, for not only does the CNS regulate endocrine activity but CNS actions are in turn influenced by hormones. Endocrinology is a rapidly changing field.

Upon this background of new information, investigation of the action of anesthetics on the endocrines has been scant, for the most part superficial and largely a product of the last 10 years. There are good reasons for this. As a rule anesthetics are not given therapeutically, but mainly to facilitate surgical procedures which occupy a small span in the course of an illness. Illness *per se* brings endocrine changes. In contrast to the effects of anesthetics on circulation and respiration which have received considerable attention because of the immediate relation to survival, the endocrine response is hardly evident except in the autonomic nervous system. In addition, practically all of the endocrine response to anesthesia is mimicked in greater degree by the surgical procedure and continues long into the postoperative period. Thus, it is hardly possible to separate the effects of anesthesia and operation, or to discern the specific effect of an inhalation anesthetic when given after premedication and administered with controlled respiration and various types of supportive therapy.

Most studies on anesthetics and endocrines naturally relate to those systems that are adaptive to a changing environment and responsive to stress for the purpose of maintaining a steady state. These are: the hypothalamic-hypophyseal-adrenal cortical axis, the sympathetic and parasympathetic divisions of the autonomic nervous system and to a lesser extent the thyroid. Information concerning the autonomic nervous response to anesthetics will appear in another chapter of this volume and additional facts on the endocrines in the *Clinical Monographs*, in the section on Central Nervous System as well as in the discussions of the Cardiovascular System, Liver, Kidney and Metabolic Effects. This dispersal of information cannot fail to demonstrate the broad relationships that exist among the endocrines. In consequence this chapter attempts a critical appraisal of the information specifically pertaining to the action of inhalation anesthetics on the endocrines. To place the studies in proper context each section will be introduced with a resumé of existing knowledge concerning the physiology of the endocrine system discussed. Most studies have failed to take into account the effects of anesthetic technique and most of the work has been done on the older inhalation anesthetics, diethyl ether and cyclopropane. As background in interpreting these reports it should be realized that there are species differences in the chemistry of the active hormones as well as their patterns of activity.

The primary purpose of a discussion on anesthetics and endocrines is the meaning of the endocrine response for the patient and therefore his survival in terms of the entire operative experience. Second, one must bear in mind how endocrine activity might affect the course of anesthesia. Lastly, the endocrinologist should be enabled to interpret the results of experimental studies when anesthetics have been employed.

Pharmacologically Active Brain Substances. Although the effects of anesthetics on centrally acting neurotransmitters has been accorded little attention, such studies would seem to be of prime importance in relation to mechanisms of anesthesia and narcosis *per se.* Perhaps of equal importance, therefore, to the regulation by the central nervous system of peripheral endocrine activity is the process by which central regulation is carried out. A number of substances have been indicted as central neurotransmitters; the evidence for the action of some undisputed — in other cases circumstantial. Prominently mentioned are acetylcholine and norepinephrine (the principle peripheral transmitters) as well as epinephrine, dopamine, serotonin (5-hydroxytryptamine), histamine, glutamic acid, γ-amino butyric acid and substance P, WAY and SUTHERLAND (1963). All have been found in brain, the reputed action excitatory or inhibitory, specific sites of action suggested and their concentrations fluctuating with varying states of neural activity. Investigation of their action has been carried out by means of micro-injection and iontophoresis, histochemistry, recording of electrical activity and determination of brain content which is an index of secretion, turnover rate and metabolism of the compound in question. The presence of choline acetylase as well as acetylcholinesterase and the demonstration of vesicles containing acetylcholine (ACh) at synaptic junctions suggests that the central neurones may be classified as cholinergic or non-cholinergic as they are in the periphery. It has been known for some time that during sleep or conditions of diminished activity, such as anesthesia, the ACh content of brain increases irrespective of the anesthetic agent — and decreases during the hyperactivity accompanying anoxia or the action of analeptic drugs.

SCHMIDT (1966) conducted a well controlled study of the effect of halothane anesthesia on regional ACh levels in rat brain, seeking a correlation between ACh content and EEG activity during light and deeper levels of anesthesia. Using guinea pig ileum for bioassay, the ACh content of brain increased with greater depth of anesthesia. Cortex showed the largest increase, upper brain stem a significant increase only in deep anesthesia (catecholamines and serotonin are believed to be the transmitters here), middle brain stem a marked increase during light anesthesia, but no further change, corresponding perhaps to depression of the reticular activating system. The latter is depressed early during the loss of consciousness associated with all general anesthetics. Finally, concentrations of ACh in lower brain stem were unchanged, a finding corresponding to the clinical signs of anesthesia wherein the viscero-motor centers, particularly respiration and circulation, seem to be spared until the 4th plane of anesthesia is reached. However, only halothane was studied here, in one species, the rat, and it is possible that other anesthetics, particularly the non-inhalational substances, could yield different results.

Since serotonin is also believed to be a central transmitter, Diaz et al. (1968), studied the effects of cyclopropane, halothane and diethyl ether on the cerebral metabolism of serotonin in the rat. Prior work had shown a twofold increase in serotonin content of brain, interpreted as evidence of CNS depression during barbiturate, ether and chloralose anesthesia as well as with other depressants such as chloral hydrate, meperidine and ethyl alcohol. But other workers had found no change. Diaz et al. using fluorometric analysis studied turnover rates during steady state kinetics. Cyclopropane resulted in a slight but significant increase, halothane a progressive decrease and diethyl ether no change in serotonin concentrations. All three anesthetics increased 5-hydroxyindoleacetic acid levels (5-HIAA), ether showing the most marked effect and the only anesthetic seeming to increase turnover rate. A rise in 5-HIAA can be interpreted as increased turnover rate, decreased rate of removal, or a combination of both. Halothane and cyclopropane blocked efflux while ether not only increased turnover but accelerated synthesis, rate of oxidation and decreased removal rate. There was no clue as to the site of action of the anesthetics.

Since anesthetics had been shown to affect serotonin metabolism in brain, Thompson and Campbell (1967) studied the effects of anesthetics upon serotonin concentrations in the jejunal mucosa of the rat. In prior studies on serotonin metabolism in the gut a possible influence of anesthetics had not been taken into account. Supramaximal anesthetic doses of ether, urethan, chloralose and sodium pentobarbital were given by various routes without regard to measurement of physiological variables such as depth of anesthesia, changes in circulation, respiration or body temperature. After exsanguination of the rat, jejunal segments were assayed for serotonin content by spectrofluorometric analysis. Elevated serotonin levels were found after the administration of all the anesthetics but only the changes after ether and urethan were significant. No information was provided on the meaning of these alterations.

In connection with endocrines and centrally acting brain substances it is of interest that Selye (1941) first showed that pharmacological doses of progesterone, desoxycorticosterone acetate and pregnanedione could induce anesthesia in the rat. The rats lost righting reflexes and abdominal operations could be performed without inducing motor activity. In 1955 hydroxydione, a pregnanediol derivative and otherwise endocrinologically inactive, was introduced as a possible useful anesthetic. This compound failed to induce effective anesthesia, but a state of somnolence and a reduction in reflex activity brought forth promise of more useful steroid derivatives to come. Thus, studies have continued on the effect of certain of the naturally occurring steroids, Heuser (1967), although shown to be not nearly as effective as the compounds noted above. Some steroids tested offer some of the attributes of anesthesia while others are convulsants. Heuser showed that steroids in low subconvulsive doses produced intermittent behavioral sedation accompanied by electrical slow wave EEG activity.

In another study Kuntzman et al. (1965) found that certain drugs and insecticides of the anticholinesterase variety adversely influenced the anesthetic action of steroids. Chronic administration of phenobarbital, chlorcyclizine, phenylbutazone, chlordane and DDT markedly decreased the central depressant effects of desoxycorticosterone and progesterone. Whether this was the result of enhanced metabolism of the steroids or a decrease in brain uptake could not be established.

In concluding this section it is perhaps worth noting that if better anesthetics are to be developed, departing from the hydrocarbon structure of the inhalation agents now in use with their many adverse properties, a suitable compound might very well be found as a congener of one of the natural occurring central inhibitors, or a competitive blocker of one of the transmitter substances.

The Hypothalamic-Hypophyseal-Adrenal-Cortical Axis. To understand the many means whereby adrenal cortical activity has been studied during anesthesia and otherwise, it is essential to outline the intricate chain of hormonal events giving rise to cortical activity. The neurohypophysis is a functional extension of the hypothalamus and the adenohypophysis is anatomically in continuity with the hypothalamus via a portal system of veins. Neurosecretory cells in the several nuclei of the hypothalamus secrete at least two known octapeptides, one, oxytocin, concerned with lactation and the other, vasopressin, with antidiuretic and vasoconstrictive properties. Each compound coupled with a carrier protein is transported via axones to the neurohypophysis. Somewhat differently, a polypeptide secreted by the hypothalamus, called adrenocorticotrophic releasing substance (CRF), circulates via the portal venous system to the adenophypophysis causing the release of adrenocorticotrophic hormone (ACTH). Similarly the gonadotrophins, thyroid stimulating hormone (TSH) and somatotrophin or growth hormone (STH, GH) are caused to be released by transmitter substances still unidentified. Norepinephrine, histamine and vasopressin are among the suspects.

Upon release, ACTH a large straight chain polypeptide, is transported via the circulation to act principally upon the *zona fasciculata* of the adrenal cortex giving rise to the formation and release of steroids that are active in intermediary carbohydrate and protein metabolism, with somewhat lesser effects on salt and water metabolism. In man the most important of the steroids is hydrocortisone (17 hydroxycorticosterone, 17 OHCS). In other species cortisone is the chief steroid liberated. Compounds with these basic metabolic characteristics are liberated in response to a variety of stresses.

ACTH is detectable in peripheral blood within several seconds of application of an appropriate stimulus and remains detectable for from 5—15 min. ACTH increases the rate of synthesis of metabolically active steroids through intermediation of cyclic AMP. Thus, the activity of the hypothalamic-pituitary-adrenal system can be measured by any of several means, including the use of blocking agents that cause intermediary non-metabolically active compounds to accumulate and the cycle of events to be interrupted. ACTH is amenable to assay; metabolically active 17 OHCS is measured in adrenal or peripheral venous blood; over a long period the excretion of both free and conjugated steroids is measured in the urine. Normally the secretion of 17 OHCS follows a diurnal rhythm, the highest rate being early in the day. It is important to know that the concentrations of 17 OHCS found in peripheral blood are not only a measure of cortical secretion but a reflection of conjugation in liver, urinary excretory rate and tissue distribution and utilization.

The several factors contributing to the effects of anesthetics on the adrenal cortex have been studied individually: preanesthetic anxiety; the effects of preanesthetic medication; influence of the anesthetic *per se* and the added effect of operation — all of these combining to provide a stress. The resulting endocrine response is more indicative of the severity of operation than action of the anesthetic agent, VANDAM and MOORE (1960), and VAN BRUNT and GANONG (1963). Reported effects of preanesthetic medication are conflicting. Preanesthetic anxiety is not a major stimulus to the cortex though there is considerable evidence that emotional upset may activate the adrenals. Some of the earlier studies measured the adrenal-cortical response according to the degree of eosinopenia found, or, in the laboratory animal, by ascorbic acid depletion of the cortex. Neither of these effects is specific for cortical activity because sympathetic nervous system stimulation alone produces indentical changes. Morphine blocks release of ACTH at the hypothalamic level, BRIGGS and MUNSON (1955), an action counteracted by narcotic antagonists. Barbiturates are uniformly depressant of cortical activity with the locus of action probably at the hypothalamic level. BARRETT and STOCKHAM (1965) found that pentobarbitone reduced hypothalamic influence as demonstrated by release of corticotrophin releasing factor. Release of ACTH as ordinarily follows administration of diethyl ether or histamine was inhibited while sensitivity of the adrenal cortex to the action of ACTH was unaltered. BERNIS and VANEK (1958) reported a stimulating effect of hydroxydione on the cortex as shown by urinary excretion of corticosteroids.

With evidence that the hypothalamic-hypophyseal-adrenal axis is activated by trauma or operation and prevented by peripheral denervation [as in the quadriplegic, HUME (1953)] it was anticipated that regional anesthesia might lessen the cortical response to operation. Almost all reports of the effects of spinal anesthesia, as measured by circulating levels of 17 OHCS, eosinopenic responses or corticoid excretion indicate that regional anesthesia effectively blocks the adreno-cortical response to operation. A similar effect of epidural anesthesia has likewise been reported, HUME (1959). In the interpretation of these findings it should be recognized that spinal anesthesia also blocks the action of the sympathetic nervous system in proportion to the extent of nerve block.

Diethyl ether and cyclopropane, to a lesser extent, cause adrenal cortical stimulation in proportion to depth of anesthesia. Peripheral blood and adrenal venous levels of corticoids have shown significant elevations in most studies. When not quite as pronounced as might have been expected, the response to ether and cyclopropane may have been blunted by preanesthetic medication or induction of anesthesia with thiopental. OYAMA et al. [1968 (1)] measured levels of ACTH and 17 OHCS in the peripheral plasma of ten patients given ether alone, followed by operation. Adrenal reserves had been shown to be normal and ACTH was measured by bioassay. ACTH levels showed remarkable increases during planes 2—3 of the third stage of ether anesthesia, while cortisol levels followed more slowly and progressively, indicating a relation to ACTH activity. The well known attribute of ether in stimulating the sympathetic nervous system again adds to the complexity of interpreting the pure effect of anesthetic action on endocrine responses. Likewise the actions of ether and cyclopropane in diminishing both hepatic and renal blood flow must be taken into account in interpretation of elevated blood levels of 17 OHCS. Finally, the significance for the patient of elevated 17 OHCS levels must be assessed. In studies on volunteers given local, spinal, diethyl ether or cyclopropane anesthesia, without accompanying operation, HAMMOND et al. (1958) found that the only measurable accompaniment of the elevated corticoid levels was a tendency toward sodium retention. Whether this response was the result of adrenal cortical stimulation or secondary to the action of these anesthetics on renal function and hemodynamics was not established.

Several studies have been carried out with the techniques already mentioned, on adreno-cortical effects of halothane and methoxyflurane. In general, however, the studies have been poorly controlled from the standpoint of maintenance of physiological variables which could influence the results, although several species were studied. By and large the halogenated hydrocarbons evince only slight, if any, stimulating effects on the adrenal cortex. For example, OYAMA et al. [1968 (2)] measured free 17 OHCS levels in peripheral venous blood of man following preanesthetic medication, after induction of anesthesia with thiopental, during a moderate depth of halothane anesthesia and during operation. Acid-base parameters, respiratory and circulatory changes and possible alterations in body temperature were not recorded. Nevertheless, during halothane anesthesia alone there was some increase in corticoid levels and during the subsequent operation a more significant increase. The conclusion was that halothane has a mild cortical stimulating effect. In another study in the dog, CARNES et al. (1961) during halothane anesthesia and cyclopropane anesthesia, found a decrease in plasma levels of epinephrine with both anesthetics and equivocal changes in 17 OHCS levels with either anesthetic. Experimental conditions were poorly controlled. STARK (1966), in a poorly controlled study, measured the effect of nitrous oxide-halothane anesthesia following dihydromorphinone and atropine premedication, on urinary excretion of aldosterone, cortisone, sodium and potassium. The study can have little meaning because measurements were made on the day after operation. As expected sodium excretion was reduced, but surprisingly no change in hormone excretion was noted.

OYAMA et al. [1968 (3)] followed the same pattern in studying methoxyflurane as had been done for halothane. Experimental conditions were poorly controlled. After preanesthetic medication, 17 OHCS levels in plasma were lower than the controls and after 30 min of an undefined level of anesthesia with methoxyflurane there was no change. However, with surgical incision, levels of 17 OHCS rose and continued to do so thereafter. The conclusion was that methoxyflurane is not a stressful agent but neither did it interfere with the response to operation.

Finally, OYAMA et al. [1968 (4)] studied the effects of γ-hydroxybutyrate on plasma 17 OHCS concentrations, the plan being the same as in the other studies by this group on anesthetics. Data were not given on the physiological state of the patients during these studies. The authors postulate that adrenocortical stimulation occurs, though it is not clear whether in relation to the intravenous administration of 200 mg/kg of body weight of γ-hydroxybutyrate or to the surgical procedure.

In an appraisal of these studies, if indeed once can accept the results, an interesting question arises. Is it wise to employ a non-stressful anesthetic, or an anesthetic that obtunds the stress response to operation, in view of the fact that alterations in metabolism and water and electrolyte are only temporarily prevented ? On the one hand we know that some degree of adrenal cortical activity is necessary for survival and that circulatory collapse can follow a minor stress in the presence of adrenal insufficiency. Furthermore, the patient with adrenal insufficiency on a sufficient maintenance regimen of steroids requires additional amounts when undergoing operation. The answer is not readily at hand. Suffice it to say that even with some hindrance to activity of the adrenal cortex, as suggested by circulating levels of 17 OHCS, patients seem to fare well during administration of anesthesia.

In concluding this section some aspects of hormonal interaction involving the adrenal cortex deserve mention. As subsequently pointed out, in addition to activation of the sympathetic nervous system, and release of glucocorticoids from the cortex, other hormones under the trophic influence of the hypophysis, both anterior and posterior divisions, are involved in the response to stress: renin; angiotensin; aldosterone and thyroxine. Of all the relationships, those of the sympathetic system and the cortex are most interdependent. Both groups of hormones exert a permissive role in the regulation of several physiological parameters: the circulation; the blood volume; and, intermediary carbohydrate and fat metabolism. For example, in the absence of adrenal cortical steroids the threshold for action of norepinephrine and epinephrine on the circulation is elevated. A hypotensive subject who does not respond with an adequate pressor response to an intravenous infusion of norepinephrine may show improvement if pharmacological doses of hydrocortisone are simultaneously given. The interaction probably takes place at the membrane interface in heart muscle and peripheral vessels, affecting sodium, potassium and calcium flux. RABB (1959) has reviewed various aspects of the interaction on the circulation of catecholamines, adrenal steroids and electrolytes.

Antidiuretic Hormone. In addition to actions on glucocorticoid secretion, anesthetics exert an influence on renal function which is a manifestation of catecholamine release, secretion of antidiuretic hormone (ADH) and a complex interplay of hormones that regulate water and salt exchange at the tubular level. A marked antidiuresis accompanies the administration of all general anesthetics in large part relating to release of ADH. In studies on renal hemodynamics employing classical clearance techniques, the antidiuretic effect must be counteracted by the administration of ethanol in order to make valid measurements based on urinary output. As noted above, the supraoptic and paraventricular nuclei of the hypothalamus synthesize vasopressin which is transmitted with a carrier protein via nonmyelinated fibers to the neurohypophysis. Vasopressin, an octapeptide (arginine-8-vasopressin in man), has a perceptible antidiuretic effect in amounts as small as $2\,\mu U$. Many types of stressful stimuli cause the release of ADH, believed to be the result either of baro- or osmoreceptor stimulation at central or peripheral sites. In addition to anesthetics, hemorrhage is a powerful stimulus. Arginine vasopressin bound to protein in the circulating blood shows a rapid turnover rate. At the renal tubular level, from the loop of Henle through the distal convoluted tubule and possibly the collecting tubule, vasopressin accelerates reabsorption of water mediated through an influence on sodium and potassium flux. Vasopressin has also been considered to be the adrenocorticotrophic releasing factor. Indeed, vasopressin has proved useful in the evaluation of pituitary adrenal function, TUCCI et al. (1968).

KIVALO (1966) studied the effects of anesthetics on diuresis and hypothalamohypophyseal neurosecretion in the rat. Ether, thiopental and hydroxydione were administered and the response determined by measurement of urinary output and estimation of neurosecretory material and volume of neurosecretory cells in the hypothalamus. Increasing duration and depth of ether anesthesia led to prolonged antidiuresis as well as increase in neurosecretory material in the infundibular process. Thiopental caused no changes in doses of 20—40 mg/kg and a decrease in neurosecretory material in the 60 mg/kg range. Hydroxydione caused a reduction both in diuresis and neurosecretory material. Unfortunately, circulatory and other physiological parameters were not measured and the author admits that changes in renal function otherwise mediated could have been responsible for the changes observed.

In addition to an antidiuretic effect several recent reports describe a nephropathy presumably induced by methoxyflurane in which there is inappropriate diuresis. A vasopressin challenge test suggested, however, that the disorder arose not as a result of insufficiency of endogenous ADH but from a defect at the tubular level, CRANDELL and MacDONALD (1968).

Renin, Angiotensin and Aldosterone. The glucocorticoids also exert a minor influence on water and salt balance. However, the adrenal cortex secretes an extremely potent steroid primarily concerned with sodium and potassium balance, namely, aldosterone. Although to some extent responsive to the action of ACTH, aldosterone secretion results from a more intricate series of hormonal events possibly originating in the kidney at the juxtaglomerular body and evoking a number of neurogenic receptor mechanisms elsewhere. In response to alterations either in blood vessel tone or sodium concentration at the juxtaglomerular body or similar changes elsewhere, the kidney secretes renin. Renin in turn reacts with a circulating protein to form angiotensin, an octapeptide. In addition to a strong vasoconstrictive action, angiotensin acts on the adrenal cortex to cause release of the steroid, aldosterone. In keeping with other endocrine regulating mechanisms, angiotensin exerts a negative feed back influence over renin release which seems to be independent of changes in renal arterial pressure or aldosterone secretion.

In consort with the other adaptive endocrine responses, the renin-angiotensin-aldosterone response is activated by many stimuli of a stressful nature, particularly changes in blood volume and hemodynamic changes at large. Thus, it is not surprising that anesthesia, so far only demonstrated during the administration of cyclopropane, has been found to be associated with elevated plasma renin levels. DEUTSCH et al. (1967) measured cyclopropane effects on renal function in normal volunteers. At steady state conditions with partial reversal by ethanol of the anti-diuresis produced by cyclopropane, glomerular filtration rate decreased by 39%, renal blood flow decreased by 42% and renal vascular resistance increased by 84%. Changes in water and salt excretion consisted of the following: a reduction in urine volume with increased osmolality; an increased $Uosm/Posm$ ratio and negative free water clearance. The latter findings, consistent with an intense antidiuresis of ADH origin, were only partially countered by infusion of ethanol. The finding of increased afferent and efferent arteriolar constriction was in part explained by the prominent sympathetic stimulating property of cyclopropane. However, the discovery of increased peripheral venous levels of renin suggests another means whereby the renal hemodynamic changes could have occurred: that is, formation of angiotensin, a potent vasoconstrictor with demonstrable effects on renal vascular tone. Renin release could have been triggered as a result of increased sympathetic tone in the renal vessels, possibly as an aftermath of changes in sodium concentration. Finally, although the action of ADH may have been partially blocked, changes in water and salt excretion could be attributed to the action of aldo-sterone. This complex humoral response to the administration of cyclopropane, affecting renal performance, clearly demonstrates the degree of interaction among the several endocrine systems prominently concerned in circulatory and metabolic homeostasis.

Thyroid. In the regulation of thyroid activity, thyroid stimulating hormone (TSH), a glucoprotein, is probably secreted by the basophilic cells of the adeno-hypophysis. However, hypothalamic centers are again dominant, secreting a trans-mitter substance which circulates to the adenohypophysis via the pituitary portal venous system. In some manner TSH acts on the thyroid gland so that thyroxin is ultimately produced — secretion being accompanied by inhibition of water and sodium, increased oxygen and glucose usage, increased vascularity and iodine trapping. Iodine is trapped by the gland (a measure of this is the I^{131} uptake), and tyrosine is iodinated with sequential formation of monoiodotyrosine, di-iodotyro-sine with two molecules of the latter forming thyroxine. These compounds are stored in the form of thyroglobulin. TSH in circulating blood is measurable by radioimmunoassay. The neural mechanism whereby thyroid activity is increased by exposure to cold is not known, but there is negative feed-back control between thyroid and adenohypophysis, with superimposed control at the hypothalamic level.

Thyroxin is by far the chief component of the circulating thyroid hormones, bound to protein (protein bound iodine test). Falsely high PBI levels resulting from the ingestion of iodine or the use of radiodiagnostic contrast media can be differentiated by the butanol iodine extraction test. Unbound thyroxine is also measurable and several other tests of thyroid activity are available. At any rate, there is no major organ system not influenced by thyroid hormone and it would be surprising therefore if thyroid activity were not in some manner influenced by anesthetics and operation. Thyroid hormone influences central nervous activity, body growth, the circulation, lipid metabolism, muscle activity and oxygen consumption by all cells, at the mitochondrial level.

Studies of the effect of anesthetics on thyroid function are few in number and admittedly poorly controlled. Greene and Goldenberg (1959) studied the effects in 18 patients of preanesthetic medication, spinal and nitrous oxide-ether anesthesia on thyroid activity. Changes in protein bound iodine were expressed as conversion ratios. Data were not supplied on depth of anesthesia, changes in body temperature, circulation or respiration. No changes took place after preanesthetic medication, immediately after induction of anesthesia or during anesthesia and operation. The type of anesthesia and the nature of the operation seemed irrelevant although there was a tendency for patients under the age of 50 to show higher conversion ratios. Since circulating cortisol levels were significantly elevated, the authors drew the conclusion that neurosecretory centers influencing output of thyroxine do not respond to peripheral afferent stimulation in the same manner as does ACTH.

Oyama (1957) performed a series of studies on anesthetics and thyroid function in man and in the rat, employing ether, cyclopropane, halothane and methoxyflurane. Several types of assay, including PBI and the I^{131} resin sponge uptake, were employed. None of the studies were well controlled from the standpoint of steady state conditions, depth of anesthesia, circulation, respiration, hydration and body temperature. It seems unlikely that clear-cut conclusions can be drawn from this type of study.

Growth Hormone. There is only one study of the effects of anesthetics on the release of growth hormone. Schalch and Reichlin (1966) measured the influence of diethyl ether on the level of plasma GH levels in the rat using a radioimmunoassay technique. Since ether (given under poorly controlled conditions) lowered growth hormone levels in the male rat and similar changes had been observed by the authors in the monkey given thiopental, the authors drew the conclusion that the central nervous system must be continually active in the regulation of GH.

Oxytocin. Yokoyama and Ota (1965) examined the effects of cyclopropane on milk yield and maintenance of lactation both in the goat and rat. Cyclopropane did not alter milk yield in the goat.

Insulin. The effects of anesthetics on the action of insulin will have been discussed in the chapter on Metabolic Effects where the interaction with the sympathetic nervous system is shown to play a prominent role. For example, during ether anesthesia (a recognized sympathetic stimulant) in man Henneman and Vandam (1960) noted a blockage of the hypoglycemic action of insulin which they attributed to alteration in phosphorylating mechanisms and failure of transport of insulin across the cell membrane.

Parathyroid Hormone. Although the biochemical changes secondary to both hyper- and hypoparathyroidism can profoundly influence the response of the body to anesthetics, there are no studies specifically related to anesthetics and parathyroid activity.

Summary

Endocrinology is a rapidly changing field with new concepts arising and new hormonal substances discovered from time to time. The interaction among hormones becomes more and more evident as physiological processes are clarified. Despite considerable investigation in other areas, studies relating to the effects of anesthetics on endocrine systems are few in number and generally inconclusive. The reasons for the paucity of interest seem evident. Anesthesia is a small part of a surgical illness and the endocrine response to operation is not only qualitatively similar, but far greater in magnitude. The consequences of andocrine stimulation by anesthetics are neither major nor clearly defined. Most studies done relate to anesthetics and the stress response involving the hypothalamic-hypophyseal-adrenal-cortical axis. The importance of any studies on the endocrines during anesthesia lies in patient survival and the possible effects of endocrine alterations on the course of anesthesia.

References

BARRETT, A. M., STOCKHAM, M. A.: The response of the pituitary-adrenal system to a stressful stimulus — the effect of conditioning and pentobarbitone treatment. J. Endocrinol. 33, 145—152 (1965).

BERNIS, R., VANEK, R.: Excretion of total urinary reducing corticoids in surgical stress. Influence of various methods of anesthesia. Acta anaesth. belg. 9, 116—138 (1958).

BRIGGS, F. N., MUNSON, P. L.: Studies on mechanism of stimulation of ACTH secretion with aid of morphine as blocking agent. Endocrinology 57, 205—219 (1955).

BUTCHER, R. W.: Role of cyclic AMP in hormone actions. New Engl. J. Med. 279, 1378—1384 (1968).

CARNES, M. A., McPHAIL, J. L., FABIAN, L. W., HARDY, J. D.: Adrenergic and adrenocortical responses to Fluothane and cyclopropane. Am. J. Surg. 27, 223—229 (1961).

CRANDELL, W. B., MacDONALD, A.: Nephropathy associated with methoxyflurane anesthesia. A follow-up report. J. Am. Med. Assoc. 205, 798—799 (1968).

DIAZ, P. M., NGAI, S. H., COSTA, E.: The effects of cyclopropane, halothane and diethyl ether on the cerebral metabolism of serotonin in the rat. Anesthesiology 29, 959—963 (1968).

DEUTSCH, S., PIERCE, E. C., JR., VANDAM, L. D.: Cyclopropane effects on renal function in normal man. Anesthesiology 28, 547—558 (1967).

GREENE, N. M., GOLDENBERG, I. S.: The effect of anesthesia on thyroid activity in humans. Anesthesiology 20, 125—126 (1959).

HAMMOND, W. G., VANDAM, L. D., DAVIS, J. M., CARTER, R. D., BALL, M. R., MOORE, F. D.: IV-Studies in surgical endocrinology; anesthetic agents as stimuli to change in corticosteroids and metabolism. Ann. Surg. 148, 199—211 (1958).

HENNEMAN, D. H., VANDAM, L. D.: Effect of epinephrine, insulin and tolbutamide on carbohydrate metabolism during ether anesthesia. Clin. Pharmacol. Therap. 1, 694—702 (1960).

HEUSER, G.: Induction of anesthesia, seizures and sleep by steroid hormones. Anesthesiology 28, 173—183 (1967).

HUME, D. M.: Neuroendocrine response to injury: present status of problem. Ann. Surg. 138, 548—557 (1953).

— BELL, C. C.: Secretion of epinephrine, norepinephrine and corticosteroid in adrenal venous blood of the human. Surg. Forum 9, 6—12 (1959).

KIVALO I.,: Effect of some anesthetic agents on diuresis and hypothalamo-hypophysial neurosecretion in the rat. Ann. Med. Exp. et Biol. Fenniae 44 Supp. 5, 1—60 (1966).

KUNTZMAN R., SANSUR, M., CONNEY, A. H.: Effect of drugs and insecticides on the anesthetic action of steroids. Endocrinology 77, 952—954 (1965).

OYAMA, T.: Effects of anesthesia on thyroid function of rats. Anesthesiology 18, 719—722 (1957).

— KUDO, T., SHIBATA, S., MATSUMOTO, F.: (4) Effects of gamma-hydroxybutyrate on plasma hydrocortisone concentration in man. Anesthesia and Analgesia, Current Researches 47, 350—354 (1968).

— SAITO, T., ISOMATSU, T., SAMEJIMA, N., UEMURA, T., ARIMURA, A.: (1) Plasma levels of ACTH and cortisol in man during diethyl ether anesthesia and surgery. Anesthesiology 29, 559—564 (1968).

— SHIBATA, S., MATUSMOTO, F., TAKIGUCHI, M., KUDO, T.: (2) Effects of halothane anaesthesia and surgery on adrenocortical function in man. Canad. Anaesth. Soc. J. 15, 258—266 (1968).

— — — MATSUKI, A., KIMURA, K., TAKAZAWA, T., KUDO, T.: (3) Adrenocortical function related to methoxyflurane anaesthesia and surgery in man. Canad. Anaesth. Soc. J. 15, 362—368 (1968).

Rabb, W.: Transmembrane cationic gradient and blood pressure regulation. Am. J. Cardiol. **4**, 752—884 (1959).

Schalch, D. S., Reichlin, S.: Plasma growth hormone concentration in the rat determined by radioimmunoassay — influence of sex, pregnancy, lactation, anesthesia, hypophysectomy and extrasellar pituitary transplants. Endocrinology **79**, 275—280 (1966).

Schmidt, K. F.: Effect of halothane anesthesia on regional acetylcholine levels in the rat brain. Anesthesiology **27**, 788—792 (1966).

Selye, H.: Anesthetic effect of steroid hormones. Proc. Soc. Exptl Biol. Med. **46**, 116—121 (1941).

Stark, G.: The effect of anesthesia on the excretion of aldosterone, cortisone and cortisol as well as sodium and potassium. Anaesthetist **15**, 4—6 (1966).

Thompson, J. H., Campbell, L. B.: The effect of several anaesthetic agents upon the 5-hydroxytryptamine concentration in the jejunal mucosa of the Sprague-Dawley rat. Arch. intern. pharmacodynamic **169**, 1—5 (1967).

Tucci, J. R., Espiner, E. A., Jagger, P. I., Lauler, D. P., Thorn, G. W.: Vasopressin in the evaluation of pituitary-adrenal function. Ann. Internal Med. **69**, 191—202 (1968).

Van Brunt, E. E., Ganong, W. F.: The effects of preanesthetic medication, anesthesia and hypothermia on the endocrine response to injury. Anesthesiology **24**, 500—514 (1963).

Vandam, L. D., Moore, F. D.: Adrenocortical mechanisms related to anesthesia. Anesthesiology **21**, 531—552 (1960).

Way, E. L., Sutherland, V. C.: Pharmacologically active brain substances and their relation to endocrine effects. Anesthesiology **24**, 543—562 (1963).

Yokoyama, A., Ota, K.: The effect of anaesthesia on milk yield and maintenance of lactation in the goat and rat. J. Endocrinol. **33**, 341—351 (1965).

4.9. The Action of Inhalation Anesthetics on the Gastrointestinal Tract

Donald R. Bennett and Paul Bass

With 5 Figures

I. Introduction

Investigations of the action of inhalation anesthetics on the gastrointestinal tract have not kept abreast with studies on other organ systems. There are several reasons for this neglect. The unanesthetized state is usually the preferred control condition for a study of an anesthetic drug. Technically it is difficult to assess gastrointestinal functions in the unanesthetized animal. This is a major reason for the paucity of available data. In addition, when an anesthetic is used in the laboratory, it is used more to immobilize the animal than to study the anesthetic. Inhalational anesthetic agents are not popular because of; the relative ease of laboratory use of intravenous anesthetics, the cost of necessary equipment, the potential flammability of some agents, and the need for adequate ventilation. Thus, the paucity of data referred to for anesthetic agents is particularly true for inhalation anesthetic agents.

The acute cardiovascular and respiratory actions of anesthetic agents are more life-threatening than comparable actions on the gastrointestinal tract. The latter actions are principally a matter of discomfort to the patient. There is an exception to the last statement and that relates to vomiting and aspiration of gastric contents during anesthetic induction. This can be a serious hazard since aspiration of vomit is responsible for one-third to one-half of the anesthetic deaths in the United States (Parker, 1956). Thus, it is not surprising that of the references available on gastrointestinal tract and anesthetic studies, a large percentage are related to emesis and gastric content aspiration.

A. Potential Spectrum of Gastrointestinal Activity

The literature on anesthetic agents frequently carries the generalized and meaningless statement that "anesthetic agent X depresses the gastrointestinal tract". The term *gastrointestinal activity* when used by gastroenterologists brings to mind a spectrum of parameters including at least *absorption, secretion,* and *contractile activity.* We shall use the term motility in this chapter to refer to integrated smooth muscle contractions. An investigator who determines the action of inhalation anesthetic agents on gastrointestinal activity must keep in mind the potential sites of action where such chemicals can act. The ultimate effector elements of gastrointestinal activity where drug action occur are connective tissue, smooth muscle, epithelial, secretory, and intrinsic nerve cells. In addition, other sites or mechanisms of regulation of such effector elements where chemicals can act include blood supply, hormones, extrinsic nerve activity and local chemical regulation of the bowel. Subcellular sites of action and biochemical functions may play an essential role in the *modus operandi* of a drug and as such also serve as a basis for classification of chemical action on the gut. An author may not be able to state whether a chemical which specifically depresses gut motility acts on effector elements, e.g., by a) altering excitability or inotropism of smooth muscle cells, b) altering excitability or conduction of nerve cells, or c) interfering with the generation of an essential cofactor, etc. However, it is inappropriate to label an agent a gut depressant if the author does not at least differentiate between the functions of absorption, secretion, or motility, and in addition does not at least differentiate between stomach, small, and large intestine as a site of action.

Under each of the subheadings in this chapter, a brief review of some of the current ideas on the physiology or pathophysiology of the area under discussion is included. The authors hope this information will stimulate the type of research which will lead to new and challenging theories on the sites and mechanisms of anesthetic action on the gastrointestinal tract.

II. Esophagus

A. Physiology

The effects of anesthetics on the pressures and contractile properties of the esophagus and the gastroesophageal sphincter have received only a minimum of attention in animals and man. Observations by CODE (1969) and LEVITT et al. (1965) indicate that anesthesia eliminates some of the important components of the motor actions of the esophagus. Both the pharyngoesophogeal and gastroesophogeal sphincter pressures and swallowing reflexes are difficult to detect or are often eliminated by anesthetics. It is surprising that the physiological factors controlling the above loci have not been comprehensively studied by anesthesiologists since emesis and regurgitation are two phenomena that are of vital concern to them. Extensive normal and abnormal functions of this portion on the gastrointestinal tract have been characterized by relatively simple techniques that are currently available. A review by INGELFINGER (1958) provides complete coverage of the historical and modern literature up to 1958. More recent reviews have also been published by INGELFINGER (1963) and KRAMER (1965). An excellent atlas by CODE et al. (1958) is also available showing the normal and abnormal patterns that may be recorded from this area of the tract by intraluminal devices.

Several techniques have proved useful as methods for studying the esophagus and its sphincters. The use of intraluminal pressure detecting devices (small balloons or open-tip catheters), cineradiography, electromyography and intraluminal pH recordings have contributed to basic information about this organ. The combination of several types of sensors offers the broadest coverage for monitoring the sequence of motor events. Studies combining cineradiography and intraluminal pressure recordings have been decsribed by RINALDO (1966) and SOKOL et al. (1966).

1. Pharyngoesophageal Sphincter

Deglutition is the normal stimulus to caudal transport. Though deglutition is voluntary, once initiated it sets in motion a complex series of involuntary events. The oral and pharyngeal components are involved in the initial portion of swallowing. This follows the sequence of first closing the mouth, then the passage between the mouth and nose and finally the entry into the trachea. Caudal transport is accomplished by orderly, sequential contractions of the muscles of the tongue and pharynx with coordinated relaxation and subsequent contraction of the pharyngoesophageal sphincter. The sequence of pressure changes are presented in Fig. 1. The relaxation of the sphincter occurs before the arrival of the pharyngeal peristaltic contraction. The bolus propelled by the contraction passes through the sphincter after which the sphincter contracts. The contraction produces pressures of 70—100 cm of water above atmosphere which lasts 2—4 sec then returns to

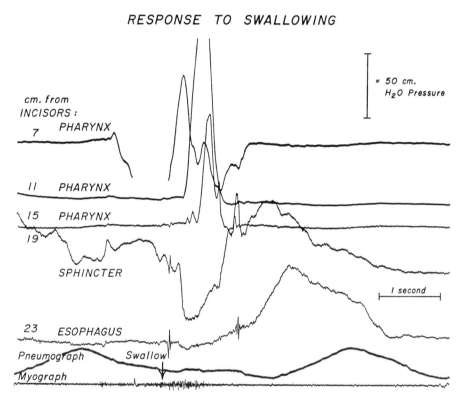

Fig. 1. Simultaneous recording of pressure in the mouth, pharynx, pharyngoesophageal sphincter, and esophagus during a swallow in a healthy person. A decisive increase of pressure due to muscular contraction started in the mouth and swept in a peristaltic fashion through the pharynx and the sphincter into the esophagus. From CODE and SCHLEGEL (1968)

resting pressures which range from 18—60 cm water above atmosphere (CODE and SCHLEGEL, 1968).

2. Esophagus

The muscular wall of the esophagus of man, monkey and cat is unique in that the "conduit" contains a junction between skeletal and smooth muscle fibers. Other unique features of the esophageal skeletal muscle are that it is under involuntary control, is innervated by the vagus nerve, and is in juxtaposition to the intrinsic plexi of Auerbach. These features raise questions on the action that drugs may have on this unique structural arrangement.

The normal motor pattern in the esophagus is a peristaltic wave of 40—80 cm water pressure which is propagated in a sequential manner down the esophagus. It is initiated by swallowing or by distention of the esophagus. The peristaltic wave, consisting of a band of contracting fibers, is normally behind the bolus. The velocity of progress of the peristaltic wave is different in different parts of the esophagus and it changes depending upon the material swallowed. The amplitude and duration of the pressure wave is, however, less in the upper portion of the esophagus where the skeletal muscle fibers are located (HIGHTOWER, 1959; KANTROWITZ et al. 1966; CODE and SCHLEGEL, 1968).

Normal resting pressure of part of the esophagus is subatmospheric because it is in the pleural cavity. In humans, it ranges from -12 to -15 cm with inspiration, -1 to -2 with expiration and -5 to -6 cm water pressure between breaths. Violent efforts like coughing can lead to pressure changes ranging between 150 to -65 cm water. This should be of vital concern to anesthesiologists since these pressures can be influenced by upper esophageal obstruction, respiratory obstruction, or changes in the gastroesophageal pressure differential.

3. Gastroesophageal Sphincter

The gastroesophageal junction plays an important role in preventing regurgitation. No definitive studies have been done on this area with anesthetics. Anesthetics conceivably could be selective in not affecting, relaxing, or ideally increasing the pressure of this area, which in the resting esophagus is normally closed. Normally, the lower esophageal sphincter represents a zone of elevated pressure relative to the stomach that extends 1—2 cm both above and below the hiatus of the diaphragm. This zone demonstrates intrinsic sphincteric mechanisms without identifiable anatomical counterparts. The anatomy and function of this area have been extensively reviewed (INGELFINGER, 1958; ATKINSON, 1962; JOHNSON, 1966; JOHNSON and LAWS, 1966). The resting pressure in the lower esophageal sphincter can be 10 cm of water above the pressure in the fundus of the stomach when recorded with an open-tip catheter. This pressure differential can vary depending upon respiration and the type of recording units used for detection (RINALDO and LEVEY, 1968; CODE and SCHLEGEL, 1968). Using several techniques, it has been shown that below the hiatus, end-expiratory pressure exceeds end-expiratory pressure; the reverse is true above the hiatus. Also, at the end-inspiration, the axial extent of the pressure zone is shorter than at end-expiration. Because of the pressure properties, gastric reflux and regurgitation are most likely to occur at end-inspiration (CREAMER, 1955; FORSHALL, 1955). Changing the position of the subject from upright to sitting, to supine, or the head down position changes the pressure in the fundus of the stomach. Concurrently, the sphincter pressure is also changed to maintain a small but consistently higher level of pressure than that recorded from the stomach (FYKE et al., 1956). It should be emphasized that the abdominal portion of the esophagus and the "resting" stomach are subject to the same intraperitoneal pressures. Thus, any positional changes or alterations of abdominal muscle activity alter the external pressures on both organs and only a slight sphincteric pressure is needed to retain gastric contents.

In response to deglutition, the lower esophageal sphincter pressure usually decreases 1.5—2.5 sec after the initiation of swallowing and remains relaxed for 5—12 sec (Fig. 2). Thus, the sphincter is relaxed 3 or more sec before the esophageal peristaltic wave approaches it. Closing of the sphincter is coordinated with the esophageal wave so that the orad portion of the sphincter is in peristaltic sequence with that of the esophagus. This closing pressure can reach 20 or more cm

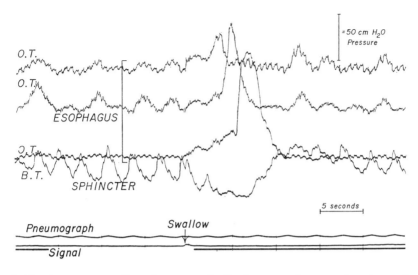

Fig. 2. Simultaneous recording of pressures in the lower esophagus and gastroesophageal sphincter. Note the relaxation and then contraction of the gastroesophageal sphincter during swallowing. During the break in the signal line 5 ml of water was held in the mouth and then swallowed. O.T., open tip; B.T., balloon tip. From CODE and SCHLEGEL (1968)

of water, can last for 7—10 sec and gradually returns to its residual resting pressure of 10 cm of water.

B. Pathophysiology

1. Nausea, Retching and Emesis

Orad transport of material up the esophagus can occur during vomiting, regurgitation, or eructation (belching). The vomiting act is a complex procedure that is controlled centrally and with some of the afferent inputs located in the gastrointestinal tract (BORISON and WANG, 1953). With the onset of retching, the gastroesophageal sphincter and the esophagus relax. Increased intraabdominal pressure and contractions of the antrum of the stomach force contents into the esophagus. If these antral contractions are forceful, emesis can occur. The nasal and respiratory passages are closed during the action (LASKIEWICZ, 1956). The role of the pharyngoesophageal sphincter has not been defined in this action. Possibly, it may retain the esophageal contents during retching.

Pressure changes for the gastroesophageal sphincter have been well documented during ingestion of material. Yield pressures at the lower sphincter for the movement of material from the stomach are vague. In general, there is a great resistance to flow in an orad direction. KELLING (1901) observed that in cadavers, air placed in the stomach may escape easily by the esophagus in some, while other stomachs will burst before gastroesophageal closure will yield. As explained above, abdominal pressures will not initiate reflux since a portion of the gastroesophageal sphincter is intra-abdominal. The explanation for the maintained competence of the sphincter during increased intragastric pressures is not readily available. During thiopental anesthesia in man, manual compression of the stomach to pressures of 90 cm water could not empty gastric contents into the espohagus (O'MULLANE,

1954). In unanesthetized dogs, an intragastric pressure of 25 cm water was sufficient to induce eructation, but during chloroform anesthesia pressures of 50 to 70 cm water were not effective (KELLING, 1901). These studies argue against the presence of an intrinsic sphincter mechanism in the esophagus. However, a reflex may be present in the upper portion of the stomach, which when stimulated, could conceivably decrease the sphincteric pressure. The presence of such a reflex has not been investigated, but if present, the two above studies would suggest that anesthetics depress the reflex. Evidence has also been presented that the gastroesophageal sphincter slips into the thoracic cavity during eructation and vomiting in both dog and man (JOHNSON, 1966; JOHNSON and LAWS, 1966). Under these conditions, the increase in abdominal pressure becomes a very effective orad propulsive force since the sphincter is no longer subject to the increased abdominal pressure. Clearly, more studies should be conducted on this sphincter to clarify its mechanisms of response to intragastric pressures and changes induced by anesthetics.

2. Regurgitation

Regurgitation in either unanesthetized or anesthetized individuals has not been studied extensively. Regurgitation is defined as a passive process in which fluid passes from the stomach to the pharynx as a gravitational effect if the upper and lower ends of the esophagus are sufficiently relaxed (MORTON and WYLIE, 1951). The exact pressures in the esophagus or gastroesophageal junction have not been measured during regurgitation. O'MULLANE (1954) noted that resting gastric pressures in people in the supine position with distended abdomens, e.g., gravid uterus, differed from people with "concave" abdomens. The gastric pressures in these two groups were different during thiopental anesthesia, the administration of relaxant drugs such as d-tubocurarine or succinylcholine, and different positions (Table 1). Neither group demonstrated regurgitation. The application of the local

Table 1[a]. *Average gastric tone (cm H_2O)*

Group	Awake[b]	Light[b]	Deep[b]	Total paralysis			
		Anesthesia		Supine	Foot-down 20%	20° Trendelenburg	Lithotomy
Pregnant n = 10	+5 to +18	+2 to +18	+5 to +15	+9	+6	+12	+15
Nonpregnant n = 12	+2 to +5	−2 to +5	−2 to +3	−3	−5	+2	−2

[a] Modified from O'MULLANE (1954).
[b] Range of pressure. Anesthetic was thiopental; relaxant agents were d-turbocurarine or succinylcholine.

anesthetic tetracaine to the cardia region or administration of ganglionic blocking drugs such as hexamethonium or trimethaphan did not enhance the tendency to regurgitate. Following deep anesthesia with cyclopropane and distention of the stomach with saline, saline did enter the esophagus during inspiration. Proper manometric and radiological studies are needed to validate objectively the actions of drugs in this area. Regurgitation could also be induced by distending a balloon in the esophagus. This could induce repeated secondary peristalsis which would lead to a continuously open sphincter and corresponding regurgitation. Distention of the stomach with air or other materials initiates an adjustment of smooth muscle of the stomach and striated muscle of the anterior abdominal wall to adapt reflexly, i.e., receptive relaxation, such that no large pressures are generated. Under these conditions, the gastroesophageal sphincter remains competent in the face of gastric distention (MCNALLY et al., 1964).

The pharyngoesophageal sphincter could be relaxed in man with deep cyclopropane anesthesia and a muscle relaxant to the point where fluid (200 cc) placed in the esophagus would enter the pharynx. Conversely, fluid in the mouth did not readily enter the esophagus when the patient was under the influence of thiopental and a muscle relaxant (O'MULLANE, 1954). This response is difficult to interpret because the same anesthetics were not used in the two experiments.

3. Eructation

Belching or eructation denotes the transport of gas from the stomach to the esophagus and possibly into the pharynx and mouth. Gas can be brought from the stomach into the esophagus during inspiration. If the abdominal muscles contract, the gas is expelled into the pharynx and mouth through a relaxed pharyngoesophageal sphincter. If the somatic muscles do not contract, the distended esophagus excites a normal peristaltic wave which moves the gas back into the stomach (MCNALLEY et al., 1964). Belching of air from the esophagus is accompanied at will by relaxation of the pharyngoesophageal sphincter and an increase in intrathoracic pressure. The latter is accompanied by closing the glottis and slight straining. Thus in man, the gas is not expelled from the esophagus by an antiperistaltic action but by increased intrathoracic pressure.

4. Clinical Considerations

BONICA et al. (1958), BELLVILLE (1961), and RIDING (1963) have reviewed the major factors which are responsible for postoperative nausea and emesis. The factors include: *sex difference* — where there is a three-fold greater incidence in the female up to age 70; *age* — the adolescent has a greater susceptibility than the adult; *depth and particularly duration of anesthesia* — augments incidence; *type of anesthesia* — regional has less incidence than general; *type of operation* — intraabdominal and intrathroacic have the greatest incidence; *pre-anesthetic medication* — particularly where narcotics are used in large doses, augments incidence; *metabolic state of the individual* — nutritional, electrolyte, and fluid status may effect incidence adversely; and *hypoxia* — especially associated with *hypercapnia*, augments incidence. BONICA et al. (1958) concluded that "the *inhalational anesthetic* is one of the most important factors" in postoperative nausea and emesis. However, the anesthetic agent may be less of a factor since the recent advent of the newer halogenated hydrocarbons (*vide infra*).

BONICA (1967) has presented a review of the factors involved in regurgitation and aspiration. The competency of the gastroesophageal sphincter is, of course, fundamental. In addition, factors of consideration are the pressure gradients between the stomach and esophagus as well as the intraperitoneal and intrathoracic cavities, alteration of the gastroesophageal angle by gastric distention, and certain disease states, e.g., hiatus hernia. Upper abdominal operations are more predisposing than other types of surgery (MARSHALL and GORDON, 1958). The presence of a cough reflex does not guarantee protection and may even predispose to regurgitation (BANNISTER and SATILLARO, 1962). A general discussion of silent regurgitation and aspiration is available (STEVENS, 1964), and recent

statistics concerning incidence can be found in CULVER et al. (1951) and MUCKLOW
and LARARD (1963).

A universal method to prevent regurgitation and aspiration of emesis is, of
course, not available. DINNICK (1957) states "... that the skill of the anaesthetist
is of greater importance than the method he employs" and this is probably still
true. Papers concerned with proponents of esophageal intubation (GIUFFRIDA and
BIZZARRI, 1957), endotracheal intubation following topical anesthesia of the oropharynx (WEAVER, 1964), endotracheal intubation in the left lateral head-down
position (BOURNE, 1962), and the routine use of apomorphine (HOLMES, 1957) are
available. HAMELBERG and BOSOMWORTH (1965) have written a recent paper on
the prevention and therapy of aspiration pneumonia.

C. Pharmacology

BANNISTER and SATILLARO (1962) in their review note that no experiments
have been devised to determine the comparative effects of general anesthetics on
the vomiting center. The deficiency has not been corrected to date. No single
clinical comparison or continuing studies conducted by the same group under
similar clinically controlled conditions have been reported for nitrous oxide,
diethyl ether, chloroform, divinyl ether, trichloroethylene, cyclopropane, fluroxene,
halothane or methoxyflurane. The incidence of postoperative nausea and vomiting
for any one agent may vary considerably among clinical groups (e.g., diethyl ether
from 33—56.5% incidence) even where the depth and duration of anesthesia, as
well as the surgical procedure, is similar (HAUMANN and FOSTER, 1963). The likely
major factors responsible for such variation in results are the lack of a precise
definition and subjective grading of postoperative nausea and vomiting as well as
the type and amount of preanesthetic medication used (BEECHER, 1952; KNAPP
and BEECHER, 1956; BELLVILLE, 1961).

After examining what clinical data is available; ARTUSIO et al. (1960), ARTUSIO
(1963), BODMAN et al. (1960), BONICA et al. (1958), BURTLES and PECKETT (1957),
DAVIES (1941), DENT et al. (1955), DORNETTE et al. (1962), HAUMANN and FOSTER
(1963), LEE and ATKINSON (1964), NOVOA (1960), RIDING (1963), ROBBINS (1958),
and WATERS (1936), the following conclusions regarding emesis seem appropriate.
Diethyl ether and chloroform are the worst offenders with diethyl ether being
given the number one position by the majority of the investigators. Following
close behind are cyclopropane and trichloroethylene and again these two are
occasionally reversed. Nitrous oxide is in a class by itself in that it is less provocative than the preceding four but more so than intravenous thiopental. Halothane
is similar to or less active than thiopental and, in fact, appears to have an anti-
emetic action in its own right (CHANG et al., 1957; ABAJIAN et al., 1959; NOVOA,
1960; RIDING, 1963). The latter action may be of no consequence except where
high doses of preanesthetic opiate drugs are used (DUNDEE, 1968); however, the
low incidence of emesis with halothane is certainly an important property in its
acceptance by patients. The mechanism of this antiemetic action of halothane
against nitrous oxide, trichloroethylene, and morphine is said to be a depression
of the vomiting center (NOVOA, 1960). No references or experimental evidence to
substantiate the claim were given in that communication. To the best of the
authors' knowledge, methoxyflurane has not been specifically compared to halothane under similar conditions. Initial clinical impressions would appear to place
it in a category with halogenated inhalation anesthetics like halothane rather than
chloroform or trichloroethylene (ARTUSIO, 1963).

The search for inhalation anesthetic agents with only minimal emetic activity would appear to be more fruitful than the use of anti-emetic drugs pre- or post-operatively. The adverse effects (KNAPP and BEECHER, 1956), cost and minimal benefit (SIMONSEN and VANDEWATER, 1962) preclude the routine use of anti-emetic drugs. BELLVILLE (1961) feels the benefit of such drugs outweighs the risks; however, anesthesiologists that use or plan to use anti-emetic medication should review the pharmacologic principles of drug dosage and action set forth in Bellville's study.

D. Special Clinical Considerations

The administration of anesthetics to infants and young children requires special attention to the esophageal area. The details of the pressure changes of the esophagus in the unanesthetized state are well documented (GRYBOSKI et al., 1963). Similar studies under anesthesia have not been carried out. In general, the gastroesophageal sphincter zone is poorly defined during the first 6 days of life but increases significantly thereafter through the first year of life. In the majority of children, the sphincter is located at or above the level of the diaphragm and an intra-abdominal segment cannot be detected.

The obstetrical patient is a special problem because of the frequent emergency nature of the case, possibly coupled with a full stomach, an increased incidence of emesis, an increased intragastric pressure, and an increased incidence of hiatus hernia. BONICA (1967) considers the above factors as predisposing, while the anesthetic agent is the precipitating factor.

The anesthesiologist should be aware that certain disease states can alter the motor function of the esophagus and the competence of the sphincters. Neurological lesions resulting from conditions of midbrain strokes, poliomyelitis, or from myasthenia gravis can affect the pharynx and pharyngoesophageal sphincter. Achalasia and hiatal hernia alter the characteristics of the gastroesophageal sphincter. The reader is referred to reviews for more details on this topic (CREAMER, 1968).

III. Gastric Emptying

A. Physiology

Both animal models, dog (WEISBRODT et al., 1969) or rat (REYNELL and SPRAY, 1957) and clinical methods (CHANG et al., 1968; GEORGE, 1968; GRIFFITH et al., 1966; HUNT, 1959) have been developed to assess gastric emptying. There are 4 ways of measuring the rate of gastric emptying (HUNT and KNOX, 1968):

A. Measurement of the volume of efflux past the gastroduodenal junction.

1. Measurement of the amount of an unabsorbed isotope or marker in the intestines.

2. Drainage of duodenal contents through a fistula or tube passed through the mouth.

B. Measurement of the volume of gastric contents.

3. By assessment of the amount of radioopaque or radiation emitters *in situ*.

4. By withdrawal of the gastric contents through a tube.

Through the use of various techniques, it is established that the stomach empties its contents in an exponential manner. In man, food begins to leave the stomach 2 or 3 min after it has been swallowed and continues following an orderly pattern into the duodenum. This exponential property has been established to be independent of the viscosity of the test meal (HUNT, 1954). This exponential property of gastric emptying has been established in man and verified in dog (Fig. 3). The choice of the test meal can lead to rapid emptying (trisodium citrate), intermediate (glucose) or slow emptying (trisodium citrate with 10 mN oleic acid). The control of emptying has been attributed to the presence of at least three types of receptors located in the duodenum. 1. The osmoreceptor has the widest range of stimuli and the lowest sensitivity. 2. The receptors sensitive to fat are more specific, being most sensitive to fatty acids with chain lengths of 12—18 carbon atoms. 3. The acid-sensitive receptors are not related to the dissociation constants of the acid. Hydrochloric and acetic acids are the most potent inhibitors, while citric acid is the least potent inhibitor of stomach emptying. A closer correlation is obtained between decreased stomach emptying rates and acid type by comparing

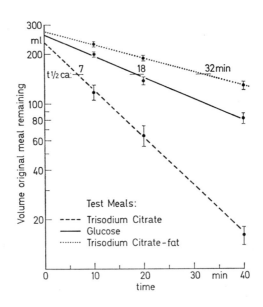

Fig. 3. Gastric emptying of 300 ml of three test meals. Vertical bars denote standard error. Each mean represents 15 test meals. A total of 135 test meals were used. From Weisbrodt et al. (1969)

stomach emptying with the molecular weight of the anions of the acid. This has been interpreted as being due to the slower rate of diffusion of the larger anions to the receptor site (Hunt and Knox, 1969).

The relationship between antral-duodenal motility and gastric emptying has been established in dogs by Weisbrodt et al. (1969). These studies indicate that the body of the stomach acts as a reservoir regardless of the test meal, and that emptying is controlled by the relationship of antral to duodenal motility. Maximal gastric emptying, as indicated by a citrate test meal, occurs when the antrum is actively contracting and the duodenum is quiescent. Conversely, the presence of a fatty acid leads to slower emptying because antral contractions are reduced while the duodenum is contracting (Fig. 4). Whether the motility patterns generated by different test meals are hormonally or neurogenically controlled awaits elucidation.

It should be emphasized that in the above presentation no reference was made to the pyloric sphincter exerting any controlling influence. Both histological and

electrical studies (BASS et al., 1961; HORTON, 1928) have failed to demonstrate
the presence of any specialized muscle in the gastroduodenal area. In fact quite
the contrary is true. There is a complete separation of circular muscle and only
approximately 30% of the longitudinal muscle bridges the two organs. This hypo-
muscular segment is not capable of exerting a sphincteric influence. Pharmacological studies have also revealed that all of the antrum responds as a homogeneous organ either relaxed by catecholamines (McCoy and BASS, 1963) or

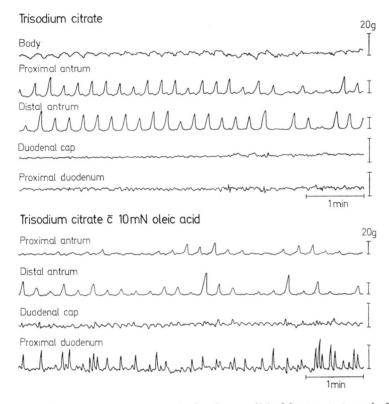

Fig. 4. Contractile pattern of the gastroduodenal area elicited by two test meals. The records were obtained from the same animal 5 min post-administration. Note the relatively
high antral to low duodenal activity elicited by the citrate test meal (upper record) and the
reversed relationship induced by the addition of fat (lower record. From WEISBRODT et al.
(1969)

stimulated by 5-hydroxytryptophan (ANDERSON et al., 1968). Thus, stomach
emptying is more dependent on antral-duodenal contractile relationships rather
than on any specific sphincteric mechanisms.

It had been suggested that gastric emptying utilizing barium is not delayed in
labor (CRAWFORD, 1956), however, when barium is mixed with food a delay is
observed (HYTTEN and LEITCH, 1963). In any event, 4 h does not appear to be a
sufficient time for gastric emptying in many clinical cases (BODMAN et al., 1960)
and besides, food in the stomach is not essential for regurgitation or aspiration
(WYLIE and CHURCHILL-DAVISON, 1966).

B. Pharmacology

CANNON and MURPHY (1907) concluded that "etherization, either one-half or one and one-half hours was found not to delay to any marked degree the discharge of food from the stomach." It is probably important to note that the test meal was bismuth subnitrate and carbohydrate (mashed potato). The most comprehensive and last study reported on the comparative effects of inhalation anesthetic agents on the emptying time of the stomach in the dog was published by SLEETH and VAN LIERE (1938). Four normal dogs were conditioned so as to determine their gastric emptying time fluoroscopically with a test meal consisting of hamburger, bread, milk and barium sulfate. The animals were lightly anesthetized (surgical plane) for 15 min in the morning. The test meal was fed 20 min after anesthesia was discontinued. Four days were allowed to elapse between tests after anesthesia to make certain no irreversible change or alteration of control had taken place. A summary of their results is shown in Table 2. Unfortunately, nitrous

Table 2[a]

Agent	Mean gastric emptying time (h)	% Prolonged over control
Normal	5.14	—
Chloroform	8.47	64
Diethyl ether	7.22	40
Nitrous oxide	5.91	15
Ethylene	5.49	7
Divinyl ether	5.49	7
Cyclopropane	5.62	9

[a] Data from SLEETH and VAN LIERE (1938).

oxide was administered at a 95% concentration for 15 min so that a definite element of hypoxia was likely present. In view of the careful design of the study and the comparative results, it is unfortunate that the authors assumed that their findings would also hold true for the small intestine. More recent data presented later in this chapter will suggest that small intestine transit time is not nearly as prolonged as gastric emptying time following surgery.

IV. Secretion

The digestive secretions derived from the salivary, gastric, pancreatic, biliary and intestinal juices amount to 5 l/24 h in man. Since the greater part of these secretions is derived from the blood, conditions of metabolic alkalosis or acidosis affect the character of the secretion. Also, the absorptive process of the gut must be as efficient as the kidney or marked electrolyte disturbances would result. The details on mechanism of secretion of the various digestive glands has not been completely elucidated. Current studies have been directed more to the control of secretion. Neural control is most prominent for the salivary glands. Conversely, humoral control assumes more of a role in the secretory functions of the stomach pancreas and other secretory glands in the lower gastrointestinal tract.

A. Salivary Secretion

Saliva is secreted by the major paired salivary glands and the numerous small labial, buccal and palatal glands. In most species, at least one of the glands has a continuous flow without extraglandular stimuli. This basal secretion keeps the mucous membranes moist at all times (SCHNEYER and SCHNEYER, 1967). When a number of different organs supplied with parasympathetic nerves are compared, the response of the salivary glands to nerve stimulation is particularly easy to abolish with atropine (HENDERSON, 1923). Quantitative evaluation of salivary flow reflexly induced by inhalation anesthetics has been studied by ROBBINS (1935) in dogs. Ether and chloroform were definitely irritant, cyclopropane slightly irritant, and ethylene and nitrous oxide were not irritant. Cocainization of the oropharynx blocked the response to diethyl ether. Pilocarpine-induced secretions were not blocked by ether, thus supporting the concept that ether reflexly induces salivary secretion. Deep surgical anesthesia with ether suppresses this ether-induced reflex secretion by an action of the anesthetic on the medullary center (ROBBINS, 1935). The introduction of muscle relaxants and endotracheal intubation has decreased considerably the amount of salivary secretions induced by certain inhalation anesthetic agents. Two reports based on qualitative clinical impressions suggest that fluroxene (DORNETTE et al., 1962) and the recently introduced halogenated hydrocarbons (ARTUSIO et al., 1960) stimulate salivary secretion less than ether, cyclopropane and chloroform. Electrical stimulation of the chorda nerve is markedly blocked by 0.5%, intensely blocked by 1.0% and completely blocked by 2.5% halothane although carbachol-induced salivary secretion was unaffected (RAVENTÓS, 1961). Thus halothane may reflexly stimulate salivary secretion like other halogenated hydrocarbons; however, its ganglionic blocking action nullifies the reflexly-induced secretion as well as the secretion normally present during anesthesia. Some of the barbiturates block the salivary reflex by acting centrally or as ganglionic or parasympathetic effector blocking agents (STAVRAKY, 1931; MONTGOMERY, 1935; EMMELIN, 1941; GUIMARAIS et al., 1955; BRÅHAMMAR and EMMELIN, 1942).

B. Gastric Secretion

The gastric mucosa is penetrated by gastric pits into which several types of cells secrete. These secretions enter the lumen of the stomach which is lined by mucous secreting cells. The secretion output of the stomach which can normally be collected as a mixture are the products from four cell types, i.e., parietal, chief, mucus neck and surface mucus secreting cells. Various theories have been developed to explain the mechanism of secretion of the various cell types, particularly that of the parietal cell which produce the hydrogen ion. These have been presented and elegantly summarized by HUNT and WAN (1967).

A major development in understanding the control of gastric secretion has evolved with the isolation, identification and synthesis of the antral hormone, gastrin. The elucidation of the mechanism of release and action of gastrin has shown that the vagus nerve exerts its influence on secretion by at least two routes: (1) Release of gastrin from the gastric antrum, and (2) a direct control and interaction of gastrin and other hormones on the parietal cell.

Current evidence indicates that acid secretion is modulated by many stimulatory and inhibitory factors and that the final interplay determines the secretion output. The histamine system and substances that inhibit histidine decarboxylase alter secretion. Serotonin inhibits hydrogen ion output. The sympathetic nervous system mediators and drugs that can prolong the half-life of these mediators decrease secretory output (BASS and PATTERSON, 1966). A series of biologically active poly-peptides like bradykinin, Substance P, or the prostaglandin series (ROBÉRT et al., 1967) exert potent affects on secretion.

No comparative clinical data on the action of inhalation anesthetics on gastric, intestinal and pancreatic secretions during or following anesthesia are available. Secretion of bile and gall bladder activity is said to require 24 h for recovery follo-wing diethyl ether anesthesia (ROBBINS, 1958). A reference to gastric secretion of acid depressed by 0.75% halothane completes the information available at present (RAVENTÓS, 1961). For comparative purposes it should be stated that subanesthetic doses of pentobarbital did not depress gastric secretion in the spider monkey (WOO and BROOKS, 1963). POWELL and HIRSCHOWITZ (1967) found, however, that water, hydrogen, and chloride ion secretion were depressed by pentobarbital in anesthetic doses regardless of whether the secretion was spontaneous or induced by histamine, alcohol, insulin, sham feeding, or barbituric acid derivatives which stimulate secretion. MERENDINO (1948) was not able to block this pentobarbital depression of gastric secretion by denervation of the stomach.

The isolated frog gastric mucosa has been extensively used to study acid and other ion movements. VILLEGAS (1969) has adapted this method to demonstrate that amobarbital can inhibit the hydrogen ion secretion, chloride transport and the water flux of the gastric mucosa. Methoxyflurane, chloroform and halothane can also inhibit the hydrogen ion and chloride movements of the gastric mucosa (MACKRELL and SCHWARTZ, 1969; SCHWARTZ and MACKRELL, 1969). These authors feel that these actions may be due to the anesthetics entering the "channels" of the gastric mucosa membrane and impeding hydrogen and chloride ion flow.

V. Absorption

The homeostasis of the body is intimately involved with the bidirectional flux of water and electrolytes in the gut. The normal and pathological patterns of absorption have been well documented in the literature. It has been demonstrated that the small bowel of man is capable of normal bidirectional movement of water within 24 h after various operative procedures (TINCKLER and KULKE, 1963). In contrast, the stomach and colon have a decreased capacity for absorbing water after various major operative procedures or traumatic injury (HOWARD, 1955; DRAWHORN and HOWARD, 1957).

No clinical studies involving a comparison of the action of inhalation anesthetic agents on absorption of water and/or ion, carbohydrate, protein, or lipid deriv-atives in either the stomach, small intestine or colon are available. The effects of anesthetics on the various absorptive mechanisms in different portions of the alimentary tract are a necessary and important study. Clinical or laboratory studies involving absorption might give some insight into a better choice of an anesthetic agent in situations where assimilational or nutritional status is marginal. Significant, rather than subtle differences may be the reward of such proposed studies, for qualitative and not just quantitative differences have been observed in animal studies.

Diethyl ether significantly depressed the absorption of glucose but not iodide in the upper gastrointestibal tract of the rat (REYNELL and SPRAY, 1957), while pentobarbital at a comparable anesthestic level did not interfere with the absorp-tion of either substance. Chloroform also depressed absorption of glucose in the rat (CORDIER and CHANEL, 1948). A study by HELLER and SMIRK (1932) demonstrated that chloroform and diethyl ether significantly decreased absorption of orally administered water. However, this could be related to an altered stomach emptying time induced by the two anesthetics. A study on the effects of xenon on isolated cecum of rat indicated that this agent alters water transport (BERGER et al., 1968). Anesthetic doses of pentobarbital sodium in dogs did not alter the bidirectional movement of sodium or water in the ileum or the exsorption (movement from blood to gut) in the duodenum (CODE et al., 1960). Pentobarbital sodium had no effect on calcium absorption from the small intestine of dogs (exact portion of intestine studied was not indicated) (CRAMER et al., 1967). Halothane prolongs DNA synthesis in the epithelial cells of the small intestine of the rat (BRUCE and TRAURIG, 1969). This susceptibility of the cells to halothane could alter the absorptive function of the gut. This latter point is need of further study, particularly with other anesthetics.

VI. Motility

A. Physiology

Concepts based on gastrointestinal electric and motor activity are establishing new relations among smooth muscle contractions, pressure wave activity, propulsion and rate of transit through the tract (CODE, 1968). The small bowel of man has a frequency gradient of electric activity, 11.7 in the proximal and 9.5 cycles per min in the distal end. The cyclic electric phenomena, called the basic electric rhythm, determines the maximal frequency of contractions for both longitudinal and circular smooth muscle. This pattern of frequency gradients is similar in all species studied; however, the absolute values may vary among species. Local conditions along the tract and integrated nerve plexi activity throughout the tract determine whether and to what degree smooth muscle contractions take place. Thus, the alimentary canal has pacemaker activity inherent to the smooth muscle and nerve receptors which influence contractile activity. The coordination of both intrinsic and extrinsic mechanisms effect the contractions of the smooth muscle.

The majority of pressure waves recorded from the small intestine result from circular muscle activity [BASS and WILEY, 1965 (1, 2)]. These circular muscle contractions slow aboral or oral movement of contents by increasing resistance although allowing for maximal mixing and absorption of chyme. This type of activity has been described as rhythmic segmentation (CANNON, 1911). Chyme is moved down the small intestine, and regulated by at least two principles: (1) the maximal frequency of electric and motor activity is higher in the upper than in the lower small bowel. This tends to move chyme in the aboral direction; (2) a flow-resistance relationship exists which moves material in an orad or aboral direction from a high zone of activity (rhythmic segmentation) to a area of low activity. The latter principle was discussed and demonstrated under *Gastric emptying*. Based on these principles, morphine exerts its constipating action by increasing tone and stimulating rhythmic segmentation (increased resistance) simultaneously throughout all areas of the small intestine (VAUGHAN-WILLIAMS, 1954). In contrast, saline cathartics act by decreasing resistance to flow throughout the small bowel (BASS, 1969). Diarrhea is associated with a quiet sigmoid colon and constipation with a active sigmoid colon (CONNELL, 1962).

Considerable difficulty in understanding flow through the alimentary tract occurs in concepts which are based on propulsion being equated to "peristalsis". This term has ambiguous meanings when applied to the small intestine. In physiological studies, a continuous stripping or conducting motor wave which has been called "peristalsis" is not seen in normal dog's or man's small intestine. Peristalsis may be adequate to describe the brief colonic contractile event during defecation but not the normal mixing and slow aboral movement of chyme in the small and large intestine.

Two physiological conditions of the gastrointestinal tract exist which are the interdigestive (fasting) and the digestive (fed) states. The motor characteristics for these two states have been characterized in the dog (REINKE et al., 1967).

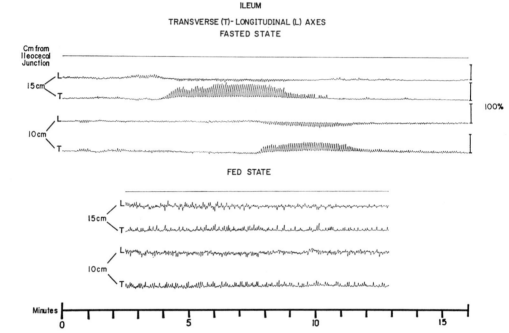

Fig. 5. Ileal contractile activity patterns from dog. Examples of three patterns of contractile activity obtained simultaneously from circular and longitudinal muscle layers. Fasted-state record (at top) after 20-hour fast. Fed-state record (at bottom) obtained from same animal 4 hours after meal of canned dog food. One hundred percent represents maximum contractile force attained for each lead, T indicates transverse axis; L, longitudinal axis. From REINKE etal. (1967)

An example of the motor patterns during fed and fasted states in the ileum of dog are shown in Fig. 5. During the interdigestive state, the predominant contractile pattern is *basal* activity interrupted by *burst* activity. The digestive state is dominated by *intermediate* activity. Thus, control patterns of activity must be established before drug evaluation.

B. Preanesthetic Medication

This monograph relates specifically to the actions of volatile inhalational anesthetic agents in man. The authors have considered experiments performed in laboratory animals since the preanesthetic medicants, e.g., atropine, promethazine, morphine and anesthetics affect gastrointestinal motility in clinically effective doses (GOLDEN and MANN, 1943; JOHNSON and MANN, 1942; MARSHALL et al., 1961; PUESTOW, 1940; RAVENTÓS, 1961; REINKE et al., 1967; ROSS et al., 1963; WEISEL et al., 1938).

Drugs used for their primary effects on other systems frequently markedly alter gut function. Neostigmine in clinical doses used to antagonize curariform muscle paralysis also affects gastrointestinal activity (MARSHALL et al., 1961; PUESTOW, 1940; REINKE et al., 1967). The clinical investigator who desires analgesia in his patient "overdoses" the gastrointestinal tract with morphine because the gut is more sensitive than the central nervous system. The laboratory investigator markedly "overdoses" the gastrointestinal tract with morphine (> .5 mg/kg), since he is trying to put his animal in a state of gross central nervous system depression. One need only recall that the gastrointestinal action of paregoric can occur at an oral dose of 20 μg/kg (one-sixth grain in a 50 kg person). With these observations in mind, we can proceed to evaluate the data available on the action of inhalation anesthetics on gastrointestinal motility.

C. Pharmacology

1. Gastric and Intestinal Contractile Activity

An early roentgenographic observation established that diethyl ether and chloroform depressed stomach movements in the dog (BÁRON and BÁRSONY, 1914). A more precise quantitative study was conducted by MILLER (1926). Following surgical preparation of dogs with a stomach fistula, a Thiry-Vella loop of small bowel and an appendicostomy, the animals were allowed to recover and trained to lie quietly on a table. Contractile activity was determined by insertion of a rubber balloon into the appropriate fistula. MILLER was careful to prove that this type of balloon did not appear to stimulate contractile activity. He observed that ether and chloroform in stage I and II slightly depressed gastric contractile amplitude and tone. Stage III was characterized by an almost complete inhibition of amplitude and tone. The stomach was slow to recover (ca. 5 h) with either anesthetic, although the small intestine and colon recovered much more rapidly. Ethylene had little if any effect even in a comparable surgical plane. BISGARD and JOHNSON (1939) in a similar experiment, except that gastric contractile activity was recorded via a Pavlov pouch, confirmed the finding of MILLER with regard to ether. Nitrous oxide was also noted to depress gastric, intestinal and colonic contractile amplitude, however, cyclopropane produced an actual stimulation of contractile amplitude. The stimulation induced by cyclopropane was also noted by BURSTEIN (1938) in chronic Thiry-Vella loop dogs. Gastric contractile activity was not studied. Tone and amplitude were stimulated in plane I and II, but contractile amplitude was depressed while tone remained elevated in plane III. Ether depressed both amplitude and tone throughout all planes of stage III. BISGARD and JOHNSON (1939) also observed that oxygen stimulated and carbon dioxide depressed gastric, intestinal and colonic contractions. It is perhaps worth emphasizing that, like preanesthetic medication, hypoxia and hypercapnia may also be factors to be critically controlled when studying inhalation anesthetics on the gut. Carbon dioxide accumulation is also suspected to augment the emetic action of anesthetics (DORNETTE et al., 1962). In an extended study involving the stomach of the dog, JOHNSON and MANN (1942) surgically prepared Mann-Bollman fistulas in which a segment of ileum is used to make a passage from the gastric body to the anterior abdominal wall. An air-filled balloon was used to record contractility. The period of induction was not studied, only a steady 15-min state after reaching plane II. Ether was depressant to gastric contractile amplitude and tone and recovery required up to 10 h. Cyclopropane was also similar to ether. As quoted by LEECH (1939), Seevers showed that 6% cyclopropane depressed gastric contractile amplitude in man. JOHNSON and MANN also observed only transient depression with nitrous oxide, ethylene, Avertin (tribromoethanol in amylene hydrate) and thiopental. They concluded that the depth of anesthesia was the most critical factor with regard to depression of gastric contractile activity. Further, they were able to demonstrate that the duration of anesthesia (75 vs. 15 min) at the same depth did not appreciably prolong the transient depression of gastric contractile activity depression. Thus on termination of anesthesia, we might conclude that loss of the above four anesthetics from the gastrointestinal tract takes place rapidly. Finally double vagotomy and/or double splanchnicectomy did not alter the results presented for JOHNSON and MANN's work. MARSHALL et al. (1961) observed that halothane depressed gastric and intestinal contractile amplitude and tone. The stomach was completely intact in this study and an esophageal tube with a balloon was used to record gastric contractile activity. BLACK (1965) also noted similar actions for halothane.

A few studies have been conducted to determine the site and mechanism of action of inhalation anesthetics on the gastrointestinal tract. BURN and EPSTEIN (1959) initially presented evidence that halothane was a ganglionic blocking agent and had a direct relaxing action on intestinal smooth muscle in vitro. Shortly thereafter, RAVENTÓS (1961) in an extensive and well-designed study demonstrated that various ganglia exhibited different sensitivities to halothane. Mesenteric ganglia were most sensitive (.5—.75% halothane); stellate ganglion (1%) and superior cervical ganglion (2%). He also showed that intestinal contractility induced by vagal stimulation in the animal was blocked by 1% halothane but not that of intestinal contractile activity induced by methacholine. However, MARSHALL et al. (1961) did demonstrate that halothane antagonized both methacholine and barium chloride induced intestinal contractile activity in acute canine preparations. This latter study indicated perhaps that halothane had the potential to act as a direct smooth muscle depressant.

SPEDEN (1965) compared the action of inhalation agents on the transmurally stimulated guinea pig ileum. Although this is an in vitro technique, the study is particularly informative because SPEDEN used bath concentrations for the various anesthetics which fell within the ranges of the blood concentrations of the same anesthetics found during surgical anesthesia. Diethyl ether, halothane, chloroform, methoxyflurane and trichloroethylene all depressed the response of the ileum stimulated either electrically, or by acetylcholine or potassium chloride. All anesthetics also slowed the rate of relaxation following an electrically-induced twitch. The ED_{50} for depression of the electrically-induced twitch for halothane, chloroform and methoxyflurane were well within their respective blood concentration ranges required for surgical anesthesia. Trichloroethylene was slightly higher and ether was considerably higher in concentrations needed to depress the electrically stimulated bowel. Further, ether and trichloroethylene invariably depressed the response to acetylcholine to the same extent or more than the electrically induced twitch, while halothane, methoxyflurane and chloroform usually had less effect on the response to acetylcholine than on the twitch. Ether and trichloroethylene were slightly stimulant to the preparation initially. Chloroform produced a definite stimulation of contractile activity which was not blockable by the anticholinergic, atropine or by lachesine. Although SPEDEN did not comment on the possibility, we feel that such stimulation may be due to darmstoff possibly being extracted from the intestine by the chloroform (BASS and BENNETT, 1968).

The Biebl loop is a more "natural" preparation than the Thiry-Vella loop in that intestinal continuity is not compromised and a more normal chyme of either the fasted or fed state is present within the lumen. The Biebl loop is an uninterrupted intestinal segment four to six inches long, exteriorized, and enclosed in a skin flap. It has the appearance of a suitcase handle on the abdomen. GOLDEN and MANN (1943) prepared chronic dogs with Biebl loops of jejunum (close to the duodenum) or ileum (close to the ileocecal junction). Two animals had both loops. Contractile activity was determined via a small balloon. They compared a number of anesthetic agents during a steady state period of 15 min in plane II. Feeding response were also determined for each animal as soon as the animal recovered from anesthesia. Such feeding responses were undoubtedly mediated through extrinsic nervous activity or were of hormonal origin rather than through local intrinsic reflexes, as the responses occurred in the jejunal loop within 3 and the ileal loop within 8 min. Contractile activity was depressed and the feeding response blocked by both morphine (1 mg/kg) or atropine (.6 mg total dose), but these doses are high compared to the human preanesthetic medication dose on a per kilogram basis. Diethyl ether, ethylene, and cyclopropane all depressed contractile activity in both loops and none of the agents affected the feeding response. They differed only in their duration of action in that ether persisted 10—25 min, ethylene 5 min, and cyclopropane recovery was immediate on cessation of anesthesia. Ether's degree and duration of depression of contractile activity was the same whether a 15 or 75 min steady state of plane II was chosen. This confirms results when a different method of study was employed (JOHNSON and MANN, 1942). It is interesting to note in GOLDEN and MANN's study that contractile activity depression induced by intravenous thiopental was related to the speed of injection. It persisted 8—12 min if given rapidly or had no effect if given slowly. This effect would certainly parallel the time course of the anticipated hypotension induced by rapid intravenous thiopental. The subsequent reflex sympathetic stimulation was likely the cause of the depression of contractile amplitude. One cannot overemphasize the necessity of considering all actions of a chemical when examining any one of its actions on a particular physiological system. This obviously includes all reflexly-induced responsed whether they tend to reinforce or to counteract the final measured response(s).

2. Gastrointestinal Transit

Contractile activity is not always directly correlated with propulsive motility (CONNELL, 1961; GIUS and PETERSON, 1944). Intestinal propulsive motility can be recorded in a Thiry-Vella loop of intestine in one way by placing a bolus (cotton wool) in one end and determining transit time through the loop. WEISEL et al. (1938) utilized such a preparation in eleven chronic dogs in which the loops were either normal or denervated. Their results were the same whether the loops were normal or denervated. Some of the animals were premedicated with large doses of morphine (1 mg/kg), and/or scopolamine (.6—1.2 mg total). Initial stimulation of contractile amplitude and tone was observed for morphine while scopolamine depressed such activity. However both depressed propulsive motility. Cyclopropane also initially stimulated contractile activity but not propulsive motility — see also VAN LIERE et al. (1947). Depressed contractile activity induced by a higher concentration of cyclopropane was only partially effective in blocking a stimulating dose of morphine. Considerably more information is obtained from a study of propulsive motility coupled with contractile activity, and helps to resolve apparent differences between ether and cyclopropane noted when only contractile activity is studied.

At the turn of the century, it was generally accepted that anesthesia per se did not affect the gastrointestinal tract. Investigators, as cited by Sleeth and van Liere (1938), then began to present evidence that this was not the case. From approximately 1925—1940, studies were extended to compare the capacity of different inhalational anesthetic agents to alter gastrointestinal activity (Emerson, 1937; Luckhardt and Lewis, 1923; Miller, 1926; Peoples and Phatak, 1935; Sleeth and van Liere, 1938; van Liere et al., 1947) generally under the same conditions of depth and duration of anesthesia. The pharmacology of the anesthetic gases prior to 1938 was reviewed by Seevers and Waters (1938). Some information on the actions of nitrous oxide, ethylene and cyclopropane on the gastrointestinal tract was included in this review. In the last three decades, clinical as well as laboratory studies have stressed the importance of such a comparison at the same level of the gastrointestinal tract. Following surgery, gastric and colonic motility was found to be much more affected than small intestine motility regardless of the anesthetic agent employed (Baker et al., 1964; Baker and Webster, 1968; Rothnie et al., 1963; Tinckler, 1965; Wells et al., 1961, 1964). When water, glucose or radioopaque drug absorption rather than motility was used as the index of activity, similar parallels were observed (Drawhorn and Howard, 1957; Tinckler and Kulke, 1963). Consequently, advocates of early feeding postoperatively are increasing if fluid can be assured to reach the small intestine (Rothnie et al., 1963; Ross et al., 1963; Wells et al., 1961, 1964).

VII. Gas

The subject of gastrointestinal gas has been extensively discussed in a symposium (Berk, 1968) and in a review (Calloway, 1968). Gas of varying constituents is a normal substance in the alimentary tract, particularly the stomach and colon. The tract normally contains 115 ± 23 ml (Bedell et al., 1956). This volume is based on 23 observations on 13 normal subjects. There is no corresponding study in people who are awaiting surgery, where apprehension, preanesthetic medication or the influence of a host of other variables could readily alter the gas content of the gut.

Gas in the alimentary canal can arise from several sources. The major source is swallowed air. Other contributing sources are fermentation, passage from blood to gut and intraluminal CO_2 arising from acidic gastric effluent with salivary, biliary and pancreatic bicarbonates. In normal individuals a bolus of swallowed air is rapidly transported through the gastrointestinal tract. This was demonstrated by Magnusson (1931), who self-administered 0.75 l of air and radiologically noted that the air moved from stomach to cecum in from 6—30 min and to the rectum in 36 min. This rapid passage of air has been confirmed in nine people by Maddock et al. (1949). Gas in the gastrointestinal tract can exchange with the environment, with other material in the lumen and with surrounding blood and tissues. The physiological basis for these exchanges are reviewed by Forster (1968). Clinical aspects of intestinal gas have also been presented by Andersen and Ringsted (1943), and Hood (1966).

The exchange of gas (anesthetics) from blood to gastrointestinal lumen may be a factor in anesthetic dynamics. This factor has not been evaluated. In a study in cats anesthetized with amobarbital (50 mg/kg), 50 cc of various gases (oxygen, nitrogen, hydrogen, methane, hydrogen sulphide, carbon dioxide or air) when placed in the small intestine, showed differences in the rate of diffusion [McIver et al., 1926 (2)]. It is conceivable that different anesthetics may diffuse at different rates across the bowel wall.

Though not common, acute dilatation of the stomach can represent a potentially lethal situation during the administration of anesthetic. The exact cause and physiological mechanism of the acute gastric dilatation has not been elucidated, though McIver (1927) and Morris et al. (1947) demonstrated that this condition is due to swallowed air. Experimental studies suggest that arterial hypotension which accompanies acute gastric dilatation is a result of decreased venous return and may be a cause of death (Engler et al., 1967).

Some degree of stomach distention, though not life threatening, may be present during and after anesthetics. Studies in cats, anesthetized with chloralose, showed that 60—90 cc of air injected into the stomach stimulated motility but the air was not expelled [McIver et al., 1926 (1)]. Sectioning the vagus nerve did not alter the situation. Sectioning the vagus and the splanchnic nerves resulted in the gas readily passing into the small bowel. The retention of this air in the stomach also suggests that the gastroesophageal sphincter may not relax normally under anesthesia. Clinical observations made by McIver et al. [1926 (1)] suggest that as many as 26 of 107 patients had some degree of postoperative stomach distention. These patients had received ether, preceded by nitrous oxide. The authors observed that in three patients receiving ether that during induction there were 115, 67 and 54 swallows, respectively. Presumably, current techniques of handling patients markedly reduce the incidence of distention though a study in 1945 indicated that air swallowing is still common during the induction of anesthesia (Davis and Hanson, 1945). The problem of air swallowing was quantified by Maddock et al. (1949). In a study of 23 patients receiving a variety of anesthetics, and morphine (10 mg) and atropine (4 mg), the swift induction with modern anesthetics resulted in very few swallowing movements (e.g., 1.5 swallows per patient) and minimal amounts of gas in the stomach (Table 3). The only incidence of stomach distention was when positive pressure was used to augment respiration (Table 3).

Table 3. *Air ingestion during anesthesia*

	No. of patients	Induction period			Operative period		
		time min	swallows	gas cc	time min	swallows	gas cc
Spinal and thiopental	7	16.7	0.0	0.0	133.9	0.6	179.3
NO_2 or C_2H_4 or $C_3H_6 + O_2$ + ether	6	6.7	1.7	21.7	95.0	0.6	45.8
Cyclopropane and curare	5	5.6	0.6	0.0	103.6	0.0	31.0
Cyclopropane and curare + augmented positive pressure	5	5.8	2.2	41.0	144.8	0.0	952.0

Modified from Maddock et al. (1949).

An inherent danger to the patient as well as to the anesthesiologist is the accumulation of combustible gas in the stomach or colon. Several cases of this type of gas accumulation are presented by Galley (1954).

Alterations in gastric pressure may be induced with adjunct drugs used with anesthetics. Andersen (1962) reported that succinylcholine when used in combination with thiopental anesthesia led to increased gastric pressures in 3 of 10 patients which coincided with the time of most pronounced twitching. A conflicting study in 25 patients (Roe, 1962), who were administered succinylcholine at the time of thiopental anesthesia, showed no consistent marked change in intra-gastric pressure. In any event, any abdominal muscle activity which leads to changes of gastric pressure would also exert an equal pressure on the abdominal portion of the gastroesophageal sphincter and would not necessarily mean that regurgitation was inevitable.

Summary

The actions of anesthetics on the gastrointestinal tract have been reviewed. Emphasis was placed on current physiological concepts. These concepts are essential for the design and interpretation of the action of anesthetics on the gastrointestinal tract. The actions of anesthetics were assessed for their actions on the various gastrointestinal parameters. The gastrointestinal functions discussed were areas that should be of some concern to the practicing anesthesiologist.

The paucity of quantitative data on actions of anesthetics on the gastrointestinal tract is emphasized. Extensive research is necessary to answer pertinent questions on the actions of anesthetics on the gastrointestinal tract. These answers would lead to better prophylactic treatment of patients that develop problems before, during or in the recovery period.

References

ABAJIAN, J., Jr., BRAZELL, E. H., DENTE, G. A., MILLS, E. L.: Experience with halothane (Fluothane) in more than five thousand cases. J. Am. Med. Assoc. 171, 535—540 (1959).
ANDERSEN, K., RINGSTED, A.: Clinical and experimental investigations on ileus with particular reference to the genesis of intestinal gas. Acta Chir. Scand. 88, 475—502 (1943).
ANDERSEN, N.: Changes in intragastric pressure following the administration of suxamethonium. Brit. J. Anaesthesia 34, 363—367 (1962).
ANDERSON, J. J., BOLT, R. J., ULLMAN, B. M., BASS, P.: Differential response to various stimulants in the body and antrum of the canine stomach. Am. J. Digest. Diseases 13, 147—156 (1968).
ARTUSIO, J. F.: Halogenated anesthetics. Philadelphia, Pennsylvania: F. A. Davis Co. 1963.
— VAN POZNAK, A., HUNT, R. E., TIERS, F. M., ALEXANDER, M.: A clinical evaluation of methoxyflurane in man. Anesthesiology 21, 512—517 (1960).
ATKINSON, M.: Mechanism protecting against gastro-oesophageal reflux: A review. Gut 3, 1—15 (1962).
BAKER, L. W., JONES, P. F., DUDLEY, H. A. F.: Intestinal activity after operation. Proc. Roy. Soc. Med. 57, 391—394 (1964).
— WEBSTER, D. R.: Postoperative intestinal motility. Brit. J. Surg. 55, 374—378 (1968).
BANNISTER, W. K., SATILLARO, A. J.: Vomiting and aspiration during anesthesia. Anesthesiology 23, 251—264 (1962).
BÁRON, A., BÁRSONY, T.: Über die Einwirkung der Chloroform- und Äthernarkose auf die motorischen Magenfunktionen. Arch. ges. Physiol., Pflüger's 158, 464—477 (1914).
BASS, P.: Personal observations (1969).
— BENNETT, D. R.: Local chemical regulation of motor action of the bowel-substance P and lipid-soluble acids. In: Handbook of physiology, Sec. 6: Alimentary canal, Vol. 4. Washington, D.C.: Amer. Physiol. Soc. 1968.
— CODE, C. F., LAMBERT, E. H.: Electric activity of gastro-duodenal junction. Am. J. Physiol. 201, 587—592 (1961).
— PATTERSON, M. A.: Gastric secretory responses to drugs affecting adrenergic mechanisms in rats. J. Pharmacol. Exptl Therap. 156, 142—149 (1966).
— WILEY, J. N.: (1) Effects of ligation and morphine on electric and motor activity of dog duodenum. Am. J. Physiol. 208, 908—913 (1965).
— — (2) Electrical and extraluminal contractile-force activity of the duodenum of the dog. Am. J. Digest. Disease 10, 183—200 (1965).
BEDELL, G. N., MARSHALL, R., DU BOIS, A. B., HARRIS, J. H.: Measurement of the volume of gas in the gastrointestinal tract. Values in normal subjects and ambulatory patients. J. Clin. Invest. 35, 336—345 (1956).

BEECHER, H. K.: Experimental pharmacology and measurement of subjective response. Science 116, 157—162 (1952).

BELLVILLE, J. W.: Postanesthetic nausea and vomiting. Anesthesiology 22, 773—780 (1961).

BERGER, E. Y., PECIKYAM, F. R., KANZAKI, G.: Anesthetic gases and water structure. The effect of xenon on tritiated water flux across the gut. J. Gen. Physiol. 52, 876—886 (1968).

BERK, J. E. (Ed.): Gastrointestinal gas. Ann. N.Y. Acad. Sci. 150, 1—190 (1968).

BISGARD, J. D., JOHNSON, E. K.: The influence of certain drugs and anesthetics upon gastro-intestinal tone and motility. Ann. Surg. 110, 802—822 (1939).

BLACK, G. W.: A review of the pharmacology of halothane. Brit. J. Anaesthesia 37, 688—705 (1965).

BODMAN, R. I., MORTON, H. J. V., THOMAS, E. T.: Vomiting by out-patients after nitrous oxide anaesthesia. Brit. Med. J. 1960 I, 1327—1330.

BONICA, J. J.: Aspiration of gastric contents. In: Principles and practice of obstetric anal-gesia and anesthesia. Philadelphia, Pennsylvania: F. A. Davis Co. 1967.

— CREPPS, W., MONK, B., BENNETT, B.: Postanesthetic nausea, retching and vomiting. Evaluation of cyclizine (Marezine) suppositories for treatment. Anesthesiology 19, 532 to 540 (1958).

BORISON, H. L., WANG, S. C.: Physiology and pharmacology of vomiting. Pharmacol. Revs 5, 193—230 (1953).

BOURNE, J. G.: Anaesthesia and the vomiting hazard. A safe method for obstetric and other emergencies. Anaesthesia 17, 379—382 (1962).

BRÅHAMMAR, N. S., EMMELIN, N.: The effect of narcotics, especially barbiturates, on salivary secretion, elicited through chorda stimulation or parasympathomimetic drugs. Acta Physiol. Scand. 3, 182—184 (1942).

BRUCE, D. L., TRAURIG, H. H.: The effect of halothane on the cell cycle in rat small intestine. Anesthesiology 30, 401—405 (1969).

BURN, J. H., EPSTEIN, H. G.: Hypotension due to halothane. Brit. J. Anaesthesia 31, 199 to 204 (1959).

BURSTEIN, C. L.: Effect of cyclopropane anesthesia on intestinal activity in vivo. Proc. Soc. Exptl Biol. Med. 38, 530—532 (1938).

BURTLES, R., PECKETT, B. W.: Postoperative vomiting. Some factors affecting its incidence. Brit. J. Anasthesia 29, 114—123 (1957).

CALLOWAY, D. H.: Gas in the alimentary canal. In: Handbook of physiology, Sec. 6: Alimen-tary canal, Vol. 5. Wahington, D.C.: Amer. Physiol. Soc. 1968.

CANNON, W. B.: The mechanical factors of digestion. London: Arnold 1911.

— MURPHY, F. T.: Physiologic observations on experimentally produced ileus. J. Am. Med. Assoc. 49, 840—843 (1907).

CHANG, C. A., McKENNA, R. D., BECK, I. T.: Gastric emptying rate of the water and fat phases of a mixed test meal in man. Gut 9, 420—424 (1968).

CHANG, J., MACARTNEY, H. H., GRAVES, H. B.: Clinical experience with Fluothane, a new non-explosive anaesthetic agent. Canad. Anaesth. Soc. J. 4, 187—206 (1957).

CODE, C. F. (Ed.): Handbook of physiology, Sec. 6: Alimentary canal, Vol. 4. Washington, D.C.: Amer. Physiol. Soc. 1968.

— Personal communication (1969).

— BASS, P., McCLARY, G. B., Jr., NEWNUM, R. L., ORVIS, A. L.: Absorption of water, sodium and potassium in small intestine of dogs. Am. J. Physiol. 199, 281—288 (1960).

— CREAMER, B., SCHLEGEL, J. F., OLSEN, A. M., DONOGHUE, F. E., ANDERSEN, H. A.: An atlas of esophageal motility in health and disease. Springfield, Illinois: C. C. Thomas 1958.

— SCHLEGEL, J. F.: Motor action of the esophagus and its sphincters. In: Handbook of physi-ology, Sec. 6: Alimentary canal, Vol. 4. Washington, D. C.: Amer. Physiol. Soc. 1968.

CONNELL, A. M.: The motility of the small intestine. Postgrad. med. J. 37, 703—716 (1961).

— The motility of the pelvic colon. Part II. Paradoxical motility in diarrhoea and consti-pation. Gut 3, 342—348 (1962).

CORDIER, D., CHANEL, J.: Influence des anésthésiques volatils et des barbituriques sur la vitesse du transit gastrique et l'absorption intestinale des solutions de glucose chez le rat. Compt. rend. soc. biol. 142, 1120—1122 (1948).

CRAMER, C. F., SADLER, S. J., SCHULZ, R. G.: A plastic-cannulated intestinal loop to study effects of anesthesia on Ca absorption. J. Appl. Physiol. 22, 1149—1150 (1967).

CRAWFORD, J. S.: Some aspects of obstetric anaesthesia. Brit. J. Anaesthesia 28, 201—208 (1956).

CREAMER, B.: Oesophageal reflux. Lancet 1955 I, 279—281.

— Motor disturbances of the esophagus. In: Handbook of physiology, Sec. 6, Vol. 4. Washing-ton, D.C.: Amer. Physiol. Soc. 1968.

CULVER, G. A., MAKEL, H. P., BEECHER, H. K.: Frequency of aspiration of gastric contents by the lungs during anesthesia and surgery. Ann. Surg. 133, 289—292 (1951).

322 D. R. Bennett and P. Bass

Davies, R. M.: Some factors affecting the incidence of postanesthetic vomiting. Brit. Med. J.
1941 II, 578—580.
Davis, H. H., Hansen, T. M.: Investigation of the cause and prevention of gas pains following
abdominal operation. Surgery 17, 492—497 (1945).
Dent, S. J., Ramachandra, V., Stephen, C. R.: Post-operative vomiting: Incidence,
analysis and therapeutic measures in 3,000 patients. Anesthesiology 16, 564—572 (1955).
Dinnick, O. P.: Some aspects of general anaesthesia. Proc. Roy. Soc. Med. 50, 547—552
(1957).
Dornette, W. H. L., Miller, G. L., Sheffield, W. E., Cavallaro, R. J., Poe, M. F.:
Clinical experiences with trifluoroethyl vinyl ethe anesthesia. Anesthesia & Analgesia 41,
605—614 (1962).
Drawhorn, C. W., Howard, J. M.: Further studies on the absorption and equilibration of
water (deuterium oxide) from the gastro-intestinal tract. Ann. Surg. 146, 239—245 (1957).
Dundee, J. W.: Evaluation of the effect of halothane on postoperative vomiting. Brit. J.
Anaesthesia 40, 633—634 (1968).
Emerson, G. E.: Intestinal motility in rats anesthetized with ether. Amer. J. Digest. Disease
4, 255—256 (1937).
Emmelin, N.: Evipan and the parasympathetic nervous system. Acta Physiol. Scand. 2, 289
to 310 (1941).
Engler, H. S., Kennedy, T. E., Ellison, L. T., Purvis, J. G., Moretz, W. H.: Hemo-
dynamics of experimental acute gastric dilatation. Am. J. Surg. 113, 194—198 (1967).
Forshall, I.: The cardio-esophageal syndrome in childhood. Arch. Disease Childhood 30,
46—54 (1955).
Forster, R. E.: Physiological basis of gas exchange in the gut. In: Gastrointestinal gas
(Berk, Ed.). Ann. N.Y. Acad. Sci. 150, 4—12 (1968).
Fyke, F. E., Jr., Code, C. F., Schlegel, J. F.: The gastroesophageal sphincter in healthy
human beings. Gastroenterologia 86, 135—150 (1956).
Galley, A. H.: Combustible gases generated in the alimentary tract and other hollow viscera
and their relationship to explosions occurring during anesthesia. Brit. J. Anaesthesia 26,
189—193 (1954).
George, J. D.: New clinical method for measuring the rate of gastric emptying: The double
sampling test meal. Gut 9, 237—242 (1968).
Giuffrida, J. G., Bizzarri, D.: Intubation of the esophagus. Am. J. Surg. 93, 329—334
(1957).
Gius, J. A., Peterson, C. G.: Postoperative ileus and related gastrointestinal complications.
Surg. Gynecol. Obstet., Abstr. Suppl. 79, 265—291 (1944).
Golden, R. F., Mann, F. C.: The effects of drugs used in anesthesiology on the tone and
motility of the small intestine: An experimental study. Anesthesiology 4, 577—595 (1943).
Griffith, G. H., Owen, G. M., Kirkman, S., Schields, R.: Measurement of rate of gastric
emptying using chromium-51. Lancet 1966 I, 1244—1245.
Gryboski, J. D., Thayer, W. R., Jr., Spiro, H. M.: Esophageal motility in infants and
children. Pediatrics 31, 382—395 (1963).
Guimarais, J. A., Malafaya-Baptista, A., Garrett, J., Osswald, W.: Barbituriques et
sécrétion salivaire antagonisme de l'effet inhibiteur sécrétoire. Arch. intern. pharmacodynamie. 102, 235—248 (1955).
Hamelberg, W., Bosomworth, P. P.: Inhalation of gastric contents. GP, J. Am. Acad. Gen.
Pract. 32, 130—134 (1965).
Haumann, J. le R., Foster, P. A.: The anti-emetic effect of halothane. Brit. J. Anaesthesia
35, 114—117 (1963).
Heller, H., Smirk, F. H.: Studies concering the alimentary absorption of water and tissue
hydration in relation to diuresis. Part IV. The influence of anaesthetics and hypnotics on
the absorption and excretion of water. J. Physiol. (London) 76, 292—302 (1932).
Henderson, V. E.: On the sensitivity of different nerve endings to atropine. J. Pharmacol.
Exptl Therap. 21, 99—102 (1923).
Hightower, N. C., Jr.: Motility of the alimentary canal of man. In: Disturbances in gastric
intestinal motility: diarrhea, constipation, biliary dysfunction. Springfield, Illinois: C. C.
Thomas 1959.
Holmes, J. M.: The prevention of inhaled vomit during obstetric anaesthesia. Proc. Roy. Soc.
Med. 50, 556 (1957).
Hood, J. H.: Clinical considerations of intestinal gas. Ann. Surg. 163, 359—366 (1966).
Horton, B. T.: Pyloric musculature with special reference to pyloric block. Am. J. Anat. 41,
197—225 (1928).
Howard, J. M.: Studies of the absorption and equilibration of water (deuterium oxide) from
the gastrointestinal tract following injury. Surg. Gynecol. Obstet. 100, 69—77 (1955).

HUNT, J. N.: Viscosity of a test-meal, its influence on gastric emptying and secretion. Lancet **1954 I**, 17—18.
— Gastric emptying and secretion in man. Physiol. Revs **39**, 491—533 (1959).
— KNOX, M. T.: Regulation of gastric emptying. In: Handbook of physiology, Sec. 6: Alimentary canal, Vol. 4. Washington, D.C.: Amer. Physiol. Soc. 1968.
— — The slowing of gastric emptying by nine acids. J. Physiol. (London) **201**, 161—179 (1969).
— WAN, B.: Electrolytes of mammalian gastric juice. In: Handbook of physiology, Sec. 6: Alimentary canal, Vol. 2. Washington, D.C.: Amer. Physiol. Soc. 1967.
HYTTEN, F. E., LEITCH, I.: The physiology of human pregnancy. Philadelphia, Pennsylvania: F. A. Davis Co. 1963.
INGELFINGER, F. J.: Esophageal motility. Physiol. Revs **38**, 533—584 (1958).
— The esophagus, March 1961 to February 1963. Gastroenterology **45**, 241—264 (1963).
JOHNSON, C. R., MANN, F. C.: Effects of gastric tonus and motility with special reference to acute gastric dilatation. Surgery **12**, 599—614 (1942).
JOHNSON, H. D.: The fluid mechanics of the control of reflux. Lancet **1966 II**, 1267—1268.
— LAWS, J. W.: The cardia in swallowing, eructation, and vomiting. Lancet **1966 II**, 1268 to 1273.
KANTROWITZ, P. A., SIEGEL, C. I., HENDRIX, T. R.: Differences in motility of the upper and lower esophagus in man and the its alteration by atropine. Bull. Johns Hopkins Hosp. **118**, 476—491 (1966).
KELLING, G.: Über den Mechanismus der akuten Magendilatation. Arch. klin. Chir. **64**, 393 to 417 (1901).
KNAPP, M. R., BEECHER, H. K.: Postanesthetic nausea, vomiting, and retching. Evaluation of the antiemetic drugs dimenhydrinate (Dramamine), chlorpromazine and pentobarbital sodium. J. Am. Med. Assoc. **160**, 376—385 (1956).
KRAMER, P.: The esophagus. Gastroenterology **49**, 439—463 (1965).
LASKIEWICZ, A.: Vomiting and eructation with regard to its upper respiratory organs. Acta Oto-Laryngol. **46**, 27—34 (1956).
LEE, J. A., ATKINSON, R. S.: A synopsis of anaesthesia, 5th ed. Baltimore, Maryland: Williams and Wilkins Comp. 1964.
LEECH, P. N.: The present status of cyclopropane—Report of the Council on Pharmacy and Chemistry. J. Am. Med. Assoc. **112**, 1064—1070 (1939).
LEVITT, M. N., DEDO, H. H., OGURA, J. H.: The cricopharyngeus muscle, an electromyographic study in the dog. Laryngoscope **75**, 122—136 (1965).
LUCKHARDT, AB., LEWIS, D.: Clinical experiences with ethylene-oxygen anesthesia. J. Am. Med. Assoc. **81**, 1851—1857 (1923).
MACKRELL, T. N., SCHWARTZ, M.: Electrophysiological effects of methoxyflurane (Penthrane) on frog gastric mucosa. Am. J. Physiol. **216**, 572—576 (1969).
MADDOCK, W. G., BELL, J. L., TREMAINE, M. J.: Gastro-intestinal gas. Observations on belching during anaesthesia, operations and pyelography; and rapid passage of gas. Ann. Surg. **130**, 512—535 (1949).
MAGNUSSON, W.: On meteorism in pyelography and on the passage of gas through the small intestine. Acta Radiol. **12**, 552—561 (1931).
MARSHALL, B. M., GORDON, R. A.: Vomiting, regurgitation and aspiration in anaesthesia, I. Canad. Anaesth. Soc. J. **5**, 274—281 (1958).
MARSHALL, F. N., PITTINGER, C. B., LONG, J. P.: Effects of halothane on gastrointestinal motility. Anesthesiology **22**, 363—366 (1961).
McCOY, E. J., BASS, P.: Chronic electrical activity of gastroduodenal area: effects of food and certain catecholamines. Am. J. Physiol. **205**, 439—445 (1963).
McIVER, M. A.: Acute dilatation of the stomach occurring under general anesthesia. Ann. Surg. **85**, 704—712 (1927).
— BENEDICT, E. B., CLINE, J. W., Jr.: (1) Postoperative gaseous distension of the intestine: an experimental and clinical study. Arch. Surg. **13**, 588—604 (1926).
— REDFIELD, A. C., BENEDICT, E. B.: (2) Gaseous exchange between the blood and the lumen of the stomach and intestines. Am. J. Physiol. **76**, 92—111 (1926).
McNALLY, E. F., KELLY, J. E., Jr., INGELFINGER, F. J.: Mechanism of belching: effects of gastric distention with air. Gastroenterology **46**, 254—259 (1964).
MERENDINO, K. A.: Pharmacological aspects of gastric secretion. Part V. The effect of phenobarbital on the gastric secretions in dog and man. Gastroenterology **10**, 531—539 (1948).
MILLER, G. H.: The effects of general anesthesia on the muscular activity of the gastrointestinal tract: a study of ether, chloroform, ethylene and nitrous oxide. J. Pharmacol. Exptl Therap. **27**, 41—59 (1926).
MONTGOMERY, M. F.: Effect of amytal upon pilocarpine-induced submaxillary and gastric secretion. Proc. Soc. Exptl. Biol. Med. **32**, 1287—1290 (1935).

MORRIS, C. R., IVY, A. C., MADDOCK, W. G.: Mechanism of acute abdominal distention. Arch.
  Surg. 55, 101—124 (1947).
MORTON, H. J. V., WYLIE, W. D.: Anaesthetic deaths due to regurgitation or vomiting.
  Anaesthesia 6, 190—205 (1951).
MUCKLOW, R. G., LARARD, D. G.: The effects of the inhalation of vomitus on the lungs:
  Clinical considerations. Brit. J. Anaesthesia 35, 153—159 (1963).
NOVOA, R. R.: The anti-emetic action of Fluothane: A comparative study in obstetrical
  anaesthesia. Canad. Anaesth. Soc. J. 7, 109—115 (1960).
O'MULLANE, E. J.: Vomiting and regurgitation during anaesthesia. Lancet 1954 I, 1209—1212.
PARKER, R. B.: Maternal death from aspiration asphyxia. Brit. Med. J. 1956 II, 16—19.
PEOPLES, S. A., PHATAK, N. M.: Effect of cyclopropane on isolated intestinal muscle. Proc. Soc.
  Exptl Biol. Med. 33, 287—289 (1935).
POWELL, D. W., HIRSCHOWITZ, B. I.: Sodium pentobarbital depression of histamine- or
  insulin-stimulated gastric secretion. Am. J. Physiol. 212, 1001—1006 (1967).
PUESTOW, C. B.: Intestinal motility of the dog and man. Urbana, Illinois: University of
  Illinois Press 1940
RAVENTÓS, J.: The action of fluothane on the autonomic nervous system. Helv. Chir. Acta
  28, 358—371 (1961).
REINKE, D. A., ROSENBAUM, A. H., BENNETT, D. R.: Patterns of dog gastrointestinal con-
  tractile activity monitored in vivo with extraluminal force transducers. Amer. J. Digest.
  Disease 12, 113—141 (1967).
REYNELL, P. C., SPRAY, G. H.: The effect of ether and pentobarbitone sodium on gastro-
  intestinal function in the intact rat. Brit. J. Pharmacol. 12, 104—106 (1957).
RIDING, J. E.: The prevention of postoperative vomiting. Brit. J. Anaesthesia 35, 180—188
  (1963).
RINALDO, J. A., Jr.: Some observations concerning the physiology of the distal esophagus
  with comments on hiatal hernia. Henry Ford. Hosp. Bull. 14, 77—83 (1966).
— LEVEY, J. F.: Correlation of several methods for recording esophageal sphincteral pressures.
  Am. J. Digest. Disease 13, 882—892 (1968).
ROBBINS, B. H.: Effect of various anesthetics on salivary secretion. J. Pharmacol. Exptl.
  Therap. 54, 426—432 (1935).
— Cyclopropane anesthesia, 2nd ed. Baltimore, Maryland: Williams and Wilkins Co. 1958.
ROBÉRT, A., NEZAMIS, J. E., PHILLIPS, J. P.: Inhibition of gastric secretion by prostaglandins.
  Am. J. Digest. Disease 12, 1073—1076 (1967).
ROE, R. B.: The effect of suxamethionium on intragastric pressure. Anaesthesia 17, 179—181
  (1962).
ROSS, B., WATSON, B. W., KAY, A. W.: Studies on the effect of vagotomy on small intestinal
  motility using the radiotelemetering capsule. Gut 4, 77—81 (1963).
ROTHNIE, N. G., HARPER, R. A. K., CATCHPOLE, B. N.: Early postoperative gastrointestinal
  activity. Lancet 1963 II, 64—67.
SCHNEYER, L. H., SCHNEYER, C. A.: Inorganic composition of saliva. In: Handbook of
  physiology, Sec. 6, Vol. 2. Washington D.C.: Amer. Physiol. Soc. 1967.
SCHWARTZ, M., MACKRELL, T. N.: A confirmation of electrogenicity of frog gastric mucosa by
  using methoxyflurane. Proc. Soc. Exptl. Biol. Med. 130, 1048—1051 (1969).
SEEVERS, M. H., WATERS, R. M.: Pharmacology of the anesthetic gases. Physiol. Revs 18,
  447—479 (1938).
SIMONSEN, L. E., VANDEWATER, S. L.: Postoperative vomiting: A review and present status
  of treatment. Canad. Anaesth. Soc. J. 9, 51—60 (1962).
SLEETH, C. K., VAN LIERE, E. J.: A comparative study of the effects of various anesthetic
  agents on the emptying time of the stomach. J. Pharmacol. Exptl Therap. 63, 65—69
  (1938).
SOKOL, E. M., HEITMANN, P., WOLF, B. S., COHEN, B. R.: Simultaneous cineradiographic and
  manometric study of the pharynx, hypopharynx and cervical esophagus. Gastroenterology
  51, 960—974 (1966).
SPEDEN, R. N.: Effect of some volatile anesthetics on transmurally stimulated guinea pig
  ileum. Brit. J. Pharmacol. 25, 104—118 (1965).
STAVRAKY, G. W.: Effect of amytal on the autonomic nervous system as indicated by the
  salivary glands. J. Pharmacol Exptl Therap. 43, 499—508 (1931).
STEVENS, J. H.: Anaesthetic problems of intestinal obstruction in adults. Brit. J. Anaesthesia
  36, 438—450 (1964).
TINCKLER, L. F.: Surgery and intestinal motility. Brit. J. Surg. 52, 140—150 (1965).
— KULKE, W.: Post-operative absorption of water from the small intestine. Gut 4, 8—12
  (1963).
VAN LIERE, E. J., STICKNEY, J. C., NORTHUP, D. W.: Camparative study of anesthetic agents
  on propulsive motility of the small intestine. Gastroenterology 8, 82—89 (1947).

VAUGHAN-WILLIAMS, E. M.: The mode of action of drugs on intestinal motility. Pharmacol. Revs **6**, 159—190 (1954).

VILLEGAS, L.: Inhibition by amytal of water movements in gastric mucosa. Biochim. et Biophys. Acta **173**, 348—350 (1969).

WATERS, R. M.: Present status of cyclopropane. Brit. Med. J. **1936 II**, 1013—1017.

WEAVER, D. C.: Preventing aspiration deaths during anesthesia. J. Am. Med. Assoc. **188**, 971—975 (1964).

WEISBRODT, N. W., WILEY, J. N., OVERHOLT, B. F., BASS, P.: A relation between gastro-duodenal muscle contractility and gastric emptying. Gut **10** 543—548 (1969).

WEISEL, W., YOUMANS, W. B., CASSELS, W. H.: Effect on intestinal motility of cyclopropane anesthesia alone and after morphine-scopolamine premedication. J. Pharmacol. Exptl Therap. **63**, 391—399 (1938).

WELLS, C., RAWLINSON, K., TINCKLER, L., JONES, H., SAUNDERS, J.: Ileus and postoperative intestinal motility. Lancet **1961 II**, 136—137.

— TINCKLER, L., RAWLINSON, K., JONES, H., SAUNDERS, J.: Postoperative gastrointestinal motility. Lancet **1964 I**, 4—10.

WOO, C., BROOKS, F. P.: The effect of subanesthetic doses of sodium pentobarbital on gastric content of spider monkeys (Ateles). Gastroenterology **45**, 239—240 (1963).

WYLIE, W. D., CHURCHILL-DAVISON, H. C.: Anaesthesia and the gastrointestinal tract. In: A practice of anaesthesia, 2nd ed. Chicago, Illinois: Year Book Med. Pub. 1966.

Section 5.0.

Absorption, Distribution and Excretion

5.1. Kinetics

W. W. MAPLESON

With 12 Figures

A. A Simple Analogue

Consider the system shown in Fig. 1. A number of open cylindrical vessels are interconnected by pipes. Water flows continuously and rapidly into the first vessel so that it is always liberally overflowing. When the lower tap is opened water flows into the second vessel where the water level begins to rise. Therefore a pressure head develops between the second vessel and the remaining vessels and water flows on into the remaining vessels where also the water levels begin to rise. The closer the water levels approach the constant head of water in the first vessel the slower becomes the rate of rise but, eventually, the water levels in all vessels come into equilibrium with the constant level in the first vessel.

This system is an analogue of the way in which an inhaled anesthetic is taken up by and distributed within the body. The water represents the anesthetic itself; the constant head of water in the first vessel represents a constant inspired partial pressure, or tension, of the anesthetic; the gradually-rising levels of water in the other vessels represent the gradually-rising tensions of anesthetic in different parts of the body. The second vessel represents the lungs and the remaining vessels

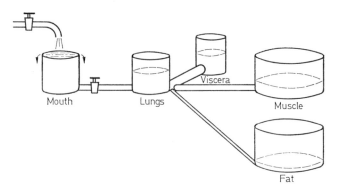

Fig. 1. The water analogue. A system of cylindrical vessels interconnected by pipes. With certain reservations (see text) the distribution of water in this system mimics the distribution of inhaled anesthetics in the body. (From MAPLESON: In: Proceedings of the 4th World Congress of Anesthesiologists, 1969)

represent various groups of organs and tissues. The pipe connecting the first two vessels represents the ventilation which conducts the anesthetic from the mouth to the lungs. The remaining pipes represent the blood flows which conduct the anesthetic from the lungs to the various body tissues.

B. Quantitation of the Analogue

The equivalence between properties of the analogue and properties of the body and of the anesthetic can be expressed quantitatively as follows.

Let
$$\text{volume of water} \propto \text{quantity of anesthetic,} \qquad (1)$$
and
$$\text{height of water} \propto \text{tension of anesthetic.} \qquad (2)$$

Now,
$$\text{volume of water in a cylinder}$$
$$= \text{height of water in cylinder} \times \text{cross-sectional area of cylinder.}$$

Therefore,
$$\text{cross-sectional area of cylinder}$$
$$= \frac{\text{volume of water in cylinder}}{\text{height of water in cylinder}}.$$

Therefore, substituting from (1) and (2),
$$\text{cross-sectional area of cylinder}$$
$$\propto \frac{\text{quantity of anesthetic in tissue}}{\text{tension of anesthetic in tissue}}. \qquad (3)$$

Multiplying and dividing the numerator of the right-hand side of this equation by the same quantity will not alter the validity of the equation. Therefore,
$$\text{cross-sectional area of cylinder}$$
$$\propto \frac{\text{volume of tissue} \times \dfrac{\text{quantity of anesthetic in tissue}}{\text{volume of tissue}}}{\text{tension of anesthetic in tissue}}.$$

But
$$\frac{\text{quantity of anesthetic in tissue}}{\text{volume of tissue}} = \text{concentration of anesthetic in tissue;}$$
and
$$\frac{\text{concentration of anesthetic in tissue}}{\text{tension of anesthetic in tissue}} = \text{solubility of anesthetic in tissue.}$$

Therefore,
$$\text{cross-sectional area of cylinder}$$
$$\propto \text{volume of tissue} \times \text{solubility of anesthetic in tissue.} \qquad (4)$$

Again,
$$\text{rate of flow of water from mouth vessel to lung vessel}$$
$$= \frac{\text{height difference between mouth and lung vessels}}{\text{resistance between mouth and lung vessels}}.$$

Assuming laminar flow of water in the pipe,
$$\text{resistance} \propto \frac{1}{\text{pipe-bore}^4}.$$

Therefore,
$$\text{rate of flow of water from mouth vessel to lung vessel}$$
$$\propto \text{height difference between mouth and lung vessels} \times \text{pipe-bore}^4. \qquad (5)$$

However, with certain reservations (see below),

net rate of uptake of anesthetic from mouth to lungs

= tension difference between mouth and lungs (alveoli) × alveolar ventilation.   (6)

Therefore, since

height difference α tension difference,

if rate of flow of water from mouth vessel to lung vessel is to be proportional to net rate of uptake of anesthetic

pipe-bore^4 must be α alveolar ventilation.   (7)

Similarly,

rate of flow of water into a tissue vessel

α height difference between lung vessel and tissue vessel × pipe-bore^4.   (8)

But,

net rate of uptake of anesthetic into tissue

= concentration difference between arterial and venous blood × blood flow to tissue,

= tension difference between arterial and venous blood
× solubility of anesthetic in blood × blood flow to tissue.   (9)

Therefore, in so far as arterial tension = alveolar tension, and in so far as tension in venous blood = tension in tissue from which the blood drains,

net rate of uptake of anesthetic into tissue

= tension difference between lungs (alveoli) and tissue
× solubility of anesthetic in blood × blood flow to tissue.   (10)

Therefore, comparing Eqs. (8) and (10), if rate of flow of water into a tissue vessel is to be proportional to net rate of uptake of anesthetic into tissue,

pipe-bore^4 must be α blood flow to tissue × solubility of anesthetic in blood.   (11)

In summary, therefore, the movement of water in the analogue in Fig. 1 will (with certain reservations) be quantitatively equivalent to the movement of anesthetic in the body, provided that the following proportionalities are observed.

The cross-sectional area of each cylindrical vessel must be proportional to the capacity of the corresponding tissue to store anesthetic (3), that is, to the volume of the tissue multiplied by the solubility of the anesthetic in the tissue (4).

The size of the pipe connecting the mouth vessel to the lung vessel (strictly speaking the fourth power of its bore) must be proportional to the alveolar ventilation (7), and the size (bore^4) of the pipe leading to each tissue vessel must be proportional to the blood flow to that tissue multiplied by the solubility of the anesthetic in blood (11).

Now it is possible to explain the proportions of the model in Fig. 1. Ideally, a separate vessel would be used for every part of every tissue in the body, but it has been shown [MAPLESON, 1963 (1)] that, for most purposes, little error results from combining tissues into three groups on the basis of the richness of their blood supply in relation to their storage capacity for anesthetic.

Thus, the vessel labelled "viscera" represents all the well-perfused organs (principally heart, brain, liver, kidneys) which together constitute a small fraction of the total body volume but account for a large fraction of the cardiac output. Therefore the visceral vessel has a relatively small cross-sectional area but is supplied by a relatively wide-bore pipe.

The vessel labelled "muscle" represents mostly muscle and skin which constitute a large fraction of the body volume but which, at rest, have a relatively poor blood supply. Therefore the muscle vessel has a relatively large cross-sectional area but is supplied by a relatively narrow-bore pipe.

Fat constitutes a moderate fraction of the body volume, but all inhaled anesthetics are more soluble in fat than in aqueous tissues. Therefore the fat vessel
also has a large cross-sectional area and, for some anesthetics, should be considerably larger than the muscle vessel. However, the blood supply to fat is very
poor and therefore is represented by a very narrow pipe. The size relationship
between the lung vessel and the tissue vessels and between the ventilation pipe
and the blood-flow pipes is considered below.

C. Comparison with Experiment

So far in this chapter the validity of the system in Fig. 1, as an analogue of the
uptake and distribution of inhaled anesthetics, has been argued on theoretical
grounds. Now it is necessary to test it against experimental observation. For this
it is necessary to use the analogue in a fully quantitative manner to predict the
pattern of uptake in circumstances which have been studied experimentally and
to compare the predictions with experimental measurements.

From the detailed description of the analogue it is evident that, in order to
make it fully quantitative, it is necessary to know the following:

Total body volume and how this is shared amongst the different tissues.

Alveolar ventilation.

Total cardiac output and how this is shared amongst the tissues.

Solubility of the anesthetic in blood and tissues.

Some of these factors have been directly measured in the subjects of experimental
observations of uptake; the other factors have to be estimated from "normal"
values.

Although the water analogue of Fig. 1 is very convenient for visualizing the
distribution of anesthetics, it is very inconvenient for accurate quantitative work.
For quantitative work, therefore, it is preferable to use an electric analogue
[MAPLESON, 1961, 1963 (1, 2), 1964; SEVERINGHAUS, 1963] which obeys the same
mathematical equations as the water analogue. Then a test of the electric analogue
shows how valid the water analogue is.

Fig. 2 shows both computed and experimental values for the rate of uptake
of anesthetic by the body (the total rate of flow of water into all vessels of the
analogue) against time (on a logarithmic scale) for three different inhalational
agents. A range of muscle and skin blood flows has been used because of uncertainty over the "normal" values. Nevertheless, it is evident that, with the
intermediate flow, the computed curves come within plus or minus twice the
standard error of most of the experimental means, although the fit might be
improved by a somewhat higher flow in the case of cyclopropane and a somewhat
lower flow in the case of nitrous oxide and halothane. These possible improvements
may be reflections of the fact that the subjects of the cyclopropane measurements
were not anesthetized, whereas those of the nitrous oxide and halothane measurements were.

In view of the good agreement between analogue and measurement in Fig. 2
it is clear that the analogue provides a good approximation to reality, at least in
some circumstances. However, there are a number of processes involved in the
distribution of inhaled anesthetics in the body which are known from theory, or
experiment, or both, but which are not represented by the simple water analogue.

These processes are considered in some detail at the end of this chapter but,
generally speaking, their effects on the patterns of distribution are essentially those

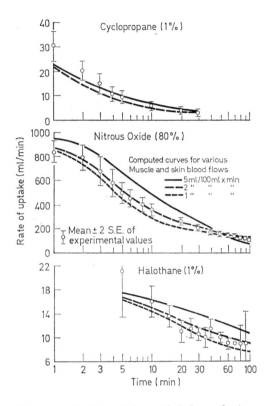

Fig. 2. Comparison of the rates of uptake of three inhaled anesthetics as measured in human subjects with the rates computed from an electrical equivalent [Mapleson, 1961, 1963 (1)] of the water analogue shown in Fig. 1. Experimental data for cyclopropane from Sechzer et al. (1959), for nitrous oxide from Severinghaus (1954), and for halothane from Mapleson (1962). [From Mapleson: In: Uptake and distribution of anesthetic agents, p. 110 (Papper and Kitz, Eds.). New York: McGraw-Hill 1963]

of correction factors. Therefore, it is of value to study the behaviour of the simple analogue of Fig. 1 in some detail, knowing that the results will represent a good approximation to the distribution of anesthetics in the body.

D. The General Pattern of Distribution

When the lower tap in Fig. 1 is opened, water begins to flow into the lung vessel; when the face mask is applied to the patient, or when the vaporizer is turned on, anesthetic is conducted by the ventilation to the lungs. As the water level in the lung vessel rises, water flows on into the other vessels; as the tension of anesthetic in the lungs rises, anesthetic is conducted by the circulation to the body tissues.

The viscera are represented by a small vessel supplied by a large pipe. Therefore the water level in the visceral vessel follows the rise in the lung vessel quickly; the tension in heart, brain, liver, kidneys is never far behind that in the lungs. On the other hand, the large capacity of the muscle vessel and its small blood-

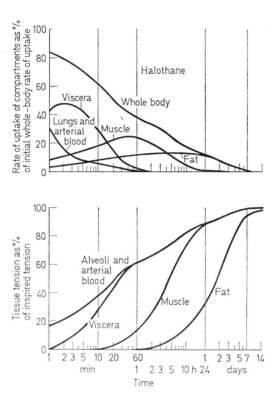

Fig. 3. Rates of uptake and tensions of anesthetic in the various body compartments during the administration of a constant inspired tension of halothane. Curves computed on the electric equivalent of the water analogue in Fig. 1. Note logarithmic time scale. [From MAPLESON: In: Uptake and distribution of anesthetic agents, p. 112 (PAPPER and KITZ, Eds.). New York: McGraw-Hill 1963]

supply pipe mean that the water level in that vessel can rise only slowly and must lag far behind the level in the lung vessel. In the fat vessel the same is true only more so. Thus the water levels indicated in Fig. 1 represent the anesthetic tensions to be expected in the various compartments of the body after the anesthetic has been administered for a certain period of time. If administration is continued for long enough, the levels in all compartments rise until they come into equilibrium with the constant level at the mouth.

In order to demonstrate the pattern of distribution quantitatively the approach to equilibrium in a "standard man" [MAPLESON, 1963 (1)] has been computed in detail for one anesthetic agent, halothane. This was done on what was the electrical equivalent of the water analogue in Fig. 1. The results (Fig. 3) are given in terms, both of the way in which the rate of uptake of each compartment, and of the whole body, varies with time, and also of the way in which the tension in each compartment approaches the inspired tension. (If the shapes of the curves are found to be at all puzzling, it should be noted that a logarithmic time scale has been used in order to keep the curves well separated from each other.)

Having established the general pattern of distribution, the effect of changes of various parameters can be considered.

E. The Effects of Different Inspired Tensions

Having observed in the water analogue the approach to equilibrium described above, suppose the approach is repeated, but with the inspired tension reduced to a half — cut off the top half of the mouth vessel. Now there will be only half the head of pressure driving water into the system, giving half the initial flow. However, at equilibrium, lung and tissue vessels will be only half as full. Thus, with only half the driving force, and only half the quantity of anesthetic to be driven into the body, it might be expected that the two halves would cancel and that the time to reach equilibrium would be independent of the inspired tension.

This is precisely true for the water analogue but, in the body, one of the correction factors mentioned above (and considered at the end of the chapter) comes into play. As a result, the approach to equilibrium is in fact somewhat faster at high inspired tensions. EGER (1963) called this phenomenon the "concentration effect". In this context "high" is used, not in relation to the clinically effective level, but in an absolute sense — say an inspired concentration of more than 20%. In practice, therefore, its importance is almost confined to nitrous oxide and perhaps rapid induction with di-ethyl ether.

F. The Effects of Different Solubilities

Since the solubilities of an anesthetic in blood and tissues affect the sizes of pipes and vessels in the analogue, this property can be expected to have a marked effect on the pattern of distribution. Accordingly, a list of solubilities of the common inhaled anesthetics in blood is given in Table 1. It may be noted that the solubilities cover a range of almost 100 to 1.

Solubilities in aqueous tissues, for a given anesthetic, are often about the same as the solubility in blood, but may range up to about three times as high. Compared with the very wide differences between agents, therefore, it is not far from the truth to say that the solubility of any agent in any aqueous tissue is about the same as its solubility in blood. Solubility in fat, on the other hand, ranges from a minimum of about three times the solubility in blood (nitrous oxide) to a maximum of over 100 times (methoxyflurane).

Fig. 4 shows two versions of the water analogue, one for an anesthetic of low solubility in blood and aqueous tissue and the other for one of high solubility. In the version which represents a low-solubility anesthetic, all the tissue compart-

Table 1. *Ostwald solubility coefficients*[a] *of various inhaled anesthetics in blood at 37 to 38 °C*

Ethylene	0.14
Cyclopropane	0.46
Nitrous oxide	0.47
Halothane	2.3
Trichloroethylene	9
Chloroform	10.3
Di-ethyl ether	12
Methoxyflurane	13

[a] That is, cc of "pure" anesthetic vapour (measured at ambient pressure and temperature and regarding the vapour as through it behaved as an ideal gas) per cc of blood per atmosphere of partial pressure of anesthetic with which the blood is in equilibrium. Values from LARSON et al. [1926 (2)] except for halothane [LARSON et al., 1962 (1)], di-ethyl ether (EGER et al., 1963) and methoxyflurane (EGER and SHARGEL, 1963).

ments are relatively small; in the version which represents a high-solubility agent they are all relatively large. But the relative sizes within each version are maintained: small for viscera, large for muscle and large for fat.

Similarly, all the blood-flow pipes are relatively large for the high-solubility anesthetic and relatively small for the low-solubility one, but the relative sizes are maintained: wide for viscera, medium for muscle, narrow for fat. The lung vessel is shown to be a little larger for the high-solubility anesthetic because it represents lung tissue as well as the gas in the lungs.

Now the approach to equilibrium for these two cases can be considered. In order to achieve equilibrium in the low-solubility case, only a small quantity of anesthetic has to go into the system whereas, in the high-solubility case, a much

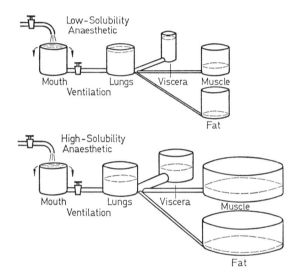

Fig. 4. Two versions of the water analogue representing anesthetics of low and high solubility. For both anesthetics, the solubility in all aqueous tissues has been taken to be the same as that in blood, and the solubility in fat has been taken to be about three times that in blood. (From MAPLESON: In: Proceedings of the 4th World Congress of Anesthesiologists, 1969)

larger quantity has to go in for the same inspired tension. In the high-solubility case, the blood-flow pipes are larger (but only proportionately so in terms of their ability to transport anesthetic) while the ventilation pipe is the same size. Thus the much larger quantity of anesthetic has to go through the same-sized ventilation pipe and, therefore, to reach equilibrium takes longer.

However, the tensions of anesthetic in muscle and fat are of little direct importance to the anesthetist: the tensions in brain and other vital organs are of much greater importance. For both low- and high-solubility agents, the blood-flow pipe to the visceral vessel is large in relation to the size of the vessel so that, in both cases, the brain tension follows the lung tension quite closely with only a short lag (see, for instance, Fig. 3). In the low-solubility case, the pipes to the muscle and fat vessels are small in relation to the ventilation pipe so that drainage to these compartments from the lungs is slow; therefore the lung tension, and with it the brain tension, can get quite close to equilibrium with the inspired tension, long before complete equilibrium has been achieved. In the high-solubility case, on the other hand, the pipes to the muscle and fat vessels are comparable in size to the ventilation pipe, so that the lung tension, and with it the brain tension, is held down to some level intermediate between that at the mouth and those in muscle and fat. Therefore, in the high-solubility case, not only is complete equilibrium slow, but also the lung and brain tensions cannot approach equilibrium until the whole body is nearly equilibrated.

G. The Approach to Equilibrium for Specific Agents

In order to make these differences clear in a quantitative way, the approach to equilibrium has been computed for a number of anesthetics. Again, this was done on the electrical equivalent of the water analogue.

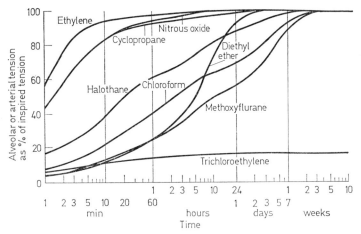

Fig. 5. The approach of the lung tension (alveolar or arterial) towards equilibrium with a constant inspired tension for various inhaled anesthetics. Curves computed on the electric equivalent of the water analogue. [From MAPLESON: In: Uptake and distribution of anesthetic agents, p. 113 (PAPPER and KITZ, Eds.). New York: McGraw-Hill 1963]

The results are shown in Fig. 5. As in Fig. 3, a logarithmic time scale has been used but, in this figure, for the sake of clarity, only the lung tensions are shown. It is clear that, with the low-solubility anesthetics (ethylene, nitrous oxide, cyclopropane), the lung tension does indeed approach equilibrium in quite a short time, although full equilibrium is not finally achieved for several hours. On the other hand, with the high-solubility anesthetics, equilibrium is not even approached unless the administration is continued for many hours or even days.

The curve for trichloroethylene is shown as never reaching equilibrium with the inspired tension. This is because, in computing the curve, account was taken of the fact that trichloroethylene was known to be broken down at a fast rate [CLAYTON and PARKHOUSE, 1962; MAPLESON, 1963 (2)]. Since these curves were first published, it has become apparent that most, if not all, inhaled anesthetics are broken down in the body to some extent (see section 5.2). If this were taken into account, all the lung-tension curves would flatten out at some limit less than the inspired tension but probably very much closer to it than is the case for trichloroethylene. Breakdown or bio-transformation of an agent can be represented in the water analogue simply by making a hole in the bottom of the vessel in which the breakdown is supposed to occur. If the breakdown occurs at a rate which is proportional to the tension of anesthetic at the site of breakdown, the representation may be made quantitative by connecting a pipe of suitable bore to the hole, in order to regulate the outflow.

The curves of Fig. 5 are of interest in showing what a very long time it takes with some agents to achieve equilibrium with a constant inspired tension. However, as far as the more-soluble agents are concerned, the curves are somewhat unrelated to clinical practice. The anesthetist does not administer a constant inspired tension, equal to the tension he needs to produce in the brain to achieve surgical anesthesia, and then wait for equilibrium. If he did, induction of anesthesia with di-ethyl ether might well take 24 h. Instead, he starts by administering an inspired tension which is much higher than that which he wishes to produce in the brain. The consequences of this procedure are now considered.

H. The Use of "Overpressure"

The procedure is illustrated by the version of the analogue shown in Fig. 6. From this it is evident that the desired brain tension will be achieved when the system is only a small part of the way towards equilibrium with the extra-high inspired tension. By means of this "overpressure", as E. I. EGER has called it, induction of anesthesia can be achieved in a matter of minutes, even with a high-solubility anesthetic.

It is also evident from Fig. 6 that, once the desired depth of anesthesia has been achieved, the inspired tension must be reduced to prevent the patient becoming too deeply anesthetized. The level to which the inspired tension must be reduced is not the same as that which has been achieved in the brain. Instead it is a level, shown by the dotted line in Fig. 6, just sufficiently in excess of the lung tension to provide an uptake into the lungs which just balances the drainage out of the lungs into the muscle and fat. Furthermore, as time passes, the muscle and

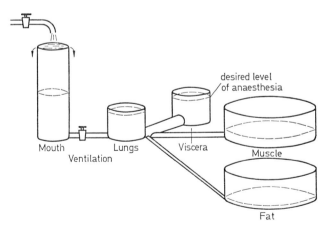

Fig. 6. A version of the water analogue which illustrates the use of an inspired tension much higher than that required to be produced in the brain (an "overpressure") in order to achieve rapid induction of anesthesia with a highly-soluble agent. (From MAPLESON: In: Proceedings of the 4th World Congress of Anesthesiologists, 1969)

fat tensions gradually rise, so that their uptake gradually becomes less; therefore the inspired tension must be progressively reduced in order to maintain the lungs and the brain "floating" between them at the desired level.

On the assumption that the objective is to raise the brain tension quickly to a specified level and then to maintain it constant, the necessary variation of inspired tension has been computed for the most soluble inhalational anesthetic, methoxyflurane, using the electrical equivalent of the analogue in Fig. 6. The results are plotted in Fig. 7. It is noteworthy that, even after prolonged anesthesia, the inspired tension is still higher than the tension being maintained in the brain.

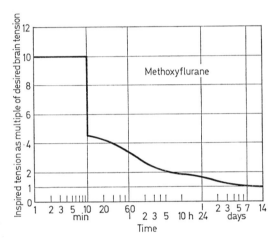

Fig. 7. The way in which the inspired tension of methoxyflurane needs to be varied with time in order to achieve a given brain tension in 10 min and then to maintain it constant. Curve computed on the electrical equivalent of the analogue shown in Fig. 6. (Modified from MAPLESON: In: Proceedings of the symposium on methoxyflurane at the Royal Society of Medicine, 1963)

J. The Effects of Changes of Ventilation and Circulation

So far in this chapter it has been assumed that the patient has been a passive "standard man" unaffected by the anesthetic or any other circumstances. In practice, the ventilation and the circulation may be very much "non-standard" in some patients and may be altered by the anesthetic itself. The general nature of the effects of these "non-standard" conditions can readily be deduced from the water analogue but it is necessary to consider induction and maintenance separately.

Induction. During induction, the objective is to raise the brain tension to the desired level, usually as quickly as is conveniently possible. From any of the versions of the analogue above, it is evident that the factors which aid the transfer of anesthetic to the brain are a large ventilation and a large blood supply to the brain. Therefore, anything which increases these factors will increase the speed of induction. This explains two elements in the rationale of administering carbon dioxide during an ether induction: the carbon dioxide increases the ventilation, and the raised arterial carbon-dioxide tension increases the blood flow to the brain. The third element in the rationale is that the increased ventilation permits the use of a higher inspired tension of ether without any risk of coughing.

In a somewhat similar way induction can be made more rapid, not by a direct increase in the blood flow to the brain but, instead, by a decrease in the blood flow to the other compartments. To make this clear it is necessary to separate out the brain from the rest of the viscera as in Fig. 8. From this figure it can be deduced that any reduction in blood flow to muscle and to the other viscera will leave more of whatever anesthetic reaches the lungs to go on preferentially to the brain.

An alternative way of expressing this is to say that the reduced drainage of anesthetic, to the other viscera and the muscle, allows the tension in the lungs to rise more rapidly; therefore the tension in the brain, with its normal blood flow, also rises more rapidly. It is probably this process which explains why induction is more rapid in a shocked patient, in whom the total circulation is reduced but the blood supply to the brain is probably fairly well maintained.

This situation has recently been the subject of some computations by MUNSON et al. (1968) on a digital computer programmed in such a way as to make it the mathematical equivalent of the water analogue in Fig. 8 (apart from some slight differences in the grouping of tissues into compartments). MUNSON and his colle-

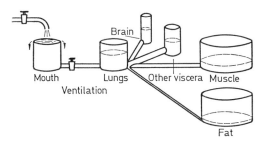

Fig. 8. A version of the water analogue showing the brain and its blood supply separately from the rest of the viscera. (From MAPLESON: In: Proceedings of the 4th World Congress of Anesthesiologists, 1969)

agues also examined the converse case of an excited patient, in whom peripheral blood flow is above normal so that the brain gets less than its usual supply of anesthetic and induction is slower.

Maintenance. The above remarks on induction are valid for both low- and high-solubility anesthetics although MUNSON et al. have shown that the effects of shock and excitement are more marked in the latter case. In considering what happens during maintenance, however, it is essential to treat the two cases separately.

In the low-solubility case it can be seen from Fig. 4 that, for much of the duration of anesthesia (while the muscle and fat compartments are filling up), the brain and lungs are already virtually at the inspired tension and, short of respiratory arrest, changes in ventilation and circulation have little effect.

In the high-solubility case, on the other hand, the lung tension, and with it the brain tension, is precariously "floating" somewhere between the inspired tension and the muscle tension. Therefore, any increase in ventilation puts the lungs into better communication with the mouth so that the lung tension, and with it the brain tension, is raised, and the patient becomes more deeply anesthetized. Conversely, any decrease of ventilation makes the patient become more lightly anesthetized. Thus, so long as the patient is breathing spontaneously, this operates as a negative-feedback system, protecting the patient, to some extent, from inappropriate inspired tensions.

If the patient is on controlled respiration, this negative-feedback system is, in effect, switched off. In these circumstances, any reduction in blood flow tends to cut off the lungs from the body and to allow the lung tension to rise towards the inspired tension. Now the brain, because of its separate perfusion-regulating mechanism, probably maintains its blood supply almost unaltered; therefore the brain tension follows the lung tension upwards. Hence, a reduction in cardiac output leads to a deepening of anesthesia, and probably also to an increase in tension in the heart as well, and therefore, quite possibly, to a further fall in circulation, and a further rise in tension. In other words, there is now a positive-feedback system in which the situation may get rapidly worse and worse to the point of cardiac arrest — unless the inspired tension is reduced.

K. Elimination during Recovery

For recovery the inspired tension is reduced to zero. In general, the low-solubility anesthetic, since it went in fast, comes out fast; conversely, the high-solubility anesthetic, since it went in slowly, comes out slowly. During recovery, in the high-solubility case, there is no equivalent to raising the inspired tension to a high level: there is no such thing as a negative inspired tension of anesthetic to suck the anesthetic out.

For a closer study of the process of elimination it is useful to distinguish two stages of recovery.

It was said above that, during maintenance, the lung tension, and with it the brain tension, floats somewhere between the inspired tension and the muscle tension. Even in the low-solubility case this can be said to be so, but then the lung tension is very close to the inspired tension. Exactly the same is true during recovery: when the inspired tension is reduced to zero the lung tension, and with it the brain tension, falls fairly rapidly until it reaches a new "floating" level, somewhere between the new (zero) inspired tension and the muscle tension. In the low-solubility case the lung "floats" very nearly at zero tension and recovery is virtually complete very quickly. In the high-solubility case on the other hand, the lung tension simply moves from a little above the muscle tension to a little below it. In other words there is an initial rapid recovery which, for the low solubility anesthetic, is almost complete but, for the high-solubility anesthetic, is only very small in extent. The second stage of recovery, full recovery, with the lung and brain tension falling virtually to zero, can be achieved only when the muscle compartment has almost completely emptied. With a high-solubility anesthetic this takes a very long time.

It was remarked above that there is no such thing as a negative inspired tension to accelerate recovery. However, it is possible to achieve some acceleration of recovery by increasing the ventilation so that the lung tension falls more rapidly than otherwise. There are two possible disadvantages to this.

Firstly, if the hyperventilation is produced by controlled respiration, without any addition of carbon dioxide, the resultant fall in arterial carbon-dioxide tension will diminish the blood flow to the brain. Therefore, although the lungs are put in better communication with the mouth, the brain tends to be cut off from the lungs. Consequently, although the lung tension falls faster than otherwise, the brain tension may not do so. From the water analogue, it can be seen that increasing the ventilation is most likely to speed recovery when the ventilation represents the biggest resistance to the outflow of anesthetic from the brain, that is, when the ventilation pipe is small compared with the blood-flow pipes. This is the case for the agents of higher solubility. The quantitative theoretical study by MUNSON and BOWERS (1967) of the equivalent problem in induction is in agreement with this and suggests that, with the low-solubility agents, increasing the ventilation without the addition of carbon dioxide, may actually delay recovery.

The second disadvantage to the use of hyperventilation arises if, at the end of the process, the muscle tension is higher than the lung tension — as is quite likely to be the case after prolonged anesthesia with one of the high-solubility agents. In these circumstances, when the ventilation is allowed to return to normal, the lung tension, and with it the brain tension, may well "float" up towards the higher muscle tension and the patient may become re-anesthetised.

L. The Effects of Processes not Represented by the Simple Analogue

It was mentioned above that, although the simple analogue of Fig. 1 generally gave a good approximation to reality, there were a number of known processes which it failed to reproduce. The effects of breakdown of an anesthetic, and the way in which this could be built into the analogue, have already been mentioned. The effects of other processes can now be considered. Before doing so, however, it is opportune to stress that the curves of Figs. 2, 3, 5 and 7 were computed without taking account of these other processes.

The concentration effect. The first process is involved in equation (6) above. This states that the net rate of uptake of anesthetic, from mouth to lungs, is equal to the product of the tension difference between mouth and lungs and of the alveolar ventilation. This equation suggests that alveolar ventilation is unaffected by uptake, or at least is the same in inspiration as in expiration. However, anesthetic in the lungs dissolves in the blood flowing through the lungs. The rate of solution is represented in the analogue by the sum of the rates of flow of water into the tissue vessels. This solution of anesthetic in blood tends to diminish the gas volume in the lungs. To prevent this occuring the inspired alveolar ventilation must exceed the expired alveolar ventilation; this may occur in one of three ways.

1. It may occur as a result of the inspired ventilation rising above what it would otherwise be (as is likely when ventilation is primarily controlled by the excretion of carbon dioxide).

2. It may occur as a result of the expired ventilation falling below what it would otherwise be (as is likely when ventilation is primarily controlled by the uptake of oxygen).

3. It may occur as a result of a combination of these processes (as may occur when ventilation is controlled by certain types of automatic ventilator).

Thus there may be an increase in the inflow of anesthetic to the lungs in each inspiration (1), or a decrease in the outflow in each expiration (2), or a mixture of the two (3); but in all three cases there will be an increase in the net rate of inflow of anesthetic to the lungs, over and above what it would be if the inspired ventilation were the same as the expired ventilation. The effect of this extra inflow is discussed below but it can be seen now that the effect will be important only when the difference between inspired and expired ventilation is appreciable, that is, only when the rate of solution in the blood is an appreciable fraction of the alveolar ventilation. This can occur only if the anesthetic has at least a moderate solubility in blood (as is true of all the common inhaled agents) and if it is administered at a fairly high inspired concentration, say at least 20%. Therefore, in practice, the effect is commonly of importance only for nitrous oxide and, perhaps, in rapid induction with di-ethyl ether.

22*

The process is not represented by the water analogue in Fig. 1. An indirect method of incorporating the process accurately into an electric analogue has been described (MAPLESON, 1964) and has been used to compute the curves of Fig. 9 which give an idea of the magnitude of the effect. This indirect method could be applied to the water analogue to give an accurate representation of the process. However, the object of the water analogue is to help in visualizing the processes of distribution, so that an indirect representation would be of no value. Instead, suppose the greater inflow of anesthetic to the lungs, consequent upon solution of the anesthetic in the blood flowing through the lungs, is imagined to be due to a simple increase in mean alveolar ventilation instead of to a difference between

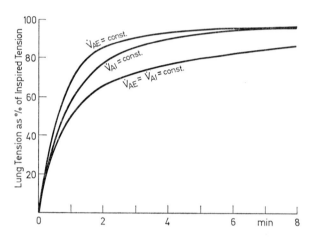

Fig. 9. The "concentration effect". This figure shows the extent to which the approach of the lung tension of nitrous oxide towards equilibrium with the inspired tension is more rapid at 75% inspired tension than at 1%. The figure also shows that the increased rapidity depends on whether it is the inspired ($\dot{V}_{AI}$) or the expired ($\dot{V}_{AE}$) alveolar ventilation which remains constant. Computed values from an electric analogue (MAPLESON, 1964) which is more complex than the equivalent of the water analogue of Fig. 1. [From MAPLESON: J. Appl. Physiol. **19**, 1193—1199 (1964)]

inspired and expired ventilation. This would be only an approximation to the true state of affairs but it could be represented directly in the water analogue if the ventilation pipe were imagined to dilate in accordance with the rate of flow of water from the lung vessel to the tissue vessels.

The second-gas effect. The way in which the solution of anesthetic in the blood flowing through the lungs causes the inspired ventilation to exceed the expired ventilation has a second consequence: the uptake of one anesthetic can influence the uptake of another. For instance, if 1% halothane is administered in air or oxygen, the rate at which the halothane dissolves in the blood has a negligible effect on the ventilation. However, if the halothane is carried in 75% nitrous oxide, the solution of the nitrous oxide causes a substantial increase in inspired ventilation (or decrease in expired ventilation) which increases the rate of input of halothane to the lungs, so that the lung tension of halothane builds up more rapidly. This process has been called the "second-gas" effect (EPSTEIN et al., 1964). Like the concentration effect it can be represented accurately in the electric analogue, from which the curves of Fig. 10 were computed, but the effect cannot be represented in any helpful way in the water analogue.

Deviations from Henry's law. EGER (1969) has recently argued theoretically that inhaled anesthetics may not obey Henry's law, that is, that the concentration of anesthetic dissolved in blood or tissue may not be proportional to the tension in the medium. Furthermore, he has shown experimentally that important deviations from Henry's law do occur with cyclopropane. So far as tissues are concerned, this effect could be more easily represented in the water analogue than in the electric analogue: since solubility decreases with increasing tension, it follows from equations (2) and (4) above that the cross-sectional area of a vessel should decrease

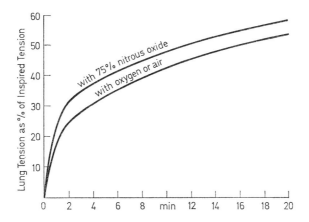

Fig. 10. The "second-gas" effect. This figure shows the extent to which the rise in lung tension of halothane is more rapid when the halothane is carried in nitrous oxide than when it is carried in air. (Computed as in Fig. 9. Expired alveolar ventilation constant.) [From MAPLE-SON: J. Appl. Physiol. **19,** 1193—1199 (1964)]

with increasing height. In other words, the vessels should not be perfect cylinders but should taper inward toward the top to some extent.

Alveolar-arterial tension differences; shunts. In deriving equation (10) above it was assumed that alveolar tension was equal to arterial tension. This is probably very nearly true in normal lungs. In patients, however, it is by no means uncommon for there to be an uneven distribution of ventilation and perfusion in the lungs. Then "mixed" alveolar tension (that is, end-tidal tension) is not the same as arterial tension and the pattern of uptake is modified. This process has been studied by EGER and SEVERINGHAUS (1964) with an electric analogue which represented the two lungs separately. A fixed cardiac output was shared equally between the two lungs; a fixed overall ventilation was shared in proportions varying between (a) equal amounts going to each lung, and (b) all the ventilation going to one lung and none to the other. They found that increasing the unevenness of distribution led to generally higher levels of end-tidal tension and lower levels of arterial tension. With low-solubility anesthetics the dominant effect was the lowering of the arterial tension so that induction would be delayed. With high-solubility anesthetics the dominant effect was the raising of the end-tidal tension with very little effect on arterial tension and hence little effect on induction time.

It would not be difficult to draw, or even to construct, the water-analogue equivalent of the EGER and SEVERINGHAUS circuit. However, the result might be rather too complex to help much in visualizing the effects. An alternative approach is to consider the situation in which there are three regions of the lungs: (1) a region in which ventilation and perfusion are evenly distributed, (2) a region which is ventilated but totally unperfused, (3) a region which is perfused but totally unventilated. It seems likely that this may give as good an approximation to real situations as the arrangement used by EGER and SEVERINGHAUS. Region (1) is already represented in the analogue. Region (2) is also represented already in that it is merely an addition to the dead space ventilation which is represented by its absence! (The size of the pipe connecting mouth and lungs is related to only the effective part of the ventilation.) Region (3), perfused but not ventilated, can be represented as in Fig. 11 which is, in effect, an extreme case of the EGER and SEVERINGHAUS model. The pipes connecting the vessel which corresponds to the unventilated parts of the lungs to each tissue vessel represent each tissue's share of the shunt flow, which is at mixed-venous tension. To understand this model it

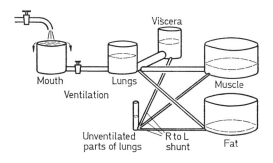

Fig. 11. A version of the water analogue which incorporates a representation of a right to left shunt of blood past the lungs

is best to compare it with a model representing a patient with the same alveolar ventilation, and with an (evenly-distributed) cardiac output which is equal to the non-shunt part of the cardiac output in Fig. 11. In other words, the shunt in Fig. 11 is best regarded as something added to an otherwise constant, non-shunt cardiac output; that is, it is best to regard the shunt as an extra burden on the heart, rather than as a reduction in effective pulmonary blood flow. (If, in fact, the effect of the shunt is to reduce the effective pulmonary blood flow, then this reduction should be considered as a separate effect first.) Having adopted this approach, Fig. 11 makes it clear that the effect of the shunt is to act as a sort of "mixer of tissues", in that it tends to reduce the differences of tension which develop between them: the extent to which the tension in the well-perfused tissues rises above that in the poorly-perfused ones is reduced because the shunt is equivalent (both from the mathematical, and the analogue, point of view) to a direct connection from the well-perfused to the poorly-perfused tissues.

Tissue-venous tension differences; diffusion within tissue. The other assumption made in deriving Eq. (10) was that venous tension was equal to the tension in the tissue from which the blood drained. Even if this is true at the capillary level, it will not be true at the "compartment" level if compartments contain tissues with too wide a range of "blood flows per unit storage capacity". A study of the

effects of different kinds of grouping of tissues into compartments has already
been referred to [MAPLESON, 1963 (1)]. At the capillary level it used to be considered that diffusion within the tissue was sufficiently rapid for it to be reasonable
to regard tissue as effectively "well-stirred". However, the recent work of HILLS
(1967) has shown that diffusion in tissue is very much slower than previously
suspected, so that there will not, in general, be the same tension of anesthetic
throughout a tissue as assumed here. An approximate representation of this in
the water analogue would be given by replacing the single vessel for each tissue
by a row of vessels (of the same total cross-sectional area) each connected to its
neighbour by a pipe of suitable size and only the vessel at one end of the row
connected by the blood-flow pipe to the lungs. A limited version of this, in which
the tissue compartments are merely sub-divided into intra-cellular-fluid and extra-
cellular-fluid sections, is shown in Fig. 12.

Diffusion between tissues. Finally, there is the work of RACKOW et al. (1965)
and PERL et al. (1965) which appears to show that there is some direct diffusion
of anesthetic from one compartment to another, independent of the blood supply.

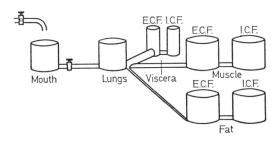

Fig. 12. A version of the water analogue which includes a simplified representation of intra-
tissue diffusion. ECF= extra-cellular fluid. ICF= intra-cellular fluid

A crude, qualitative way of showing this in the analogue is to add some narrow
pipes which directly interconnect the different tissue vessels.

References

CLAYTON, J. I., PARKHOUSE, J.: Blood trichloroethylene concentrations during anaesthesia
under controlled conditions. Brit. J. Anaesthesia 34, 141—148 (1962).
EGER, E. I., II: Applications of a mathematical model of gas uptake. In: Uptake and distribution of anesthetic agents, pp. 88—103 (PAPPER, E. M., KITZ, R. J., Eds.). New York:
McGraw-Hill 1963.
— Implications of some simple concepts of partition coefficients. In: Progress in Anesthe-
siology: Proceedings of the 4th World Congress of Anesthesiologists, Sep 1968, pp. 400—
404 (BOULTON, T. B., et al., Eds.). Amsterdam: Excerpta Medica Foundation 1970.
— SEVERINGHAUS, J. W.: Effect of uneven pulmonary distribution of blood and gas on
induction with inhalation anesthetics. Anesthesiology 25, 620—626 (1964).
— SHARGEL, R.: Solubility of methoxyflurane in human blood and tissue homogenates.
Anesthesiology 24, 625—627 (1963).
— — MERKEL, G.: Solubility of diethyl ether in water, blood and oil. Anesthesiology 24, 676
—678 (1963).
EPSTEIN, R. M., RACKOW, H., SALANITRE, E., WOLF, G. L.: Influence of the concentration
effect on the uptake of anesthetic mixtures: the second gas effect. Anesthesiology 25,
364—371 (1964).
HILLS, B. A.: Diffusion versus blood perfusion in limiting the rate of uptake of inert non-polar
gases by skeletal rabbit muscle. Clin. Sci. 33, 67—87 (1967).

LARSON, C. P., Jr., EGER, E. I., II, SEVERINGHAUS, J. W.: (1) Solubility of halothane in blood and tissue homogenates. Anesthesiology 23, 349—355 (1962).
— — — (2) Ostwald solubility coefficients for anesthetic gases in various fluids and tissues. Anesthesiology 23, 686—689 (1962).
MAPLESON, W. W.: Simple analogue for the distribution of inhaled anaesthetics about the body. In: Abstracts of contributed papers, International Biophysics Congress, p. 81. Stockholm 1961.
— Rate of uptake of halothane vapour in man. Brit. J. Anaesthesia 34, 11—18 (1962).
— (1) An electric analogue for uptake and exchange of inert gases and other agents. J. Appl. Physiol. 18, 197—204 (1963).
— (2) Quantitative prediction of anesthetic concentrations. In: Uptake and distribution of anesthetic agents, pp. 104—119 (PAPPER, E. M., KITZ, R. J., Eds.). New York: McGraw-Hill 1963.
— Inert gas-exchange theory using an electric analogue. J. Appl. Physiol. 19, 1193—1199 (1964).
MUNSON, E. S., BOWERS, D. L.: Effects of hyperventilation on the rate of cerebral anesthetic equilibrium. Calculations using a mathematical model. Anesthesiology 28, 377—381 (1967).
— EGER, E. I., II, BOWERS, D. L.: Effects of changes in cardiac output and distribution on the rate of cerebral anesthetic equilibration. Calculation using a mathematical model. Anesthesiology 29, 533—537 (1968).
PERL, W., RACKOW, H., SALANITRE, E., WOLF, G. L., EPSTEIN, R. M.: Intertissue diffusion effect for inert fat-soluble gases. J. Appl. Physiol. 20, 621—627 (1965).
RACKOW, H., SALANITRE, E., EPSTEIN, R. M., WOLF, G. L., PERL, W.: Simultaneous uptake of N_2O and cyclopropane in man as a test of compartment model. J. Appl. Physiol. 20, 611—620 (1965).
SECHZER, P. H., DRIPPS, R. D., PRICE, H. L.: Uptake of cyclopropane by the human body. J. Appl. Physiol. 14, 887—890 (1959).
SEVERINGHAUS, J. W.: Rate of uptake of nitrous oxide in man. J. Clin. Invest. 33, 1183—1189 (1954).
— Role of lung factors. In: Uptake and distribution of anesthetic agents, pp. 59—71 (PAPPER, E. M., KITZ, R. J., Eds.). New York: McGraw-Hill 1963.

5.2. Biotransformation

RUSSELL A. VAN DYKE

I. Introduction

The concept that anesthetics are biochemically inert and are eliminated from the body unchanged was held from the early work of HAGGARD (1924) until 1962 (VAN DYKE, 1963). HAGGARD studied the absorption, distribution, and elimination of diethyl ether and found that he could account for 87% of the anesthetic in the expired air. On this basis it was decided that anesthetics were not metabolized. HAGGARD's techniques and studies were commendable but we now know that much of the 13% of unrecovered material had been metabolically altered.

From the studies made to date on the volatile anesthetics, it has become clear that mammals have enzyme systems which are capable of chemically altering these materials. The exact nature of these enzyme systems has not been uncovered but those bits and pieces which are known will be presented in later sections of this chapter. The evidence suggests that the enzyme systems which catalyze the biotransformation of the volatile anesthetics are probably the same as certain of those systems which metabolize drugs (microsomal electron transport system) and perform certain steroid interconversions.

Why study the metabolism of the volatile anesthetics? We now know that metabolism of these compounds does not give rise to products which are anesthetics, so why look further? This can be answered in four parts. First, the knowledge gained in these studies is useful in developing new anesthetics. It allows us to predict how a particular compound will react when placed in a biologic system.

Second is the question of the toxic side-effects. This question is best answered by understanding the route and mechanism by which metabolism of an anesthetic is accomplished. It is likely that the intermediates in the metabolism are the materials which give rise to the occasional toxic side-effects. In this regard, each anesthetic must be considered independently, and no sweeping generalities can be made as to the reason for the toxicity.

Third, aside from the question of toxicity of the anesthetics, the behavior of these materials when placed in a biologic system is of academic interest. As a group they have diverse but unique chemical compositions and therefore a study of their biotransformation involves some very interesting biochemistry. It allows the investigator to study new enzyme systems or new uses for known systems as well as new mechanisms of enzyme action.

Fourth is the role that this metabolism plays in clinical circumstances. Because of the biochemical reactivity of these anesthetics, their metabolism may interfere with the metabolism of other drugs. This becomes important when one considers that metabolism is one way the body has of limiting the duration of action of a drug. Furthermore, because of this reactivity these volatile anesthetics are good

Mayo Clinic and Mayo Foundation: Section of Surgical Research (Anesthesia).

This investigation was supported in part by NIH Contract PH 43-67-666 from the National Institutes of Health, Public Health Service.

enzyme-inducing agents for the enzyme systems which metabolize drugs and steroids.

Many of these questions remain to be answered but, in the sections of this chapter which follow, it is evident that a good start has been made.

II. Chloroform

Chloroform was one of the first anesthetics to be used but was one of the first to be discarded as the newer anesthetics were introduced. It provides inexpensive and fair anesthesia but the possibility of producing liver toxicity makes it a very poor choice as an anesthetic agent.

The evidence indicates that the toxic side-effects of chloroform may be the result of its metabolism. Whipple (1912) and Dawkins (1963) have shown that the liver damage produced by chloroform and carbon tetrachloride (although carbon tetrachloride is not used as an anesthetic, it will be discussed with chloroform because its biochemistry is very similar) in adults does not occur in newborns (within the first 7 days of life). In addition, Fouts and Hart (1965) have shown that little or no metabolism of drugs occurs in these young animals. If chloroform is metabolized by the drug-metabolizing system, then it is possible that either a product of or an intermediate in the metabolism of chloroform by this route is toxic but the parent molecule is not. Attempts to learn the identity of this toxic material have not been successful to date.

The exact mechanism by which chloroform is metabolized is not known. There are several possible routes, but basically it is either enzymatic or nonenzymatic. Chloroform is unstable in alkaline conditions and, because the mammalian system is slightly basic, this nonenzymatic route may account for a portion of the degradation. It involves a direct conversion of chloroform to carbon dioxide as follows:

$$\begin{array}{ccccc} & \text{Cl} & & \text{Cl} & \\ & | & & | & \\ \text{Cl}-\!\!&\text{C}&\!\!-\text{H} \longrightarrow \text{Cl}-\!\!&\text{C}&\!\!\cdot \xrightarrow{\;O_2\;} CO_2 \; . \\ & | & & | & \\ & \text{Cl} & & \text{Cl} & \end{array}$$

Butler (1961) and Paul and Rubinstein (1963) reported that they were able to find chloroform but not dichloromethane in the expired air of dogs which had been given carbon tetrachloride. Thus, chloroform apparently follows an oxidative route of breakdown rather than the reductive route to dichloromethane.

Wood et al. (1968) reported that chloroform is one of several chlorinated hydrocarbons that will bind to the cobalt in cobalamin (vitamin B_{12}). As this binding occurs, a chloride is released. This binding can be reversed by light. The contribution that this reaction makes to the metabolism of chloroform is probably of little consequence since the evidence suggests that the major portion of the metabolism of chloroform is carried out by the microsomal drug-metabolizing system. (This enzyme system will be discussed in later sections of this chapter.) In whole-animal studies it was found that 2% of a dose of chloroform was expired as CO_2 and 4% appeared as unidentified urinary metabolites (van Dyke, 1963).

Ordinarily, when one does an *in vivo* metabolic study it is assumed that the urinary products, CO_2, and exhaled unchanged anesthetic, all collected for a period of 24—48 h, represent the total metabolic pattern. Experiments based on recovery of all anesthetic and metabolites eliminated by the body suffer from extreme lack of precision. If recovery percentages are low, it is easy to assign it to poor technique or experimental error. Thus, little effort has been made to determine what, if anything, remains in the body at the end of the recovery period. However, COHEN and HOOD (1969) utilized an autoradiographic technique to investigate the distribution of chloroform with time *in vivo* in the rat and found that not all the metabolites were excreted in the period of the study. For this study they used ^{14}C-labeled chloroform and low temperature whole-body autoradiography. The amount of radioactivity in the liver increased during the postanesthetic period. A liver extract at this time showed two nonvolatile chloroform metabolites. In spite of the fact that these metabolites have not been identified, this study points out that perhaps not all the metabolites appear immediately in the urine and expired air but are excreted very slowly over a period of several days or possibly weeks. It raises questions as to whether these metabolites represent the toxic elements in chloroform metabolism and also as to why they accumulate in the liver.

III. Diethyl Ether

As referred to previously in this chapter, HAGGARD (1924) studied the uptake, distribution, and elimination of diethyl ether in dogs and was able to account for 87% of the administered dose. In addition, he found that the duration of anesthesia did not influence the percentage recovery.

We now know that diethyl ether is metabolized by mammals (VAN DYKE et al., 1964). This metabolism is not unusual, considering what we know about metabolism of other drugs. Many drugs are transformed *in vivo* by the removal of a methyl or ethyl group from N or O to yield the corresponding amine or phenol. This is classified as N-dealkylation or O-dealkylation. The O-dealkylation can be considered as an ether cleavage of a chemically complex ether. The O-de-ethylation of diethyl ether would be an ether cleavage of a chemically simple ether, and the evidence suggests that this is catalyzed by the same enzyme system that O-dealkylates the more complex ethers. One would expect, therefore, that the cleavage of the ether would result in the formation of ethanol and acetaldehyde. These metabolites would be quickly oxidized to carbon dioxide, and one should expect that, of the amount metabolized, most, if not all, should appear as carbon dioxide. This is the case. VAN DYKE et al. (1964) found that 2—4% of a dose of diethyl ether appeared as carbon dioxide within 24 h and that there were no detectable amounts of urinary metabolites. The urinary metabolites, if present, would represent those materials which are metabolized slowly or not at all.

Very recent work by COHEN et al. (1969) revealed that metabolism of diethyl ether gives rise to metabolites which accumulate in the liver and kidney. At 2 h after administration of the anesthetics, these metabolites accounted for 3.6% of the administered dose. They found that there were four metabolites which accumulated and that at least one of these was a glucuronide. These metabolites will in all probability eventually be excreted but questions remain as to how long it will take and whether these metabolites in any way interfere with the normal biochemistry of the organs.

IV. Halothane

Halothane ($CF_3CHClBr$) has been the most extensively studied volatile anesthetic with regard to its metabolic breakdown. The first studies on halothane were performed in rats (VAN DYKE et al., 1964). The halothane used in that study was labeled with carbon-14 in the trifluoromethyl carbon, and the results were that very little, if any, of this carbon was converted to carbon dioxide. Thus, the trifluoromethyl group is quite stable biochemically. On the other hand, a considerable amount of radioactivity appeared in the urine, but not as halothane.

Subsequent work performed *in vitro* in rat liver preparations [van Dyke and Chenoweth, 1965 (2)] has shown that less than 1% of halothane is oxidized to carbon dioxide. This is consistent with some work (G. A. Snow, personal communication) in which rats were administered halothane by either exposing them to 1% vapor for 3 h or injecting 0.25 ml intraperitoneally and then the urine was examined for fluoride. The amount of metabolism based on the urinary fluoride output was 0.77%. This agrees well with the data on the oxidation of the trifluoromethyl group to carbon dioxide. When less than 1% metabolism occurs, the significance of the data is open to question, particularly since a large portion of the fluoride found may have come from impurities in the halothane. Thus, the trifluoromethyl group may be considered to be one of the most biochemically stable groups. This obviously is not an important route for the metabolism of halothane.

The only other portion of the molecule which can be attacked is the chlorobromomethyl group. *In vitro* studies carried out with ^{36}Cl-labeled halothane have indicated the existence of an enzyme system capable of releasing the chlorine [van Dyke and Chenoweth, 1965 (2)]. (This enzyme system will be discussed in later sections of this chapter.) It is not known if the chlorine is released before the bromine but, if there is an oxidative attack on that carbon atom, it is a moot point since both the chlorine and the bromine will be released as their respective ions and the remainder of the molecule will appear as trifluoroacetic acid or trifluoroethanol. Stier (1964) has convincingly shown that trifluoroacetic acid is the main urinary metabolite of halothane. In order for difluoroacetic or monofluoroacetic acid to appear there must be a reductive defluorination. This is highly unlikely because the evidence indicates that, when halogens are removed, it is by an oxidative reaction.

Rehder et al. (1967) studied the metabolism of halothane in humans and found that this can be followed by quantitating the urinary output of trifluoroacetic acid or inorganic bromide. Based on the amount of trifluoroacetic acid which was excreted postoperatively for 13 days, at least 12% of the absorbed halothane was metabolized. If the percentage metabolism was based on the bromide output (Stier et al., 1964), the extent of metabolism was 16—20%. This discrepancy suggests that either trifluoroacetic acid has a longer half-life *in vivo* than bromide or that a small amount of the trifluoroacetate is metabolized very slowly and thus does not appear in the urine. Regardless of which value is used, the point is that humans metabolize halothane extensively and seemingly to a greater extent than do other species.

V. Methoxyflurane

Early *in vivo* studies in rats (van Dyke et al., 1964) indicated that methoxyflurane ($CH_3OCF_2CHCl_2$) is extensively metabolized. The anesthetic was labeled with carbon-14 in the methyl portion of the ether, and it was found that the ether linkage could be broken. This was shown by the fact that ^{14}C-labeled CO_2 appeared in the expired air (2% in 24 h). In addition to the oxidation to CO_2, other metabolites were formed which appeared as urinary metabolites (4—8% in 24 h). These have not been identified but, by using chromatographic techniques, it was shown that there were at least four distinguishable metabolites.

In *in vitro* experiments [van Dyke and Chenoweth, 1965 (2)] to study the ether cleavage and the dechlorination in detail, it was found that both were carried out by enzyme systems found in the endoplasmic reticulum. The ether cleavage was of the O-dealkylation type, such as described for the cleavage of diethyl ether, and this system was different in several respects from the enzyme system catalyzing the release of the chlorine. The latter system was the same as that which catalyzed the release of chlorine from halothane. (The nature of the enzyme systems and the means of distinguishing between them will be discussed in later sections.)

CHENOWETH (CHENOWETH, personal communication) has shown that the fluoride content of the bones increased significantly in animals subjected to prolonged exposure to methoxyflurane. However, any defluorination is probably the result of the ether cleavage. Thus, there appear to be several possible pathways of metabolism of methoxyflurane. The following scheme represents some of these possibilities:

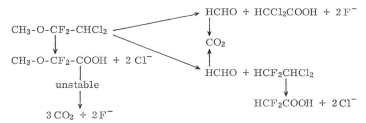

VI. Trichloroethylene

Trichloroethylene (CCl_2= CHCl) was found, as early as 1933, to undergo metabolism (BRÜNING and SCHNETKA), and the main metabolite, trichloroacetic acid, was isolated and identified in 1939 (BARRETT and JOHNSTON). In spite of this fact, the idea persisted that other volatile anesthetics were not metabolized.

The use of trichloroethylene has decreased in the United States, but study of its metabolism has continued because it represents some very interesting biochemistry.

The fact that trichloroethylene is converted to trichloroacetic acid implies that a chlorine has migrated from one carbon to another or that there has been a dechlorination of one carbon followed by a chlorination of the other carbon. The data support the former, but the mechanism is not known. DANIEL (1963) has shown that there is no mixing of the chlorine atoms of trichloroethylene with the body chloride pool and, therefore, there must be a migration of the chlorine from one carbon to another. In addition to trichloroacetic acid, which has been found in the blood and urine of humans after exposure to trichloroethylene (POWELL, 1945), trichloroethanol (SOUČEK and VLACHOVÁ, 1960) has been found in human urine. The trichloroethanol is excreted as the glucuronide.

BUTLER (1949) postulated that the first step in the metabolism of trichloroethylene was its conversion to chloral hydrate. This material then rearranged to yield trichloroethanol or trichloroacetic acid. However, he was unable to find any chloral hydrate after the administration of trichloroethylene. Subsequently, BYINGTON and LEIBMAN (1965) obtained evidence that chloral hydrate is formed as the intermediate product.

It has been proposed that a chlorine bridge may form to facilitate the movement of the chlorine atom from one carbon to the other [VAN DYKE and CHENOWETH, 1965 (1)]. This was proposed as a replacement to the theory that an epoxide was the intermediate. Assuming this to be the case, a pathway was proposed (Byington and Leibman, 1965) for the metabolism of trichloroethylene and is presented here with certain modifications:

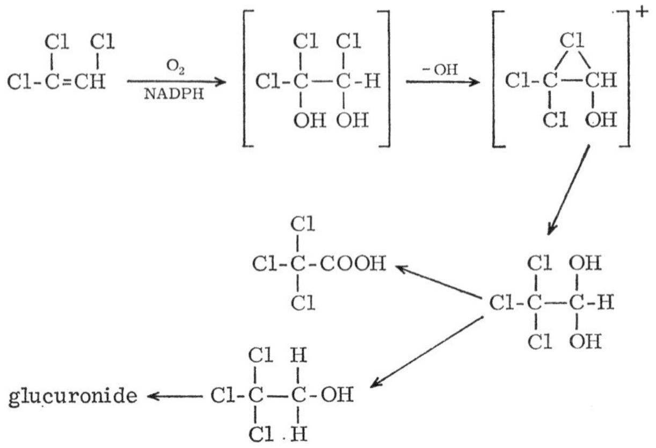

Monochloroacetic acid was found to represent 4% of a given dose of trichloroethylene (Souček and Vlachová, 1954, 1960) and probably arises by an alternate breakdown of one of the proposed intermediates. However, Daniel (1963) was unable to find any monochloroacetic acid in his studies.

The appearance of trichloroacetic acid in the blood is delayed until a few hours after the end of the administration of trichloroethylene. This has been found by several investigators (Ahlmark and Forssman, 1951; Paykoç and Powell, 1945). A similar delay in excretion of metabolites occurs in the case of halothane (Stier, 1968): the trifluoroacetic acid does not appear in the urine until several hours after administration. The reason for this is not clear but various possibilities have been proposed, such as storage in cell nuclei (Stier, 1968), slow diffusion out of the cell (Powell, 1945), or binding to proteins or erythrocytes (Bardoděj and Vyskočil, 1956; Fabre and Truhaut, 1952).

VII. Fluroxene

Blake et al. (1967) reported that fluroxene ($CF_3CH_2OCH= CH_2$) is metabolized to a variety of end products in mice and dogs. These investigators found that this anesthetic was metabolized to trifluoroethanol glucuronide, trifluoroacetic acid, and CO_2:

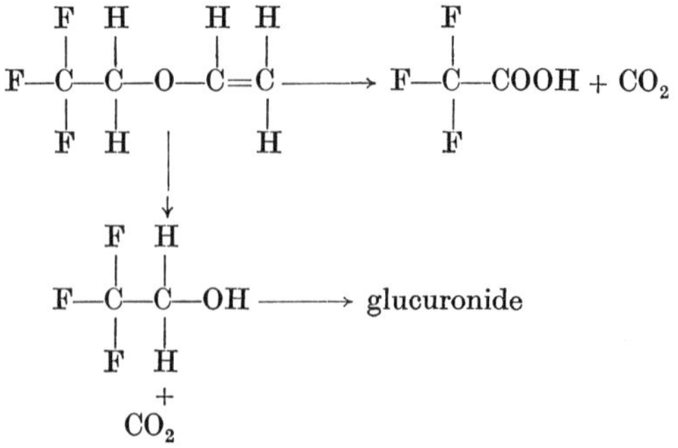

As with halothane, the trifluoromethyl group is not enzymatically broken down to a significant extent. This carbon when labeled with carbon-14 does not yield radioactivity in the expired CO_2 but it does yield radioactive trifluoroacetate and trifluoroethanol.

These authors reported that fluroxene acted to inhibit its own breakdown, so that, as the amount of anesthetic administered was increased, the percentage of metabolites formed decreased. Since the anesthetic was injected intraperitoneally, the decreasing percentage of metabolite with increasing dosage represents a more rapid release of unaltered anesthetic at higher doses. This raises the point that the body can retain low levels of anesthetic for considerable periods and it is during this period of retention that metabolism of these anesthetics is important.

VIII. Other Anesthetics

It is unfortunate that nitrous oxide, the most widely used agent, must be placed in this category but nothing is known about its disposition in the body. The problem in studying nitrous oxide is the fact that the probable products of its metabolism would be nitrates and nitrites, and these are difficult to detect in a system already rich in nitrogen-containing compounds. Furthermore, nitrous oxide cannot be labeled with radioactive isotopes as the other anesthetics have been and which has greatly facilitated their study.

Nitrous oxide is not biochemically inactive because much is known about its reactivity in the reticuloendothelial system. Biosynthesis of nitrous oxide occurs in microorganisms (MATSUBARA and MORI, 1968). It is interesting to speculate whether its activity is the result of the reactivity of the parent compound or of an intermediate or product of its metabolism.

Cyclopropane has been studied (VAN DYKE, unpublished results) but without success. Once again, to be studied the material must be labeled with carbon-14 and it was found that it was impossible to obtain material of sufficiently high chemical and radioactive purity to carry out a study of this nature. The materials used for this purpose must be at least 99.9% pure. Ethylene is very seldom used as an anesthetic agent now, but it is of interest because it has recently been recognized as active in other mammalian systems (PIETSCH and CHENOWETH, 1969). Ethylene was found to be metabolized to CO_2 and urinary metabolites (VAN DYKE, unpublished results) to the extent of 4%.

IX. Enzyme Systems

There apparently are a limited number of enzyme systems in the endoplasmic reticulum which are responsible for the biotransformation of a large number of drugs and other xenobiotics. These same enzyme systems carry out the interconversions of the steroids. Thus, one gets the impression that each enzyme system of this sort is nonspecific as to the substrate requirement but is specific as to the chemistry of the conversion. The result is that the enzymes are categorized as to type of chemical transformation involved rather than on the basis of the type of substrate attacked: there are enzyme systems for O-dealkylation, N-dealkylation, aromatic hydroxylation, S-oxidation, and others.

Basically, one or both of two types of reactions occur in the metabolism of the volatile anesthetics. These are ether cleavage and dehalogenation. They are similar in that they are oxidative reactions but are different in regard to the enzyme systems.

The ether-cleaving system is probably the same as one of the O-dealkylating systems (Axelrod, 1956). Several of these systems exist in the endoplasmic reticulum, and they require oxygen and reduced NADP for activity. The ether-cleaving system also requires oxygen and NADPH. The products of the O-dealkylation are an alcohol and an aldehyde. The products of ether cleavage have not been identified but it is presumed that they would be the same — acetaldehyde and ethanol in the case of diethyl ether, and formaldehyde and dichloroethanol in the case of methoxyflurane.

The enzyme system responsible for the release of the chlorine has several points of similarity with the ether-cleaving system but enough points of dissimilarity to identify it as a separate system. The system is located in the endoplasmic reticulum and requires oxygen and NADPH for activity. In addition, this system also requires another factor which is found in the soluble portion of the cell. This factor has not been identified as yet but attempts are being made to do so. The reaction is probably an oxidation and therefore is not a replacement of the chlorine with oxygen or a hydroxyl group. It probably proceeds as described by Stier (1968) as follows:

$$
\begin{array}{ccc}
\overset{\displaystyle F}{\underset{\displaystyle F}{F-C}}\!\!-\!\!\overset{\displaystyle H}{\underset{\displaystyle Cl}{C}}\!\!-\!\!Br & \longrightarrow & \overset{\displaystyle F}{\underset{\displaystyle F}{F-C}}\!\!-\!\!\overset{\displaystyle \cdot}{\underset{\displaystyle Cl}{C}}\!\!-\!\!Br & \longrightarrow & \overset{\displaystyle F}{\underset{\displaystyle F}{F-C}}\!\!-\!\!COOH + Br^- + Cl^-\,.
\end{array}
$$

The dechlorination of methoxyflurane would proceed in a similar manner. Thus, it would appear that this is not an enzymatic attack on the carbon-chlorine bond but an oxidation of the carbon atom with a synchronous hydrolysis of the carbon-halogen bond. The dehalogenation proceeds optimally when there are two halogens and one hydrogen on a carbon (van Dyke and Wineman, in press). Completely halogenated carbons are not dehalogenated in this system.

The enzymes for these biotransformations are located principally in the liver although there is some activity in the kidney. The enzymes are membrane bound and all attempts to release them have caused the destruction of the enzyme.

The concentrations of the ether-cleaving and dechlorination enzyme systems can be increased through treatment of the animal with various drugs, hormones, and other chemicals (van Dyke, 1966). This type of enzyme induction was the subject of a review by Conney (1967).

Pretreatment of animals with phenobarbital or benzpyrene has resulted in induction of the dechlorinating activity. Exposing rats to low (subanesthetic) concentrations of methoxyflurane has resulted in the induction of the dechlorinating enzyme system but not the ether-cleaving system. Phenobarbital pretreatment will induce the ether-cleaving system. Thus, on the basis of inducibility it appears that these two enzyme systems can be considered as different.

The metabolism of trichloroethylene is inducible, as found by Leibman and McAllister (1967). This actually was an induction of the enzyme system responsible for the conversion of trichloroethylene to chloral hydrate. This conversion also takes place in the endoplasmic reticulum and requires NADPH and oxygen.

Blake et al. (1967) found that the metabolism of flsuroxene is stimulated by pretreatment of the animal with phenobarbital. They also found, as have others, that this induction is prevented if an inhibitor of protein synthesis is present during the period of the induction.

This enzyme induction is a fairly rapid process, beginning about 6 h after treatment and reaching a maximum in 24—48 h. The enzyme levels are back to normal in 2—3 weeks.

If a variety of chemicals can cause an enzyme induction, are the volatile anesthetics capable of bringing about an induction ? The answer is, "Yes." As indicated previously, methoxyflurane administered in low doses induces the dechlorinating system. Diethyl ether has been found to be an enzyme-inducing agent (REMMER, 1962). In addition, chloral hydrate is a weak inducing agent, and so is trichloroethylene. It is not known if the enzyme induction is due to the trichloroethylene itself or to the fact that it is converted to chloral hydrate which then accomplishes the enzyme induction.

Nitrous oxide has been found to induce drug-metabolizing enzymes. This is of great interest because of our lack of knowledge concerning the total disposition of nitrous oxide. The possibility exists that, to be an enzyme-inducing agent, the chemical must be metabolizable. Thus, barbituric acid is not metabolized and does not induce these enzymes; trichloroethane is not metabolized and does not induce these enzymes even though high concentrations can be achieved *in vivo*. It must be emphasized that this is only a probability; however, if it does hold up, it becomes one of the best pieces of evidence (even though indirect) that nitrous oxide is metabolized.

X. Implications of Metabolism

The question remains, Is the metabolism of the volatile anesthetics a detoxification process or an intoxification one ? Or is it neither but simply a means to hasten the departure of anesthetic from the body ? These questions are liable to be with us for some time to come. The eventual outcome will probably be that each anesthetic must be assessed individually and no broad generalities made. The problem is one of knowing the mechanism of biotransformation. The known metabolic products of this metabolism are not toxic, at least at the concentrations achieved. Therefore, if there are any toxic side-effects, they almost certainly have to come from highly reactive transient intermediates in the metabolic route. Thus, in these cases any enzyme induction would result in an increased probability of toxic side-effects.

On the other hand, if this is simply a means to hasten the departure of the anesthetic molecule from the cell, then it would be advantageous to try to speed up the whole process by inducing the enzymes necessary to carry this out. This may well be one of the most important aspects of the metabolism of the volatile anesthetics. It has recently been recognized that the volatile anesthetics remain in the body for long periods after administration. These periods may be in excess of 2 weeks. It is obvious that the cell cannot function in a completely normal manner as long as this foreign material is present and, therefore, any mechanism whereby the cell can return to normal more readily after an operation should be investigated. It should be borne in mind that patients receiving anesthetics often already have an altered biochemical status, and the presence of an anesthetic for a prolonged period may not be beneficial. Only by a detailed study of the mechanism of the metabolism of each anesthetic will this be resolved.

Since the anesthetics are now known to be metabolized by enzyme systems similar to or the same as those systems which metabolize other drugs or steroids, the possibility of competition between anesthetic and drug or steroid at the enzyme site is apparent. Anesthetics are not the only drugs administered in a clinical situation. The result of this competition is currently under study. VAN DYKE and RIKANS (unpublished data) found that halothane and methoxyflurane stimulate the hydroxylation of aniline by 100%, but diethyl ether inhibits this hydroxylation. However, methoxyflurane and halothane have no effect on the demethylation (N-dealkylation) of aminopyrine. Thus, it would appear that each combination must be studied before any conclusion can be drawn.

While the anesthetics which are presently available are excellent and allow the anesthesiologist to select the proper anesthetic for any surgical case, we should not cease the search for new anesthetics. The metabolic studies will allow us to become more sophisticated in our approach to designing these chemicals.

References

AHLMARK, A., FORSSMAN, S.: The effect of trichlorethylene on the organism. Acta Physiol. Scand. **22**, 326—339 (1951).
AXELROD, J.: The enzymic cleavage of aromatic ethers. Biochem. J. **63**, 634—639 (1956).
BARDODĚJ, Z., VYSKOČIL, J.: The problem of trichloroethylene in occupational medicine: Trichloroethylene metabolism and its effect on the nervous system evaluated as a means of hygienic control. Arch. Ind. Health **13**, 581—592 (1956).
BARRETT, H. M., JOHNSTON, J. H.: The fate of trichloroethylene in the organism. J. Biol. Chem. **127**, 765—770 (1939).
BLAKE, D. A., ROZMAN, R. S., CASCORBI, H. F., KRANTZ, J. C., JR.: Anesthesia LXXIV: Biotransformation of fluroxene. I. Metabolism in mice and dogs in vivo. Biochem. Pharmac. **16**, 1237—1248 (1967).
BRÜNING, A., SCHNETKA, M.: Über den Nachweis von Trichloräthylen und andern halogenhaltigen organischen Lösungsmitteln. Arch. Gewerbepathol. Gewerbehyg. **4**, 740—747 (1933).
BUTLER, T. C.: Metabolic transformations of trichloroethylene. J. Pharmac. Exptl Therap. **97**, 84—92 (1949).
— Reduction of carbon tetrachloride in vivo and reduction of carbon tetrachloride and chloroform in vitro by tissues and tissue constituents. J. Pharmac. Exptl Therap. **134**, 311—319 (1961).
BYINGTON, K. H., LEIBMAN, K. C.: Metabolism of trichloroethylene in liver microsomes. II. Identification of the reaction product as chloral hydrate. Mol. Pharmac. **1**, 247—254 (1965).
COHEN, E. N., HOOD, N.: Application of low-temperature autoradiography to studies of the uptake and metabolism of volatile anesthetics in the mouse. I. Chloroform. Anesthesiology **30**, 306—314 (1969).
— — Application of low-temperature autoradiography to studies of the uptake and metabolism of volatile anesthetics in the mouse. II. Diethyl ether. Anesthesiology **31**, 61—69 (1969).
CONNEY, A. H.: Pharmacological implications of microsomal enzyme induction. Pharmacol. Revs **19**, 317—366 (1967).
DANIEL, J. W.: The metabolism of ³⁶Cl-labelled trichloroethylene and tetrachloroethylene in the rat. Biochem. Pharmac. **12**, 795—802 (1963).
DAWKINS, M. J. R.: Carbon tetrachloride poisoning in the liver of the new-born rat. J. Pathol. Bacteriol. **85**, 189—196 (1963).
FABRE, R., TRUHAUT, R.: Contribution à l'étude de la toxicologie du trichloréthylène. II. Résultats des études expérimentales chez l'animal. Brit. J. Ind. Med. **9**, 39—43 (1952).
FOUTS, J. R., HART, L. G.: Hepatic drug metabolism during the perinatal period. Ann. N.Y. Acad. Sci. **123**, 245—250 (1965).
HAGGARD, H. W.: The absorption, distribution, and elimination of ethyl ether. I. The amount of ether absorbed in relation to the concentration inhaled and its fate in the body. J. Biol. Chem. **59**, 737—751 (1924).
LEIBMAN, K. C., MCALLISTER, W. J., JR.: Metabolism of trichloroethylene in liver microsomes. III. Induction of the enzymic activity and its effect on excretion of metabolites. J. Pharmac. Exptl Therap. **157**, 574—580 (1967).
MATSUBARA, T., MORI, T.: Studies on denitrification. IX. Nitrous oxide, its production, and reduction to nitrogen. J. Biochem. (Tokyo) **64**, 863—871 (1968).
PAUL, B. B., RUBINSTEIN, D.: Metabolism of carbon tetrachloride and chloroform by the rat. J. Pharmac. Exptl Therap. **141**, 141—148 (1963).
PAYKOÇ, Z. V., POWELL, JOAN F.: The excretion of sodium trichloracetate. J. Pharmac. Exptl Therap. **85**, 289—293 (1945).
PIETSCH, P., CHENOWETH, M. B.: Muscle regeneration: Enhancement by ethylene inhalation. Proc. Soc. Exptl Biol. Med. **130**, 714—717 (1969).
POWELL, JOAN F.: Trichlorethylene: Absorption, elimination and metabolism. Brit. J. Ind. Med. **2**, 142—145 (1945).

REHDER, K., FORBES, J., ALTER, H., HESSLER, O., STIER, A.: Halothane biotransformation in man: A quantitative study. Anesthesiology **28**, 711—715 (1967).

REMMER, H.: Drugs as activators of drug enzymes. In: Proceedings of the First International Pharmacological Meeting: Mode of action of drugs. Vol. 6. Metabolic factors controlling duration of drug action. New York: Macmillan Comp. 1962.

SOUČEK, B., VLACHOVÁ, D.: Dălší metabolity trichlorethylenu u člověka. Prace Lek. **6**, 330—332 (1954).

— — Excretion of trichloroethylene metabolites in human urine. Brit. J. Ind. Med. **17**, 60—64 (1960).

STIER, A.: Trifluoroacetic acid as metabolite of halothane. (Short communication.) Biochem. Pharmac. **13**, 1544 (1964).

— The biotransformation of halothane. (Correspondence.) Anesthesiology **29**, 388—390 (1968).

— ALTER, H., HESSLER, O., REHDER, K.: Urinary excretion of bromide in halothane anesthesia. Anesthesia & Analgesia **43**, 723—728 (1964).

VAN DYKE, R. A.: Discussion. In: Uptake and distribution of anesthetic agents. New York: Blakiston Company — Division of McGraw-Hill Book Company, Inc. 1963.

— Metabolism of volatile anesthetics. III. Induction of microsomal dechlorinating and ether-cleaving enzymes. J. Pharmac. Exptl Therap. **154**, 364—369 (1966).

— CHENOWETH, M. B.: (1) Metabolism of volatile anesthetics. Anesthesiology **26**, 348—357 (1965).

— — (2) The metabolism of volatile anesthetics. II. In vitro metabolism of methoxyflurane and halothane in rat liver slices and cell fractions. Biochem. Pharmac. **14**, 603—609 (1965).

— — LARSEN, E. R.: Synthesis and metabolism of halothane-1-^{14}C. (Letter to the editor.) Nature **204**, 471—472 (1964).

— — VAN POZNAK, A.: Metabolism of volatile anesthetics. I. Conversion in vivo of several anesthetics to $^{14}CO_2$ and chloride. Biochem. Pharmac. **13**, 1239—1247 (1964).

— RIKANS, L. A.: Effect of the volatile anesthetics on aniline hydroxylase and aminopyrine demethylase. Biochem. Pharmac. **19**, 1501—1502 (1970).

— WINEMAN, C. G.: Enzymatic dechlorination: In vitro dechlorination of chloroethanes and propanes. Biochem. Pharmac. (in press.)

WHIPPLE, G. H.: Pregnancy and chloroform anesthesia: A study of the maternal, placental, and fetal tissues. J. Exp. Med. **15**, 246—258 (1912).

WOOD, J. M., KENNEDY, F. S., WOLFE, R. S.: The reaction of multihalogenated hydrocarbons with free and bound reduced vitamin B_{12}. Biochemistry (N.Y.) **7**, 1707—1713 (1968).

Section 6.0

Mechanism of Anesthesia

6.1. Molecular Aspects

R. M. FEATHERSTONE

EHRLICH wrote before the turn of the 20th century that drugs are molecules and can only react with other molecules. Many inhalation anesthetics have been studied, but the intimate nature of the biological molecules which accept the anesthetic molecules and are affected by them is still almost completely unknown. Today attention is usually focused on the alteration of some biological action and the desirability or undesirability of this event. The molecules causing narcosis or anesthesia vary considerably in their structures and component atoms, and this variance has led to many studies of the correlations between the structures and properties of the anesthetic molecules and their effectiveness as anesthetic agents. Although such comparisons of properties and potency have led in the past, and will lead in the future, to a degree of predictability for the activity of new compounds or for the handling in the body of other members of a chemical series, the data so derived have been of very limited usefulness in attempts to understand the molecular aspects of the mechanism of action of inhalation anesthetics.

If one accepts this fundamental tenet about drugs reacting with molecules, it is then necessary to leave the study of the neurological effects of inhalation anesthetics to the neurophysiological pharmacologists and, likewise, to leave the study of the biochemical effects of these agents to the biochemical pharmacologists, and to allow the molecular pharmacologists to concentrate on the molecular mechanisms by which this primary event of molecule A reacting with molecule B can lead to the observed biochemical and physiological events.

A basic question is whether a molecular theory of anesthesia can be stated at this time — a theory which is not so general that it cannot be challenged by experiment. While no such theory has yet been put forward, there has been in recent years a renewed interest in this field, and workers in several laboratories are making significant steps in this direction.

Before discussing these recent studies, the earlier "theories" will be discussed and measured against the modern requirement of molecular pharmacology that "theories" will not be really useful unless they involve the molecular details of the drug, the anesthetic in this case, and of the biological system with which it interacts.

Most of the earlier "theories" dealt with the broader concept called "narcosis", or general depression produced by drugs. Anesthesia can be considered to be a special instance of this general phenomenon. A single mechanism has often been assumed in the enunciation of a theory of *the* mechanism of action. Frequently this "mechanism" related molecules and properties of complex aggregates of molecules, such as a membrane, a cell, or organ, etc. A useful way to consider all these theories is to recall SCHUELER's (1960) listing of nine levels of integration of natural systems. These levels are shown in Table 1. It can be seen that each level of integration results from interactions of combinations of units of the next lower level. The basic principles are: (1) units of any given level interact only with like units, although the effect may be expressed at higher levels, and (2) the interaction of units on one level may modify the functions of units on the next higher as well as each succeeding level. The example of death of an organism by X-ray effects can be cited: death is due to an interaction of electrons of the X-ray beam with some fundamental particles of some atom, of some molecule, of some molecular system, etc. A major experimental problem is the development of ways to allow observations of reactions on the level on which they are occurring, instead of on

Table 1. *Levels of Integration*[a]

Level	Physical units	Investigator
1. Subatomic	Electrons, Protons, etc.	Physicist
2. Atomic	Elements — combinations of electrons, protons, etc. C, H, N, O, Xe, K, Na, etc.	Physicist Physical chemist
3. Molecular	Compounds — combinations of atoms; water, glucose, cyclopropane	Physical and Organic chemists
4. Polymolecular		Biochemist, enzymologist
5. Cellular	Interacting polymolecular systems, usually bounded by membranes — red blood cells, hepatic cells, etc.	Cytologist, physiologist, histologist, pathologist
6. Tissue	System of similar cells — epithelial, endothelial, etc.	Physiologist, pathologist, histologist
7. Organ	Discrete bodies ot different kinds of cells — liver, kidney, pancreas, etc.	Physiologist, pathologist
8. Organism	Combinations of interacting organs — man, cat, dog	Physiologist, psychologist, psychiatrist
9. Society	Collective interaction of organisms — clubs, states, cities, etc.	Psychologist, psychiatrist, Sociologist, ecologist

[a] This table is adapted from F. W. SCHUELER (1960).

the level which they are obvious — usually many steps removed from the actual primary mechanism.

Most "theories" of "mechanisms" during the past century could be classified in levels 3, 4 or 5. If the above principles are accepted, those theories involving the cellular level can be dismissed as not contributing much to an acceptable statement of the mechanisms of anesthesia, but are consequences of it.

HOBER (1907), LILLIE (1923) and WINTERSTEIN (1926) all suggested that narcotics act at cell surfaces by decreasing the permeability of the cell to essential metabolites. Nothing is offered as to how or with what the narcotics interact or what metabolites do not get into the cells. Indeed, a review of literature concerned with the measurement of cell permeability to natural and synthetic compounds in the presence of an anesthetic or narcotic agent led DE BON and MUEHLBAECHER (1963) to conclude that anesthetics may or may not change permeability, and that when a change occurs, there may be increased or decreased permeability, depending on species, cell types, and compound.

In a similar manner the same criticisms may be applied to the theories of WARBURG (1910) who stated that narcotics depress cellular oxidations. The mechanisms are not elucidated and whether overall cellular oxidation is depressed depends on the system studied. These systems, as they have been studied, can only lead to recognition that the effect may be recognized at the polymolecular level if one looks there.

Even if one looks on the molecular level and theorizes about events on this level, there may be little conceptual gain. The thermodynamic approach of FERGUSON (1939) led to the statement that isonarcotic concentrations expressed as weight or volume percentages varied over a wide range, whereas a very narrow range resulted when isonarcotic concentrations were expressed in the physical-chemical unit called "activity" — involving corrections for solvent and other molecular interactions. FERGUSON suggests that this "activity" measurement is a meaningful one because it allows the measurement of the narcotic in the biophase where anesthesia occurs even though the site and nature of the biophase are not known — based on the concept that the "activity" of a substance is equal in all parts of an equilibrium system. This statement is less an explanation of mechanism than it is of emphasizing the necessity of measuring a correct chemical quantity (here, activity) instead of the usual weight-concentrations. No more can be expected of it, because thermodynamics studies are of energy differences between states and are not concerned with the mechanisms by which these states are achieved.

MULLINS (1954) added the important variable of molecular size by postulating that anesthesia occurs when a constant fraction of the total free volume of a non-aqueous phase of a cell is occupied by anesthetic molecules — a phase such as the "pores" of a cell membrane, in which transport of small ions involved in nerve conduction might be blocked. Too little is known about details of membrane structure to evaluate this suggestion. The important point to be noted here is that this concept, like FERGUSON's, uses the "phase" picture of biological systems — a far more general view than the molecular continuum concept to be developed later in this discussion.

Another general theory which has had continuing reemphasis since it was first proposed by TRAUBE (1904) is the contention that potency of narcotic effects correlates well with the degree of lowering of surface tension at an air-water interface. Because many compounds so affecting surface tension are not anesthetic, and because such interfaces are not involved in *in vivo* situations associated with anesthesia, this type of consideration, ancient or modern, can be dismissed as being of no importance in the search for molecular level explanations.

The term "phase" or "biophase" was used frequently in these "cellular" level proposals about anesthesia mechanisms. The proposers were naturally reaching to the lower levels outlined in Table 1 for their "units" of expression. At the polymolecular level of this system, "phase" is also a much used word, and there is a greater degree of definiteness about the nature of these phases, even though all proposals fall far short of being satisfactory molecular level statements.

It was in this realm that the correlations of anesthetic potency with many physical chemical properties became the pattern indulged in by almost all scientists thinking about this field, including the author of this discussion.

Even as early as 1847 BIBRA and HARLESS (cit. HENDERSON, 1910) noted that the known anesthetics were fat solvents. They pictured the anesthetics to be washing fats out of cells, thus causing anesthesia, and they based their thought on an observed blood lipid increase during anesthesia. The almost instantaneous recoveries from anesthesia are not consistent with the involvement of such an exchange of cell lipids, but the correlation of lipid solubility and anesthesia has received much attention. H. MEYER and OVERTON (1899, 1901), at first independently and later in cooperation, stated that the narcotic potency of a compound is proportional to its distribution coefficient between lipids and water, and postulated that this was the "mechanism" of anesthesia. K. H. MEYER and HEMMI (1935) restated this general idea by saying "narcosis appears if a chemically indifferent substance has penetrated into the cell lipids, more correctly, the lipoid alcohols of cell substances, to reach a definite molar concentration. The concentration is a function of the animal or of the cell but is independent of the narcotic."

These theories, like all theories, perhaps, caused many people to think about anesthesia and they caused many others to cling to the naive thought that this was an adequate explanation of a fascinating phenomenon. Many criticisms are obvious. The generalization is best for members of a homologous series. Solubilities in water and olive oil are not at all comparable to biological systems in which the lipids vary greatly in composition and where the water is probably aggregated by forces not present in the simple oil-water mixture, such as proteins, primarily. Many compounds having greater affinities for olive oil than for water are not anesthetics. Therefore, although such considerations may play an important role in determining how compounds are distributed in the body, little insight is gained from them about specific molecular mechanisms.

The same can be said about other correlations noted in the intervening years in which anesthesia has been related to a number of other properties of the effective compounds. As WULF and FEATHERSTONE have shown (1957), good correlations of anesthetic potency with boiling point, molar refraction, and VAN DER WAALS constants a and b are all relatable to the interrelated properties of substances expressed by their critical constants and their polarizabilities and molecular volumes. PAULING (1961) used a similar correlation between anesthetic potency and molar refraction in comparing the dissociation pressures of the hydrates of anesthetic gases and the partial pressures of anesthetics necessary for narcosis. PAULING was aware that the mechanism of anesthesia could not be simply the formation of hydrate crystals in the brain, because none of the hydrates of anesthetic gases is stable at physiological temperature and pressure. He proposed that there might be a simultaneous involvement of some side chains of amino acids in proteins.

It is at this point that the work of FEATHERSTONE and his colleagues SCHOENBORN, MUEHLBAECHER et al. (1961—1968) and the postulate of PAULING have a close interrelationship. This will be brought out later in the discussion of advances in molecular level knowledge of the nature of the "receptors" for anesthetic agents. At the moment, the important point is that all these correlation studies are subject to the same criticism applied to many other statements which have been labelled, either by their authors or their readers, as theories of mechanisms of anesthetic action. They are too general. They reflect a "phase" approach which does not identify the molecular nature of the biological "receptor" sites or the place(s) where these sites might exist by virtue of their being in molecules which have functions involved in the processes of maintenance of consciousness.

The concept of "phase", as the term is used in physical chemistry discussions, usually has one of two meanings, depending on the degree of chemical naivete of the one who uses it. The non-chemist biologist uses the term as if he implies cells are made up of homogenous compartments adjacent to each other. No concentration of the anesthetic molecules is usually mentioned for either the lipid or water phases, but the implication is that a 34 to 1, 20 to 1, or some other partition exists and that this is in some way important. The non-biologist chemist uses "phase" distribution as a chemist would and recognizes all possibilities for distribution between the phases, but the idea is generally conveyed that he is thinking about these systems in terms of classical treatments of solutions, in which the solute (anesthetic) is present in close to infinite dilution in the solvents. Neither seems to consider the possibility that the continuum or matrix of molecules in biological systems, whether they be in membranes, cells, or other recognizable units of biological structure, has very specific spaces where the anesthetic molecules combine with the parts of the continuum and alter the function of the system by stabilizing the part of the molecule with which they react on a saturation basis, rather than on an infinite dilution basis.

The work that has led to a more detailed visualization of the molecular associations of inhalation anesthetics began with the observation that xenon, a gas shown by CULLEN and GROSS (1951) to be anesthetic for man, combined with macromolecules (FEATHERSTONE et al., 1961; MUEHLBAECHER et al., 1963, 1966). Specifically, at 37 °C one atom of xenon was shown to combine with one molecule of hemoglobin, and almost half of the xenon carried in the blood during anesthesia was shown to be carried in combination with hemoglobin.

Thus, this combination of xenon, a remarkable model anesthetic agent due to its effectiveness and the lack of involvement of covalent, ionic, or hydrogen bonding potentials, and hemoglobin, a protein for which the knowledge of three-dimensional structures was approaching completion (PERUTZ, 1965) became the basis of studies by SCHOENBORN et al. (1965) in which the exact location of the binding of xenon in sperm whale metmyoglobin was determined using the difference electron density technique of the X-ray diffraction field.

Before describing these results, the value of having them deserves comment. Certainly myoglobin and hemoglobin cannot be easily accused of being directly involved in the chemical or physical events in the central nervous system that are related to anesthesia. However, there are no brain proteins whose atom-to-atom three-dimensional structures are known. If one assumes that an interaction between the anesthetic agent, xenon or cyclopropane, and proteins, whose structures are known, may be similar to such interactions with brain proteins, the pertinence of such studies, while not absolutely clear, is evident. Because of advances in physical techniques, the likelihood of achieving knowledge of this type is great. For example, this is particularly true following the realization of the limited number of weak bonding types involved in holding the anesthetic molecules in their specific positions inside the proteins, as discussed by SCHOENBORN and FEATHERSTONE (1967). Obviously, this is much more interesting than merely correlating physical properties or lipid solubilities with anesthetic potency.

When SCHOENBORN et al. (1965) subjected xenon-myoglobin to X-ray diffraction analysis, they were able to compare the data for the three-dimensional structure of this complex with the data of WATSON (1968) in which the three-dimensional locations of all 1260 nonhydrogen atoms of myoglobin have been located. Brief discussions of this technique are to be found in papers by SCHOENBORN and FEATHERSTONE (1967) and SCHOENBORN (1968). In the case of xenon-myoglobin, two projections gave enough information to determine the three coordinates of xenon sites in the myoglobin. Each difference electron-density map showed only one nearly circular peak corresponding to one spherical atom. Other areas of the maps were featureless indicating that the binding of the xenon atom did not disturb the positions of the other atoms and that there were no other xenon binding sites. Xenon's location in the myoglobin molecule was nearly equidistant from the heme-linked histidine, from the pyrrole ring of the heme, and from the side group atoms of several amino acids. Although the sizes of the dipoles involved in this site and the charge distribution on the heme group are not known accurately enough to allow precise calculations of the DEBYE, or dipole-induced dipole effects or the charge-induced dipole energies, the actual London energies between the xenon and the 32 atoms surrounding the xenon were calculated. A figure of about 10 kcal/mole resulted as constituting over 90% of the total bonding of the xenon in this site. This is an astonishingly large figure — approximately equivalent to two ionic bonds. Similar analyses with metmyoglobin and with reduced myoglobin gave essentially the same results.

The slightly larger cyclopropane molecule was studied in the same way. The electron-density maps showed the presence of cyclopropane in the same place occupied by xenon in xenon- myoglobin. They also showed changes corresponding to a 90° rotation of the benzene ring of phenylalanine in the native myoglobin. This shift apparently allowed the accommodation of cyclopropane. Like xenon, the cyclopropane-myoglobin complex was stabilized mainly by London forces (FEATHERSTONE, 1968).

Similar work with hemoglobin and xenon by SCHOENBORN (1965), based on work on the structure of hemoglobin by PERUTZ (1965), indicated the presence of a xenon atom in each of the two α- and β-chains of the hemoglobin molecule. The sites appeared to be within the subunits but close to their external surfaces, and therefore were quite different from those in myoglobin. However, the nearest neighbors of all the xenon sites were valine, leucine and phenylalanine, as in myoglobin, so that the primary stabilizing forces are again London interactions.

Xenon has been shown not to bind to all proteins; for example, it does not react with hen egg lysozyme, chymotrypsin, or horse heart cytochrome. Therefore, the reaction of xenon only with some regions of proteins containing nonpolar R groups indicates that very special situations must be present before this interaction occurs. Krypton, slightly smaller than xenon, does not bind at these sites (MAGNUSSON et al., 1969).

Although these well-described instances of complex formation between proteins and anesthetic agents are almost certainly not involved in an explanation of the phenomenon of anesthesia, they give considerable insight into the types of interactions these agents can and do enter. When brain proteins are characterized, these types of interactions will probably be shown to be involved in the complicated series of reactions leading to anesthesia. At the time of this writing, these experiments are the *only* ones in which there is three-dimensional knowledge of drug-protein interaction. These studies indicate the major direction molecular pharmacology must take if the goal of full knowledge of the structural and functional changes of both drug and receptor are to be attained.

The interesting and provocative clathrate and hydrate theories of PAULING (1961) and MILLER (1961) are pertinent to these protein studies. The possible association of their ideas with those of FEATHERSTONE and SCHOENBORN was emphasized by a study of the influence of xenon on protein hydration by SCHOENBORN et al. (1964). Dielectric constant measurements, using a microwave absorption technique, showed that the association of xenon with hemoglobin was accompanied by a 10—15% increase of irrotationally bound water.

The proposals by PAULING, MILLER, SCHOENBORN, and FEATHERSTONE are based on knowledge of the aggregated forms of water and of the three-dimensional structures of proteins with and without the presence of xenon or cyclopropane in cavities in the interior of the proteins. The above studies do not answer the question of the location of these associations in the biological systems of the central nervous system which are altered during the clinical phenomenon of anesthesia, but they do describe molecular level events which are possible — perhaps the only types possible — for some of the inhaled anesthetic agents.

Perhaps the era of correlating physical chemical properties with anesthetic potencies and having each new correlation labelled by many as "the" mechanism of anesthesia is past. Such correlations are interesting in that they reemphasize the interrelationships of the properties of matter to each other, but they are afflicted with "phase" thinking — thinking that implies cells are a series of compartments of pure substances, rather than a matrix of many species of molecules forming a continuum in three-dimensions. This "phase" thinking has no doubt come from the clinically practical concepts of compartments into which anesthetics enter. The management of anesthesia must rely on such a set of assumptions. Perhaps it is difficult for many to realize that, despite the elaborate lengths to which such model systems are used in clinical research on anesthesia, this type of thinking is of almost no value in the search for molecular level explanations of anesthesia mechanisms. The discussor and the listener must conceive submolecular compartments in the same manner. The group of atoms surrounding xenon or cyclopropane in myoglobin or hemoglobin make up in large measure the R groups of amino acids which are nonpolar; therefore, they constitute a lipid-like milieu for the anesthetic. However, because the rigid requirement for full knowledge of receptor molecules as well as drug molecules is not in the minds of more than a handful of researchers on anesthesia mechanisms, it becomes necessary to drop the word "lipid" from this discussion. It is too general a term in this context for 1971. Likewise, the terms "chemical", "physical", and even "solution" must be declared taboo, unless their generality and their limitations are acknowledged.

Much work must be done before the molecular mechanisms of anesthesia by inhaled molecules can be stated satisfactorily. The other inhaled agents should be studied with the X-ray diffraction techniques used with xenon and cyclopropane. The molecular make-up of the central nervous system must be ascertained, and molecular level studies involving anesthetics must be undertaken. Other new techniques, such as the use of nuclear magnetic resonance, which JARDETZKY (1965) has shown to be very useful in describing details of binding sites of drugs with proteins, and such as the refinements of the dielectric constant studies of drug effects on water associated with the other constituents of biological systems (VOGELHUT, 1962), must be exploited. Finally, there is a great need to educate many more people about the enormity of our ignorance of the molecular level details of biological systems. Far too often, writers either do not comprehend or admit the gap between their knowledge of an event and their conclusions as to how it occurs. However, this error is not as great as that made by the person who reads a "theory" of anesthesia mechanisms proposed by a person of eminence and concludes that the issue has now been settled.

The discussion offered here has not by any means dealt fully with all the papers contributing to the details of our knowledge of inhalation anesthetics at the molecular level. The suggestion has been made that this topic is very much in its infancy. The explanation of the mechanism of anesthesia — at any level — is one of the truly fundamental and foremost problems facing pharmacologists today.

References

CULLEN, S. C., GROSS, E. G.: The anesthetic properties of xenon in animals and human beings, with additional observations on krypton. Science **113**, 580—582 (1951).
DE BON, F., MUEHLBAECHER, C. A.: Mechanisms of anesthesia, management of inhalation anesthesia. Intern. Anesthesiol. Clin. **1**, 927—935 (1963).

FEATHERSTONE, R. M.: The molecular pharmacology of anesthesia: An introduction. Federation Proc. **27**, 870—871 (1968).
— MUEHLBAECHER, C. A., DE BON, F. L., FORSAITH, J. A.: Interactions of inert anesthetic gases with proteins. Anesthesiology **22**, 977—981 (1961).
FERGUSON, J.: Use of chemical potentials as indices of toxicity. Proc. Roy. Soc. B. **127**, 387 (1939).
HENDERSON, V. E.: The present status of the theories of narcosis. Physiol. Revs. **10**, 171—220 (1930).
HOBER, R.: Beiträge zur physikalischen Chemie der Erregung und der Narkose. Arch. ges. Physiol., Pflüger's **120**, 492 (1907).
JARDETSKY, O., WADE-JARDETSKY, N. G.: On the mechanism of the binding of sulfonamides to bovine serum albumin. Mol. Pharmacol. J. **1**, 214—230 (1965).
LILLIE, R. S.: Protoplasmic action and nervous action. Univ. of Chicago Press 1923.
MAGNUSSON, H., SCHOENBORN, B. P., FEATHERSTONE, R. M.: An X-ray crystallographic study of various anesthetic gases binding to myoglobin. M.S. Thesis, Univ. Calif., Dec. 1968.
MEYER, H.: Zur Theorie der Alkoholnarkose. Arch. exptl. Pathol. Pharmakol., Naunyn-Schmiedeberg's **42**, 109—118 (1899).
MEYER, H. H., GOTTLIEB, R.: Die experimentelle Pharmakologie als Grundlage der Arzneibehandlung (9th ed.). Berlin and Vienna: Urban and Schwarzenberg 1936.
MEYER, K. H., HEMMI, H.: Beitrag zur Theorie der Narkose. III. Biochem. Z. **277**, 39—71 (1935).
MILLER, S. L.: A theory of gaseous anesthesia. Proc. Natl. Acad. Sci. US **47**, 1515—1524 (1961).
MUEHLBAECHER, C. A., DE BON, F. L., FEATHERSTONE, R. M.: Interactions of lipids and proteins with anesthetic gases. Intern. Anesthesiol. Clin. **1**, 937—952 (1963).
— — — Further studies on the solubilities of xenon and cyclopropane in blood and protein solutions. Mol. Pharmacol. **2**, 86—89 (1966).
MULLINS, L. J.: Some physical mechanisms in narcosis. Chem. Revs. **54**, 289 (1954).
OVERTON, E.: Studien über die Narkose. Jena 1901.
PAULING, L.: A molecular theory of anesthesia. Science **134**, 15—21 (1961).
PERUTZ, M. F., KENDREW, J. C., WATSON, H. C.: Structure and function of hemoglobin. II. Some relations between polypeptide chain configuration and amino acid sequence. J. Mol. Biol. **13**, 666—678 (1965).
SCHOENBORN, B. P.: Binding of xenon to horse haemoglobin. Nature **208**, 760—762 (1965).
— Binding of anesthetics to protein: An X-ray crystallographic investigation. Federation Proc. **27**, 888—894 (1968).
— FEATHERSTONE, R. M.: Molecular forces in anesthesia. Advances in Pharmacol. **5**, 1—17 (1967).
— — VOGELHUT, P. O., SUSSKIND, C.: Influence of xenon on protein hydration as measured by a microwave absorption technique. Nature **202**, 695—696 (1964).
— WATSON, H. C., KENDREW, J. C.: Binding of xenon to sperm whale myoglobin. Nature **207**, 28—30 (1965).
SCHUELER, F. W.: Chemobiodynamics and drug design, p. 35. New York: McGraw-Hill Co. 1960.
TRAUBE, J.: Theorie der Osmose und Narkose. Arch. ges. Physiol., Pflüger's **105**, 541—558 (1904).
VOGELHUT, P. O.: The dielectric properties of water and their role in enzyme substrate interactions. Electronics Res. Lab. Monograph, Series 60, Issue 476, Univ. of Calif. Press 1962.
WARBURG, O.: Über die Oxydation in lebenden Zellen. Z. physiol. Chem., Hoppe-Seyler's **66**, 305—340 (1910).
WATSON, H. C.: Progr. in Stereochem. **IV** (1968) (in press).
WINTERSTEIN, H.: Die Narkose (2nd ed.). Berlin: Springer 1926.
WULF, R. J., FEATHERSTONE, R. M.: A correlation of van der Waals constants with anesthetic potency. Anesthesiology **18**, 97—105 (1957).

Additional Communications: Added by Ed.

CHERKIN, A.: Mechanisms of general anesthesia by non-hydrogen-bonding molecules. Ann. Rev. Pharmacol. **9**, 259—272 (1969).
EGER, E. I., LUNDGREN, E., MILLER, S. L., STEVENS, W. C.: Anesthetic potencies of sulfur hexafluoride, carbon tetrafluoride, chloroform and Ethrane in dogs: Correlation with the hydrate and lipid theories of anesthetic action. Anesthesiology **30**, 129—135 (1969).
— SHARGEL, R. D.: The lack of hydrate formation at a temperature of 0 °C of methoxyflurane, halothane, diethyl ether and fluroxene. Anesthesiology **30**, 136—137 (1969).
LARSEN, E. R., VAN DYKE, R. A., CHENOWETH, M. B.: Mechanisms of narcosis. In: Medicinal research: Biology and chemistry, Vol. 2 (BURGER, A., Ed.). New York: Pool. Marcel Dekker, Inc. 1967.

6.2. Neurophysiological Aspects

J. BIMAR and R. NAQUET

With 16 Figures

Introduction

During recent years some new volatile anesthetics have been synthesized; these include halothane (Fluothane) and methoxyflurane (Penthrane) which are quite novel. They are widely used clinically.

At the same time, developments in neurophysiology have established techniques for evaluating the various functions of the nervous system. These techniques apply either at the unit and cell level or in the wider sense of overall evaluation of nervous system function. Our research has been at the latter level.

Our experimental techniques, aimed at increased precision, have evolved from the cat to the primate, and suggest progressively closer and more superimposable correlations with the human (see GALINDO, Chapter 4.1).

These two volatile halogenated hydrocarbons are used in increasingly large numbers of both pharmacological and physiological evaluations because of their wide clinical use. Their narcotic "activity" and the orientation of our laboratory's research persuaded us to study them more closely and to define their action strictly at the central nervous system level.

The work on the cat (RENN, 1965; RENN et al., 1965; BIMAR and NAQUET, 1966; LE POULEUF, 1967) is described first, followed by that on the primate. In each case the effects of halothane are reported before those of methoxyflurane.

I. Experimental Work on the Cat

A. Halothane

1. The EEG Recording (Fig. 1)

The experimental study of changes in the electrocorticographic recording during inhalation of increasing concentrations of halothane in the cat reveals 7 successive stages:

1. Fast low amplitude activity of 15—25 µV at 30—40 c/sec. This activity appears after 3 or 4 min at a concentration of 0.5—1%.

2. After 10 min at a concentration of 0.5—1%, or 5—8 min at 1.5—2%, activity appears at 14 c/sec of greater amplitude (50—100 µV) and in spindles.

3. After 20 min at a concentration of 1%, or 15 min at 2%, or 7 min at 4%, the activity is greater in amplitude (100—200 µV); still fast but associated with slower spindles (8—10 c/sec).

4. This stage is difficult to achieve with 1% concentration of halothane in air and requires 20 min at 2%. On a slower background rhythm (5—6 c/sec) of

50—100 μV amplitude, paroxysmal spindles arise at the same frequency but of 300—400 μV amplitude.

5. After 25 min at 2% concentration or 20 min at 4%, a further slowing of the background activity occurs (2—3 c/sec) with a decrease in amplitude (50 μV); spindles of about 200 μV amplitude and 4—5 c/sec are superimposed.

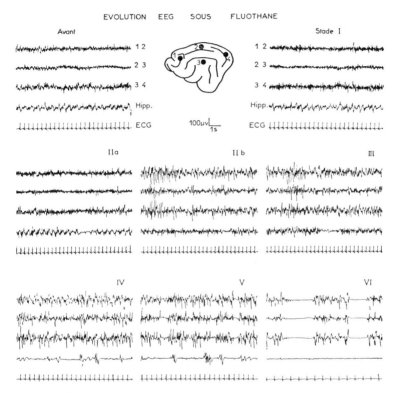

Fig. 1. Evolution of cortical and hippocampal electrical activity during inhalation of halothane in the cat (evolution EEG sous fluothane). Control: (Avant). Bipolar derivations, cortical recordings, (1—2, 2—3, 3—4) dorsal hippocampal activity recorded from bipolar: (Hipp.). Electrocardiogram: E.C.G. The stages represented here are schematic examples of the most typical changes found during halothane anesthesia (this one is with a 3% concentration). The surgical stage, according to GUEDEL, corresponds approximately to recordings III and IV

6. After 30 min at 3—4% concentration, the record contains sharp activity with amplitudes of 150 μV, which is continuous and at 3—4 c/sec, interrupted by brief pauses.

7. After 35 min at 4% the pauses become longer and longer reaching 2—4 sec, mixed with the same type of background activity.

Stages 3 and 4 may be said to correspond to the so-called "surgical" stages. It seems, therefore, that with halothane anesthesia the electrical activity characteristic of these stages is faster than that found with other anesthetics such as barbiturates, at a clinically identical "depth" of anesthesia.

Although the number of stages isolated as above is not found by all workers (RAVENTOS, 1956; STEPHEN et al., 1958; DENAVIT, 1963; etc.) nor in the other animal species used, it is, however, obvious that the recording follows the same type of evolution in relation to the depth of narcosis. All authors agree that the frequency of activity recorded is much higher than that found with other anesthetic drugs.

2. The Arousal Response (Fig. 2)

The arousal response of the neocortex and the hippocampus, effected by stimulation of the reticular formation (MORUZZI and MAGOUN, 1949) provides a way of measuring the inhibitory effect of the anesthetic agent on the ascending reticular system.

After 30 min inhalation at 1% concentration of halothane vapour in air, neocortical fast rhythms due to reticular stimulation are delayed for 1 sec but persist after the end of stimulation; at the hippocampal level, the length of the response is distinctly reduced.

After 30 min at 1.5% concentration, fast activities appear at the cortical level with 2.5 sec delay and the hippocampal response does not appear at all.

Finally, inhalation of a 2% concentration of halothane in air for 30 min produces complete abolition of the arousal response both at neocortical and hippocampal levels. By raising the stimulation voltage to 1.5 or 2 V a sketchy response is obtained but occurs late.

During recovery, an arousal response re-appears very quickly after concentrations of 1% whereas after concentrations of 2%, recovery is still not complete 30 min after finishing anesthesia.

In conclusion, it seems that halothane raises the threshold of the response without ever causing complete blocking of it, unlike the barbiturates which cause considerable rise in the threshold of the response and prevent reappearance of fast activity.

Another peculiarity of this drug is the delay in appearance of the arousal response which may sometimes extend to several seconds.

3. Evoked Potentials (Fig. 3)

a) Along the Specific Primary Pathways

Potentials evoked by photic stimulation are recorded at the retina, the optic chiasma, the lateral geniculate body and visual area I.

— At the retinal level (ERG) the evoked potential consists of an initial low amplitude, surface negative wave followed by a larger positive wave (EINTHOVEN and JOLLY, 1908; ADRIAN and MATTHEWS, 1927; etc.).

After halothane, the morphology of the ERG changes: increase in latency, decrease in amplitude of the positive wave and increase in the total duration of the potential occur.

— At the chiasma, the potential is made up of a short latency positive wave showing oscillations at the end of the positive wave which correspond to action potentials.

Halothane inhalation is accompanied here by:

— increase in latency,

— decrease in amplitude of the positive wave and a change in the morphology of the latter part of it.

— In the visual area I, the potential is seen to have two phases: the first one positive and the second negative with irregular indentation. The changes produced by halothane are exactly the same as those at the chiasma level: increase in latency, decrease in amplitude of both positive and negative waves and lengthening of the total duration of the potential.

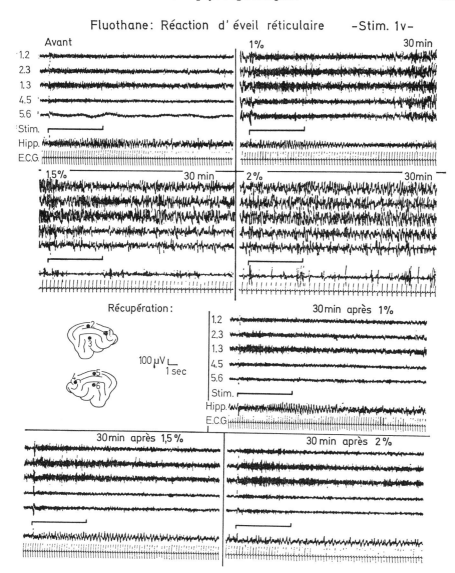

Fig. 2. Effect of halothane on the arousal response provoked by stimulation of the midbrain reticular formation in the cat (réaction d'éveil réticulaire). Cortical recordings: 1—2, 2—3, 1—3, 4—5, 5—6. Hippocampal recordings: Hipp. Electrocardiogram: E.C.G. The 1 volt stimulation of the reticular formation is indicated by an unbroken black line (Stim.). Control: (Avant). Recovery: (Récupération). During halothane anesthesia, the concentration and the duration correspond to the depth of anesthesia. After the end of anesthesia, the changes are entirely due to the concentration, inhalation having finished 30 min earlier

In summary, evoked responses all along the specific pathways are changed by the action of halothane without being abolished.

This action, which takes effect rapidly even at weak concentrations is apparent from the proto-neurone onward.

The changes consist basically of a lengthening of the latency of all the phases and in particular the late oscillatory components, and a decrease in the amplitude of the initial phase.

Although our experiments produced some results which differ from those obtained by other authors (DENAVIT, 1963) because either the animal used or the

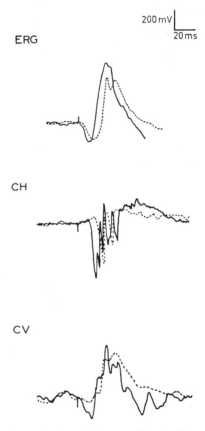

Fig. 3. Effect of halothane on visual evoked potentials in the cat. In solid lines, mean of 5 potentials before anesthesia. In dotted lines, mean of 5 evoked potentials during halothane anesthesia. The recordings obtained at each level were superimposed: — retina: ERG, — optic chiasma: CH, — primary visual cortex: CV. Changes can be seen at all levels of the primary specific pathways during halothane anesthesia: — increase in latency, — fall in amplitude of the waves at the retina and the chiasma, — damping of the oscillating after-discharge at the level of the visual cortex

stimulation was different, our findings are similar to those seen in man with photic stimulation (DOMINO et al., 1963).

b) Along the Non-specific Pathways (Fig. 4)

We investigated the effects of halothane on these conduction pathways by analyzing the potentials evoked at the level of the midbrain reticular formation, on stimulating the sciatic nerve or the bulbar reticular formation. The potential usually recorded consists of an initial positive wave followed by a low amplitude negative wave. The first wave is frequently complex. Increasing concentrations of halothane produce a decrease in the amplitude of the positive wave and virtual disappearance of the negative wave. The total length of the potential is shortened.

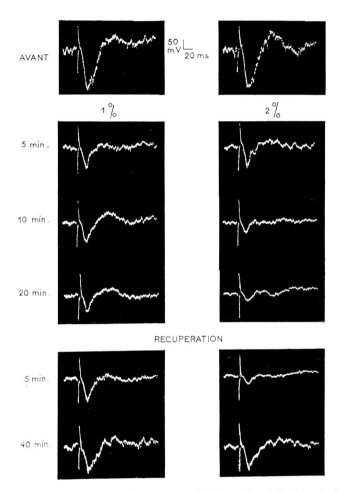

Fig. 4. Evoked potentials (potentiels évoqués) recorded from the midbrain reticular formation on single electric shock stimulation of the sciatic nerve in the cat, under halothane. Control: (Avant). Concentrations inhaled: (1 %, 2 %). Duration of the inhalation of concentration indicated: 5 min, 10 min. Evolution of the potential after the end of anesthesia. The times given indicate the period elapsed since the end of anesthesia. Recovery: (récupération 5 min, 40 min). In these oscillographic recordings one can see how the negative wave of the potential gradually diminishes and even disappears with a 2 % concentration

The multi-synaptic conduction pathways are therefore much more sensitive to the effects of halothane than are the primary specific pathways. As with many anesthetic drugs, the reticular responses seem to obey an all-or-none law. The changes appear and disappear long before the visual evoked responses show changes in their morphology.

In the limbic system, the potentials recorded in the hippocampus during stimulation of the amygdala are also greatly altered by inhalation of halothane, but here the element most affected is the latency; the amplitudes are reduced without the waves disappearing altogether (Fig. 5).

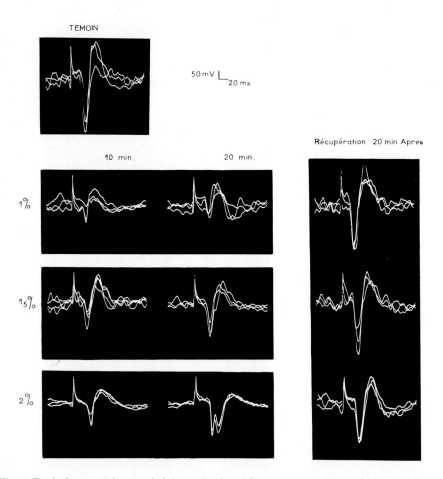

Fig. 5. Evoked potentials recorded from the dorsal hippocampus (potentiels évoqués hippocampiens), during single electric shock stimulation of the amygdala nucleus in the cat under halothane. Control: (Témoin). Concentrations inhaled: 1 %, 1.5 %, 2 %. Evolution after the end of anesthesia, 20 min after finishing with the concentration marked in the margin (Récupération 20 min après). This shows a great fall in amplitude of the evoked response and changes in its morphology as anesthesia deepens. Also the positive latency of the response elicited by the drug persists long after the end of anesthesia

4. Effect of Halothane on the Recruiting Response (Fig. 6)

This is a response of certain cortical areas to repetitive stimulation of an intralaminar thalamic nucleus, described by DEMPSEY and MORISON (1942). The two components, one stable and the other oscillating, which together produce the effect of "waxing and waning" (JASPER et al., 1955) are analyzed at the same time.

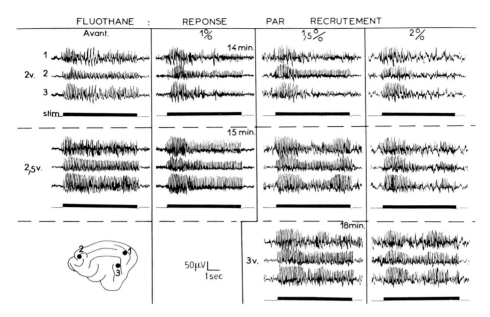

Fig. 6. Effects of halothane on the recruiting response (réponse par recrutement). Stimulation of the centralis lateralis nucleus with different voltages (2 V, 2.5 V, 3 V). The effects on the recruiting response are analyzed before each drug (Avant) and for different concentrations (1%, 1.5%, 2%) at various moments after the beginning of the inhalation

Inhalation of halothane tends gradually to banish the stable response and high concentrations give rise to the appearance of spindles. *In summary*, although it is accepted that sleep-inducing drugs facilitate the recruiting response, halothane only exerts this effect with high concentrations.

5. After-discharges

Electrical stimulation of certain rhinencephalic or neocortical structures elicits electrical after-discharges. Inhalation of halothane produces gradual disappearence of the after-discharges, at the same time abolishing the spike and wave type components.

6. Effect of Halothane on the Metrazol (Pentylene Tetrazol) Threshold

Examination of changes in this threshold confirms the anti-convulsant effect of halothane, which was to be expected considering its effect on after-discharges. However, this effect also is only transient.

7. Reactions to Dental Stimulation (Fig. 7)

We carried out electrical stimulation of the dentine with an implanted electrode and recorded the reactions to this stimulus, which may be considered as purely painful (BIMAR and VIDAL, 1968).

The electrocorticogram shows that an initial arousal response is elicited, sometimes followed by a secondary response a few seconds later, and often by a late response 50—100 sec after stimulation.

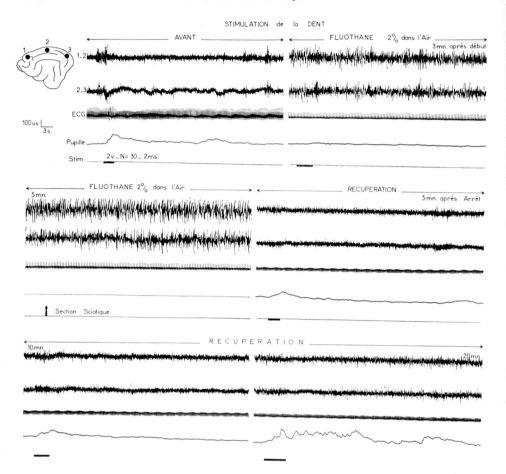

Fig. 7. Evaluation of pupillary reaction after stimulation of the dentine in the cat under halothane (stimulation de la dent). Control: (avant). Bipolar electrocorticogram: 1—2, 2—3. Electrocardiogram: (ECG). Constant photometric analysis of the pupillary dilatation: (Pupille). Stimulation of the dentine: unbroken black line: (Stim.). Before any anesthesia, stimulation of the dentine provokes an arousal response in the EEG; in the pupil, an initial dilatation at the same time as the stimulation and a delayed dilatation. Three minutes after the beginning of inhalation of a 2% concentration of halothane in air, stimulation of the dentine no longer elicits a pupillary dilatation. Five minutes after beginning halothane anesthesia, section of the sciatic nerve has no effect on pupillary dilatation (Section Sciatique). Five minutes after the end of anesthesia, stimulation of the dentine provokes a clear pupillary dilatation. The same is true 10 min after the end of anesthesia (Récupération). Finally 20 min after the end of anesthesia, the initial pupillary dilatation is followed by a long period of oscillating dilatation

In the electrocardiogram no initial change occurs but disturbances of the rhythm may appear during the delayed arousal response.

The pupillary dilatation, analyzed with a photo-electric cell, does show an initial and sometimes a secondary dilatation. The late dilatation is often very marked.

The blood pressure graph reflects the EEG and pupil changes quite faithfully.

With halothane inhalation, even before the electrical activity recorded is that of surgical sleep, the initial phenomena induced by stimulation of the tooth are greatly suppressed and the late phenomena have completely disappeared.

After 5 min inhalation of a 2% concentration of halothane in air, while the electrocorticogram still shows fast activity, the early and delayed phenomena are abolished, notably all pupil dilatation, regardless of the kind of stimulation.

As elimination of the drug progresses, the early pupillary reaction returns but the later phenomena only reappear when anesthesia has been over for 20 min.

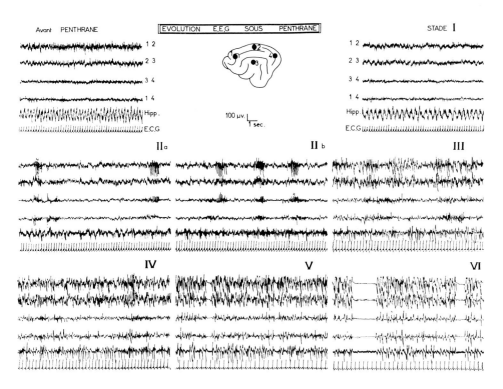

Fig. 8. Evolution of cortical and hippocampal electrical activity during methoxyflurane inhalation in the cat. Same notes as for Fig. 1. Plans 1 and 2 of the third stage of GUEDEL correspond here also to stages III and IV

B. Methoxyflurane

1. The EEG Recording (Fig. 8)

During methoxyflurane anesthesia 6 or 7 stages can be distinguished in the neocortical recording:

Stage I: Fast activity tending to be in spindle-like bursts, all of low amplitude.

Stage II: This stage can be sub-divided into two:

IIa: Spindles at 10—12 c/sec of high amplitude (200 μV) on a slowed background rhythm.

IIb: Spindles, having the same morphology as in IIa, increase in number while the background rhythm is even slower.

Stage III: The background activity is still low in amplitude but slower. The high amplitude spindles are markedly slower and almost continuous.

Stage IV: All activities are slowed, the spindles are disorganized and mixed with slow waves at 3—4 c/sec.

Stage V: With high concentrations (20 min after inhalation of 1% concentration of methoxyflurane) the recording is characterized by short electrical silences and also by paroxysmal activities which sometimes look like spikes.

Stage VI: At this stage of very deep narcosis the silences are more frequent and last longer. The paroxysmal abnormalities become accentuated but slower.

We think that stages 3 and 4 correspond in man to the first 2 parts of Guedel's stage 3.

The paroxysmal activity recorded in the stages which can be compared to those of so-called "surgical" anesthesia are much faster than with other kinds of anesthetics (barbiturates, for example).

Elimination of the drug is accompanied by a return to the alert recording, the time this takes depending on the concentration used and the length of administration: after 30 min inhalation of 1% methoxyflurane in air, it takes 60—70 min for the recording to go back to its original state.

2. Reticular Arousal Response (Fig. 9)

Stimulation of the midbrain reticular formation always produces a cortical and hippocampal arousal response during administration of 0.25% methoxyflurane.

After 15 min, a stimulus of 1 V which would have been effective before, produces no arousal response; 2 V are necessary to obtain a delayed arousal response both in the neocortex and the rhinencephalon.

With a concentration of 0.5% after 10 min, regardless of the stimulation intensity, no arousal is obtained.

Elimination of this drug is relatively slow and its recovery period is interesting. In fact, it is not until 40—60 min after the end of inhalation of 0.5% methoxyflurane in air that an arousal response reappears with a higher voltage than before starting anesthesia.

In summary, examination of the arousal response provides confirmation of the slow establishment of the anesthetic threshold and of the idea of "total quantity of drug absorbed" to reach that threshold. It is also clear that the delay before appearance of the arousal response, which is always recorded under halothane anesthesia, does not occur with this drug and that we have here a veritable "all-or-none" response.

3. Evoked Potentials

a) Changes in the Evoked Potentials along the Specific Primary Pathway under the Effect of this Drug are Seen as (Fig. 10):

— increased latency,
— increased total duration of the potential,
— no change in the amplitude of the positive wave at the retina but only in the chiasma and visual area;

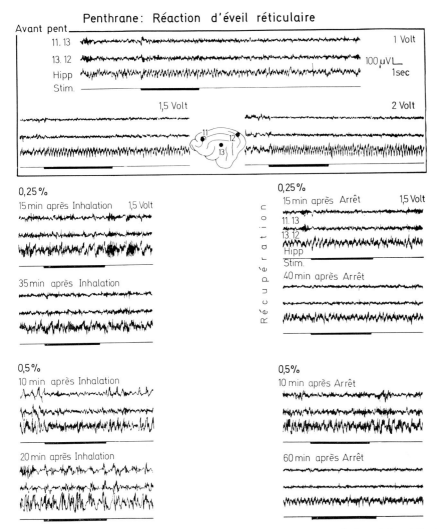

Fig. 9. Effect of methoxyflurane on the arousal response elicited by stimulation of the midbrain reticular formation in the cat (réaction d'éveil réticulaire). Cortical recordings (11—13, 13—12) as shown in the diagram. Hippocampal recording: (Hipp.). Stimulation of the reticular formation is shown by a solid black line; the voltage is given above on the right for each recording (1.5 V, 2 V). Control: in the upper frame. The recordings on the left show changes as a function of the percentage of mixture inhaled (0.25%, 0.5%) and of the length of inhalation. The recording on the right show the evolution of the arousal response during elimination of the drug (récupération). The time indicated is the period since administration of the drug ended

— damping of the negative wave which also only occurs at the chiasma and visual area.

Regardless of the cause, the modification of these response is not seen until 10 min after inhalation of 1% methoxyflurane in air.

In summary, although this drug also has an effect on latency from the proto-neurone, this seems less significant than with halothane on the amplitude of the components.

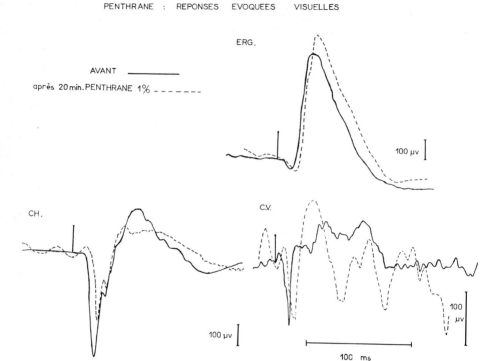

Fig. 10. Effects of methoxyflurane on the visual evoked potentials in the cat (réponses évoquées visuelles). Same key as for Fig. 3. This shows: — an increase in latency from the retina, — a decrease in amplitude of the positive peak and a dumping of the negative wave only at the chiasma, — increase in latency and facilitation of the after-discharge in the visual cortex

b) Non-specific Pathways (Fig. 11)

Using stimulation of the sciatic nerve or of the bulbar reticular formation, the potentials recorded in the midbrain reticular formation during inhalation of 1% methoxyflurane evolve in a peculiar way:
— decrease in amplitude of the positive wave,
— decrease in overall length of the evoked potential,
— transient increase of negative wave.

Fig. 11. Evoked potentials (potentiels évoqués) from the midbrain reticular formation during single electric shock stimulation of the sciatic nerve in the cat under methoxyflurane. Same key as Fig. 4, except for inhaled concentrations (0.5%) and length of waking period which goes as far as 85 min. This shows a gradual decrease in the amplitude of the positive wave as anesthesia becomes deeper. Persistence of the reticular response under deep anesthesia

Fig. 12. Evoked potentials recorded from the dorsal hippocampus (potentiels évoqués hippo-campiens) during single shock of the amygdala nucleus (pars baso-lateralis) in the cat under methoxyflurane. Same key as Fig. 5 except one concentration of inhaled mixture and in-creasing durations; the period of arousal is analysed through time and from below upwards. This shows, unlike halothane, an increase in the amplitude of the positive wave as anesthesia develops and also a decrease in latency. Forty minutes are required after the end of anesthesia before the return of morphology identical to that of the control

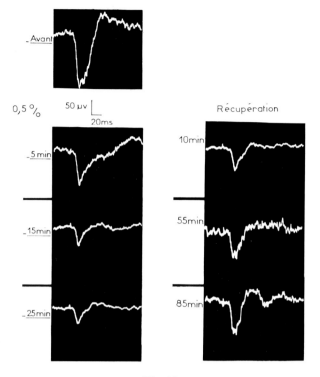

Fig. 11

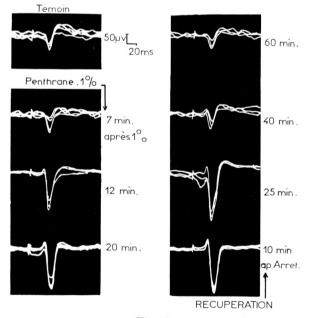

Fig. 12

To obtain a definite change in amplitude of the potential in the reticular formation the degree of anesthesia has to be deep.

In the limbic system, the potential recorded in the dorsal hippocampus during stimulation of the amygdala nucleus illustrates an activity peculiar to this drug: when the cortical activity is already made up of spindles and slow waves, the amplitude of the positive wave increases considerably while the negative wave and duration of the potential are almost unchanged (Fig. 12).

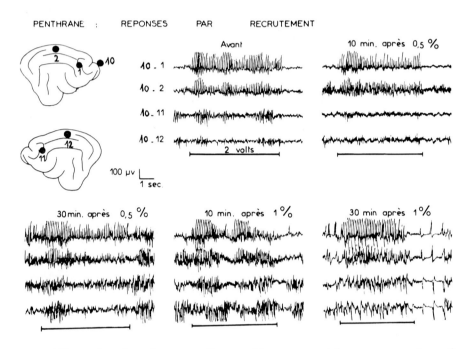

Fig. 13. Effects of methoxyflurane on the recruiting response (réponse par recrutement). Evaluation of recruiting response (Réponse par recrutement) for a 2 V stimulation of the centralis lateralis nucleus (solid black line). The examples are selected before each drug (avant), 10 min and 30 min after 1 %. The recruiting response is more limited under the effects of the different concentrations of the drug. The waxing and waning increases 10 min after 1 %

In summary, although the evoked potentials in the midbrain reticular formation seem damped and even reduced in the deep stage of methoxyflurane anesthesia, exploration of the limbic system shows facilitation which is practically unique among the actions produced by general anesthetics.

4. Effect of Methoxyflurane on the Recruiting Response (Fig. 13)

Inhalation of methoxyflurane (10 min at 0.5%) elicits a change in the recruiting response. The stable components and the waxing and waning are reduced and the spindles blocked. However, for higher concentrations the response is localized to certain cortical regions. The fall in amplitude may affect either the stable or the oscillatory part of the response.

In conclusion, since the recruiting response is never completely blocked by methoxyflurane, it can be deduced that this drug does not really obtund the thalamo-cortical tracts and is never the cause of true facilitation of waxing and waning.

5. Effects on the After-discharges and the Metrazol (Pentylene Tetrazol) Threshold

Under the effects of Methoxyflurane inhalation, repetitive stimulation of the amygdala no longer produces cortical after-discharges, although they may still persist to a reduced degree in the hippocampus.

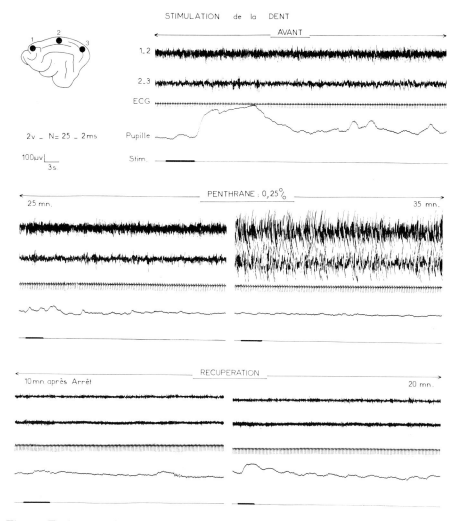

Fig. 14. Evaluation of pupillary dilatation after stimulation of the dentine in cat under methoxyflurane (Stimulation de la dent). Control: (avant). Same key as Fig. 7. This shows that it takes 35 min of anesthesia with a 0.25% concentration of methoxyflurane to abolish the pupillary reaction to dental pain. From 10 min after the end of anesthesia, the pupil reacts with a biphasic dilatation to dentine stimulation

The changes which it produces on the pentylene tetrazol threshold indicate that methoxyflurane has considerable anticonvulsant properties; what is more, this particular effect is very prolonged and persists for more than an hour after the end of a general anesthesia which has reached the surgical stage.

6. Responses to Dental Stimulation (Fig. 14)

After inhalation of 0.25% methoxyflurane in air, the pupillary dilatation induced by stimulation of the dentine becomes reduced after 25 min. It does not disappear completely until 35 min after beginning the administration of the anesthetic when the EEG corresponds to the 4th anesthetic stage of this drug. The late responses are abolished rapidly. However, the early and late responses start to appear 10 min after the end of anesthesia.

II. Primate Investigations

A more precise approach to the effects of these drugs can be made by using a primate, the Baboon *Papio papio*, as a model because of its similarity to man electroencephalographically (KILLAM et al., 1966; BIMAR et al., 1968).

Analysis of the auto-correlation functions of each channel in the form of power spectra of the principal periodic components of the EEG, gives an extremely precise measure of the relative amount of various frequencies (BRAZIER et al., 1952).

Spectral analysis demonstrates easily the individual variations in spontaneous electrocorticographic activity recorded from the various territories explored. Whenever a new animals is used it is necessary, therefore, to establish the base line spectral analysis because this may itself show changes which have nothing to do with the drug. This explains why we always present the power spectrum recorded before and after the drug (BRAZIER, 1961; WALTER, 1963; GREMY, 1967; NAQUET et al., 1968; RENN et al., 1969).

A. Halothane (Fig. 15)

a) Before the drug in the fronto-central region, the spectrum consists of several distinct peaks: the first at about 6 c/sec, the second at 15 c/sec, the third, notably smaller, at about 20 c/sec. Two other modest peaks at 25 and 30 c/sec follow the dominant activities. In the parieto-occipital region, three zones of activity can be distinguished for: 2 c/sec, 8 c/sec, and 15 c/sec; the power of the faster frequencies in this region is especially weak.

b) Effects of Inhaling 0.5% Halothane

In the fronto-central region two peaks are seen at 2 and 8 c/sec, for these frequencies, as for the intermediate ones the power is greater everywhere than before inhalation of the drug. In the parieto-occipital region, after an initial peak of slow frequencies culminating at 2 c/sec, two much smaller peaks appear at 4 and 8 c/sec; the power of the faster frequencies is virtually non-existent.

c) Effects of 1% Halothane

The power of the component frequencies of the spectrum of the fronto-central region is clearly increased. In the slow frequencies, peaks can be distinguished at 2, 6 and 8 c/sec and in the fast frequencies at 22 c/sec. In the parieto-occipital region, the suppression of the fast frequencies is further accentuated.

d) Effects of 2% Halothane

With this concentration, the power spectra continue to evolve in the same direction:
— in the frontal region, three bands of activity stand out at 6, 12 and 25 c/sec,
— in the posterior areas, only slow frequencies are present predominantly at 4 and 6 c/sec.

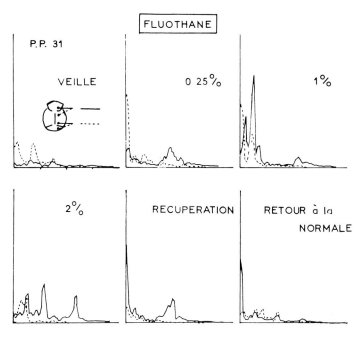

Fig. 15. Power spectra carried before, during and after inhalation of halothane in the Papio papio baboon (Spectral magnitude in arbitrary units). In this figure, the solid line represents activity recorded from the fronto-central region and the dotted line that from the parieto-occipital region. Before drug, waking animal: (Veille). Successive concentrations inhaled by the animal: 0.25%, 1%, 2%. After the end of anesthesia: (Récupération). Animal virtually returned to the waking state: (Retour à la normale). For increasing concentrations, it is seen that the power of the frequencies constituting the spectrum in the fronto-central region is clearly increased in all frequency bands but particularly in the fast frequencies. In the posterior regions, a clear reduction of the same frequencies is seen. Although halothane elicits fast frequencies at the beginning of anesthesia, these diminish gradually as anesthesia gets deeper

e) After Stopping Inhalation of Halothane

The spectra evolve in the opposite way to the preceding progression: in the fronto-central region, the power begins to deviate to the left while in the posterior region, there is an overall deviation to the right.

As a result, in the fronto-central region, the power of the frequencies above 10 c/sec dominates progressively while in the posterior region, the frequencies corresponding to alpha re-appear (12—15 c/sec).

In summary, comparative study of power carried before, during and after inhalation of halothane shows that:
— the total power of the frequencies forming the spectrum increases clearly in the anterior regions while diminishing in the parieto-occipital regions.

Halothane produces a scattering of the spectrum in the fronto-central region while tending to shrink and simplify it in the occipital regions. In the fronto-central region, additional fast frequencies are elicited by halothane (20—30 c/sec) but the slow frequencies are merely enhanced.

B. Methoxyflurane (Fig. 16)

a) Before Anesthesia

In this animal, the power is low in the anterior region, maximum activity dominating for frequencies of 5 and 9 c/sec. In the occipital region there is considerable power increasing respectively for 6, 8, 10 and 12 c/sec. Finally, there is a discrete activity at about 20 c/sec.

b) Inhalation of 0.25% Methoxyflurane

From the 6th min of inhalation of this mixture can be seen:
— in the frontal region, two well-distinguished bands of activities, one at 2 c/sec the other between 40 and 45 c/sec,
— in the occipital region, the power of the frequencies around 12 c/sec is clearly enhanced, but only two peaks persist at 2 and 22 c/sec.

Fifteen to 20 min after starting inhalation, the predominant feature in the frontal region is a very clear increase in the power of the fast frequencies: 42 c/sec at the 15th min, 45 c/sec at the 20th min, while the power of the slow frequencies fades away gradually.

In the posterior region, slow activity persists at the 15th min (5, 8 and 12 c/sec) but all frequencies decline gradually from the 20th min.

c) Inhalation of 0.5% Methoxyflurane

At this concentration, the fronto-central region shows a gradual and very large increase in the power of the fast frequencies culminating at 40 c/sec at the 6th min, 35—40 and 45 c/sec at the 10th min and 35 c/sec at the 15th min. At the same time, after 15 min a very large peak gradually appears at 8 c/sec; the total power of this peak increases as it expands towards the right at the 20th min. At this stage, still in the anterior region, the power of the fast frequencies has decreased considerably, although frequencies at 16, 32 and 45 c/sec are still distinguishable.

In the posterior region during the same period, the power of the slow frequencies is apparent at the 10th min for 8 c/sec and at the 20th min for about 5 c/sec. A few fast frequencies, although weak, are found at the 10th min and 15th min (32 and 42 c/sec). At the 20th min, some activities persist in the frequency band falling between 12 and 20 c/sec, the others being virtually non-existent.

In summary, the comparative study of the power spectra before and during inhalation of methoxyflurane in air shows that:
— Methoxyflurane encourages an increase in the total power of the spectrum and much more so in the frontal than in the occipital region.
— Methoxyflurane increases the power of the fast frequencies (30—40 c/sec) in the frontal region whereas in the occipital region it mainly augments the slow frequencies (5—8 c/sec).
— After inhalation of a certain quantity of the drug there is a noticeable decrease in the fast frequencies (20th min) while at the same time the power of the slow frequencies grows in these two regions.

It may therefore be concluded that methoxyflurane at the beginning of inhalation has a slightly preferential effect on the occipital alpha but this stage is tran-

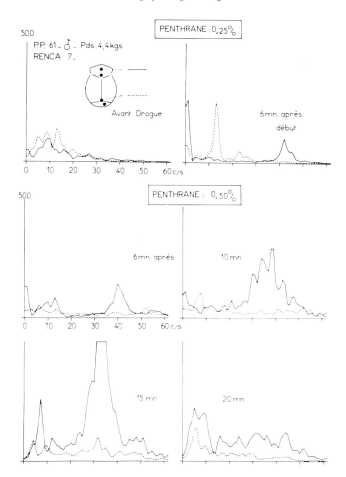

Fig. 16. Power spectra carried before and during inhalation of methoxyflurane in the Papio papio baboon (P.P. 61) (Spectral magnitude in arbitrary units). Control: (avant drogue). Six minutes after beginning: (6 min après début). Animal weighing: 4.4 kg. Magnetic tape reference: Renca 7. Same key as Fig. 15. This figure does not include analysis of the period after the end of anesthesia. This shows that inhalation of methoxyflurane produces a gradual increase in the power of the fast frequencies in the fronto-central region until the 15th min of inhalation of a 0.50% concentration. From the 20th min onward, the power of the fast frequencies decreases in the anterior and posterior regions, slow frequencies only persisting

sient and subsequently all the posterior activities decrease whatever concentration is used.

The dominant feature is the increase in power of the fast frequencies in the frontal region: from 40—50 c/sec for weak concentrations, about 30 c/sec for stronger doses.

Finally, when an even greater quantity of methoxyflurane is inhaled, only the power of the slow frequencies increases and simultaneously in the two regions, the fast frequencies gradually fading away.

This bring us back to the conclusion that at first methoxyflurane provokes a dissociation between the activities of the Rolandic and the occipital regions, the dominant feature being the deviation and increase of the spectrum towards the right in the Rolandic region. Later on a deviation of the spectrum towards the left occurs simultaneously in both regions investigated.

Conclusions

Two modern inhaled anesthetics, halothane and methoxyflurane, were assessed in laboratory animals using an experimental technique which leads to an overall appreciation of central nervous system function. The results were compared with those obtained from other inhaled anesthetics (ether, chloroform, trichloroethylene) and other neurotropic general anesthetics [thiopental, sodium gamma hydroxy-butyrate, hydroxydione ("Viadril")] and neuroleptics [chlorpromazine, "Tarac-tan" (chlorprothixene), "Valium" (diazepam)] in a recent monograph (Bimar et Naquet, 1966).

The battery of neurophysiological tests used in the cat and the accurate exploration of the spontaneous electrical activity of the baboon's cortex lead to a definition for each drug of:
— a field of action, differentiating them from the majority of neuroleptic drugs and in particular, general anesthetics.
— Common and/or differing actions which give to each of them an originality both in the type and the duration of these effects.
— Effects sufficiently oriented to suggest a preference towards one system of transmission or integration.

These two drugs possess a general anesthetic property which is quite rapidly effective and can be classified into 7 stages. However, the novelty of these two products lies in the fact that the surgical stage of anesthesia is accompanied by cortical activity which is not only ample but above all faster than that found at the same "clinical" stage with other anesthetics.

The EEG stage, consisting of slow waves and/or burst suppressions, which for thiopental and ether corresponds only to the surgical stage of anesthesia, with halothane and methoxyflurane corresponds to a narcosis which is much too deep.

Also, these two drugs alter and rapidly block the transmission of non-specific impulses and the electrographic arousal response obtained with reticular stimulation.

Their action on the specific pathways should not be overlooked since it has been shown that this takes effect from the proto-neurone as well as all along the pathways investigated.

Finally at the same stage of anesthesia, they block the transmission of painful stimuli and their neurovegetative effects.

This combination of results may be interpreted as the illustration of a balanced anesthetic action, that is to say involving narcosis, analgesia and neurovegetative protection for average concentrations.

Halothane and methoxyflurane may, however, be distinguished from each other:
— as would be expected from its physical characteristics, halothane takes effect much earlier during inhalation of a moderate concentration. At the same time, it is eliminated more rapidly, as is seen in a very early recovery of cortical electrical activity, while its action on the non-specific pathways and system may persist much longer. Methoxyflurane seems to have a much more prolonged cortical effect as illustrated by its anticonvulsant power which lasts long after the other systems, both specific and non-specific, have returned to normal function.

Finally, investigations which we carried out in primates suggest that the mode of cortical action of these anesthetics is not the same for all cortical regions. In the first stage of methoxyflurane, and almost continually with halothane, their maximum effect is restricted to the fronto-central regions. The power of the faster frequencies in this region is increased at the expense of the slow activities. On the other hand, their effect on the parieto-occipital region is minimal or acts mainly on the slow activities. A deviation of the spectrum towards the left, combined with an increase in total power in this region, distinguishes them from other inhaled anesthetics drugs: notably with ether, one never finds such effects (RENN et al., 1969). Paradoxically, similar effects are found in certain benzodiazepines and particularly diazepam (KILLAM et al., 1966; BIMAR et al., 1968). It is known that the development of the fronto-Rolandic activities is only possible when a certain degree of muscular relaxation exists, since these activities are usually blocked by movement. They may, therefore, be an even greater interest as components of the action of methoxyflurane and halothane since muscular relaxation continues to be one of the essential factors in surgical anesthesia.

References

ADRIAN, E. D., MATTHEWS, R.: The action of light on the eye. Part. 1. The discharge of impulses in the optic nerve and its relation to electric changes in the retina. J. Physiol. (London) 63, 378—414 (1927).

BIMAR, J., CACCIUTTOLO, G., RENN, C., NAQUET, R.: A comparison of different methods of utilizing the Papio papio in the evaluation of diverse group of drugs. In: The use of subhuman primates in drug evaluation, 400—424. Symposium San Antonio, University of Texas Press 1968.

— NAQUET, R. avec la collaboration de RENN, C., et LANOIR, J., LE POULEUF, N., et GERONIMI, C.: Approche neurophysiologique des mécanismes d'action de certains agents utilisés en anesthésie. Ann. Anesth. franç. VII (2), 379—452 (1966).

— VIDAL, P.: Procédé expérimental original d'évaluation de la douleur. Ann. Anesth. franç. IX (2), 213—216 (1968).

BRAZIER, M. A. B.: Computer techniques in EEG analysis: a conference. Los Angeles, October, 1960, 29—30, Elsevier Ed., 1961.

— CASBY, J. U.: Cross-correlation and auto-correlation studies in electroencephalographic potentials. Electroencephalog. and Clin. Neurophysiol. 4, 201—211 (1952).

DEMPSEY, E. W., MORISON, R. S.: The production of rhythmically recurrent cortical potentials after localised thalamic stimulation. J. Physiol. (London) 135, 293—300 (1942).

DENAVIT, M.: Action différentielle de quelques anesthésiques sur les réponses de structures alimentées par les voies spécifiques ou associatives. Anesthésie, analgésie, réanimation 10 (4), 747—809 (1963).

DOMINO, E. F., CORSSEN, G., SWEET, R. B.: Effects of various general anesthetics on the visual evoked response in man. Anesth. Analg. Cleveland 42 (6), 735—747 (1963).

EINTHOVEN, W., JOLLY, W. A.: The form and magnitude of electrical response of eye to stimulation by light at various intensities. Quart. J. Exptl Physiol. 1, 373—416 (1908).

GREMY, F.: L'analyse spectrale des tracés électroencéphalographiques. Colloque de l'I.N.S.E. R.M., 14 Déc. 1966, Ed. de l'I.N.S.E.R.M., 1967, n° 2, 17—29 (1967).

JASPER, H. H., NAQUET, R., KING, E. E.: Thalamocortical recruiting responses in sensory receiving areas in the cat. Electroencephalog. and Clin. Neurophysiol. 7, 99—114 (1955).

KILLAM, K. F., KILLAM, E. K., NAQUET, R.: Etudes pharmacologiques réalisées chez des singes présentant une activité EEG paroxystique particulière à la stimulation lumineuse intermittente. J. Physiol. (London) 58, 543—544 (1966).

LE POULEUF, N.: Etude neurophysiologique de l'éther méthylique du 2-2 dichloro-1-1 difluoroethyle. Méthoxyflurane ou Penthrane: Thèse de Doctorat en Médecine, Marseille 1967.

MORUZZI, G., MAGOUN, H. W.: Brain stem reticular formation and activation of EEG. Electroencephalog. and Clin. Neurophysiol. 1, 455—473 (1949).

NAQUET, R., KILLAM, K., BIMAR, J., GAREYTE, C., JUTIER, M.: Analyse spectrale des activités électrographiques recueillies chez le Papio papio (au cours de la veille et après différentes drogues psychotropes ou anesthésiques). Communication aux Journées sur le traitement en temps différé des informations électrophysiologiques. Colloque I.N.S.E.R.M., Paris, 14 Déc. 1966, Ed. de l'I.N.S.E.R.M., 1967, n° 2, 79—99 (1967).

Raventos, J.: The action of Fluothane. A new volatile anaesthetic. Brit. J. Pharmacol. Chemotherap. **11** (4), 394, 410 (1956).

Renn, C.: Etude neurophysiologique du 2 Bromo-2 chloro-1-1-1 trifluoroéthane (Fluothane); nouvelles données expérimentales. Thèse de Doctorat en Médecine, Marseille 1965.

— Lanoir, J., Bimar, J., Naquet, R.: Données expérimentales complémentaires sur l'action neurophysiologique du Fluothane. Compt. rend. soc. biol. **159**, 927 (1965).

— Vuillon-Cacciuttolo, G., Jutier, M., Bimar, J., Naquet, R.: Contribution de l'analyse spectrale à l'évaluation électroencéphalographique de l'action des drogues anesthésiques. Congrès français d'anesthésie-réanimation, La Baule, 1968. In: Ann. Anesth. franç. **XI**, (2) 357—382 (1970).

Stephen, C. R., Margolis, G., Fabian, L. W., Bourgeois-Gavardin, M.: Laboratory observations with Fluothane. Anesthesiology **19** (6), 770—781 (1958).

Walter, D. O.: Spectral analysis for electroencephalograms: mathematical determination of neurological relationships from records of limited duration. Exp. Neurol. **8**, 155—181 (1963).

6.3. Effects of Anesthetics on Metabolism of Brain*

B. Raymond Fink

With 1 Figure

I. Introduction

Because of the complexity and difficulty of access to the brain many of the pioneer studies on cerebral metabolism and anesthesia were done on excised tissue *in vitro*. Authoritative surveys of the results have been made by Quastel (1965) and by Hunter and Lowry (1956). For a broad view the classic discussion by Butler (1950) is still pertinent.

The present account concentrates mainly on the more recent work with functioning nervous tissue and drugs that may be administered to human beings, mostly barbiturates easy to handle in the laboratory. Regrettably, little can be said about the newer volatile anesthetics, and a general caution must be issued concerning the evidence from non-volatile and volatile anesthetics alike. The lesson of clinical anesthesiological research is that depressant drugs may cause drastic alterations to the internal environment, and that evaluation of physiological and biochemical responses must take into account the level of oxygenation, carbon dioxide tension, acid-base balance and body temperature at the time of sampling, as well as the blood or tissue level of the drug. Unfortunately this lesson generally has not yet penetrated to non-anesthesiological laboratories, and absence of such background information seriously weakens a great part of the experimental work in this field.

Extended consideration is given to oxygen and glucose because the metabolism of these substances looms very large in the comparisons of intake with output that have constituted the principal method of study *in vivo*. This is followed by an account of the work concerning the metabolic happenings to amino acids, phospholipids and neurotransmitters during anesthesia[1] which lately have received increasing attention. The discussion covers the literature to the end of 1968.

II. Oxygen and Oxidations

A. Physiological Considerations

The tenacity of the idea of a disturbance of cerebral metabolism as the basis of general anesthesia is due to the incontrovertible fact that the maintenance of normal mental function does depend on a sufficient supply of oxygen and glucose to the brain. Acute arrest of the cerebral circulation is followed within 7 sec by loss of consciousness (Rossen et al., 1943) and appearance of the delta wave in

---

* Supported by Grant GM 15991 of the U.S. Public Health Service.

[1] Anesthesia refers to a state of the nervous system observed in an animal narcosis to the condition of non-sentient systems.

the electroencephalogram. Mild hypoxia produces subtle symptoms of mental dysfunction. It is common knowledge that without oxygen the brain cannot think
for more than a few seconds (LASSEN, 1959) and fails permanently after 3 or 4 min.
The importance of oxygen to normal cerebral function is well illustrated by experiments of CARLISLE (1964) showing that temporary retinal ischemia produced
by the application of pressure to the eyeball causes loss of vision within 4 sec if
the oxygen is at ambient atmospheric pressure, whereas vision persists for as long
as 1 min with oxygen pressure at 4 atmospheres.

The early signs and symptoms of cerebral ischemia induced by hypotension
— yawning, staring, confusion — make their appearance even in the absence of
any significant change in cerebral oxygen utilization and are unquestionably due
to a decreased oxygen delivery to certain cerebral cells, since they are observed
under conditions where hypoglycemia and significant impairment of enzymatic
activity are excluded (FINNERTY et al., 1954). A reduction in internal jugular
venous oxygen saturation to 24% is incompatible with consciousness (LENNOX et
al., 1935), but even in the presence of mental symptoms produced by the inhalation of 10% O_2 no decrease in the CMR_{O_2} (cerebral metabolic rate of oxygen) can
be detected [KETY et al., 1948 (2)].

The reason for this critical need for oxygen has not been identified. On the
one hand it seems likely that electron transport takes place at a maximum rate at
oxygen partial pressures down to less than 2 mmHg, and on the other that the
normal intracellular PO_2 is low and may well approach 2 mm in some cells.

In the waking brain the mean oxygen utilization rate is 3.5 ml (156 μmol)/
100 g/min, a total of about 50 ml/min (SOKOLOFF, 1961), extracted from an
average normal cerebral blood flow of 57 ml/100 g/min.

Coma and anesthesia are generally associated with decrease in cerebral oxygen
utilization but normal sleep is not. The following CMR_{O_2} values have been reported: in uremic coma: 2.2 ml/100 g/min (HEYMAN et al., 1951); in diabetic
coma: 1.7 ml/100 g/min [KETY et al., 1948 (1)]. In monkeys, light barbiturate
anesthesia: 3.7 ml/100 g/min; areflexic: 1.7 ml/100 g/min (SCHMIDT et al., 1945).

The in vitro respiratory rate of brain slices approximates the rate in deeply
depressed living brain, or less than half the normal rate in vivo (ELLIOTT, 1952).
However, in vitro rates obtained on electrical stimulation (McILWAIN, 1951) or
cationic stimulation (QUASTEL, 1961) are comparable to the respiration rate of
physiologically resting brain in vivo. In vitro the rates from various parts of the
brain differ considerably (DIXON and MEYER, 1936; ELLIOTT and HELLER, 1957),
and blood flow studies suggest that in the functioning brain regional differences in
respiration rates also occur.

HESS (1961) estimated the oxygen uptake per cell in the eulaminate human
frontal cortex in vitro to be 34.0×10^{-6} μl O_2/h. Reasonable allowance for the
share assignable to neuroglia led to the conclusion that the average human cortical
neuron with its processes utilizes 122×10^{-6} μl O_2/h, or 16—50 times as much as
the average neuroglial cell. If eulaminate frontal cortex is representative of
eulaminate cortex in general, then the respiration of the brain as a whole is to a
large extent due to the neurons and their processes, including axons (ELLIOTT and
HELLER, 1957), in spite of the fact that the neurons are greatly outnumbered by
neuroglial cells. By the same token most of the change in cerebral O_2 uptake
produced by anesthetics is presumably also due to the neurons.

By analogy with unicellular organisms (GIESE, 1968) the high respiratory rate
of neurons may result in part from the high ratio of surface to volume. The relatively large area-to-mass ratio in the fine dendritic expansions probably means that

a disproportionately large amount of energy is needed for active transport in the plasma membrane.

B. Anesthesia

Reduced oxygen uptake by the anesthetised human brain has been observed with many, but not all, anesthetics (Table 1). Patients with severe alcoholic intoxication and a blood level of ethyl alcohol averaging 320 mg/100 ml were studied by BATTEY et al. (1953). The CMR_{O_2} in these patients averaged 2.2 ml/100 g/min, or 31% less than the CMR_{O_2} after recovery. However other patients with alcohol levels averaging 68 mg/100 ml and signs of mild inebriation did not show any changes in CMR_{O_2}.

C. Non-Volatile Anesthetics

HIMWICH et al. (1947) found that under thiopental anesthesia the oxygen consumption of the human brain diminished on the average by 36%, a value supported by subsequent observers, but the inference that oxygen utilization in the cerebral cortex is decreased more than in the lower centers has not been borne out by later work (WECHSLER et al., 1951). PIERCE et al. (1962) made measurements on human subjects anesthetized with thiopental sodium and d-tubocurarine, the total doses ranging from 10—55 mg/kg and from 0.7—1.3 mg/kg respectively, while arterial P_{CO_2} was maintained at an average of 43.8 mmHg. In the presence of clinical and electroencephalographic indications of profound anesthesia the oxygen consumption rate of the brain represented a reduction of approximately 55% from that observed in conscious normal eucapnic subjects. The cerebral respiratory quotient was unchanged, suggesting that the brain metabolism was not qualitatively altered. However, the reduction in oxygen uptake with thiopental probably does not occur uniformly throughout the brain. Autoradiographic studies with ^{131}I-labelled trifluoroiodomethane (LANDAU et al., 1955) have shown that blood flow through different areas of grey matter is remarkably non-uniform in conscious cats, but that during light anesthesia with thiopental, the differences in flow between the various cortical areas become much smaller. Perfusion through the regions of highest flow slows down almost to the rate through the more slowly perfused parts. Also pertinent in this connection is ROTH's (1963) demonstration that the concentrations of labelled thiopental in different areas of the brain varies with the local rates of blood flow at the time of injection. The greater the local blood flow, the higher the concentration of thiopental. If cerebral blood flow is autoregulated by metabolic demand, the observations by LANDAU et al. seem to indicate that thiopental reduces oxygen uptake most in those areas where oxygen uptake is highest in the conscious state. In the cat the spontaneous firing of neurons responding to peripheral stimulation is the first component of cerebral electrical activity to be depressed by thiopental sodium; some reticular neurons are more sensitive in this respect than the average cortical neuron, while others appear to be more resistant (YAMAMOTO and SCHAEPPI, 1961).

SWANK and CAMMERMEYER (1949) have evidence of a differential effect of barbiturates on large, medium and small neurons in the dog brain: the acid phosphatase of the cells is decreased, and more so in the small than in the larger neurons. Ether narcosis decreases the acid phosphatase more uniformly. In general there appears to be a direct correlation between the anesthetic depression produced by barbiturates and the depression of oxygen uptake (GLEICHMANN et al., 1962), although in schizophrenic patients seminarcosis due to thiopental is not accompanied by any change in CMR_{O_2} despite a remarkable improvement in the ability of the patients to communicate (KETY, 1948 [2]).

Table 1. *Effect of anesthetics on oxygen uptake of brain*

Species	Method	Thiopental	Anesthetic	CMRO$_2$ ml/100 g/min	Change	Reference
man			Thiopental		-36%	Himwich (1947)
man			Thiopental 0.5—1.6 g		-36%	Wechsler (1951)
man	N$_2$O		Thiopental 0.6—1.5 g	2.2 ± 0.4	-39%	Schieve (1953)
man	N$_2$O		Thiopental 1—1.5 g		-66%	Bellucci (1956)
man	N$_2$O		Thiopental	1.5 ± 0.1 SE	-55%	Pierce (1962)
man			Ether		-40%	Kety (1950)
man	N$_2$O		Alcohol 320 mg/100 ml	2.2	-31%	Battey (1953)
man			Alcohol 68 mg/100 ml	2.8	0	Battey (1953)
dog			Trichloroethylene 0.4—0.9% added to N$_2$O (60—80%)		-20%	McDowall (1964)
dog		no	N$_2$O 70%	5.59	+11%	Theye (1968)
dog		yes	Halothane 0.5% + air		-49%	McDowall (1963)
dog	^{85}Kr	no	Halothane 1% + air	2.2	-27%	Lassen (1966)
man	^{85}Kr	yes	1% Halothane + 50% N$_2$O		-27%	McHenry (1965)
man	^{85}Kr	no	1.2% Halothane	2.8 ± 0.23	-15%	Cohen (1964)
man	^{85}Kr	yes	N$_2$O (60—80%) with: Halothane 0.5%		-16%	McDowall [1965 (1)]
			Chloroform 0.5 or 1%		-10%	
			Methoxyflurane 0.5%		-13%	
		yes	N$_2$O (70%) with: 0.5% Halothane		-14%	McDowall (1967)
			2% Halothane		-33%	
dog	direct	no	0.5% Halothane (arterial)	4.77	-12% +[a]	Theye (1968)
			0.98% Halothane (arterial)	4.65	-14% +[a]	
man	^{85}Kr	no	C$_3$H$_6$—5%		-30%	Alexander (1968)

[a] Control level: 0.08% Halothane.

Another exception is the response of rat brain slices to very dilute concentrations of phenobarbital (0.2—0.5 mg-%, approximately $0.8—2 \times 10^{-5}$ M). In such an environment the respiration of the slices shows a small increase (WESTFALL, 1949).

D. Volatile Anesthetics

As regards gaseous anesthetics, it is clear that no general rule can be invoked. The data available to the end of 1968 are collected in Table 1. Some of the apparent discrepancies in the table are doubtless due to dissimilarities of technique. In many of the studies the level of anesthetic in the blood, which is a function of time as well as of the inhaled concentration, could not be measured. In others, administration of a barbiturate for induction of sleep probably added to the depression produced by the main anesthetic; also, the ^{85}Kr method, which predominantly reflects changes in the cortex, could be expected to show a greater effect of anesthetics on oxygen uptake than methods which measure the change in the brain as a whole.

KETY (1950) states that a 40% fall in CMR_{O_2} occurs with ether anesthesia in man. In the dog McDOWALL and HARPER (1965) report an insignificant fall in oxygen uptake of the cerebral cortex when chloroform is added to the previously administered nitrous oxide-oxygen mixture. The amount of chloroform added is not specified. Concerning trichloroethylene, McDOWALL et al. (1964) find that the cerebral oxygen uptake was reduced by 20% in the localized area of cerebral cortex in dogs.

Of all the volatile anesthetics, the effect of halothane is by far the best documented. COHEN et al. (1964) observe that in man 1.2% halothane causes a fall of approximately 15% in cerebral oxygen consumption in the presence of 1 °C fall in temperature, and they believe that most of the depression could be accounted for by this fall in temperature. According to the work of THEYE and TUOHY (1964) the fall in oxygen consumption observed in the brain during light halothane anesthesia in man is also found in the body as a whole. A change in the oxygen consumption of the body as a whole does not necessarily imply the same change in every organ, of course. THEYE's (1967) report that halothane produced a 17% decrease in oxygen consumption by the dog heart and only an 8% decrease in the dog as a whole is also interesting in this connection.

In their recent study THEYE and MICHENFELDER (1968 [1]) note a reduction of 17% in the rate of oxygen consumption by the brain in dogs inhaling 0—2% halothane in 70% nitrous oxide and oxygen. In a companion work (THEYE and MICHENFELDER, 1968 [2]) these authors show that nitrous oxide by itself increases, rather than decreases the cerebral demand for oxygen. That the effect of nitrous oxide is not a simple stimulation is suggested by McDOWALL's observation that nitrous oxide and halothane are synergistic in their effect on cerebral oxygen uptake. Cyclopropane also appears to have a complex effect, characterized as biphasic by ALEXANDER and colleagues. They find (ALEXANDER et al., 1968) that cerebral oxygen consumption in man is reduced to approximately 70% of normal during the inhalation of 5% cyclopropane, remains at this level during the inhalation of 13 and 37% cyclopropane but returns to nearly normal values with the inhalation of 20%. The observation of a large increase in cerebral blood flow with 20 and 37% cyclopropane in the face of 42% decline with 5% cyclopropane underlines the complexity of the response.

The data from cyclopropane argue against proportionality between the functional and metabolic depression of the nervous system induced by this anesthetic. The same group have evidence that such non-proportionality also holds for diethyl ether. Administration of 1.2 times the so-called minimum alveolar anesthetic

concentration (MAC) of ether depresses the CMR_{O_2} to 65% of normal, but administration of 2.3 times MAC is associated with a CMR_{O_2} of about 88% of normal
(H. WOLLMAN, personal communication, 1969).

E. In Vitro Studies

The effects of anesthetics on oxygen uptake by isolated organized neuronal
tissue, whether sympathetic ganglia or brain slices, have generally paralled the
in vivo effects although the ID_{50} *in vitro* is unusually high unless the metabolism
of the tissue is stimulated electrically (McILWAIN, 1953) or by increasing the
K^+/Ca^{++} ratio of the nutrient medium. The stimulated respiration is more sensitive
to inhibitory drugs but even here the concentrations in the medium usually exceed
the blood concentrations required to produce a similar inhibition in the living
brain. However some allowance must be made for the regional source of the brain
tissue (HERTZ and CLAUSEN, 1963).

In biopsied brain cortex, hypothalamus, and basal ganglia from the dog, uptake
of oxygen may be depressed to 30% of the control value by as little as 0.04%
(1.6 mM) pentobarbital added *in vitro* (WILKINS et al., 1950). Equally striking is
the behavior reported by SCHUELER and GROSS, 1950, of rat brain cortex slices
suspended in whole blood from a dog. Significant inhibition of the respiration of
the slices was observable in blood taken 3, 15, 30 and 60 min after the injection
of pentobarbital 36 mg/kg into the dog.

The mechanism of the inhibition of oxygen uptake by anesthetics may involve
several control points in the energy generating and utilizing machinery of the cell.
A summary of some current ideas is given here. Energy liberated in the metabolic
mill and stored as high energy phosphates, typified by adenosine triphosphate
(ATP), is utilized for synthesis, for transport, and for biotransformations. The rate
of energy release is controlled by many factors, among the most important being
the concentration of adenosine diphosphate (ADP) and inorganic phosphate (P_i)
available for the formation of ATP. The activity of the Na^+, K^+-sensitive ATPase
associated with active transport of ions and molecules through the plasma membrane is one of the major determinants of the level of ADP and P_i in the cell
(WHITTAM, 1961) and consequently of the rate of formation of ATP in the mitochondria. Mitochondrial formation of ATP (from ADP and P_i) is itself tightly
coupled to electron transport along the respiratory chain. Anesthetics could inhibit
oxygen utilization by inhibiting the electron transport chain at some point or by
inhibiting reactions coupled to such transport. The points of attack of course need
not be the same ones for all anesthetics.

In a model favored by QUASTEL (1965) plasma membrane Na^+, K^+-linked
ATPase is seen as one of the possible sites of anesthetic inhibition leading to
decrease of cellular oxygen uptake, on the grounds that inhibition of ATP breakdown in the plasma membrane increases the ATP:ADP ratio and consequently
decreases the ADP available for phosphorylation, at the next remove slowing
down the mitochondrial respiration because this is tightly coupled to phosphorylation.

UEDA, 1967, examined this possibility indirectly by looking for a possible effect
of general anesthetics on the ouabain-sensitive Na^+K^+-linked ATPase of microsomal fractions of rabbit brain. The result was negative: a decline in activity of
ATPase was demonstrated with ether and with halothane only when the partial
pressures were some 8 or 10 times greater than the clinical ones. However this
evidence cannot be regarded as decisive because microsomal ATPase may not be
bound to lipoprotein membrane in the same way as the Na^+, K^+-sensitive ATPase

of plasma membrane. Other data obtained with therapeutic concentrations of diethyl ether and halothane are consistent with inhibition by these anesthetics of an enzyme with ATPase activity: that of firefly luciferase (UEDA, 1965).

The work of ALDRIDGE and PARKER (1960) has shown that oxybarbiturates and thiobarbiturates differ in that the oxybarbiturates inhibit respiration whereas the thiobarbiturates inhibit respiration and in addition uncouple oxidative phosphorylation. However it should be noted that their evidence was obtained with mitochondrial preparations from rat liver; technical reasons prevented the use of mitochondria from brain tissue. Uncoupling of oxidative phosphorylation has also been demonstrated for diethylether (HULME and KRANTZ, 1955).

CHANCE et al. (1955) have shown that the site of action of an inhibitor of electron flow can be identified by the crossover point, the point in the respiratory chain where reduced cofactor accumulates upstream, and reduced forms are depleted downstream. With barbital and other oxybarbiturates this crossover point is found between reduced nicotinamide (NADH) and flavin. In the case of amobarbital a half-maximal effect is obtained with a 0.2—0.3 mM concentration (CHANCE and HOLLUNGER, 1963). Thiopental and other thiobarbiturates combine an amobarbital-like inhibition of cellular respiration with a strong uncoupling effect apparently due to mitochondrial ATPase activation. MICHAELIS and QUASTEL (1941) had earlier concluded that the effect of anesthetics on brain respiration is to inhibit a process intermediary between cytochrome oxidase and flavoprotein but FAHMY and colleagues (1962), restricting themselves to thiopental, attribute the action of this narcotic primarily to inhibition of pyruvate oxidation. In the presence of 1.3×10^{-3} M thiopental sodium, α-ketoglutaric dehydrogenase of pigeon brain, which requires the same cofactors as pyruvic dehydrogenase, was also inhibited. The various observations may be reconciled if several sites of inhibition are postulated, rather than a single one, if different anesthetics have different patterns of predilection for the various sites, and if the patterns vary somewhat according to species and tissue of origin. Few data are available in this respect for the newer volatile anesthetics.

COHEN's (1968) study of the action of halothane on the rate of phosphorylation of ADP in liver mitochondrial preparations is therefore of particular interest. It demonstrates that 50% inhibition is produced by about 1.6% halothane vapor, a a quite realistic concentration from the point of view of clinical anesthesia. The failure of succinate to reverse the inhibition suggests that halothane may interfere with the oxidation of reduced NAD by flavoprotein. Even greater sensitivity of oxidation metabolism to volatile anesthetics has been observed in certain cell culture strains (FINK and KENNY, 1968).

III. Glucose

The normal working human brain utilizes 27.8 nanomoles of glucose/100 g/min (about 70 mg/min for the whole brain), and utilizes 5.5 mM of oxygen for every millimole of glucose taken up. Since no other substrate is taken up in significant amounts the inference has been that the brain respires almost entirely at the expense of glucose (KETY, 1957).

Consistent with this conclusion is the observation that hypoglycemia produces a definite decrease in cerebral oxygen consumption and that the decrease correlates well with the arterial blood glucose level and with the mental state (TEWS et al., 1965). Consciousness lost in hypoglycemia is restored with the intravenous administration of glucose.

In perfusion experiments *in vivo* the amount of glucose taken up from the blood by the brain is equivalent to the amount of oxygen consumed and lactic acid produced (Himwich, 1951), and in brain slices the amount of glucose disappearing is also approximately equal to that expected from the oxygen consumption (assuming complete oxidation) and from the amount of lactic acid formed by aerobic glycolysis (Dixon and Meyer, 1936), although *in vitro* a greater part of the glucose is converted to lactate than *in vivo*. However conditions *in vitro* are obviously far from physiological, the blood-brain barrier, for example, is not in operation and substrates can be taken up that do not pass the blood-brain barrier or only cross it with difficulty. In the brain *in situ* glucose is transported actively across the blood-brain barrier (Fishman, 1964) and it is now clear that this transport is assisted by insulin (Rafaelsen, 1961). An estimate has been made that about 85% of the glucose obtained by the brain from the blood is oxidized to carbon dioxide, about 13% is converted to lactate, and 20% to pyruvate (Gibbs et al., 1942).

Notwithstanding the close equivalence between the amounts of glucose and oxygen taken up and the amount of carbon dioxide produced, the statement that under normal conditions glucose is the only important fuel of the brain is subject to qualification. A large part of the glucose appears to serve as precursor of various intermediaries, such as glutamate (Sacks, 1965), on which the brain draws for oxidizable substrate. Labeled glucose carbon incorporated into the pool of an intermediary becomes diluted by the unlabeled intermediary already in the pool. During the uptake of labeled glucose, the carbon dioxide produced originates partly from the pool of intermediary, some of which is unlabeled, and partly directly from the labeled glucose. In consequence, at equilibrium the specific activity of the emerging carbon dioxide is less than would be expected if all the carbon dioxide were derived directly from the direct oxidation of glucose. More generally, a respiratory quotient of 1.0 does not necessitate that the carbon dioxide evolved by derived directly from the oxidation of carbohydrate. If the brain uses glucose to manufacture non-carbohydrate at a certain rate and burns the stored non-carbohydrate at the same rate, the net result will be a respiratory quotient of unity regardless of how much glucose is oxidized directly. In the perfused brain of the cat, where glucose is taken up at the rate of 10 mg/min/100 g of tissue (almost twice the rate in the human brain) Geiger (1958) found that under "resting" conditions 30—35% of the glucose absorbed was oxidized directly, another 20—30% was taken up and rapidly transformed into acid-soluble components, such as amino acids, and large amounts were built into lipids, proteins and other acid insoluble components. During the same time interval the amount of oxygen used by the perfused brain corresponded to that necessary to oxidize all the glucose which was taken up from the perfusing "blood". It seems clear that under the conditions of the experiments the brain oxidized non-carbohydrate substrates simultaneously with glucose and that part of the glucose taken up by the brain was used for resynthesis of these substrates.

Allweis and Magnes (1958), also working with the perfused cat brain, found that radioactive glucose was oxidized to carbon dioxide at the rate of 1.9 mg/100 g/min while the total glucose uptake was 9.0 mg/100 g brain/min. Thus only 22% of the glucose taken up from the blood was oxidized to carbon dioxide, equivalent to approximately one-fifth of the oxygen consumed. Lactate production, amounting to 6.4 mg/100 g brain/min, could account for most of the remaining glucose uptake. In view of the limited cerebral store of glucose and glycogen it had to be inferred that the major part of the unlabelled carbon dioxide produced by the brain was derived from a pool that did not become radioactive during the period of the experiment. In the brain such pools are constituted mainly by lipids and proteins.

A. Glucose Uptake during Narcosis

In recent years the changes in intermediary metabolism during anesthesia have begun to receive study. Experiments by BACHELARD et al. (1966) show that the incorporation of ^{14}C from U-^{14}C-glucose into free aminoacids in the rat brain is significantly retarded by diethyl ether and by pentobarbital anesthesia (75 mg/kg) without any significant change in the blood level or brain level of amino acids. There is good reason to believe that the labeling of brain keto-acids would be similarly affected (BACHELARD, 1965).

Results qualitatively similar to those of ALLWEIS and MAGNES, mentioned above, have been obtained by BARKAI and ALLWEIS (1966) in the intact cat narcotized with pentobarbital (after induction of anesthesia with diethyl ether). These workers have measured the specific activity of the carbon dioxide produced by the brain during continuous infusion of labeled ^{14}C-glucose. At apparent isotopic equilibrium the relative specific activity of the CO_2 produced by the brain amounted to 45%, a value somewhat higher than the 32% observed in the unanesthetized perfused cat brain. In the experiments of GEIGER et al. (1960), addition of pentobarbital to the perfusion fluid roughly doubled the amount of label appearing in the CO_2 carbon; possibly the anesthetic slowed down the incorporation of glucose into other components, leaving more glucose available for oxidation. Evidence of a substantial non-glucose source of carbon dioxide has also been obtained in the brain of intact narcotized cats, where, according to GOMBOS et al. (1963) the radioactivity in the respiratory carbon dioxide produced is equivalent to 60% of the specific activity of the glucose taken up.

On the other hand in experiments in the intact anesthetized dog GAINER et al. (1963) observed that the relative specific activity of the CO_2 produced by the brain remained at 100% for most of the 4.5 h experiment. At present it is not clear whether the difference between the results with cats and with dogs is due to species or technique, but the estimate of SACKS (1957) based on studies with ^{14}C glucose suggests that in man little more than half the cerebral CO_2 production comes directly from glucose, much of it from the 3-carbon of glucose (SACKS, 1965). While doubt remains as to the amount of non-carbohydrate substrates oxidized by the human brain during anesthesia mention should be made of work by OWEN et al. (1967) showing that during prolonged fasting the brain predominantly oxidizes hydroxybutyrate and acetoacetate, probably as a result of enzyme induction (SMITH et al., 1969). OWEN's subjects did not show any deficit on psychometric testing, and electroencephalographic tracing remained unchanged-indicating that the ketoacids adequately fulfilled the cerebral energy require, ments. In narcosis the reduction of glucose uptake has been found to parallel the reduced oxygen consumption although evidence on this point is rather scarce (Table 2). According to the study of COHEN et al. (1964) the glucose uptake, normally about 9.5 mg/100 ml of blood, averages 8.1 mg/100 ml blood during the inhalation of 1.2% halothane vapor; 92% of the glucose utilized is apparently oxidized and the remainder can be accounted for as lactate. However there are indications that the path of glucose metabolism depends to some extent on the concurrent P_{CO_2}: in hypocarbia 10% of the glucose taken up appears to be utilized by routes other than oxidation or lactate production, and in hypercarbia about 10% of the oxygen utilized goes to oxidize substrates other than glucose, although the blood glucose level is somewhat elevated.

Table 2. *Effect of anesthetics on glucose metabolism of brain in vivo*

Species	Condition	Cerebral blood flow	CMR_{O_2}	CMR_G	Reference
		ml/100 g/min			
dog	control	59.2	243	42	THEYE and MICHEN-FELDER (1968)
	halothane 0.54%	70.0	212	35.8	THEYE and MICHEN-FELDER (1968)
	halothane 0.98%	84.5	207	36.6	THEYE and MICHEN-FELDER (1968)
man	resting	57	156	31	SOKOLOFF (1961)
man	halothane 1.2%	50.8	125	23	COHEN et al. (1964)

B. Brain Level of Glucose

Glucose and glycogen are stored in the mammalian brain (KERR and GHANTUS, 1936). In man the total is probably equivalent to about 2 g of glucose, sufficient substrate for 24 min of oxidative metabolism at the normal rate. In an animal deprived of oxygen, of course, the store would be used up at five or six times this rate because of the greatly increased rate of glycolysis, a point that emerges convincingly from the measurements of MARK et al. (1968), according to which the glucose level of the brain in rats, excluding the glucose in brain blood, is 0.76 µM/g fresh weight or 15 mg/100 g fresh weight. The glucose content fell to 1.10 µM/g after 45 sec ischemia. To the anesthesiologist such a rapid fall indicates that exhaustion of substrate may be a factor in precipitating irreversible damage to the brain during circulatory arrest, especially in the newborn, where, in the case of mice, the glucose content of the brain is less than half that of the adult (LOWRY et al., 1964). Anesthesia on the contrary may be protective in this respect, since it has been shown that phenobarbital, in doses sufficient to abolish the righting reflex in mice, increases the brain concentration of glucose more than two fold (MAYMAN et al., 1964). GOLDBERG and colleagues (1966) observed a threefold increase in brain glucose after 60 min of anesthesia with 4.5% diethyl ether vapor, or with amytal 135 mg/kg or phenobarbital 225 mg/kg intraperitoneally, an increase far beyond the level expected from the diminished glycolytic flux or any possible small increase in blood sugar concentration.

The increase in glucose concentration associated with anesthesia is not uniform throughout the brain. In GATFIELD's study (GATFIELD et al., 1966) the increase ranged from 130—280%, being most merked in the cerebellar cortex and the medulla, less in the parietal cortex and least in Ammon's horn. No ready explanation for the increase is available. The simplest one, that anesthesia decreases brain metabolic rate without proportionately decreasing the rate of glucose transport from blood to brain, maybe insufficient to account for the magnitude of the rise in brain glucose. This point needs further study. Perhaps an alteration in the transport or compartmentation of glucose is responsible, although the evidence from erythrocytes is that volatile anesthetics do not affect the transport of glucose across the cell membrane (GREENE, 1965). GREENE did observe that carbon dioxide stimulates the uptake of glucose by red cells and that diethyl ether (2.3%), nitrous oxide (80%), halothane (0.7%), or methoxyflurane (0.7%) suppress this stimulation.

C. Glycogen Levels

The cerebral level of glycogen is of special interest because of the vital role of this substance as a reserve store of glucose. ESTLER and HEIM (1960), working with mice found an 18% increase in brain glycogen after anesthesia with 4.5% ether vapor for 1 h. The ATP level at this time was unchanged. Phenobarbital 150 mg/kg intraperitoneally produced glycogen increases of 19—34% (ESTLER, 1961). The increase appears to be a function of time, as shown by NELSON and co-workers (1968), who maintained anesthesia for up to 8 h in rats and mice. Following injection of phenobarbital 170 mg/kg intraperitoneally, the brain glycogen content was doubled after 2.5 h and trebled after 8 h. They confirmed that prolonged ether anesthesia also had this effect, finding an increase of about 50% in 2 h.

GEY et al. (1965) studying the brain levels of components of glycolytic pathways, also observed the effect of anesthesia on glycogen. They gave rats intraperitoneal injections of phenobarbital 100 mg/kg. The drug caused a decrease of glucose-6-phosphate and fructose-6-phosphate in the brain at the time of maximal depression of the motor activity. An accumulation of glycogen was present following the time of maximal sedation, prompting the hypothesis that central depressants suppress glycolysis in the central nervous system *in vivo* by a diminution of glucose phosphorylation.

D. Effects on Glucose Metabolism in Sympathetic Ganglia and Perfused Brain

The investigations of LARRABEE and his colleagues on excised sympathetic ganglia have made important contributions to the understanding of the effect of anesthetics on the metabolism of functioning synaptic systems *in vitro*. They have shown that some anesthetics act selectively on synaptic transmission within the ganglia, in the sense that transmission is blocked by a considerably lower concentration of anesthetic than required for block of conduction along the axons leading to and from the synapses (LARRABEE and POSTERNAK, 1952): some anesthetics interfere with ganglionic transmission in concentrations as low as those employed to depress the central nervous system during anesthesia (LARRABEE and HOLADAY, 1952). Pentobarbital sodium, in 0.2 mM concentrations (the *in vivo* serum level reported by FISHER et al., 1948 and by FORBES et al., 1949), does not affect the amplitude of the preganglionic action potential but decreases the amplitude of the postganglionic action potential by 30% and the oxygen uptake of the electrically stimulated preparation by over 10% (EDWARDS and LARRABEE, 1955); at the same time the rate of glucose consumption is increased by 30% and the production of lactate rises by an approximately equivalent amount. In the case of diethyl ether, 18 mM perfusion fluid (equivalent to the concentration attained in blood during deep anesthesia produced by the inhalation of 3.5% ether vapor) reduces the preganglionic and postganglionic action potentials respectively by 10% and 25%, but has no measurable effect on the oxygen uptake. Data on the glucose metabolism under the latter conditions are not available. The authors point out that these results do not show whether a metabolic derangement is or is not the cause of the functional disturbance but do indicate clearly that the action of the two agents cannot be explained by any single metabolic effect. It may be added here that findings in a perfused ganglion of the rat are suggestive but do not bear an established relation to events in the human brain. The human brain, as far as is known, does not respond to barbiturates by increased glycolysis. In the study by PIERCE et al. (1962) thiopental sodium reduced the CMR_{O_2} by an average of 55%, but the respiratory quotient was 0.99. As far as carbohydrate metabolism is concerned the results with excised ganglia more closely resemble those obtained with slices of brain tissue, where the increment in oxygen uptake with cationic or electrical stimulation and the increase in lactate production (WEBB and ELLIOTT, 1951) are of the same order of magnitude as in the ganglionic preparation, and have the same sensitivity to anesthetics as the latter. The isolated ganglion however, is a more stable system, showing relatively little deterioration over a period of 24 h. Investigating the fate of ^{14}C from ^{14}C-glucose, LARRABEE and KLINGMAN (1962) found that 64% appeared as CO_2, 24% as lactate and 12% was retained, results qualitatively similar to results of GEIGER with the perfused brain of the cat. The relatively high production of lactate in brain slices, excised ganglia and perfused brains, as compared with the intact brain, serves as a reminder that other metabolic changes observed in the experimental preparations may also be unrepresentative of normal. GILBOE et al. (1967) believe that simplified perfusion fluids are deficient in several factors necessary for normal glucose uptake and brain function.

In the present state of the evidence few firm conclusions can be drawn. Some anesthetics retard the cerebral utilization of glucose, apparently as part of a widespread but non-uniform depression of cerebral metabolism, but dose-effect curves *in vivo* are not available, and many important anesthetics remain untested.

IV. High Energy Phosphates

Interest in the brain levels of high energy labile phosphates during anesthesia was at one time stimulated by the hope of casting light on the role of energy metabolism in the genesis of narcosis. Depleted levels would incriminate inhibition of oxidative metabolism as the primary cause, whereas an excess would suggest that decreased oxidative metabolism is secondary to a decreased drain on the energy supply. In the event, no firm conclusions have emerged from the early work. Critical importance has become attached to experimental procedure because of the extremely rapid breakdown of labile phosphates during decapitation and prior to complete freezing of the brain, and in evaluating discordant results due weight must be given to latter-day improvements in technique.

An unchanged level of ATP, a rise in creatine phosphate (CP) level and a fall in inorganic phosphate (P_i) with anesthesia was demonstrated by STONE (1940) with pentobarbital and allobarbital ("dial"), in mice (Table 3). On the other hand, LE PAGE (1946) found that animals anesthetized with pentobarbital possessed considerably higher brain levels of ATP and CP, and lower levels of ADP and AMP, than those that had not been anesthetized. Both groups were sacrificed by immersion in liquid air. A critical investigation of methodology by WEINER (1961) indicated no change in ATP content with ether or pentobarbital anesthesia, although the higher level of CP was confirmed. Increased CP was associated with an equal rise in brain creatine. In this work rats were subjected to a deep air-ether anesthesia for 10 min or to deep narcosis with subcutaneous sodium pentobarbital 70—80 mg/kg body weight for 15—30 min.

SCHMAHL (1965) measured the ATP/ADP and CP/creatine ratios in samples of brain cortex from anesthetized cats. The samples were obtained by means of a steel punch cooled in liquid nitrogen. The ratios were higher with pentobarbital anesthesia (25 mg/kg) than with phenobarbital (100 mg/kg) administered by the intraperitoneal route, but the significance of this observation is difficult to interpret without

Table 3. *Effect of anesthetics on brain level of high energy phosphates*

Species	Drug	ATP	CP	Author
mice	pentobarbital or allobarbital	no change	increased	STONE (1940)
	pentobarbital	increased	increased	LE PAGE (1946)
rats	pentobarbital or ether	no change	increased	WEINER (1961)
cats	pentobarbital or pheno-barbital	ATP/ADP increased	CP/creatine increased	SCHMAHL (1965)
rats	pentobarbital	no change	increased	WILLIAMS, et al. (1968)

knowledge of the intensity of the ensuing anesthetic depression. KING et al. (1967) reported that in mice phenobarbital at subanesthetic levels was more effective in preserving cortical ATP and CP than secobarbital at full dosage. The mice were plunged into Freon at $-150°$ and the measurements were made in the outermost, most rapidly frozen portion of the brain. WILLIAMS and co-workers (1968) noted only a slight rise in ATP content of brain in rats that had received pentobarbital 72 mg/kg intraperitoneally.

The weight of evidence indicates a rise in CP and little or no change in ATP with narcosis. Since CP probably serves to replenish ATP in the brain it would seem most likely that anesthetized animals utilize labile phosphates at a lower rate than conscious animals and that the abovementioned agents directly or indirectly decrease the utilization of ATP rather than enhance its synthesis. The possibility remains open that inhibition of ATP synthesis in strategic local areas leads to secondary accumulation of high energy phosphate compounds in related "down-stream" regions.

V. Amino Acid and Protein Metabolism

Protein turnover in the living brain takes place at a high rate comparable to the rate of turnover in liver and secreting glands. The amino-acids necessary for the functioning of the brain are partly synthesised in the brain cells from glucose, and partly transported actively across the blood-brain barrier. Although the transport of amino-acids across the blood-brain barrier into the brain is slow, rapid turnover inside the brain is maintained by uptake from the free amino-acid pool (GAITONDE and RICHTER, 1955). GAITONDE and RICHTER (1956) have studied the metabolic activity of proteins in the brain of the rat by measuring the rate of incorporation of ^{35}S from labeled L-methionine into the proteins and come to the conclusion that all the methionine in brain proteins could be replaced in a period of twenty days. For protein molecules containing more than one methionine residue the life of a given molecule would be correspondingly shortened. The effect of anesthetics on the uptake of label seems clear-cut. In one group of rats maintained at normal body temperature (38° rectal) and kept anesthetized for 3 h with ether vapor (in unspecified concentration) the rate of uptake of intracisternal ^{35}S into brain proteins appeared to decrease by 34%. In another group, anesthetized by intraperitoneal injection of 75 mg/kg sodium pentobarbital, the uptake diminished by 24%. The decrease in specific activity was apparently greatest in the animals that were most deeply anesthetized. Not surprisingly, a fall in body temperature further slowed the rate of uptake. The mechanism of the decrease has not been determined but may well be related to the general depression of the metabolism, including depression of oxygen uptake, incident to these conditions. NECHAEVA et al. (1959) obtained generally similar results with ^{35}S-methionine and with glycine-1-^{14}C injected sub-cutaneously into rats; the narcotic used in their experiments was sodium amobarbital. They considered that the changes were due to a change in intensity of protein metabolism rather than decreased rate of intake of labelled amino-acid into the brain. On the other hand, PALLADIN (1957) could not find any effect of barbital sodium on the uptake of ^{35}S-methionine into the cerebral protein of rats.

The brain can rapidly form amino-acids from glucose, as was first demonstrated on brain slices by BELOFF and colleagues in 1955. A similar rapid labeling of free amino-acids, particularly glutamic acid and aspartic acid, has been found by BARKULIS et al. (1960) in slices of cortex taken from the perfused brain of cats. Narcosis with pentobarbital does not appreciably change the pattern of labeling or the relative rates at which carbon from perfused ^{14}C glucose and endogenous cold carbon contribute to the respiratory carbon dioxide. However, TSUJI et al. (1963) have reported decreased cortical levels of gamma-aminobutyric acid (GABA) and glutamic acid in rat brain 3 h after intraperitoneal injection of pentobarbital sodium 30 mg/kg. Cyclopropane 10—15% in oxygen also provokes a drop in the GABA level but is accompanied by a rise in glutamic acid, possibly because of interference with the formation of GABA from glutamic acid. It seems doubtful that these changes play any direct part in causing the anesthetic state since they also occur in certain conditions that do not give rise to anesthesia. The intact brain of the narcotized cat is also able to incorporate ^{14}C from glucose into glutamic acid (GOMBOS et al., 1963).

SUZUKI et al. (1964) studied the effect of pentobarbital and of halothane on the lysine-incorporating activity of microsomal systems of brain tissue from rats and human beings. These systems are sites of protein synthesis, but their lysine-incorporating activity is not altered by pentobarbital or halothane, except in pharmacologically unrealistic concentrations. LAJTHA and TOTH (1965) found that in slices of mouse brain *in vitro* the uptake of L-lysine and of cycloleucine was inhibited by phenobarbital, but that *in vivo* the uptake of lysine and cycloleucine was unaffected by pentobarbital.

The evidence reviewed in the preceding sections does not provide the basis for a general biochemical theory of narcosis. In particular, a uniform depression of energy metabolism or of intermediary metabolism is not demonstrable. Nevertheless biochemical disturbances may explain some of the differences between the secondary effects of different agents.

VI. Phospholipids

Phospholipids are present in large amounts in cerebral tissue but until recently little has been known about their function. In 1950 DAWSON and RICHTER showed that the brain phospholipids are metabolically active, the rate of turnover observed with radioactive phosphorus in the mouse brain being equivalent to that required for complete replacement every 70 h. They found this rate to be decreased by 15% by sodium pentobarbital (50 mg/kg) anesthesia.

The effect of sodium thiopental anesthesia on the rate of uptake of radioactive phosphate into individual brain phospholipids in rats has been studied by ANSELL and DOHMEN (1957). The dose of thiopental was 60 mg/kg. Over a period of three hours the incorporation of ^{32}P into phosphatidylcholine was reduced by 75% and into phosphatidylethanolamine by 67%. Diphosphoinositide synthesis was reduced by more than 80%. However, the experiments did not determine whether the primary effect was inhibition of the formation of energy rich phosphate esters required for phospholipid synthesis, or inhibition of a later step in the synthetic pathway. Further experiments (ANSELL and MORGAN, 1958) demonstrated that thiopental anesthesia had no effect on the synthesis of the phospholipid precursors, phosphatidylethanolamine or phosphatidylcholine, so it appears that a non-specific depression of phospholipid metabolism will not account for the results and that thiopental affects steps in the synthetic chain other than the simple phosphorylation of the lipid bases.

Barbiturate narcosis also impairs the turnover of monophosphoinositide in the brain of the rat (MARGOLIS and HELLER, 1966). Administration of pentobarbital 50 mg/kg intraperitoneally causes a 21% decrease in the turnover of monophosphoinositide, as measured by the rate of incorporation of ^{3}H-inositol over a period of 75 min; this decrease occurs in the presence of a 28% increase in brain acetylcholine levels. Increase in brain acetylcholine content in anesthesia thus appears to be associated with a considerable depression of phospholipid turnover, but the evidence is limited to barbiturate anesthetics administered in quantities that can produce substantial hypoventilation.

The study of the role of phospholipid synthesis in the functioning of neuronal tissues took an exciting turn when LARRABEE and co-workers found that nerve cell activity induced in a sympathetic ganglion by preganglionic stimulation increased the rate of labeling of phosphatidylinositol by ^{32}P from inorganic phosphate (LARRABEE et al., 1963). The effect has been observed *in vitro* in ganglia from rats, mice, hamsters, and guinea pigs (LARRABEE and LEICHT, 1965). It is blocked by d-tubocurarine and is not elicited by antidromic stimulation of the postganglionic nerve, leading to the conclusion that the increased labeling of phophatidylinositol is an effect of the synaptic transmitter action on the postsynaptic cell, and is not a concomitant of impulse propagation or of associated ion transport. However, LARRABEE and BRINLEY (1968) have reported that increased labeling of phosphatidylinositol is also elicited by stimulation of the excised giant axon of the squid. On the other hand, DURELL and SODD (1966) corroborate the idea that stimulated phosphatidylinositol turnover is related to synaptic transmission by demonstrating that in guinea pig cerebral hemispheres the ^{32}P$_i$ incorporation into phospholipid stimulated by acetylcholine is concentrated in the subcellular fractions of brain containing "synaptosomes" (WHITTAKER et al., 1964). LARRABEE (1968) has recently demonstrated that the increased ^{32}P labeling of phosphatidylinositol also occurs in naturally stimulated ganglia. Evidence for stimulated turnover of phosphatidylinositol in postsynaptic regions in the living brain, and the effect thereon of anesthetics will be awaited with interest, but the question as to whether any change accompanying anesthesia is a result or a cause of decreased synaptic activity will be just as difficult to resolve as the older controversy over depression of cerebral respiration. A model of a possible molecular mechanism is found in the suggestion that the lipophilic action of narcotics may derange phospholipids cementing enzymes that function together in metabolic sequences (BALL and COOPER, 1949).

VII. Acetylcholine

A. Surface Release

Acetylcholine is released continuously from the cerebral cortex (MacINTOSH and OBORIN, 1953) and from the ventral surface of the cat brain (BELESLIN, 1965). The "weeping" of ACh from the cortex decreases when the degree of anesthetic depression increases and the rate is lower when associated with a synchronized electroencephalogram pattern than with an activated electroencephalogram (CELESIA,

1966; BARTOLINI and PEPEU, 1967). In sheep lightly anesthetized with ether, cyclopropane or pentobarbital the rate of release of acetylcholine is 1.0—3.54 mg/min/cm² cortex and is roughly proportional to the electrical activity of the brain (MITCHELL, 1963). With cyclopropane anesthesia the rate of release increases linearly in the first 15 min but then reaches a plateau, suggesting that acetylcholine leaves the cortex by simple diffusion at a rate equal to its rate of formation. Chloralose, a substance used in many biochemical studies of anesthetic action, produces only a minimal release of acetylcholine, less than 0.3 mg/min/cm² of cortex.

COLLIER and MITCHELL (1967) obtained a high output of acetylcholine from the visual cortex of conscious, free moving rabbits. The rate of release was closely related to the activity and state of arousal (Fig. 1) and, in a quiet, awake animal the rate was more than three times as high as when the animal was anesthetized by

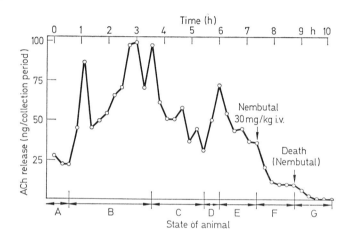

Fig. 1 A—G. Acetylcholine release from the visual cortex of a free-moving rabbit during consciousness and anesthesia. A, anesthetized after cannula implantation; B, recovered from anesthesia and continuously active; C, quiet; D, active; E, quiet; F, anesthetized; G, dead after lethal dose of "Nembutal" (pentobarbital) (COLLIER and MITCHELL, 1967; reproduced by kind permission of the Journal of Physiology)

the injection of pentobarbital 30 mg/kg intravenously. This observation is of great interest because it clearly demonstrates the relevance to the living animal of earlier more indirect evidence. For example, sleep and anesthesia induced by ether or barbiturates is accompanied by an approximately 50% increase in the content of extractable acetylcholine activity in the brain of rats (TOBIAS, 1946), cats (ELLIOTT et al., 1950), mice and rabbits (CROSSLAND and MERRICK, 1954), and dogs (MALHOTRA and PUNDLIK, 1965). Also, when these narcotic drugs are added to the medium during incubation of brain cortex slices in vitro the amount of acetylcholine released into the medium is less than during drug-free incubations (McLENNAN and ELLIOTT, 1950). Again, amobarbital sodium has been shown to reduce the presynaptic release of acetylcholine from the stimulated, perfused superior cervical ganglion of the cat (MATTHEWS and QUILLIAM, 1964). In these experiments amobarbital in a concentration of 50 mg/l in the perfusate, or approximately 0.2 mM, halved the acetylcholine output.

B. Brain Content

The acetylcholine content of the brain correlates inversely with the rate of release. As indicated in the preceding section, decreased release is accompanied by increased storage.

CROSSLAND and MERRICK (1954) investigated the acetylcholine content of several different regions of the rat brain — the cerebral hemispheres, the upper brain stem, cerebellum and the medulla and pons — under the influence of "light" and "deep" anesthesia induced with diethyl ether or with pentobarbital sodium. The effects were not the same in young rats and in adult rats. All parts of the young brain underwent an increase in acetylcholine content during light anesthesia with either agent, and a further increase during deep anesthesia. In the adult rat, light anesthesia caused only slight changes in the acetylcholine content of the various brain regions, with the exception of the medulla. SCHMIDT's (SCHMIDT, 1966) study, also on full-grown rats, shows that similar considerations apply to light and deep anesthesia with halothane.

In deep anesthesia the cerebral increase in acetylcholine concentration reaches a plateau value that is explained by the limited capacity of neural tissue to accumulate this substance. The increase is presumably due to decreased rate of utilization rather than to an increased rate of production, although a diminished rate of synthesis is not excluded. Turnover studies with labelled substrate are needed to settle this point. Inhibition of acetylcholinesterase does not seem to be responsible, but little recent evidence is available on this point (BERNHEIM and BERNHEIM, 1936). The most plausible explanation for the accumulation appears to be a decreased rate of liberation of acetylcholine from central cholinergic neurons, secondary to depressed cerebral activity accompanying anesthesia, shifting the equilibrium between synthesis and destruction in favor of synthesis. MATTHEWS and QUILLIAM (1964) suggest that interference with the normal influx of sodium ions at nerve terminals, as proposed by QUASTEL and BIRKS (1962), may play a role in preventing the mobilization of acetylcholine.

C. Enzyme-Related Studies

The brain serotonin (5-HT) level was the subject of a report by BONNYCASTLE et al. (1962); they found a twofold increase with most CNS depressants. However DIAZ et al. (1968), measuring the effect on 5-TH of three commonly used anesthetics, cyclopropane (15%), halothane (0.75%) and diethyl ether (3%), obtained little or no change, although all of the anesthetics increased the brain level of 5-hydroxy-indoleacetic acid, the main metabolite of 5-HT, presumably by preventing its removal. There was no indication of any inhibition of monamine oxidase activity.

Anesthetic depression of the activity of another enzyme involved in the biotransformation of a neuroactive substance was tested in vitro by GARDIER with cyclopropane and catecholamine-O-methyl transferase. Little effect was observed (GARDIER, 1968).

UNGAR (1965) reported that the activity of a protease from rat brain cortex is inhibited 50% by concentrations of volatile anesthetics equal to about eight times the anesthetizing concentration for goldfish.

In rats cerebral glucose 6-phosphate dehydrogenase activity is increased by various classes of depressants, including pentobarbital (20 mg/kg intraperitoneally), diethyl ether and chloroform (TAKEMORI, 1965), implying an increased utilization of glucosa via the pentose phosphate pathway.

The interactions of anesthetics and brain enzyme systems obviously invite further study.

References

ALDRIDGE, W. N., PARKER, V. H.: Barbiturates and oxidative phosphorylation. Biochem. J. **76**, 47—56 (1960).

ALEXANDER, S., JAMES, F. M., COLTON, E. T., GLEATON, H. R., WOLLMAN, H.: Effects of cyclopropane anesthesia on cerebral blood flow and carbohydrate metabolism of man. Anesthesiology **29**, 170 (1968).

ALLWEIS, C., MAGNES, J.: The uptake and oxidation of glucose by the perfused cat brain. J. Neurochem. **2**, 326—336 (1958).

ANSELL, G. B., DOHMEN, H.: The metabolism of individual phospholipids in the rat brain during hypoglycaemia, anesthesia and convulsions. J. Neurochem. **2**, 1—10 (1957).

— MORGAN, A.: The effects of thiopentone, azacyclonol (frenquel) and reserpine on rat brain phospholipid metabolism in vivo. Biochem. J. **69**, 30P—31P (1958).

BACHELARD, H. S.: Glucose metabolism and o(-keto-acids in rat brain and liver in vivo. Nature **205**, 903—904 (1965).

— GAITONDE, M. K., VRBA, R.: The effect of psychotropic drugs on the utilization of glucose carbon atoms in the brain, heart and liver of the rat. Biochem. Pharmacol. **15**, 1039—1043 (1966).

BALL, E. G., COOPER, O.: The activity of succinate oxidase in relation to phosphate and phosphorus compounds. J. Biol. Chem. **180**, 113—124 (1949).

BARKAI, A., ALLWEIS, C.: The contribution of blood glucose to the carbon dioxide produced by the narcotized brain of the intact cat. J. Neurochem. **13**, 23—33 (1966).

BARKULIS, S. S., GEIGER, A., KAWAKITA, Y., AGUILAR, V.: Study on the incorporation of ^{14}C derived from glucose into the free amino acids of the brain cortex. J. Neurochem. **5**, 339—348 (1960).

BARTOLINI, A., PEPEU, G.: Investigations into the acetylcholine output from the cerebral cortex of the cat in the presence of hyoscine. Brit. J. Pharmacol. **31**, 66—73 (1967).

BATTEY, L., HEYMAN, A., PATTERSON, J. L., Jr.: Effects of ethyl alcohol on cerebral blood flow and metabolism. J. Amer. Med. Assoc. **152**, 6—10 (1953).

BELESLIN, D., POLAK, R. L., SPROULL, D. H.: The release of acetylcholine into the cerebral subarachnoid space of anaesthetized cats. J. Physiol. (London) **177**, 420—428 (1965).

BELLUCCI, G., ROMERIA, C.: Il metabolismo cerebrale in corso di anesthesia pentotalica. Rass. studi psichiat. **45**, 47—56 (1956).

BELOFF-CHAIN, A., CATANZARO, R., CHAIN, E. G., MASI, I., POCCHIARI, F.: Fate of uniformly labelled ^{14}C glucose in brain slices. Proc. Roy. Soc. B. **144**, 22—28 (1955).

BERNHEIM, F., BERNHEIM, L. C.: Action of drugs on the choline esterase of the brain. J. Pharmacol. Exptl Therap. **57**, 427—436 (1936).

BONNYCASTLE, D. D., BONNYCASTLE, M. F., ANDERSON, E. G.: The effect of a number of central depressant drugs upon brain 5-hydroxytryptamine levels in the rat. J. Pharmacol. Exptl Therap. **135**, 17—20 (1962).

BUTLER, T. C.: Theories of general anesthesia. Pharmacol. Revs **2**, 121—160 (1950).

CARLISLE, R., LANPHIER, E. H., RAHN, H.: Hyperbaric oxygen and persistence of vision in retinal ischemia. J. Appl. Physiol. **19**, 914—918 (1964).

CELESIA, G. G., JASPER, H. H.: Acetylcholine released from cerebral cortex in relation to state of activation. Neurology **16**, 1053—1063, 1070 (1966).

CHANCE, B., HOLLUNGER, G.: Inhibition of electron and energy transfer in mitochondria. J. Biol. Chem. **278**, 418—431 (1963).

— WILLIAMS, G. R., HOLMES, W. F., HIGGINS, J.: Respiratory enzymes in oxidative phosphorylation V. A. mechanism for oxidative phosphorylation. J. Biol. Chem. **217**, 439—451 (1955).

COHEN, P. J., MARSHALL, B. E.: Effects of halothane on respiratory control and oxygen consumption of rat liver mitochondria. In: Toxicity of anesthetics (FINK, B. R., Ed.). Baltimore: Williams and Wilkins 1968.

— WOLLMAN, H., ALEXANDER, S. C., CHASE, P. E., BEHAR, M. G.: Cerebral carbohydrate metabolism in man during halothane anesthesia. Anesthesiology **25**, 185 to 191 (1964).

COLLIER, B., MITCHELL, J. F.: The central release of acetylcholine during consciousness and after brain lesions. J. Physiol. (London) **188**, 83—98 (1967).

CROSSLAND, J., MERRICK, A. J.: The effect of anaesthesia on the acetylcholine content of brain. J. Physiol. (London) **125**, 56—66 (1954).

DAWSON, R. M. C., RICHTER, D.: The phosphorus metabolism of the brain. Proc. Roy. Soc. B. **137**, 252—267 (1950).

DIAZ, P. M., NGAI, S. H., COSTA, E.: Effect of oxygen on brain serotonin metabolism in rats. Am. J. Physiol. **214**, 591—594 (1968).

DIXON, T. F., MEYER, A.: Respiration of brain. Biochem. J. **30**, 1577—1582 (1936).

DURELL, J., SODD, M. A.: Studies on the acetylcholine-stimulated incorporation of radioactive inorganic orthophosphate into the phospholipid of brain particulate preparations. II. Subcellular distribution of enzymic activity. J. Neurochem. 13, 487—491 (1966).

EDWARDS, C., LARRABEE, M. G.: Effects of anaesthetics on metabolism and on transmission in sympathetic ganglia of rats: measurement of glucose in microgram quantities using glucose oxidase. J. Physiol. (London) 130, 456—466 (1955).

ELLIOTT, K. A. C.: Brain tissue respiration and glycolysis. In: The biology of mental health and disease. New York: Hoeber 1952.

— HELLER, I. H.: Metabolism of neurons and glia. In: Metabolism of the nervous system (RICHTER, D., Ed.). New York-London-Paris-Los Angeles: Pergamon 1957.

— SWANK, R. L., HENDERSON, N.: Effects of anesthetics and convulsants on acetylcholine content of the brain. Am. J. Physiol. 162, 469—474 (1950).

ESTLER, C.-J.: Der Glykogengehalt des Gehirns weißer Mäuse unter der Einwirkung von Phenobarbital und seine Beziehungen zu Blutzucker und Körpertemperatur. Med. exp. 4, 30—36 (1961).

— HEIM, F.: Der Gehalt des Gehirns weißer Mäuse and Adeninnucleotiden, Kreatinphosphat, Coenzym A, Glykogen und Milchsäure in Ätherexcitation und -Narkose. Med. exp. 3, 241—248 (1960).

FAHMY, A. R., IBRAHIM, H. H., TALAAT, M.: Inhibitory effect of thiopentone on the pyruvic dehydrogenase in brain. Can. J. Biochem. and Physiol. 40, 477—483 (1962).

FINK, B., KENNY, G. E.: Metabolic effects of volatile anesthetics in cell culture. Anesthesiology 29, 505—516 (1968).

FINNERTY, F. A., WITKIN, L., FAZEKAS, J. F.: Cerebral hemodynamics during cerebral ischemia induced by acute hypotension. J. Clin. Invest. 38, 1227—1232 (1954).

FISHER, R. S., WALKER, J. T., PLUMMER, C. W.: Quantitative estimation of barbiturates in blood by ultra-violet spectrophotometry II experimental and clinical results. Am. J. Clin. Pathol. 18, 462—469 (1948).

FISHMAN, R. A.: Carrier transport of glucose between blood and cerebrospinal fluid. Am. J. Physiol. 206, 836—844 (1964).

FORBES, A., BATTISTA, A. F., CHATFIELD, P. O., GARCIA, J. P.: Refractory phase in cerebral machanisms. Elektroencephalogr. and Clin. Neurophysiol. 1, 141—175 (1949).

GAINER, H., ALLWEIS, C. L., CHAIKOFF, I. L.: Precursors of metabolic CO_2 produced by the brain of the anaesthetized intact dog: the effect of electrical stimulation. J. Neurochem. 10, 903—908 (1963).

GAITONDE, M. K., RICHTER, D.: The uptake of ^{3}-S into rat tissues after injection of (^{35}S) methionine. Biochem. J. 59, 690—696 (1955).

— — The metabolic activity of the proteins of the brain. Proc. Roy. Soc. B. 145, 83—99 (1956).

GATFIELD, P. D., LOWRY, O. H., SCHULZ, D. W., PASSONNEAU, J. V.: Regional energy reserves in mouse brain and changes with ischaemia and anaesthesia. J. Neurochem. 13, 185—195 (1966).

GEIGER, A.: Correlation of brain metabolism and function by the use of a brain perfusion method in situ. Physiol. Rev. 38, 1—20 (1958).

— KAWAKITA, Y., BARKULIS, S. S.: Major pathways of glucose utilization in the brain in brain perfusion experiments in vivo and in situ. J. Neurochem. 5, 323—338 (1960).

GEY, K. F., RUTISHAUSER, M., PLETSCHER, A.: Suppression of glycolysis in rat brain in vivo by chlorpromazine, reserpine, and phenobarbital. Biochem. Pharmacol. 14, 507—514 (1965).

GIBBS, E. L., LENNOX, W. G., NIMS, L. F., GIBBS, F. A.: Arterial and cerebral venous blood: arterial-venous differences in man. J. Biol. Chem. 144, 325—332 (1942).

GIESE, A. C.: Cell physiology 3rd ed. Philadelphia-London-Toronto: W. B. Saunders 1968.

GILBOE, D. D., GLOVER, M. B., COTANCH, W. W.: Blood filtration and its effect on glucose metabolism by the isolated dog brain. Am. J. Physiol. 213, 11—15 (1967).

GLEICHMANN, U., INGVAR, D. H., LASSEN, N. A., LUBBERS, D. W., SIESJO, B. K., THEWS, G.: Regional cerebral cortical metabolic rate of oxygen and carbon dioxide, related to the EEG in the anesthetized dog. Acta Physiol. Scand. 55, 82—94 (1962).

GOLDBERG, N. D., PASSONEAU, J. V., LOWRY, O. H.: Effects of changes in brain metabolism on the levels of citric acid cycle intermediates. J. Biol. Chem. 241, 3997—4003 (1966).

GOMBOS, G., OTSUKI, S., SCRUGGS, W., WHITNEY, G., SCHMOLINSKE, A., GEIGER, A.: Brain metabolites of normal intact narcotized cats. Federation Proc. 22, 633 (1963).

GREENE, N. M.: Glucose permeability of human erythrocytes and the effects of inhalation anesthetics, oxygen, and carbon dioxide. Yale J. Biol. and Med. 37, 319—330 (1965).

HERTZ, L., CLAUSEN, T.: Specificity of the potassium-stimulated respiration to certain areas of the brain. Biochem. Pharmacol. 12, 162—163 (1963).

HESS, H. H.: The rates of respiration of neurons and neuroglia in human cerebrum. In: Regional neurochemistry (KETY, S. S., ELKES, J., Eds.). New York- Oxford-London-Paris: Pergamon 1961.

HEYMAN, A., PATTERSON, J. L., JR., JONES, R. W.: Cerebral circulation and metabolism in uremia. Circulation 3, 558—563 (1951).

HIMWICH, H. E.: Brain metabolism and cerebral disorders. Baltimore: Williams and Wilkins 1951.

— HOMBURGER, E., MARESCA, R., HIMWICH, H. E.: Brain metabolism in man: unanesthetized and in pentothal narcosis. Am. J. Psychiat. 103, 689—696 (1947).

HULME, N. A., KRANTZ, J. C.: Anesthesia. XLV: Effect of ethyl ether on oxidative phosphorylation in the brain. Anesthesiology 16, 627—631 (1955).

HUNTER, F. E., Jr., LOWRY, O. H.: The effects of drugs on enzyme systems. Pharmacol. Revs 8, 89—135 (1956).

KERR, S. E., GHANTUS, M.: The carbohydrate metabolism of brain II. The effect of varying the carbohydrate and insulin supply on the glycogen, free sugar, and lactic acid in mammalian brain. J. Biol. Chem. 116, 9—10 (1936).

KETY, S. S.: The general metabolism of the brain in vivo. In: Metabolism of the nervous system (RICHTER, D., Ed.). New York-London-Paris-Los Angeles: Pergamon 1957.

— Circulation and metabolism of brain. Am. J. Med. 8, 205—217 (1950).

— POLIS, B. D., NADLER, C. S., SCHMIDT, C. F.: (1) The blood flow and oxygen consumption of the human brain in diabetic acidosis and coma. J. Clin. Invest. 27, 500—510 (1948).

— WOODFORD, R. B., HARMEL, M. H., FREYHAN, F. A., APPEL, K. E., SCHMIDT, C. F.: (2) Cerebral blood flow and metabolism in schizophrenia. The effects of barbiturate seminarcosis, insulin coma and electroshock. Am. J. Psychiat. 104, 765—770 (1948).

KING, L. J., LOWRY, O. H., PASSONNEAU, J. V., VENSON, V.: (1) Effects of convulsants on energy reserves in the cerebral cortex. J. Neurochem. 14, 599—611 (1967).

— SCHOEPFELE, G. M., LOWRY, O. H., PASSONNEAU, J. V., WILSON, S.: (2) Effects of electrical stimulation on metabolites in brain of decapitated mice. J. Neurochem. 14, 613—618 (1967).

LAJTHA, A., TOTH, J.: The effects of drugs on uptake and exit of cerebral amino acids. Biochem. Pharmacol. 14, 729—738 (1965).

LANDAU, W. M., FREYGANG, W. H., ROLAND, L. P., SOKOLOFF, L., KETY, S. S.: The local circulation of the living brain: values in the unanesthetized and anesthetized cat. Trans. Am. Neurol. Assoc. 80, 125—129 (1955).

LARRABEE, M. G.: Transynpatic stimulation of phosphatidylinositol metabolism in sympathetic neurons in situ. J. Neurochem. 15, 803—808 (1968).

— BRINLEY, F. J.: Incorporation of labelled phosphate into phospholipids in squid giant axons. J. Neurochem. 15, 533—545 (1968).

— HOLADAY, D. A.: Depression of transmission through sympathetic ganglia during general anesthesia. J. Pharmacol. Exptl Therap. 105, 400—408 (1952).

— KLINGMAN, J. D.: Metabolism of glucose and oxygen in mammalian sympathetic ganglia at rest and in action. Neurochem., 2nd ed. (ELLIOT, K. A. C., PAGE, I. H., QUASTEL, J. H., Eds.). Springfield: Thomas 1966.

— — LEICHT, W. S.: Effects of temperature, calcium and activity on phospholipid metabolism in a sympathetic ganglion. J. Neurochem. 10, 549—570 (1962).

— LEICHT, W. S.: Metabolism of phosphatidylinositol and other lipids in active neurones of sympathetic ganglia and other peripheral nervous tissues. The sits of the inositide effect. J. Neurochem. 12, 1—13 (1965).

— POSTERNAK, J. M.: Selective action of anesthetics on synapses and axons in mammalian sympathetic ganglia. J. Neurophysiol. 15, 91—114 (1955).

LASSEN, N. A.: Cerebral blood flow and oxygen consumption in man. Physiol. Revs 39, 183—238 (1959).

— CHRISTENSEN, S., HOEDT-RASMUSSEN, K., STEWARD, B. M.: Cerebral oxygen consumption in Down's syndrome. Arch. Neurol. Psychiat. 15, 595—602 (1966).

LENNOX, W. G., GIBBS, F. A., GIBBS, E. L.: Relationship of unconsciousness to cerebral blood flow and to anoxemia. Arch. Neurol. Psychiat. 34, 1001—1013 (1935).

LEPAGE, G. A.: Biological energy transformations during shock as shown by tissues analyses. Am. J. Physiol. 146, 267—281 (1946).

LOWRY, O. H., PASSONNEAU, J. V., HASSELBERGER, F. X., SCHULZ, D. W.: Effect of ischemia on known substrates and cofactors of the glycolytic pathway in brain. J. Biol. Chem. 239, 18—30 (1964).

MALHOTRA, C. L., PUNDLIK, P. G.: The effect of some anaesthetics on the acetylcholine concentrations of different areas of dog brain. Brit. J. Pharmacol. 24, 348—351 (1965).

MARGOLIS, R. U., HELLER, A.: The effect of cholinergic and other pharmacologic agents on brain monophosphoinositide turnover in vivo. J. Pharmacol. Exptl Therap. **151**, 307—312 (1966).
MARK, J., GODIN, Y., MANDEL, P.: Glucose and lactic acid content of the rat brain. J. Neurochem. **15**, 141—143 (1968).
MATTHEWS, E. K., QUILLIAM, J. P.: Effects of central depressant drugs upon acetyl-choline release. Brit. J. Pharmacol. **22**, 415—440 (1964).
MAYMAN, C. I., GATFIELD, P. D., BRECKENRIDGE, B. M.: The glucose content of brain in anaesthesia. J. Neurochem. **11**, 483—487 (1964).
MCDOWALL, D. G.: The effects of clinical concentrations of halothane on the blood flow and oxygen uptake of the cerebral cortex. Brit. J. Anaesthesia **39**, 186—196 (1967).
— HARPER, A. M.: Blood flow and oxygen uptake of the cerebral cortex of the dog during anaesthesia with different volatile agents. Acta Neurol. Scand. Suppl. **41**, 146—151 (1965).
— — JACOBSON, I.: Cerebral blood flow during trichloroethylene anesthesia: a comparison with halothane. Brit. J. Anaesthesia **36**, 11—18 (1964).
MCHENRY, L. C., JR., SLOCUM, H. C., BIVENS, H. E., MAYES, H. A., HAYES, G. J.: Hyperventilation in awake and anesthetized man. Arch. Neurol. Psychiat. **12**, 270—277 (1965).
MCILWAIN, H.: Metabolic response in vitro to electrical stimulation of sections of mammalian brain. Biochem. J. **49**, 382—393 (1951).
— The effect of depressants on the metabolism of stimulated tissues. Biochem. J. **53**, 403—412 (1953).
MCLENNAN, H., ELLIOTT, K. A. C.: Effect of convulsant and narcotic drugs on acetylcholine synthesis. J. Pharmacol. Exptl Therap. **103**, 35 (1951).
MICHAELIS, M., QUASTEL, J. H.: The site of action of narcotics in respiratory processes. Biochem. J. **35**, 518—533 (1941).
MITCHELL, J. F.: The spontaneous and evoked release of acetylcholine from the cerebral cortex. J. Physiol. (London) **165**, 98—116 (1963).
NECHAEVA, G. A., SADIKOVA, N. V., SKVORTSEVICH, V. A.: Renewal of amino acids of protein under different functional states. Chem. Abstr. **53**, 1500 (1959).
NELSON, S. R., SCHULZ, D. W., PASSONNEAU, J. V., LOWRY, O. H.: Control of glycogen levels in brain. J. Neurochem. **15**, 1271—1279 (1968).
OWEN, O. E., MORGAN, A. P., KEMP, H. G., SULLIVAN, J. M., HERRERA, H. G., CAHILL, G. F.: Brain metabolism during fasting. J. Clin. Invest. **10**, 1589—1595 (1967).
PALLADIN, A. W.: Der Stoffwechsel im Gehirn bei verschiedenem funktionellem Zustand. Wien. klin. Wschr. **66**, 473—477 (1954).
PIERCE, E. C., JR., LAMBERTSEN, C. J., DEUTSCH, S., CHASE, P. E., LINDE, H. W., DEIPPS, R. D., PRICE, H. L.: Cerebral circulation and metabolism during thiopental anesthesia and hyperventilation in man. J. Clin. Invest. **41**, 1664—1671 (1962).
QUASTEL, D. M. J., BIRKS, R. I.: Effect of sodium ions on acetylcholine metabolism in a sympathetic ganglion. Abst. 5th Meet. Canad. Fed. Biol. Sci., p. 64 (1962).
QUASTEL, J. H.: Effects of drugs on metabolism of the brain in vitro. Brit. Med. Bull. **21**, 49—56 (1965).
— QUASTEL, D. M. J.: The chemistry of brain metabolism in health and disease. Springfield: Thomas 1961.
RAFAELSEN, O. J.: Action of insulin on glucose uptake of rat brain slices and isolated rat cerebellum. J. Neurochem. **7**, 45—51 (1961).
ROSSEN, R., KABAT, H., ANDERSON, J. P.: Acute arrest of cerebral circulation in man. Arch. Neurol. Psychiat. **50**, 510—528 (1943).
ROTH, L. J.: Uptake and distribution of anesthetic agents (PAPPER, E. M., KITZ, R. J., Eds.). New York: McGraw Hill 1963.
SACKS, W.: Cerebral metabolism of isotopic glucose in normal human subjects. J. Appl. Physiol. **10**, 37—43 (1957).
— Cerebral metabolism of doubly labeled glucose in humans in vivo. J. Appl. Physiol. **20**, 117—130 (1965).
SCHIEVE, J. F., WILSON, W. P.: The influence of age, anesthesia and cerebral vascular activity to CO_2. Am. J. Med. **15**, 171—174 (1953).
SCHMAHL, F. W.: Effects of anesthetics on regional cerebral blood flow and the regional content of some metabolites of the brain cortex of the cat. Acta Neurol. Scand. Suppl. **41**, 156—159 (1965).
SCHMIDT, C. F., KETY, S. S., PENNES, H. H.: The gaseous metabolism of the brain of the monkey. Am. J. Physiol. **143**, 33—52 (1945).
SCHMIDT, K. F.: Effect of halothane anesthesia on regional acetylcholine levels in the rat brain. Anesthesiology **27**, 788—792 (1966).
SCHUELER, F. W., GROSS, E. G.: The effect of nembutalized blood upon the in vitro respiration of brain. J. Pharmacol. Exptl Therap. **98**, 28—29 (1950).

Smith, A. L., Satterthwaite, H. S., Sokoloff, L.: Induction of brain D(--)-B-hydroxy-butyrate dehydrogenase activity by fasting. Science **163**, 79—81 (1969).

Sokoloff, L.: Local cerebral circulation at rest and during altered cerebral activity induced by anesthesia or visual stimulation. Regional Neurochem. (Kety, S. S., Ed.). New York: Pergamon 1961.

Stone, W. E.: Acid-soluble phosphorus compounds and lactic acid in the brain. J. Biol. Chem. **135**, 43—50 (1940).

Suzuku, K., Korey, S. R., Terry, R. D.: Studies on protein synthesis in brain microsomal system. J. Neurochem. **11**, 403—412 (1964).

Swank, R. L., Cammermeyer, J.: The selective effect of anesthetics and picrotoxin on the cerebral cortex of the dog: an electroencephalographic and histochemical study. J. Cellular Comp. Physiol. **34**, 43—70 (1949).

Takemori, A. E.: Effect of central depressant agents on cerebral glucose C-phosphate dehydrogenase activity of rats. J. Neurochem. **12**, 407—415 (1965).

Tews, J. K., Carter, S. H., Stone, W. E.: Chemical changes in the brain during insulin hypoglycaemia and recovery. J. Neurochem. **12**, 679—693 (1965).

Theye, R. A.: Myocardial and total oxygen consumption with halothane. Anesthesiology. **28**, 1042—1047 (1967).

— Michenfelder, J. D.: (1) The effect of halothane on canine cerebral metabolism. Anesthesiology **29**, 1113—1118 (1968).

— — (2) The effect of nitrous oxide on canine cerebral metabolism. Anesthesiology **29**, 1119—1124 (1968).

— Tuohy, G. F.: Oxygen uptake during light halothane anesthesia in man. Anesthesiology **25**, 627—633 (1964).

Tobias, J. M., Lipton, M. A., Lepinat, A. A.: Effect of anesthetics and convulsants on brain acetylcholine content. Proc. Soc. Exptl Biol. Med. **61**, 51—54 (1946).

Tsuji, H., Balagot, R. C., Sadove, M. S.: Effect of anesthetics on brain γ-aminobutyric and glutamic acid levels. J. Am. Med. Assoc. **183**, 133—135 (1963).

Ueda, I.: Effects of diethylether and halothane on firefly luciferin bioluminescence. Anesthesiology **26**, 603—606 (1965).

— Mietani, W.: Microsomal ATPase of rabbit brain and effects of general anesthetics. Biochem. Pharmacol. **16**, 1370—1374 (1967).

Ungar, G.: Inhibition of a brain protease by general anaesthetics. Nature **207**, 419—420 (1965).

Webb, J. L., Elliott, K. A. C.: Effects of narcotics and convulsants on tissue glycolysis and respiration. J. Pharmacol. Exptl. Therap. **103**, 24—34 (1951).

Wechsler, L., Dripps, R. D., Kety, S. S.: Blood flow and oxygen consumption of the human brain during anesthesia produced by thiopental. Anesthesiology **12**, 308—313 (1951).

Weiner, N.: The content of adenine nucleotides and creatine phosphate in brain of normal and anaesthetized rats: a critical study of some factors influencing their assay. J. Neurochem. **7**, 241—250 (1961).

Westfall, B. A.: Effects of phenobarbital on oxygen consumption of brain slices. J. Pharmacol. Exptl Therap. **96**, 193—197 (1949).

Whittaker, V. P., Michaelson, I. A., Kirkland, R. J. A.: The separation of synaptic vesicles from nerve-ending particles "synaptosomes". Biochem. J. **90**, 293—303 (1964).

Whittam, R.: Active cation transport as a pace-maker of respiration. Nature **191**, 603—604 (1961).

Wilkins, D. S., Featherstone, R. M., Schwidde, J. T., Brotman, M.: Studies on the depression of brain oxidations. J. Lab. Clin. Med. **35**, 411—420 (1950).

Williams, S., Paterson, R. A., Heath, H.: The effect of B, B-iminodiproprionitrile and anaesthesia on some adenine nucleotides of rat brain and retina. J. Neurochem. **15**, 227 to 233 (1968).

Yamamoto, S., Schaeppi, V.: Effects of pentothal on neural activity in somatosensory cortex and brain stem in cat. Electroencephalog. and Clin. Neurophysiol. **13**, 248—256 (1961).

Section 7.0

Exploratory and Newer Compounds

T. H. S. Burns and A. Bracken

With 1 Figure

In writing a chapter on "Exploratory and Newer Compounds" in a book concerned with anesthesia, the authors feel that it is most important to have a clear idea of the aims of their work. The "Why?" must never be lost sight of, in the excitement of the "How?".

Prior to 1956, it was felt by many that the progress of anesthesia and surgery was being held up by the flammability of two of the most popular anesthetic agents — ether and cyclopropane. Not only was the surgeon denied the use of the diathermy when these drugs were in use, but precautions to eliminate the risk of a spark's arising in any of the many pieces of apparatus which were being introduced into the operating theatre in greater and greater numbers, were restricting the design of theatres and equipment.

In England, in 1956, a Ministry of Health Working Party on Anaesthetic Explosions published its Report (Report 1956). One of its recommendations was that the Medical Research Council should set up a committee to encourage the production and use of an anesthetic drug which should have the desirable properties of ether and cyclopropane, without being flammable, and without having such undesirable properties as the irritant effect of ether vapour, or the nausea often associated with cyclopropane.

The introduction of halothane in 1956 went a long way to meet these criteria (Raventos, 1956). It was certainly a major advance. However, in some patients, halothane can cause anxiety for the anesthetist by its effects on blood pressure, pulse rate, heart rhythm or respiration. Respiration can be depressed, or a tachypnoea may be produced. The blood pressure may fall, the pulse rate slow, and arrhythmias have been shown to occur (Brennan et al., 1957). These appear to occur more frequently if epinephrine is used (Brindle et al., 1957; Forbes, 1966).

I. Aim

The aim of the investigation of new compounds, following the introduction of halothane was, therefore, to find a drug which would produce the sort of anesthesia obtained with halothane and be equally non-flammable. It should not depress respiration or blood pressure, and should not encourage cardiac arrhythmias in the presence of epinephrine. One of the biggest disappointments of the authors, in this field, was to find that although hexafluorobenzene was an anesthetic and that it appeared to meet most of these requirements, it proved to be flammable in oxygen at 6% (Imperial Smelting, 1966). The desirable properties of hexafluorobenzene have been confirmed by other workers (Garmer and Leigh, 1967), but all efforts to reduce its flammability have proved unavailing (Imperial Smelting, 1966). It is non-flammable in air, and the possibility of using it with air, as ether has been used in the past, was investigated. It was felt, however, that modern operating conditions demand the ability to give extra oxygen to the patient, and the possibility that an explosion would result if extra oxygen were added to the hexafluorobenzene/air mixture, could not be ruled out.

Hexafluorobenzene therefore remains a tantalisingly attractive new anesthetic, which has an unexpected undesirable property. The discovery of a drug with so many desirable features and yet one not acceptable for modern anesthesia serves to emphasise the need to be quite clear in one's mind *why* one is looking for new drugs and techniques, and what is acceptable and what is not.

An anesthetic drug or technique is necessary for two main reasons. The protective reflexes of a patient must be interfered with, in order that the surgeon may have access to the part on which he wishes to operate and the pain, which

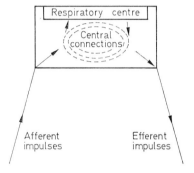

Fig. 1. The three main divisions of a protective reflex

would otherwise result for the patient, must be prevented as far as possible; and all this must be done with the minimum of risk to the patient.

The mechanisms whereby a person is reflexly protected from injury or surgery may be thought of in three parts. An afferent path, an efferent path, and central connections, as shown in diagram 1.

A painful stimulus will travel up afferent nerves and produce an efferent response, the most notable feature of which, to a surgeon, is muscular tone. At the same time various "centres" are stimulated, with a resultant increase in blood pressure, pulse rate, and respiration. At the same time, pain is felt.

Good operating conditions can be obtained by modifying some or all of the main divisions of this reflex. For example, curare will prevent any efferent signal from reaching muscle, thus abolishing its tone. A local anesthetic will prevent the passage of pain impulses to the brain, and in suitable concentration will also block motor nerve impulses. General anesthetics such as ether or halothane, may be regarded as "intoxicating" the central connections and preventing afferent stimuli from producing their normal reflex efferent response. Doses which produce this effect also produce loss of consciousness and so the patient has no sensation of pain. Some general anesthetics, such as ether and halothane also have a curare effect, in addition to this "Central intoxication" (Karis et al., 1967).

It is convenient to consider the shortcomings of existing drugs and techniques according to which part of the reflex arc they modify, and then to decide along which lines they could be improved. Local anesthesia requires considerable special knowledge, is time consuming, and is not always effective. There is a danger of sepsis, overdosage, and complications due to the apparatus used. A major break through would be achieved if some method of interrupting the passage of nerve impulses, locally, could be discovered, which would not involve the injection of substances into accurately defined parts of a patient. It might be possible to produce an electrical "field" which would have this effect.

General anesthetics at present interfere with more reflexes than is desirable. In fact the patient is very much "at risk" during general anesthesia. The anesthesiologist has to see to it that the reduction of reflex activity which he produces does not allow the patient to be harmed or produce pharmacologically undesirable effects.

Relaxant drugs can produce complications if they are not combined with adequate analgesics or narcotics and recovery from their effects is not always straightforward.

II. History

When it was shown that xenon, then believed to be chemically inert, could produce anesthesia (CULLEN and GROSS, 1951; BRACKEN et al., 1956), it was hoped that some other relatively inert compound could be discovered, which would meet all the requirements of an anesthetic, without harm to the patient. Harmful effects of a general anesthetic may be divided into those due to a permanent chemical damage to some organ, such as the liver or kidney, and those due to a pharmacological effect on, for example, the cardiovascular system.

Nitrous oxide approximates these goals, but does not produce sufficient interference with reflex activity to be useful as a "single agent" anesthetic. If it were possible to introduce a *single* drug which would allow an anesthesiologist to produce good access for the surgeon with safety and pain relief for the patient, this would represent a major advance. The combination of two or more drugs can produce complications which are more difficult to understand than those of a single drug.

At present, halothane comes closest to being the chemically inert compound with the desired properties. It will produce relaxation and unconsciousness and is excreted without detectable chemical damage to the patient, and until recently, was not thought to involve the body in its breakdown processes (DUNCAN and RAVENTOS, 1959; STIER, 1964). However, it is not the complete answer, since anxiety can still be caused by its effects on respiration, blood pressure, pulse rate and heart rhythm.

The pharmacological desiderata of a new anesthetic are fairly clearly understood, but the type of compound to be investigated is much less obvious. Questions which need to be answered are:

1. What chemical structure should it have?

2. How pure should it be?

3. How non-flammable should it be?

4. How inert as far as metabolism in the patient is concerned should it be? This raises what is possibly the most difficult question of all: what advance claimed for a new drug is sufficient to justify the risk of using it on a human patient?

1. Chemical Structure

A voluminous literature exists in which courageous attempts are made to forecast from chemical and physical data whether a given substance or class of substances will show anesthetic properties. Some of the most recent results confirm some of the earliest theories. K. W. Miller et al. [1967] and Eger et al. (1965) indicate that oil solubility is, after all, the most important single property possessed by a volatile anesthetic. This supports Meyer (1899) and Overton (1901) rather than Pauling (1961) and S. L. Miller (1961), for both these last authors expressly referred to the aqueous phase in their "ice-crystal" and "ice-

Table 1. A "League Table" of Anesthetics after K. W. Miller et al. [1967 (1)]

Substance	Chemical fomula	Molecular weight	Boiling point °C	Best estimate for righting data (mice) (atm)	MAC[a] (dogs) atm
1. Chloroform	$CHCl_3$	119.4	61.3	0.008	—
2. Halothane	C_2HF_3ClBr	197.4	50.2	0.017	0.008
3. Ether	$C_4H_{10}O$	74	35.8	0.032	0.03
4. Cyclopropane	C_3H_6	42	− 32.9	0.11	0.115
5. Arcton 12	CF_2Cl_2	121	− 30	0.4	—
6. Acetylene	C_2H_2	26	− 83.8 (sublimes)	0.85	—
7. Ethylene	C_2H_4	28	− 103.9	1.1	—
8. Xenon	Xe	131.3	− 108.12	1.1	1.19
9. Nitrous oxide	N_2O	44	− 88.46	1.5	—
10. Krypton	Kr	83.7	− 153.4	3.9	—
11. Methane	CH_4	16	− 161.5	5.9	—
12. Sulphur hexafluoride	SF_6	146	− 63.8 (sublimes)	6.9	—
13. Carbon tetrafluoride	CF_4	88	− 128	19	—
14. Argon	Ar	39.9	− 185.86	24	—
15. Nitrogen	N_2	28	− 195.8	35	1.88
16. Hydrogen	H_2	2	− 252.8	85	—
17. Neon	Ne	20.2	− 246.0	110	—
18. Helium	He	4	− 268.9	190	—

[a] MAC is the minimum alveolar concentration required to prevent gross muscular movements in dogs in response to a painful stimulus. The concentration is normally given by volume, but tensions may also be used, as above (Merkel and Eger, 1963).

berg" theories of anesthesia. K. W. Miller et al. have come to the conclusion that benzene most nearly approaches the solvent characteristics of whatever lipid interface anesthetics are involved with. They have produced a most interesting analysis of recorded estimates of anesthetic potencies for mice. We take the liberty of using the same list of substances, turning their Table upside-down and adding other properties. Thus we arrive at a "League Table of Anesthetics".

Miller et al. used the righting reflex for mice in assessing anesthetic potency. In dogs, Eger's school (Merkel and Eger, 1963) used the minimum alveolar concentration. Where they apply, Eger's figures fit quite well into our Table based on Miller et al.

How to measure anesthetic potency is a problem, but it is surprising how, over all, assessments using differing techniques and animals are not often widely at variance. It is much more difficult to correlate physical and chemical properties with anesthetic properties. PAULING (1961) excluded ether from his hydrate theory of anesthesia because it is exceptional in its not forming a hydrate although it produces anesthesia.

Substances of high molecular weight tend to have high boiling points and be among the more potent anesthetics. This is shown in the table by the position of halothane, although as will be discussed later, one may observe a fluorine compound as very exceptional, namely No. 12, sulphur hexafluoride, which has the second highest molecular weight and yet is in the lower half of the table. It is possible to go a little further than this by considering those substances with molecular weights below 45. If this is done it includes the last five and also numbers 4, 6, 7, 9 and 11. One then makes up a series where fall in molecular weight leads in general to a fall in anesthetic potency. The substances left out are krypton (10), and two of the fluorine compounds, sulphur hexafluoride (12) and carbon tetrafluoride (13) where high molecular weights are associated with low potency.

The misplacing of two fluorine compounds in the table is almost to be expected since those compounds rarely fit theories of anesthesia based on physical properties of substances [K. W. MILLER et al., 1967(1)]. This reflects their unusual properties, which are dictated by a low cohesive force between the molecules, this being due to the very powerful forces within the molecules. So one finds in fluorine compounds, low surface tension, high coefficient of thermal expansion, low boiling point and high vapour pressure. On the other hand, the intense intramolecular forces tend to produce the other characteristic properties of high density, low refractive index, low dielectric constant, small molecular size, and low polarizability. Some of these aspects will be referred to again later. Finally, since any chemical reactions of fluorine compounds involve bonds other than C–F, then the more heavily fluorinated a substance is, the less its chemical reactivity. As will be seen later, the less also will be its anesthetic activity.

In any compound, replacing each hydrogen atom (atomic weight 1) with fluorine (atomic weight 19) increases the molecular weight by 18. At first, as each atom is replaced, the boiling point and molecular weight increase together. Finally, when the characteristic fluorine properties begin to predominate, the boiling point falls until the fully fluorinated compound of highest molecular weight in the series has the lowest boiling point. These points can be illustrated in the diethyl ether series. Diethyl ether, $C_4H_{10}O$, molecular weight 74, boiling point 35.8 °C passes, on fluorine substitution, through hexafluorodiethyl ether $C_4H_4F_6O$ molecular weight 182, boiling point 63.9 °C to become decafluorodiethyl ether $C_4F_{10}O$, molecular weight 254, boiling point 0 °C. The pharmacological activity changes from a potent anesthetic through the hexafluoro compound (the convulsant "Indoklon") to the decafluoro ether, which is inert. Thus rise in molecular weight has decreased boiling point and anesthetic potency, reversing what one might expect by simply studying molecular weight.

The convulsant activity of the intermediate substance hexafluorodiethyl ether $C_4H_4F_6O$ tends to support the suggestion of MULLINS (1954) that anesthetic and convulsant activity are independent. Perhaps they act on different parts of the brain or on different cells within the same region of the brain.

The inertness of the lower boiling decafluorodiethyl ether, contrasted with the potency of diethyl ether, shows a better correlation with the general principle that substances of high vapour pressure are less potent than those of low pressure. EGER et al. (1965) found the correlation between vapour pressure and potency in the volatile drugs they tested to be the next best to oil solubility (see also SACHS, 1968; EGER, 1968).

We have come across two substances which are striking in their high molecular weight, relatively low boiling point, and yet complete inertness. Perfluoro-n-hexane, C_6F_{14} (BURNS et al., 1968) boiling point 57 °C and perfluoromethylcyclohexane, C_7F_{14} (BURNS et al., 1964) boiling point 75 °C were complete by inert in tests on mice, yet their molecular weights 338 and 350 respectively approach twice that of halothane. These two substances were odourless, and this is a convenient point to digress for a moment to this most characteristic property of inhalational anesthetics — their smell.

On consulting the "League table", it will be observed that the property of odour is found only amongst substances in the top half of the table, that is, amongst the anesthetics. Nitrous oxide, in the middle of the table, has a faint smell, but none of the gases below it has any. Our colleague Dr. J. G. BOURNE, of Salisbury, England, has observed that if a substance possesses "pungency", which he likens to the sensation felt in the nose after drinking soda water, or in the throat on aspirating strong ether vapour [BOURNE, 1968 (1)] it will have high tissue solubility, so that a considerable quantity will be required to produce saturation. This is related to a slow induction of anesthesia. If a substance has little pungency, its solubility will be low. Then it will be rapid in its induction. Chloroform is at one extreme, cyclopropane and nitrous oxide at the other. Substances with no odour, such as perfluoro-n-hexane, and perfluoromethylcyclohexane, will be inert or, if active at all, quick in their induction. Oil solubility is a well-known characteristic of highly odorous volatile substances (BEST and TAYLOR, 1955) and has for long been associated with anesthetic potency.

Thus odour, pungency and anesthetic activity are all properties of the heavier molecules. Whilst the exceptions to the use of molecular weight as a guide are too numerous for it to be used except cautiously, it can be said that if a substance has a high molecular weight, this could be an additional reason for trying it as an anesthetic, especially if it has a pleasant, distinct odour.

Molecular size, rather than molecular weight, is a better guide as to whether a substance can be expected to be an anesthetic. BENSON and KING (1965) state that the molecular size and polarizability are the two most important attributes of a volatile anesthetic.

The polarizability of a molecule is a measure of the ease with which charges within it can be displaced by an applied electric field to produce a dipole. The molecule then comes to resemble a bar magnet with a positive pole at one end and a negative pole at the other. Polarizability is directly proportional to the molar refraction (and is indeed obtained experimentally from the refractive index) and has units corresponding to a volume measurement. When so expressed, the value of polarizability is nearly the same as that of molecular size. In this case one can examine size and polarizability together for any molecule. Hydrogen, helium and neon have the lowest polarizability of the gases and are the least anesthetising. These gases also support the "hydrate" theory of anesthesia in which e.g. PAULING (1961) drew attention to the correlation between the partial pressure necessary to form hydrate crystals, and that necessary for anesthesia. A good anesthetic readily forms hydrates. Hydrogen, helium and neon do not form hydrates and are at the bottom of the table. MILLER's proposed "icebergs" or "ice covers" (1961) differ from PAULING's microcrystals in being smaller and non-crystalline, but he also stresses that the reaction of anesthetics is primarily with water molecules in the aqueous portions of the brain rather than with the molecules of lipids. BENSON and KING, however, revert to lipids in cell membranes. An easily polarizable molecule is more likely to be electrically disturbed and adsorbed on any charged site on such a membrane than a molecule like that of hydrogen with a lower polarizability. Such a molecule will be preferentially adsorbed by an essentially electrostatic force on to some specific site. This will change the surface potentials at the interface between the aqueous solution of salts and other electrolytes within the cell, and the outer, non-conducting, organic cell wall. The conduction of charges across the interfaces, essential for nerve conduction, will be impeded and anesthesia will follow. This is an attractive model for the action of anesthetics, including as it does, oil solubility, the size and polarizability of the molecule, and the fact that substances not forming hydrates can yet be anesthetics.

If the above theory of BENSON and KING is valid it implies a purely physical beginning to anesthetic action. That there is also a more chemical aspect of anesthesia, possibly in what follows absorption, seems likely. It is, of course, doubtful whether there is a simple chemical reaction with a given protein complex such as an enzyme system to explain the phenomena of anesthesia. The biochemistry of anesthetic action remains completely obscure and we can only look for hints at the present time. One such hint may follow an examination of the lower part of the "League table". Helium and neon are the least chemically reactive of the noble gases, helium, neon, argon, krypton, and xenon. They have the lowest polarizbility values, do not form hydrates, and are not anesthetics in small animals, even at pressures where mechanical failure of tissues commence (K. W. MILLER et al., 1967). Helium was not an anesthetic for mice at pressures up to 125 atm and was lethal at 135—145 atm because of the effect of hydrostatic pressure. Similar results were obtained with neon in tests with newts *(Triturus Italicus)* instead of mice. Argon, krypton and xenon can show anesthetic activity. Indeed, under pressure xenon is quite potent (PITTINGER et al., 1955) and in general its position is not far from that of nitrous oxide in the table. But it is also significant that xenon was the first and the easiest of the noble gases to be induced into genuine chemical combinations. Here the much larger atom suggests that the outer electrons may be involved more easily in chemical reactions. If this is so, one would expect xenon to be the most anesthetizing of the noble gases. In this limited series of noble gases all the "rules" are obeyed. Molecular weight, boiling point, solubility, molecular size, and polarizability all steadily rise with the anesthetic potency as one progresses from helium to xenon. This could suggest that in anesthesia due to xenon there is a chemical undertone. It is not impossible that living systems can carry out chemical changes involving the noble gases which have not yet been achieved in vitro. SCHREINER et al. (1965) report that the mould *Neurospora crassa* shows 50% inhibition of growth for the following pressures of noble gases:

helium	300 atm,
neon	35 atm,
argon	3.8 atm,
krypton	1.6 atm,
xenon	0.8 atm.

Isolated enzyme systems and tissue culture cells behave similarly suggesting that all the noble gases can show biological activity. It is well known that helium cannot be used by divers below about 1500 feet, because it begins to show narcotic effects. At greater depths they use hydrogen, which on this count should be No. 18 in the "League table". This agrees with its molecular weight being the lowest.

It is possible to begin to examine substances as possible anesthetics by examining a number of properties together. Molecular weight alone is a poor guide, but coupled with odour is much better. The "League table" grades substances in many ways apart from anesthetic potency. As one passes down the table, the tendency is for molecular weight, molecular size, polarizability, odour, boiling point and water solubility to decrease.

One would expect on reasoning like this to find fully fluorinated substances amongst the non-anesthetics despite their relatively high molecular weight. If other atoms and groupings are considered the following points emerge:

Substances containing both hydrogen and fluorine are often convulsants and otherwise toxic, and the following compounds illustrate how the ethylenic double bond also often confers a measure of toxicity.

Six perfluoro cyclobutanes tried as anesthetics

$$\begin{array}{cc} CF_2—CF_2 \\ | \quad\quad | \\ CF_2—CF_2 \end{array}$$

1. Perfluorocyclobutane B.P. − 6 °C
(Clayton, 1967)

$$\begin{array}{cc} CF_2—CF \\ | \quad\quad \| \\ CF_2—CF \end{array}$$

2. Hexafluorocyclobutene B.P. + 3 °C
[Burns et al., 1961 (1)]

$$\begin{array}{cc} CF_2—CH \\ | \quad\quad \| \\ CF_2—CF \end{array}$$

3. 1,H-pentafluorocyclobut-1-ene B.P.
26 °C [Burns et al., 1961 (1)]

$$\begin{array}{cc} CF_2—CFH \\ | \quad\quad | \\ CF_2—CFH \end{array}$$

4. 1,H:2,H-hexafluorocyclobutane B.P.
63 °C (Burns et al., 1964)

$$\begin{array}{cc} CF_2—CFH \\ | \quad\quad | \\ CF_2—CFH \end{array}$$

5. Another 1,H:2,H-hexafluorocyclobutane
B.P. 26 °C [Burns et al., 1961 (1)]

$$\begin{array}{cc} CF_2—CFCl \\ | \quad\quad | \\ CF_2—CFCl \end{array}$$

6. 1,2-dichlorohexafluorocyclobutane
B.P. 59 °C [Burns et al., 1961 (1)]

Of these compounds, Nos. 2, 3 and 6 were toxic convulsants. No. 1 was inert. Nos. 4 and 5 were anesthetics but No. 4 less satisfactory than No. 5.

In the series of ring compounds below, some are aromatic, some aliphatic. Those compounds having only one double bond are toxic and may be convulsants too. Introduction of hydrogen or methyl maintained toxicity. Introducing a double bond or hydrogen made the cyclopentane and cyclobutane derivatives toxic. No. 3. Hexafluorobenzene, an aromatic compound, was a good anesthetic as also was the monohydrogen derivative, No. 4. With the next compound No. 5 where a CF_3 is inserted instead of this hydrogen, a non-toxic substance is converted into a toxic one. (One might note that in the hydrogen analogues toluene is not as toxic as benzene.) If one considers that the aromatic ring seems to confer non-toxicity on fluorine compounds, the toxicity of octafluorotoluene is surprising, and conflicts with Banks et al. (1954) who state that fluorocarbons when very pure are non-toxic. The introduction of an ether grouping shown in the last two compounds, whether this is fluorinated (No. 10) or not (No. 9) does not prevent toxicity being present, and the aromatic ring becomes a toxic one as the aromaticity is removed by fluorinating double bonds. Thus both octafluorocyclohexadiene and decafluoro-cyclohexene, in which the double bonds in the hexafluorobenzene molecule are saturated one at a time by fluorine, are toxic.

Full fluorination is variable in its effects in reducing the boiling points of hydrogen-containing substances. Thus in the above series benzene and perfluoro-benzene have the same boiling points, but toluene B.P. 110 °C has a boiling point about 7 °C higher than its perfluoro analogue. An interesting example of a much greater reduction is shown by perfluoropiperidine $C_5F_{11}N$ referred to again later, whose boiling point of 48 °C contrasts with that for piperidine itself, $C_5H_{11}N$ B.P. 106 °C although the molecular weight has risen from 85 to 283 on fluorina-

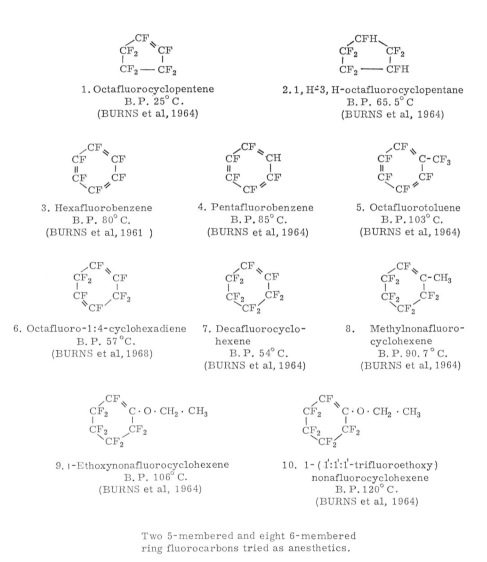

1. Octafluorocyclopentene
B.P. 25° C.
(BURNS et al, 1964)

2. 1, H≙3, H-octafluorocyclopentane
B.P. 65.5° C
(BURNS et al, 1964)

3. Hexafluorobenzene
B.P. 80° C.
(BURNS et al, 1961)

4. Pentafluorobenzene
B.P. 85° C.
(BURNS et al, 1964)

5. Octafluorotoluene
B.P. 103° C.
(BURNS et al, 1964)

6. Octafluoro-1:4-cyclohexadiene
B.P. 57°C.
(BURNS et al, 1968)

7. Decafluorocyclo-
hexene
B.P. 54° C.
(BURNS et al, 1964)

8. Methylnonafluoro-
cyclohexene
B.P. 90.7° C.
(BURNS et al, 1964)

9. 1-Ethoxynonafluorocyclohexene
B.P. 106° C.
(BURNS et al, 1964)

10. 1-(1':1':1'-trifluoroethoxy)
nonafluorocyclohexene
B.P. 120° C.
(BURNS et al, 1964)

Two 5-membered and eight 6-membered
ring fluorocarbons tried as anesthetics.

tion. This is a good example of the reduction of intramolecular bonding forces by fluorination.

To some extent solubility of gases tends to be a property related, not to the solvent, but the boiling point of the gas. Thus gases of low boiling point (hydrogen, oxygen) tend to have low solubilities in water, oil and organic solvents generally, whilst gases of higher boiling point (nitrous oxide, xenon) tend to have higher

Table 2. *Anesthetic activities of fluorinated derivatives of n-butane, n-butene and n-butyne*

Name	Formula	B.P. (°C)	Remarks	Source
A. Saturated compounds				
Perfluoro-n-butane	$CF_3(CF_2)_2CF_3$	—5 to —2	Poisonous to mice	1
1,4-dichlorooctafluoro-n-butane	$Cl \cdot CF_2CF_2CF_2CF_2Cl$	68	Not anesthetic	3
1,4-dihydrooctafluoro-n-butane	$H \cdot CF_2CF_2CF_2CF_2 \cdot H$	44	Good anesthetic	3
2,2,4,4,4-pentafluoro-butane	$CF_3CH_2CF_2CH_3$	40	Anesthetic in mice	2
2,2,3,3-tetrafluoro-butane	$CH_3(CF_2)_2CH_3$	17	Unsatisfactory as anesthetic	2
2,3,3-trifluoro-2-chloro-butane	$CH_3CF_2CFCl\,CH_3$	53	Good anesthetic	2
1,1-dichloro-3,3-di-fluorobutane	$CH_3CF_2CH_2CHCl_2$	117	Delayed deaths	2
1,2-dichloro-3,3-di-fluorobutane	$CH_3CF_2CHCl\,CH_2Cl$	120	Unsatisfactory anesthetic	2
2-Chloro-3,3-difluoro-butane	$CH_3CF_2CHCl\,CH_3$	71.4	Fairly good anesthetic	2
2-Chloro-2-fluorobutane	$CH_3CH_2CFCl\,CH_3$	67	Good anesthetic	2
2,2-difluorobutane	$CH_3CH_2CF_2CH_3$	30.8	Anesthetic in mice	2
B. Unsaturated compounds				
Perfluoro-2-butene	$CF_3CF{=}CF \cdot CF_3$	1.2	Moderately toxic	5
Perfluoroisobutene	$(CF_3)_2C{=}CF_2$	6.5	Toxic	5
2,3-dichloro-1,1,1,4,4,4-hexafluorobutene-2 trans	$CF_3 \cdot CCl{=}CCl \cdot CF_3$	66[a]	Mild anesthetic but toxic	4,8
2,3-dichloro-1,1,1,4,4,4-hexafluorobutene-2 cis	$CF_3 \cdot CCl{=}CCl \cdot CF_3$		Similar to trans but 3 x less toxic	4
2-chloro-1,1,1,4,4,4-hexafluorobutene-2 trans	$CF_3CH{=}CCl \cdot CF_3$	35	Convulsant, not anesthetic	4
2-bromo-1,1,1,4,4,4-hexafluorobutene-2 trans	$CF_3CH{=}CBrCF_3$	52	Convulsant, not anesthetic: toxic	4
2H-heptafluorobutene-2	$CF_3CF{=}CH \cdot CF_3$	7—8	Very toxic	6
Perfluoro-2-butyne	$CF_3C{\equiv}C \cdot CF_3$	24.6	Toxic: not anesthetic	7

[a] B.P. of cis-trans mixture containing about 14% of cis form.

1. Struck and Plattner (1940).
2. Robbins (1946).
3. Burns et al. (1966).
4. Raventos and Lemon (1965).
5. Matheson (1961).
6. Clayton (1966).
7. Lu et al. (1953).
8. Danishevskii, S. L., Kochanov, M. M. (1961).

solubilities. McAULIFFE's report (1966) on water solubilities of hydrocarbons is thus relevant for he states that this solubility is increased by

> ring formation;
> increasing unsaturation of ring or chain;
> increasing molar volume.

This last relates to molecular weight, polarizability and other properties and suggests that knowledge of water solubility alone is better than nothing in assessing whether a substance could be an anesthetic. We agree with Dr. BOURNE however (BOURNE, 1967) that if one is studying solubility one should consider blood solubility as of vital significance.

To the above points one adds the chemical characteristics conferred by atoms other than carbon and hydrogen, i.e. oxygen, nitrogen, sulphur, and the halogens. Full fluorination tends to produce an inert substance, and physiological activity increases with the introduction of hydrogen, ethylenic double bonds, chlorine, bromine and iodine in that order.

However, it is typical of the fluorine series of compounds that one no sooner propounds a set of rules than one finds exceptions. Trifluoroethylene $CHF:CF_2$ contains a double bond and hydrogen with fluorine. It is completely inert to mice (BURNS et al., 1961), and furthermore differs from its chlorine analogue, $CHCl:CCl_2$ in being flammable in air with a lower limit of flammability of 17.4% v/v and an upper limit lying between 25% and 30% v/v.

Two normal butanes showed unusual anesthetic activity when tested by us in that perfluoro 1:4-dihydro-n-butane was an anesthetic whereas the 1:4-dichloro compound was not (BURNS et al., 1966). This led us to look at other butanes and the result of a brief survey of the literature is given in Table 2. This shows that double bonds alone can confer toxicity, hydrogen and a cyclic structure not being essential. *Also shown is the separation in some cases of convulsant or other toxic symptoms from anesthetic action.*

From this brief survey it becomes apparent that any chemical substance has its own characteristics, boiling point, volatility, chemical nature, molecular arrangements and interactions with its environment, and all of these have to be taken into account in assessing whether a given substance might be an anesthetic. A chemist does not merely introduce a fluorine atom or a double bond into a molecule. He produces a new individual compound with its own character. This creates a glorious uncertainty in the quest for a new anesthetic. The study of the chemical and physical properties of a new substance is essential, but tests for anesthesia should not wait upon laborious physico-chemical investigations. However, three properties are of particular importance — the compound must be of known purity; its flammability characteristics must be known; and it must be stable to alkali. These properties can usefully be investigated at the same time or immediately after tests for anesthesia.

The failure of purely physical tests may be illustrated by some unpublished, because negative, investigations carried out some years ago. It seemed to us that if a liquid could be found whose anesthetic potency was very high, say twice that of chloroform, it could be almost non-volatile and yet be useful. If such a liquid had a boiling point around 150 °C its saturation vapour pressure would be so low that the vapour concentration in oxygen at near room temperature would never reach the lower limit of flammability in oxygen, an aspect of flammability to be discussed later. Two such liquids came to our attention. One was a vinyl ether of boiling point 147 °C, the other a somewhat exotic substance, cyclo-octatetraene,

27*

B.P. 142—143 °C. The structures of these substances follow with that of benzene to which the latter is related:

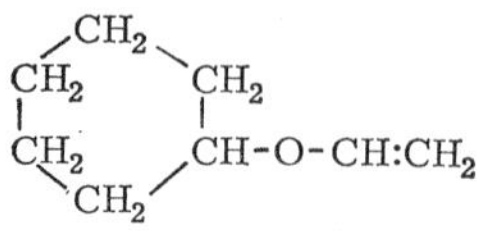

| Cyclohexyl vinyl ether B. P. 147° C. | Cyclo-octatetraene (COT) B. P. 142-143° C. | Benzene (cyclo-hexatriene) B. P. 80. 4° C. |

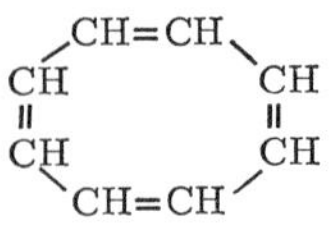

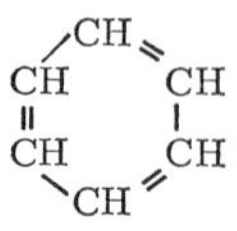

It was felt that animal experiments might be avoided by a study of the chemistry and physics of the compounds.

Benzene is flammable in air and is a dangerous poison (cf. WINEK et al., 1967). It is the parent of the aromatic series of compounds. Cyclo-octatetraene was of interest to chemists because it is the next highest member of the cyclic dienes and to know whether it was aromatic in its chemical nature was of interest. COT is not, in fact, aromatic. Both the vinyl ether and COT possessed tolerable odours and a stream of oxygen bubbled through them gave a non-flammable mixture. Examination of the water solubilities and olive oil/water partition coefficients are summarized in the following table.

Solubilities of two possible anesthetics compared with those of chloroform and nitrous oxide

Substance	Aqueous solubility mg/ml	Oil/water partition co-efficient
Cyclo-hexyl vinyl ether	3.96	29.3, 60.4
Cyclo-octatetraene	0.26	1080, 1525
Chloroform	6.2	100
Nitrous oxide	0.76	3.2

It must be said that the work involved in producing the above figures was considerable, and the reliability was not of a high order. The low aqueous solubility of COT could well imply rapid action if any anesthetic potency were present and the high oil/water partition coefficient, could indicate considerable potency. In an (unpublished) quick assessment carried out with Dr. W. E. ORMEROD, then at St. Mary's Hospital Medical School, London, it was shown that the substances were quite inert to mice except that they seemed to dislike the smells. The general conclusion reached was that it was more difficult to determine those physical characteristics which could lead to selecting a possible anesthetic, than to carry out simple tests on animals.

The view of the present authors is to give half answers to the questions posed above by giving certain indications of properties which could produce a good anesthetic. Almost all the following statements can be challenged [especially 7 (Ed.)], but they are also incorporated in one or other of potent anesthetics in use today.

1. Chemically stable especially to alkali.
2. Non-flammable in air, oxygen and nitrous oxide.

3. Water solubility low, oil solubility high.
4. Pleasant quite pronounced aroma.
5. Boiling point over 100° C need not exclude a substance.
6. There should be no ethylenic double bonds in the molecule.
7. The presence of hydrogen with fluorine should be avoided.
8. Cyclic compounds are more likely to be toxic than non-cyclic ones.
9. The molecular weight should be relatively high.
10. Polarizability (molar refraction) should be high.

A study of which substances agree with and which contradict the above specifications starting with the "League table" presented earlier, will reveal much about modern inhalation anesthetics.

It is possible to follow BOURNE [1968 (2)] and insist that the measurement of the inhaled concentration of an anesthetic is not a measure of intrinsic potency. For this one needs to find the concentration in the brain. In our work, however, it is a grading of anesthetics in a preliminary way by methods close to those prevailing in the operating theatre, which engages our attention. Simple volume/volume concentrations in the anesthetic circuit are then all that is required.

In this connection, the arrangements which have developed, over a number of years, for the investigation of new compounds on behalf of the Medical Research Council appear to be worth description.

The Chemistry Department of Birmingham University produces compounds which are technically feasible, and which it is hoped will have anesthetic properties. The initial screening is carried out by the authors, one of whom is attached to a Medical School, while the other is employed by an industrial concern. By this arrangement it is hoped that the academic side will prevent undue commercial pressure from being applied to the introduction of a new drug, while the industrial side will prevent the research from losing sight of its main goal.

The initial screening aims at determining the purity of the compound, its stability to soda lime, its flammability and its anesthetic activity. In practice, the first test carried out is to determine whether or not the substance is an anesthetic for mice. This can be done quickly, and the physical tests follow. It is our experience that these take longer, and are more complicated than the simple mouse tests for anesthesia. In addition to deciding whether or not a compound is an anesthetic, it has been possible with several substances, to note such things as gross lung damage, or convulsions. Indeed, we are by no means the first to comment on the close structural relationship between drugs which depress and those which stimulate the central nervous system.

It might be objected that mice are not the best animals to use for this work since, for example, nitrous oxide will not anesthetise mice. However, the need is for a compound more potent than nitrous oxide and it is considered very unlikely that a useful new anesthetic would be undetected by this system.

The administration of compounds to mice by inhalation can only demonstrate the presence or absence of anesthetic properties and of toxic effects. Experiments on larger animals not only allow a more accurate evaluation of these properties but also permit a detailed study of the pharmacological activity of the compound to be made.

Those compounds which produce anesthesia, and are acceptable as regards their physical properties, are therefore passed to Dr. L. W. HALL and his colleagues of the Cambridge School of Veterinary Medicine.

In the initial phase of their studies a compound which has appeared to show anesthetic properties when administered to mice is given to decerebrate and spinal preparations as well as to animals already lightly anesthetised with agents such as chloralose and pentobarbital. The object of these experiments is to measure the effects, if any, of various inspired concentrations of the compound on the cardiovascular and respiratory systems. At the same time any undesirable irritant properties of the compound on the respiratory tract become obvious. Compounds which appear in these tests to be satisfactory anesthetic agents, are then administered to animals under conditions nearer to those of clinical practice. Attempts are made to determine the inspired concentrations necessary for the production and maintenance of unconsciousness and the speed and smoothness of both induction and recovery are observed. In all these studies the effects of the compound are compared with those of an accepted inhalation agent such as halothane. These investigations are designed to screen out compounds whose properties would seem, from the results obtained, to warrant further study.

Further studies include the effects of the compound on the cardiac output, peripheral resistance and response to sympathoadrenal stimulation, as well as on respiratory efficiency and general acid-base balance.

The choice of methods and experimental animals used in these trials is limited by three considerations. First, only a small quantity of the compound is generally available for the initial tests. Secondly, it is essential that the exact concentration administered should be known. Finally, because some of the compounds may have toxic properties the methods for administration used must be designed to ensure the safety of the laboratory personnel. These considerations are usually met by the choice of a laboratory animal such as the cat or rabbit and the use of a non-rebreathing valve which permits the animal to inhale a known concentration of the compound prepared in a gas-tight bag via a cuffed endotracheal tube or tracheal cannula, and allows the exhalations to be conducted to the outside air directly or through an exhaust system.

The choice of the cat as the experimental animal is open to objection, but in general it is to be preferred to the rabbit because the larger blood volume enables blood sampling for the determination of oxygen and carbon dioxide tensions and acid-base status to be carried out more frequently without exsanguination of the animal. Moreover, the cat has been a standard laboratory animal for pharmacologists for very many years so that its natural characteristics are well known. However, it is recognised that different toxic and side-effects may predominate in different species of animal and when supplies of compounds permit, the experiments are always repeated first in dogs and later in animals closer to man such as pigs and the smaller primates.

While certain toxic effects may be immediately obvious from simple observation of the progress of the experiment and a study of the measurements made during its course, others may be overlooked unless every experimental animal is subject to a detailed post mortem examination. Therefore, all animals used in acute experiments are examined after death, particular care being taken to look for histological changes in the lungs, liver and kidneys. Animals which are used in recovery studies are also destroyed and examined at a post mortem at a later date.

Only if a compound passes all these tests is it considered for clinical trial. Hexafluorobenzene alone of the 83 substances tested has approached consideration for clinical trial, and even this was turned down because of flammability in oxygen. It did, however, pass the test of offering real pharmacological advantages over halothane in that it appeared to stimulate breathing, maintain blood pressure, and, possibly the most interesting of all its properties, it did not appear to sensitize the heart to epinephrine (Garmer and Leigh, 1967).

The fact that hexafluorobenzene was an anesthetic was quite unexpected. In fact, it was only tested because of a shortage of samples of drugs which had been requested for an investigation into a chemical series of compounds. It emphasises that there are exceptions to all the suggested criteria relating physical or chemical properties to anesthetic effect. As long ago as 1949 NISBETT in a review of anesthetics (NISBETT, 1949) referred to the possibility of changes in selective permeability of membranes or re-orientation of dipoles and changes in the resting state of nerves as possible contributions to the mode of action of anesthetics. With this went a statement that much more information is needed about the nature of the biological system and the physical chemistry of nerve action. Today, 20 years later these remarks appear strangely modern in that no advance has been made. It is almost as if we need to wait for some discovery on the scale of the identification of bacteria as the cause of infectious diseases. We seem to lack the knowledge of the existence of some system which can be modified by drugs to produce anesthesia. Indeed, after summarising all the generally accepted ideas of the relationship of composition to pharmacological effect, we find ourselves in the same position as KRANTZ, who says "there are exceptions to each of these statements" (KRANTZ and RUDO, 1966).

All that can usefully be said today is that some compounds when introduced into the body, interfere with the action of the Central Nervous System, in an apparently reversible way, to produce a reduction in protective reflex activity, associated with unconsciousness.

There is no good reason why any compound whose physical and chemical properties allow it to be introduced into animals should not be tested for anesthetic properties. It happens that for some years, attention has been focussed on fluorine compounds (J. KRANTZ, JR.). This arose originally from the great interest shown in fluorinated hydrocarbons during the second World War owing to their chemical inertness, and more recently has been encouraged by the success of halothane. Trifluoro-ethyl vinyl ether, methoxyflurane, teflurane, Comp. 347, and hexafluorobenzene all suggest that this type of compound should be fully investigated as soon as possible.

It is interesting that, since ROBBINS described his investigations of 46 compounds in 1946, the production of new compounds has been the limiting factor, rather than their testing. Even if we were able to design a molecule which we should expect to be a good anesthetic, there is no guarantee that it would be possible to produce the substance.

The investigation of new anesthetics, is, therefore, still very much a matter of trial and error.

Without doubt, the most interesting compound discovered recently has been halothane $CF_3CHClBr$ a potent anesthetic. Its success has naturally renewed interest in ethanes as anesthetics. Indeed teflurane, CF_3CHFBr B.P. 8 °C where the chlorine atom in the halothane molecule is replaced by fluorine (ARTUSIO and VAN POSNAK, 1961) is interesting in this connection. We went further with halothane fluorination and tried pentafluoroethane, CF_3CF_2H, B.P. −50 °C but this was inert to mice even at a concentration of 93% v/v (BURNS et al., 1962). Other substances related to halothane have been shown to be anesthetics in mice. These were: 1,1,1-trifluoro-2,2-dichloroethane (CF_3CHCl_2, B.P. 27 °C) where the bromine atom in the halothane molecule is exchanged for chlorine; and 1,1,2-trifluoro-1-bromo-2-chloroethane (CF_2Br. $CHClF$, B.P. 50 °C), where the bromine atom is moved within the molecule, the halogen atoms being the same in number and kind as they are in halothane. Looking back on our work we now suspect that we were a little cavalier in our rejection of these two compounds (BURNS et al., 1962).

The structural relationships among these compounds are set out in the following scheme, together with some other related ethanes. The halogen analogues of teflurane, No. 4, where the bromine atom is replaced by chlorine, No. 5, (van Poznak and Artusio, Jr., 1960) and that in which it is replaced by iodine No. 6 (Cascorbi et al., 1962) are both anesthetics. Thus in the ethane series $CF_3CHF \cdot X$ where X is any of the halogens fluorine, chlorine, bromine or iodine, all have been tried as anesthetics and only the fluorine analogue is inert. The last substance in the scheme, pentafluoroiodoethane (No. 8), CF_3CF_2I B.P. 13 °C [Krantz and Rudo, 1961 (2)] is also an anesthetic and contrasts with pentafluoroethane (No. 7).

$$\begin{array}{ccc} & F & H \\ & | & | \\ F & -C-C- & Cl \\ & | & | \\ & F & Br \end{array}$$

1. 1,1,1-trifluoro 2-bromo-2-chloroethane (halothane) B.P. 50 °C

$$\begin{array}{ccc} & F & H \\ & | & | \\ Br & -C-C- & F \\ & | & | \\ & F & Cl \end{array}$$

2. 1,1,2-trifluoro 1-bromo-2-chloroethane B.P. 50 °C (Burns et al., 1962)

$$\begin{array}{ccc} & F & H \\ & | & | \\ F & -C-C- & Cl \\ & | & | \\ & F & Cl \end{array}$$

3. trifluorodichloroethane B.P. 27 °C (Burns et al., 1962)

$$\begin{array}{ccc} & F & H \\ & | & | \\ F & -C-C- & F \\ & | & | \\ & F & Br \end{array}$$

4. tetrafluorobromoethane (teflurane) B.P. 8 °C [Artusio, Jr. and van Poznak, 1961 (1)]

$$\begin{array}{ccc} & F & H \\ & | & | \\ F & -C-C- & F \\ & | & | \\ & F & Cl \end{array}$$

5. tetrafluorochloroethane B.P. −12 °C (van Poznak and Artusio, Jr., 1960)

$$\begin{array}{ccc} & F & H \\ & | & | \\ F & -C-C- & F \\ & | & | \\ & F & I \end{array}$$

6. tetrafluoroiodoethane B.P. 39 °C (Cascorbi et al.. 1962)

$$\begin{array}{ccc} & F & H \\ & | & | \\ F & -C-C- & F \\ & | & | \\ & F & F \end{array}$$

7. pentafluoroethane B.P. − 50 °C (Burns et al., 1962)

$$\begin{array}{ccc} & F & F \\ & | & | \\ F & -C-C- & F \\ & | & | \\ & F & I \end{array}$$

8. pentafluoroiodoethane B.P. 13 °C (Cascorbi et al., 1962)

Prior to the introduction of halothane, attention had been concentrated in finding out whether a non-explosive "ether" could be produced by substituting fluorine atoms for the hydrogen in the diethyl ether molecule. Thus arose the first fluorinated compound to be tried in man, namely fluroxene ("Fluoromar"), trifluoroethyl vinyl ether, $CF_3 \cdot CH_2 \cdot O \cdot CH=CH_2$, B.P. 42.7 °C (Krantz et al., 1953). Methoxyflurane, 2,2-dichloro-1,1-difluoroethylmethyl ether $CHCl_2CF_2OCH_3$ B.P. 104 °C followed in 1960 (Artusio et al., 1960). Both of these are in use today. Roflurane, 1,1,2-trifluoro-2-bromoethyl methyl ether $CBrFH \cdot CF_2O \cdot CH_3$ B.P.

88.8 °C was reported as being successfully used in man [ARTUSIO and VAN POZNAK, 1961 (2)] but seems not to have come into wide use. The latest addition to fluorine compounds used clinically is also an ether, namely Ohio Chemical Company's Compound 347 (VIRTUE et al., 1966; McDOWELL et al., 1968) which is 2-chloro-1,1,2-trifluoroethyl difluoromethyl ether $CF_2HO \cdot CF_2CClFH$, B.P. 56.5 °C (clinically evaluated by DOBKIN et al., 1968). This compound is now known as Ethane.

The presence of the ether grouping does not by itself confer freedom from toxicity, at least not in the six-membered ring compounds noted earlier. On the other hand one ether was quite a fair anesthetic and was genuinely non-flammable because of its high boiling point. This was the compound pentafluorophenyldifluoromethyl ether, $C_6F_5O \cdot CHF_2$, B.P. 128 °C. It is interesting in having hydrogen and fluorine only attached to carbon but showed no signs of convulsant activity. Studies on it carried out since our report (BURNS et al., 1966) have shown that it is too weak to be of value clinically. It may be suggested that the boiling point of methoxyflurane, 104 °C is approaching the maximum possible for a volatile anesthetic. A substance of higher boiling point would need an unusually high vapour pressure to give a useful vapour concentration.

Some other ethers tried [BURNS et al., 1961 (3)], namely a homologous series $CFClH \cdot O \cdot R$, where R was methyl, (CH_3) ethyl (CH_2CH_3) isopropyl $[CH \cdot (CH_3)_2]$ or n-propyl, $(CH_2CH_2CH_3)$ had the correct gradation in boiling points, 69, 88, 100 and 109 °C respectively appropriate to molecular weight increase but their anesthetic potencies, though considerable, did not. Thus the methyl and n-propyl ethers were comparable and were not unpromising at first, a promise not confirmed on further tests, whereas the ethyl and iso-propyl compounds were unsatisfactory.

The attached Chronological List of Developments in fluorinated anesthetics shows how development has quickened with the years. The patent literature is summarized in a second attached list.

The field of organic fluorine chemistry is almost limitless. Virtually every organic substance can be prepared with hydrogen replaced by fluorine in stages right up to complete replacement. Thus a new organic chemistry based on C–F rather than C–H has been called into existence; any one of thousands of substances might be an inhalation anesthetic. However, there are certain limitations which restrict the choice. Amongst these are that the molecular weight must not be too high if the substance is to be volatile, it must be stable to light, and especially to hot alkali, and the substance must not be known to be toxic or unpleasant in other ways (odour). Many compounds can be prepared, however, all likely to meet the above requirements, and it is desirable to examine as many of these as possible as quickly as possible. Many are variants on existing molecules where one inserts fluorine atoms at a different place in the molecule.

It is just as important, however, to consider quite different types of compounds, for example those containing nitrogen, oxygen, and sulphur. Simple fluorinated nitrogen-containing substances such as nitrogen trifluoride, NF_3 (B.P. -120 °C) are inert and HASZLEDINE (1952) has reported that this inertness is carried forward into the fluorinated methyl and ethyl derivatives.

As examples: perfluorotrimethylamine $(CF_3)_3N$ B.P. -6—7 °C; perfluorotriethylamine $(C_2F_5)_3N$ B.P. 69.8—71 °C; and perfluoroethyldimethylamine $C_2F_5(CF_3)_2N$, B.P. 20—22 °C resemble the fluorocarbons in stability, and show no basic properties. The presence of nitrogen and oxygen in the same molecule is also possible. Perfluoro-N,N-dimethylacetamide, $CF_3CON(CF_3)_2$ has B.P. 29.5 to 30 °C and bis (trifluoromethyl) carbamyl fluoride boils at 15—20 °C (YOUNG et al., 1956). Some Russian work in this field deserves notice. ENGLIN et al. (1966) describe preparations of two chloroethyldifluoramines, $CH_3CHCl NF_2$, B.P. 40 to

42 °C and $CH_2Cl \cdot CH_2 \cdot NF_2$, B.P. 80—82 °C and YAKUBOVICH et al. (1966) have synthesized fluorovinyl compounds.

Of more complex products, especially ring compounds, the differences between pyridine C_5NH_5 and its fully fluorinated derivative C_5NF_5 are most striking, reflecting the fascination of fluorine chemistry. Pyridine is a foul smelling, water soluble, basic, substance not even to be thought of as an anesthetic. Pentafluoro-pyridine (BURDON et al., 1960; BANKS et al., 1961), has almost no smell, a much lower boiling point (83 °C compared with 114 °C for pyridine), is non basic, and differs also from pyridine in being almost insoluble in water, although miscible with many organic solvents. Similar differences are shown in the corresponding saturated compounds piperidine C_5NH_{11} and perfluoropiperidine, C_5NF_{11} (SIMMONS et al., 1957). This latter is a stable low boiling liquid (B.P. 49—50 °C) with a characteristic musty smell (HASZLEDINE, 1950), non-basic, and having a 1-fluoromethyl analogue boiling at 66 °C (SIMMONS et al., 1957).

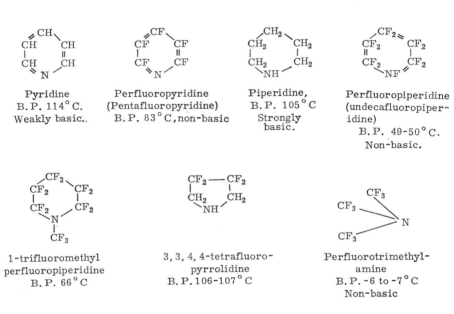

We have tested one of these ring containing substances, 3,3,4,4-tetrafluoro-pyrrolidine, but it proved to be lethal in 40 min to the four mice who inhaled it in oxygen. One would hesitate to exclude them all on this account, since in the cyclohexane series the presence of hydrogen atoms in the molecule led to pronounced toxicity (BURNS et al., 1966).

Whether the above compounds will prove to be anesthetics can be shown only by experiment. On their general stability one can deduce from the method of preparation that they are stable to alkali, but it is fatal to argue by analogy in organic chemistry. For example, the substance 2,4,6-trifluoro-s-triazine has a remarkably reactive fluorine atom on carbon 4, far more so than the corresponding chloro compound. This is thus a remarkable exception to the general rule that the C–F bond is more stable than the C–Cl bond (KOBER and GRUNDMANN, 1959).

Of more interest as possible anesthetics are certain derivatives of nitrogen which also carry an ether oxygen atom. BARR and HASZLEDINE (1955) described perfluoro-2-methyl-1:2-oxazetidine:

$$CF_3 - N - O \qquad\qquad C_3F_7 - N - O$$
$$\quad\ \ |\quad\ \ | \qquad\qquad\qquad\quad |\qquad\ |$$
$$\ \ \ CF_2 - CF_2 \qquad\qquad\qquad CF_2 - CF_2$$

Perfluoro-2-methyl-1:2-oxazetidine   Perfluoro-2-n-propyl-1:2-oxazetidine

as a colourless gas of B.P. $-6.8\ ^{\circ}C$, unaffected by water, aqueous alkali or acid or U.V.-light. They later described the n-propyl analogue, B.P. $50.5\ ^{\circ}C$, again unaffected by water or aqueous alkali. These may be viewed as cyclic ethers. Similar products are reported by YOUNG and DRESDNER (1958).

Two of these are perfluoro-oxazolidines:

$$
\begin{array}{cc}
\begin{array}{c}
CF_2 - O \\
|\qquad | \\
CF_2\ \ \ CF_2 \\
\diagdown N \diagup \\
| \\
CF_3
\end{array}
&
\begin{array}{c}
CF_3 \\
\diagdown \\
\quad N - CF - O \\
CF_3 \diagup \quad |\qquad | \\
\qquad\ \ CF_2\ \ CF_2 \\
\qquad\ \ \diagdown N \diagup \\
\qquad\qquad | \\
\qquad\qquad CF_3
\end{array}
\end{array}
$$

B.P. $21\,^{\circ}C.$ B.P. $81\,^{\circ}C.$

Their relatively high molecular weights 249, and 382 respectively suggest that they might be anesthetics, and their stability to alkali likewise renders them attractive.

The same authors (DRESDNER and YOUNG, 1959) refer to sulphur-bearing fluorocarbon derivatives, some of which are in a suitable boiling range, and can be regarded as derivatives of the non-toxic, inert sulphur hexafluoride SF_6. Amongst these products are:

$$CF_3 \cdot SF_4 \cdot C_2F_5 \qquad\text{B. P. } 47.1^{\circ}C.$$
$$C_2F_5 \cdot SF_4 \cdot C_2F_5 \qquad\text{B. P. } 70-70.5^{\circ}C.$$

and the cyclic sulfur-bearing ether:

$$
\begin{array}{c}
\diagup O \diagdown \\
CF_2 \qquad CF_2 \\
|\qquad\qquad | \\
CF_2 \qquad CF_2 \\
\diagdown SF_4 \diagup
\end{array}
$$

B.P. $80.3\,^{\circ}C.$

One would need to be satisfied on stability and flammability as well as pharmacology of such compounds, but once sulphur and oxygen are introduced into the molecule an enormous variety of combinations becomes possible. For example, why restrict oneself to only one sulphur atom? The substance:

$$CF_3 \cdot SF_4 \cdot CF_2 \cdot SF_5$$

has a boiling point of 87.8—88.1 °C which would be acceptable. The parent sulphur hexafluoride has the low boiling point (actually a sublimation point) of -63.8 °C, so that the entire range of boiling points can be covered within this field of sulphur bearing fluorocarbons.

The compounds which have been most interesting to us have been: $CCl_2F \cdot CClFH$, $CClF_2 \cdot CClFH$. The ethanes $CBrF_2 \cdot CClFH$ and $CF_3 \cdot CCl_2H$, as already mentioned, we may well have rejected on insufficient evidence. The other ethanes, $CClF_2 \cdot CCl_2F$ and $CCl_2F \cdot CCl_2F$, and the butane $C_4F_8H_2$, and the ether, pentafluorophenyl difluoromethyl ether C_7HOF_7, and, of course, hexafluorobenzene have also shown considerable promise.

Another ether, investigated recently by VIRTUE et al. (1966) and DOBKIN et al. (1968) is compound 347 (CF_2H-O-CF_2CClFH). This is said to produce good conditions in man, without cardiac arrythmias, unless epinephrine is used, and to produce rapid induction and recovery. Blood pressure and respiration tend to be depressed.

It has been said that newer compounds should be chemically inert, and therefore non-flammable, and non-reactive with body systems, apart from the central nervous system. They should be obtainable pure and capable of producing good relaxation. But these are not clearly defined goals. The investigations into hexafluorobenzene posed the question *"how* non-flammable ?" It is possible to ignite even halothane, in conditions which could not be produced in normal operating conditions. STIER (1964) has shown that although it was originally thought that halothane was excreted through the lungs unchanged (DUNCAN et al., 1959), significant amounts may be broken down in the body. Although it is claimed that no analytical chemical is more pure than halothane, modern analyzing techniques have shown traces of impurities (see below). Neither the breakdown products nor the impurities appear to upset the safety of halothane; but they do emphasize the need to specify what constitutes purity, flammability and lack of chemical reaction with the body.

2. Purity

The purity of any drugs tested as anesthetics should be high. Even for preliminary tests the level of impurity should not exceed 1%, a suitable standard being that set by preparative gas chromatography. Drugs should be independently tested for purity before being used in animal tests, and this can conveniently be combined with the test for stability to soda lime. The sample is first examined by gas chromatography. A small quantity is next sealed with soda lime in a glass tube and heated for 3 h in a water bath held at 70 °C. Afterwards the sample is again subjected to gas chromatography, any change in composition *showing* that hot soda lime has produced *volatile* impurities (GLOVER and HODGSON, 1961). This procedure shows up another important aspect of purity when working with fluorine compounds. Glass can be sealed for the above test only by fusion in a flame. Great care must be taken not to allow any vapour to be present in the area heated by the sealing flame. With fluorine compounds the pyrolytic decomposition products are certain to be highly toxic including as they must, hydrogen fluoride, and unsaturated fluorine compounds produced by "cracking". Because fluorine compounds often possess abnormally high volatilities, new compounds are frequently sealed in glass tubes. It is essential therefore to take similar precautions to avoid decomposition when sealing the tube. This is achieved by maintaining the sample in acetone-solid carbon dioxide (-78 °C) at which temperature its vapour pressure is substantially zero and then sealing while the tube is highly evacuated.

One must consider in some detail the importance of impurities in test substances. Most of these are obtained in the laboratory as a fraction in a distillation procedure. They may or may not be further purified by preparative gas chromatography or in some other way. This further purification is somewhat tedious, time consuming, and therefore expensive. In the absence of any guide to anesthetic potency from considerations of structure it is often possible to short circuit this final purification. In such cases samples may be tested having over 10% of impurity, and this despite the comments of authorities such as BANKS et al. (1954) who have stated that the presence of impurities invalidates any tests for anesthetic potency. It may be suggested, however, that useful information can be obtained from tests on impure substances so long as the level of impurities is known. If the whole substance is non-toxic none of the impurities is likely to be toxic. If it is also anesthetic then further purification is called for. If the substance proves to be toxic, without producing anesthesia, then it is questionable whether it is justifiable to undertake the work of separation, although impurities of the order of 10% may mask anesthetic action.

If the impure substance should be a good anesthetic and further purification is very difficult this may again be avoided. The sample will be a constant boiling mixture, an azeotrope, so that in eventual anesthetic practice it would be treated as a single substance. Its use would then recall that of the azeotrope of ether and halothane. The test for stability to soda lime can also be useful if the sample is impure, because a change in composition of the vapour phase may suggest a method of purification or preparation as well as a possible reason for rejecting the sample.

The danger in using impure test samples lies in their being used in the absence of knowledge concerning purity. This was the point made by BANKS et al. (1954) and repeated by us (BURNS et al., 1964) and could apply to many substances of which even today valid purity checks are not reported. We had a result confirming the views of BANKS et al. Perfluoromethylcyclohexane was tested by us some years ago, but not reported upon, because the tests showed that it was toxic and flammable in oxygen. Later tests (BURNS et al., 1964) on a known pure sample showed it to be inert to mice.

The question of purity of anesthetics is of topical interest in view of the suspected importance of impurities in halothane.

The standard of purity set in 1956 by Imperial Chemical Industries Ltd., was 0.1% w/w for total volatile impurities and 0.05% for any particular individual. Recently, advances in methods of purification have reduced this figure to below 0.0075% w/w (less than 75 parts per million). Each single saturated impurity is held below 20 ppm and any single unsaturated impurity below 5 ppm (RAVENTOS and LEMON, 1965). A later publication by CHAPMAN et al. (1967) reported that 16 impurities were present down to the 1 ppm level as shown by gas chromatography, nuclear magnetic resonance, and combined mass and infra red spectrometry. It was the unsaturated compounds which were toxic. BANKS et al. (1954) made the point that fluorocarbon vapours are non-toxic when impurities are at a sufficiently low level. This appears to be true for saturated fluorocarbons but not when they are unsaturated. Thus perfluorotoluene C_7F_8 is toxic (BURNS et al., 1964). The introduction of hydrogen can confer toxicity and the tendency of chlorine and bromine in the molecule to do so is well known (BURNS et al., 1966).

It must be confessed that the standard of purity for halothane which makes it one of the purest of drugs, is not likely to be reached in the range of newer and exploratory compounds mentioned by the present writers. It is not impossible that we have rejected a compound as toxic which contains up to 1% of a toxic impurity. However, since we are concerned only with a rapid assessment it is not a justifiable exercise to purify rigorously down to the 100 ppm range (0.01% w/w) every substance tested, most of which will be rejected.

3. Flammability

In the same way there is a certain reluctance to purify before testing for flammability. One aspect of flammability has been touched upon already. Cyclo-octatetraene (COT) burns in air when an ignited match is held to an exposed surface sufficiently long to raise the local temperature above the flash point. Halothane does not burn however heated the liquid may become. On the other hand, if nitrous oxide is bubbled through halothane, an explosive mixture can be produced, whereas COT, similarly treated gives a vapour/gas mixture which is completely safe. Which is now the flammable liquid?

Almost any substance can be regarded as flammable in the sense that it can be made to enter into a chemical reaction evolving heat and light. Oxygen is non-flammable but supports combustion. By this is meant that a flammable gas such as cyclopropane will burn in an oxygen atmosphere.

Some substances are formed from their constituent elements with the absorption of heat and are hence known as "endothermic compounds". They can undergo a spontaneous decomposition with the evolution of heat. (In some cases this energy is sufficiently large to produce heat and light, i.e. a flame without any supporting atmosphere. Thus ethylene oxide, hydrazine $NH_2 \cdot NH_2$, and hydrogen peroxide in vapour form in a tall vertical column can be "ignited" and "burn" in the absence of any supporting atmosphere, a "flame front" passing up the column.)

Nitrous oxide is another endothermic compound since its decomposition leads to the evolution of heat as well as an oxygen rich atmosphere: $2 N_2O \longrightarrow 2 N_2 + O_2$ (33% oxygen compared with air's 21% oxygen). Nitrous oxide is sometimes more active than oxygen as a supporter of combustion of vapours. It has hitherto been accepted that halothane burns in pure nitrous oxide (lower limit 3.8% v/v) but not in pure oxygen or in nitrous oxide/oxygen atmospheres in which the oxygen concentration is over 67% v/v (SEIFLOW, 1957). However, a recent German report (SCHÖN and STEEN, 1968) states that flammable mixtures of halothane are readily obtainable with nitrous oxide/oxygen mixtures currently used in anesthesia and proposes a sequence of actions for minimising the danger of halothane explosions when using a mixture of 10% v/v halothane in 40% nitrous oxide and 50% oxygen.

Thus it is not possible to speak of halothane as a non-flammable agent without qualification. The present investigations aim to find a substance having better pharmacological properties than those possessed by halothane but whose flammability should not be any greater. Hexafluorobenzene C_6F_6, was reported as early as 1961 [BURNS et al., 1961 (2)] to be a satisfactory anesthetic for mice. Later trials using cats (GARMER et al., 1967) to a large extent confirmed its safety. However, the flammability picture was less satisfactory since it could be induced to burn in oxygen at 6% concentration (v/v) or nitrous oxide at 4% v/v. These concentrations might be used in anesthesia, although they would seem to be high and difficult to realise in practice, since its saturation vapour pressure at 20 °C is about 8.5% v/v (BURNS et al., 1968) compared with 7.9% v/v for trichloroethylene. Further, the energy needed to ignite mixtures in oxygen and nitrous oxide appears to be high, and the general stability to light, heat and storage is extremely high, whilst the cost could be relatively low. At the time, unfortunately, the clinical advantages did not appear great enough to our colleagues and ourselves to overcome the disadvantage of flammability and encourage the numerous animal trials which would be required before it was used on human subjects. Yet it is non-flammable in air, and a good anesthetic.

There is no doubt that in the present climate of anesthetists' opinions any new drug must be as non-flammable as halothane to stand a chance of being received. This may be a pity because useful substances may be discarded because of it. It is reasonable to ask how much increased danger there would be in the theatre if, for example, hexafluorobenzene replaced halothane. It could be offset by the greater clinical safety for the patient.

The situation is especially interesting if one calls into question the wide use of trichloroethylene on the grounds that it is flammable in oxygen at a concentration of 10% v/v or in nitrous oxide at 5% v/v. These mixtures are achievable (admittedly with difficulty) in a theatre but only one somewhat doubtful case of an explosion involving trichloroethylene has been recorded (FORRESTER, 1959). So of the three agents, halothane, trichloroethylene and hexafluorobenzene, only the last is at present being excluded from use on account of its flammability. The important point is how real is the risk to the patient if a given substance is used. If an anesthetic can be made to burn, but the experimental conditions for combustion are far removed from those prevailing during an operation — and this would appear to be the case with both halothane and trichloroethylene — it should not be excluded on the grounds of its flammability unless it can be shown to ignite more readily than our tests have so far indicated hexafluorobenzene does. Further thought needs to be given to the subject of flammability of anesthetics in its relation to patient safety.

4. Chemical Inertness

This is probably the most difficult factor to evaluate and where the greatest risk lies in introducing a new drug. A compound should only be given a clinical trial if it claims to offer genuine qualitative or really significant quantitative advances over existing drugs. When halothane was introduced, the greatest thing it had to fight was the 100 years of experience with ether, which had enabled anesthesiologists to provide good, safe anesthesia. Major advances such as those claimed for halothane, in the form of non-flammability and less upset to the patient's metabolic processes, must be accompanied by rigorous animal testing to exclude every possible undesirable reaction. Only then should a drug be offered for clinical trial, and even then there is always the risk of a completely unforeseen complication, as in the case of thalidomide. Thalidomide was a great improvement on existing tranquillizers but its teratogenic effects were quite unexpected, and ruled out its further use as a routine tranquillizer.

The toxic activity of volatile anesthetics is a biological property which could indicate their mode of action. ALDRETE and VIRTUE (1967) report that the teratogenic activity of nitrous oxide, previously reported by LASSEN et al. (1956) and confirmed by PARBROOK (1967) among others, is not unique. Ethylene, acetylene, cyclopropane, and xenon all damaged the hematopoietic system in rats exposed to them for 6 days. Xenon as an example produced 30% leucopenia, 18% erythropenia, and a moderate diminution of granulocytes of the bone marrow. Other side reactions of anesthetics may well indicate a mode of action, because in the case quoted, helium, neon and argon showed no activity. It is possible to state that "cellular toxicity of inhalational anesthetics is directly related to anesthetic activity" (SMITH, 1967). What is the link between cellular toxicity in the bone marrow and narcotizing activity in the brain?

Some of the greatest advances in surgery in the last 30 years have been due to the use of new anesthetic drugs. It would be tragic if patients were to suffer death or injury just for the sake of introducing a drug which was only marginally better than existing, well tested ones. What the authors continue to look for is a drug which can produce anesthesia as deep as halothane but which encourages a normal heart rhythm, pulse rate and respiration. An additional advantage, although only a marginal one, would be a lower solubility in blood and body tissues generally, to achieve an even quicker recovery.

Chronological List of Some Key References in the Development of Fluorinated Anesthetics

1932
Booth, H. S., Bixby, E. M.: Fluorine derivatives of chloroform. Ind. Eng. Chem. 24, 637—641. (The first use of organic fluorine compounds was as refrigerants, despite the title of this publication.)
1939
Henne, A. L., Renoll, M. W., Leicester, H. M.: Aliphatic difluorides. J. Amer. Chem. Soc. 61, 938—940. (Chemical studies, still not of a medical nature.)
1940
Struck, H. C., Plattner, E. B.: A study of the pharmacological properties of certain saturated fluorocarbons. J. Pharmacol. Exptl Therap. 68, 217—219. (First studies of anesthetic properties of fluorine compounds.)
1946
Robbins, B. H.: Preliminary studies of the anesthetic activity of fluorinated hydrocarbons. J. Pharmacol. Exptl Therap. 86, 197—204. (A classic in the field of fluorinated anesthetics.)
1953
Krantz, J. C., Jr., Carr, C. J., Lu, G., Bell, F. K.: Anesthesia XL. The anesthetic action of trifluoroethyl vinyl ether. J. Pharmacol. Exptl Therap. 108, 488—495. (The first clinical use of a fluorine compound.)
1955
Burgeson, R. M., O'Malley, W. E., Heisse, C. K., Forest, J. W., Krantz, J. C., Jr.: Anesthesia XLVI. Fluorinated ethylenes and cardiac arrhythmias induced by epinephrine. J. Pharmacol. Exptl Therap. 114, 470—472. (An important contribution to theoretical understanding of why fluorine compounds have their biological properties.)
1956
Bryce-Smith, R., O'Brien, H. D.: "Fluothane", a non-explosive volatile anaesthetic agent. Brit. Med. J. 2, 969. (A significant advance in anesthesia.)
Raventos J.: The action of Fluothane: a new volatile anaesthetic. Brit. J. Pharmacol. 11, 394. (Announces halothane.)
1957
The following publications in 1957/58 indicate how the pace was quickening, especially the interest in halothane.
Burn, J. H., Epstein, H. G., Feigan, G. A., Paton, W. D. M.: Some pharmacological actions of Fluothane. Brit. Med. J. 2, 479—490.
Dundee, J. W., Linde, H. W., Dripps, R. D.: Observations on trifluoroethyl vinyl ether. Anesthesiology 18, 66—72.
Krantz, J. C., Jr., Truitt, E. B., Jr., Ling, A. S. C., Speers, L.: Anesthesia LV. The pharmacological response to hexafluorodiethyl ether (Indoklon) J. Pharmacol. Exptl Therap. 121, 362—368.
Park, C. S., Truitt, E. B., Jr., Krantz, J. C., Jr.: Anesthesia LI. A comparative study of ethyl vinyl and trifluoroethyl vinyl ethers. Anesthesiology 18, 250—256.
Seiflow, G. H.: The non-inflammability of Fluothane. Brit. J. Anaesthesia. 29, 438—439. (Halothane behaves as an inert diluent.)
Suckling, C. W.: Some chemical and physical factors in the development of Fluothane. Brit. J. Anaesthesia 29, 466—472.
1958
Krantz, J. C., Jr., Park, C. S., Truitt, E. B., Jr., Ling, A. S. C.: Anesthesia LVII. A further study of the anesthetic properties of 1,1,1-trifluoro-2,2 bromochloroethane (Fluothane). Anesthesiology 19, 38—44.
Raventos, J., Spinks, A.: The development of halothane, Part II. Manch. Univ. Med. School Gaz. 37, 55—59.

SUCKLING, C. W.: Halothane — The chemical approach to non-explosive volatile anaesthetic agents. Anaesthesia 13, 194.

1959

DOBKIN, A. B.: Anaesthesia with the azeotropic mixture of halothane and diethyl ether. Brit. J. Anaesthesia 31, 53—65. (A novel approach to overcoming flammability — only partly successful.)

1960

ARTUSIO, J. F., JR., HUNT, R. E., TIERS, F. M., ALEXANDER, M.: A clinical evaluation of methoxyflurane in man. Anesthesiology 21, 512—517.

FABIAN, L. W., DE WITT, H., CARNES, M. A.: Laboratory and clinical investigation of some newly synthesized fluorocarbon anesthetics. Anesthesia and Analgesia, Current Researches 39, 456—462.

VAN POZNAK, A., ARTUSIO, J. F., JR.: Anesthetic properties of a series of fluorinated compounds II. Fluorinated ethers. Toxicol. Appl. Pharmacol. 2, 374—378. (This led to methoxyflurane being tried on man.)

1961

ARTUSIO, J. F., JR., VAN POZNAK, A.: Laboratory and clinical studies with 1,1,2-trifluoro-2-bromoethyl methyl ether. Federation Proc. 20, (1), 312. (Roflurane, which seems to have fallen by the wayside.)

BURNS, T. H. S., HALL, J. M., BRACKEN, A., GOULDSTONE, G.: An investigation of new fluorine compounds in anaesthesia (3). The anaesthetic properties of hexafluorobenzene. Anaesthesia 16, 333—339. (A fluorinated anaesthetic of a completely new type.)

1962

CHENOWETH, M. B., HAKE, C. L.: The smaller halogenated aliphatic hydrocarbons. Ann. Rev. Pharmacol. 2, 363—398. (Halothane is such a compound and this surveys the others.)

1963

COHEN, E. N., BELLVILLE, J. W., BUDZIKIEWICZ, H., WILLIAMS, D. H.: Impurity in halothane anaesthetic. Science 141, 899. (This publication has had far-reaching repercussions.)

KRANTZ, J. C., JR., LU, G. G., SPEERS, L., RUDO, F. G., CASCORBI, H. F.: Anesthesia LXV. The anesthetic properties of 2,2,2-trifluoroethyl iodide. Anesthesia and Analgesia, Current Researches 42, 12—18. (Iodine is also a halogen and iodides can be anesthetics.)

SALMAN, K. N.: A new anesthetic compound, 2,2-dichloro-1,1-difluoroethyl methyl sulphide. Univ. of Maryland, College Park, Univ. Microfilms Order No. 64-11, 109. (Sulphur has not previously been included in the molecules of anesthetics.)

STACEY, M.: Biological properties of organic fluorine compounds. Mfg. Chemist 34 (3), 96—98.

1965

RAVENTOS, J., LEMON, P. G.: The impurities in fluothane; their biological properties. Brit. J. Anaesthesia 37, 716—737.

TOMLIN, P. J.: Methoxyflurane. Brit. J. Anaesthesia 37, 688—705.

1966

INAGAKI, M., YUSA, T., AOBA, Y., IWATSUKI, K.: Azeotropic mixture of Fluoromar and Freon 113. Tohoku J. Exptl Med. 89 (2), 143—150.

KRANTZ, J. C., JR., RUDO, F. G.: The fluorinated anesthetics. Ch. 10 in Handbook of Experimental Pharmacology. Berlin-Heidelberg-New York: Springer. (The most comprehensive recent survey.)

NEAL, M. J., ROBSON, J. M.: The analgesic and anaesthetic action of tetrafluorobenzene. Brit. J. Pharmacol. 26 (2), 482—493. (The fluorinated aromatic ring system contains several anesthetics.)

VIRTUE, R. W., LUND, L. O., PHELPS M., JR., VOGEL, J. H. K., BECKWITT, H., HERON, M.: Difluoromethyl-1,1,2-trifluoro-2-chloroethyl ether anaesthetic agent. Results with dogs and a preliminary note on observations with men. Canad. Anesth. Soc. J. 13 (3), 233—241. (The latest fluorinated anaesthetic "Compound 347".)

1967

CLAYTON, J. W., JR.: Fluorocarbon toxicity and biological action. Fluorine Chem. 1 (2), 197 to 252.

GARMER, N. L., LEIGH, J. M. Some effects of hexafluorobenzene in cats. Brit. J. Pharmacol. 31 (2), 345—350.

Patent List of Fluorinated Anaesthetics

a) British Patents

1. B.P. 742,083 (to Air Reduction Co.) Dec. 21, 1955.
   Fluoro alkyl vinyl ethers e.g.

$CF_3CHCH_3O\ CH:CH_2$	61.5 °C.
$CF_3CH_2O\ CH:CH_2$	57.8 °C.
$C_3F_7CH_2O\ CH:CH_2$	75—77.5 °C.

These are claimed to be suitable for anaesthetic use.

2. B.P. 767,779 (to I.C.I.) Feb. 6, 1957.
Preparation of 1,1,1-trifluoro-2-bromo-2-chloroethane, claimed to be suitable as an inhalation anaesthetic (halothane).

3. B.P. 782,477 (to Air Reduction Co.) Sept. 4, 1957.

Preparation of fluorovinyl ethers e.g.	CF_3CH_2O $CF:CHCl$	84 °C.
	$C_2H_5 \cdot O \cdot CF:CCl_2$	121 °C.
Some of these ethers are stated	$CF_3 \cdot CH_2O \cdot CF:CCl_2$	154 °C.
to be inhalational anaesthetics.	$CF_3CH_2O \cdot CF:CFCl$	75 °C.
	$CF_3 \cdot CH_2O \cdot CF:CH_2$	43 °C.
	$C_2H_5 \cdot O \cdot CF:CHCl.$	89 °C.

4. B.P. 805,764 (to I.C.I.) Dec. 10, 1958.
Preparation of inhalation anaesthetic $CHBrCl \cdot CF_3$ (Halothane) and $CHBrCl \cdot CF_2Cl$.

5. B.P. 894,823 (to I.C.I.) Apr. 26, 1962.
Preparation of 1,1,1,3,3,3-hexafluoro-2-chloropropane B.P. 15 °C and the corresponding 2 bromopropane B.P. 31 °C. Both stated to be inhalation anaesthetic.

6. B.P. 908,110 (to I.C.I.) Oct. 17, 1962.
Preparation of 1,1,3,3,3-pentafluoro-1-bromopropane, an inhalation anaesthetic.

7. B.P. 908,290 (to I.C.I.) Oct. 17, 1962.
Method of manufacture of halothane.

8. B.P. 999,762 (to I.C.I.) Jul. 28, 1965.
Describes preparation of 3-bromo-3-chloro-1,1,2,2-tetrafluoropropane, a non-flammable anaesthetic of low toxicity and high margin of safety. B.P. 99 °C.

9. B.P. 1,004,637 (to I.C.I.) Sept. 15, 1964.
Describes preparation of 3-bromo-3-chloro-2,2-difluoropropane, a non-flammable inhalation anaesthetic.

10. B.P. 1,021,275 (to I.C.I.) Mar. 2, 1966.
Preparation of 1,1-dichloro-2,2-difluoropropane as described. Suitable as an anaesthetic.

b) U. S. Patents

1. U.S.P. 2,951.102 (to Dow Chemical Co.) Aug. 30, 1960.
Preparation of 2-chloro-1,1,1,2-tetrafluoroethane is described. The gas (B.P. -12^0 to -8 °C) is claimed to be non-explosive and shows good promise as an anesthetic.

2. U.S.P. 2,971,990 (to Dow Chemical Co.) Feb. 14, 1961.
Preparation of 2-bromo-1,1,1,2-tetrafluoroethane (B.P. 5—6 °C) is described. Stated to be non flammable, non-explosive and to have anesthetic properties in humans and dogs when administered with oxygen.

3. U.S.P. 3,027.299 (to Air Reduction Co. Inc.) Mar. 7, 1962.
2,2,2-trifluoroethyl vinyl ether is mixed with 1,1,2-trichloro-1,2,2-trifluoroethane to reduce the flammability of the former and yet retains its efficacy as an anesthetic.

4. U.S.P. 3,034.959 (to du Pont) May 15, 1962.
3-Bromo-1,1,2,2-tetrafluoropropane (I) is a member of a series of compounds represented by the formula $H(CF_2)_n\text{-}CH_2Br$ where n is an integer. Only (I) is suitable for use as an inhalation anesthetic.

5. U.S.P. 3,080,430 (to du Pont) Mar. 5, 1963.
3-chloro- and 3-bromo-1,1,2,2-tetrafluoropropane are claimed to be suitable as inhalation anesthetics.

6. U.S.P. 3,261,748 (to Dow Chemical Co.) Jul. 19, 1966.
1,1,1,2-tetrafluoroethane (B.P. -29 °C) is claimed to be suitable as an inhalation anaesthetic but mixtures with $> 30\% \ O_2$ are inflammable.

7. U.S.P. 3,264,356 (to Dow Chemical Co.) Aug. 2, 1966.
2,2-Dichloro-1,1-difluoroethyl methyl ether, free from contaminants is stable for practically unlimited periods of time under normal storage conditions and is entirely satisfactory as an anesthetic (Methoxyflurane).

8. U.S.P. 3,314,850 (to Allied Chemical Corp.) Apr. 18, 1962.

$$CH_2 \underset{\underset{\displaystyle CH_2 - O}{|}}{\overset{\overset{\displaystyle O}{\diagup}}{}} C \overset{\diagup CF_3}{\diagdown CF_3}$$

Preparation of 2,2-Bis-(trifluoromethyl)1,3-dioxolane is described. This substance is stable, of low inflammability and is suitable for use as an inhalation anesthetic.

9. U.S.P. 3,324,145 (to Dow Chemical Co.) Jun. 6, 1967.
   Preparation of fluorinated dioxolanes is described. In addition to the dioxolane mentioned in U.S.P. 3,314,850 above the Dow patent also mentions 4-methyl-2,2-bis-(trifluoromethyl)1,3 dioxolane as being suitable for use as an inhalation anesthetic.

10. U.S.P. 3,346,448 (to Allied Chemical Corp.) Oct. 10, 1967.
    The preparation of hexafluoroisopropyl methyl and ethyl ethers (B.P. 50—50.5 °C and 64—65 °C, respectively) is described. Both are claimed to be suitable for use as inhalational anesthetics.

11. U.S.P. 3,362,874 (to Baxter Laboratories Inc.) Jan. 9, 1968.
    The preparation of 2-chloro- and 2-bromo-1,1,3,3-tetrafluoropropane is described. Both are stated to be useful anesthetics.

c) Other Patents

1. German Patent 1,175,825 (to du Pont) Aug. 13, 1964.
   Preparation of 1,1,2,2,3,3,4,4-octafluoro-5-chloro- and 5-bromopentanes. These produced convulsions.

2. Japanese Patent 21,323 (to Daikin Kogyo Co. Ltd.) Oct. 21, 1967.
   Preparation of ethyl-1-bromotetrafluoroethyl ether, B.P. (624 mm) 76.5 °C. This compound is claimed to be a useful anesthetic.

Patent Information Concerning Fluorinated Compounds not Specifically Claimed to be Anesthetics

a) British Patents

1. B.P. 839,034 (to W. T. Miller) Jun. 29, 1960.
   Preparation of 13-perfluoro- or perchlorofluoro-hydrocarbons.

2. B.P. 921,254 (to Union Carbide Corp.) Mar. 20, 1963.
   Preparation of vinylfluoride and 1,1-difluoroethane.

3. B.P. 945,017 (to Union Carbide) Dec. 18, 1963.
   Preparation of 5 chlorofluoropropanes.

b) U. S. Patents

1. U.S.P. 2,452,975 (to I.C.I.) Nov. 2, 1948.
   Preparation of a number of fluorochloroethanes is described.

2. U.S.P. 2,456,027 (to Minnesota Mining and Manuf. Co.) Dec. 14, 1948.
   Preparation of fluorinated hydrocarbons from CF_4 to C_7F_{11}.

3. U.S.P. 2,461.142 (to du Pont) Feb. 8, 1949.
   Preparation of 1,1,2-trichloroethane.

4. U.S.P. 2,462,402 (to du Pont) Feb. 22, 1949.
   Preparation of a number of chlorofluoropropanes.

5. U.S.P. 2,466,189 (to du Pont) Apr. 5, 1949.
   Preparation of various chlorofluoropropanes.

6. U.S.P. 2,486,023 (to Purdue Research Foundation) Oct. 25, 1949.
   Preparation of 1,1-difluoro-1-chloropropane.

7. U.S.P. 2,490,764 (to Kinetic Chemicals Inc.) Dec. 13, 1949.
   Preparations of some highly fluorinated compounds ranging from $H(CF_2)_4F$ to $H(CF_2)_{13}F$.

8. U.S.P. 2,578,721 (to Purdue Research Foundation) Dec. 18, 1951.
   Preparation of fluoro-pentachloroethane and other fluorinated saturated halocarbons.

9. U.S.P. 2,578,913 (to du Pont) Dec. 18, 1951.
   Preparation of some fluoromethanes.

10. U.S.P. 2,644,845 (to Purdue Research Foundation) Jul. 7, 1953.
    Preparation of number of bromo and chloro fluorocarbons.

11. U.S.P. 2,842,603 (to Minnesota Mining and Manuf. Corp.) Jul. 8, 1958.
    Straight chain and cyclic perhalofluoro-olefins.

12. U.S.P. 2,880,248 (to Minnesota Mining & Manuf. Corp.) Mar. 31, 1959.
    Preparation of perhalogenated fluoalkanes containing one Br. atom.

13. U.S.P. 2,965,683 (to Hooker Chemical Corp.) Dec. 20, 1960.
    Preparation of 2,2,3-trichloroheptafluorobutane.

14. U.S.P. 2,972,637 (to du Pont) Feb. 21, 1961.
    Preparation of bromofluoromethanes.

15. U.S.P. 3,046,304 (to R.N. Haszeldine) Jul. 24, 1962.
    Covers the preparation of a large number of halogenated fluorocarbons both saturated and unsaturated.

16. U.S.P. 3,067,263 (to Dow Chemical Co.) Dec. 4, 1962.
    Preparation of 3,3,3-trifluoropropene.

17. U.S.P. 3,080,428 (to du Pont) Mar. 5, 1963.
    Preparation of a number of symmetrical polyhalopropyl ethers.

c) Miscellaneous

1. French Patent 1,319,071 (to Allied Chem. Corp.) Feb. 22, 1963.
   Preparation of 1,2-dichloro-1,1,2,3,3,3-hexafluoropropane.

References

Aldrete, J. A., Virtue, R. W.: Prolonged inhalation of inert gases by rats. Anesthesia and Analgesia, Current Researches 46, 562—564 (1967); — Smith, B. E.: Discussion. Anesthesia and Analgesia, Current Researches 46, 564—565 (1967).

Artusio, J. F., Jr., Van Poznak, A.: Laboratory and clinical investigation of teflurane, 1,1,1,2-tetrafluoro-2-bromoethane. Federation Proc. 20, (1) 312 (1961).

— — Hunt, R. E., Tiers, F. M., Alexander, M.: A clinical evaluation of methoxyflurane in man. Anesthesiology 21, 512—517 (1960).

Banks, A. A., Campbell, A., Rudge, A. J.: Toxicity and narcotic activity of fluorocarbons. Nature 174, 885 (1954).

Banks, R. E., Ginsberg, A. E., Haszledine, R. N.: Heterocyclic polyfluoro-compounds — Part I. Pentafluoropyridine. J. Chem. Soc. 1961,1740—1743.

Barr, D. A.: Perfluoroalkyl derivatives of nitrogen. Part III. Heptafluoronitrosopropane, perfluoro-2-n-propyl-1:2 oxazetidine, perfluoro (methylene-n-propylamine), and related compounds. J. Chem. Soc. 1956, 3416—3428.

— Haszledine, R. N.: Perfluoroalkyl derivatives of nitrogen — Part I. Perfluoro-2-methyl-1:2 oxazetidine and perfluoro (alkylene-alkylamines). J. Chem. Soc 1955, 1881—1889.

Benson, S. W., King, J. W., Jr.: Electrostatic aspects of physical adsorption. Implications for molecular sieves and gaseous anesthesia. Science 150, 1710—1713 (1965).

Best, C. H., Taylor, N. B.: The physiological basis of medical practice, 6th Ed. p. 1220. Baltimore, Md.: Williams and Wilkins Comp. 1955.

Bourne, J. G.: (1) Personal communication (1968).

— (2) The anaesthetic pressures of certain fluorine-containing gases. Brit. J. Anaesthesia 40, 142 (1968).

— Studies in anaesthetics including intravenous dental anaesthesia. London: Lloyd-Luke (Medical Books) Ltd. 1967.

Bracken, A., Burns, T. H. S., Newland, D. S.: A trial of xenon as a non-explosive anaesthetic. Anaesthesia 11, 40—49 (1956).

Brennan, H. J., Hunter, A. R., Johnstone, M.: Halothane. A clinical assessment. Lancet 1957, II, 453—457.

Brindle, G. F., Gilbert, R. G. B., Millar, R. A.: The use of Fluothane in anaesthesia for neurosurgery: a preliminary report. Canad. Anaesth. J. 4, 265—281 (1957).

BURDON, J., GILMAN, D. J., PATRICK, C. R., STACEY, M., TATLOW, J. C.: Pentafluoropyridine. Nature **186**, 231—232 (1960).

BURN, J. H., EPSTEIN, H. G., GOODFORD, P. J.: The properties of the anaesthetic substance 1,1,2-trifluoro-1,2-dichloroethane. Brit. J. Anaesthesia **1959**, 518—529.

BURNS, T. H. S.: (2) An investigation of new fluorine compounds in anaesthesia (3). The anaesthetic properties of hexafluorobenzene. Anaesthesia **16**, 333—339 (1961).

— (3) An investigation of new fluorine compounds in anaesthesia (4). Examination of an ethane and four ethers. Anaesthesia **16**, 440—444 (1961).

— Fluorine compounds in anaesthesia (5). Examination of six heavily halogenated aliphatic compounds. Anaesthesia **17**, 337—343 (1962).

— Fluorine compounds in anaesthesia (7). Examination of two derivatives of normal butane and nine heavily halogenated ring compounds. Anaesthesia **21**, 42—50. (1966).

— Unpublished data (1968).

— HALL, J. M., BRACKEN, A., GOULDSTONE, G.: Fluorine compounds in anaesthesia (6). Examination of fourteen heavily halogenated ring compounds. Anaesthesia **19**, 167—176 (1964).

— — — — NEWLAND, D. S.: (1) An investigation of new fluorine compounds in anaesthesia (1). Anaesthesia **16**, 3—18 (1961).

CASCORBI, H. F., KRANTZ, J. C., JR., RUDO, F. G.: Unpublished data (1962). Quoted in KRANTZ, J. C., JR., RUDO, F. C. (q.v.) p. 538.

CHAPMAN, J., HILL, R., MUIR, J., SUCKLING, C. W., VINEY, D. J.: Impurities in halothane: their identities, concentrations and determination. J. Pharm. and Pharmacol. **19**, 231—239 (1967).

CLAYTON, J. W., JR.: The mammalian toxicities of organic compounds containing fluorine. Handbook of Experimental Pharmacology, Vol. XX/I, p. 490. Berlin-Heidelberg-New York: Springer 1966.

— Perfluorocyclobutane non-toxic. Chem. Eng. News **45**, 8 (1967).

CULLEN, S. C., GROSS, E. G.: The anaesthetic properties of xenon in animals and human beings, with additional observations on krypton. Science **113**, 580—582 (1951).

DANISHEVSKII, S. L., KOCHANOV, M. M.: Toxicity of some fluoro-organic compounds. Gigiena Truda i Professional. Zabolevaniya **5** (3), 3—8 (1961).

DOBKIN, A. B., HEINRICH, R. G., ISRAEL, J. S., LEVY, A. A., NEVILLE, J. F., OUNKASEM, K.: Clinical and laboratory evaluation of a new inhalation agent: Compound 347 ($CHF_2 \cdot O \cdot CF_2 \cdot CHFCl$). Anesthesiology **29**, 275—287 (1968).

DRESDNER, R. D., YOUNG, J. A.: Some new sulphur bearing fluorocarbon derivatives. J. Am. Chem. Soc. **81**, 574—577 (1959).

DUNCAN, W. A. M., RAVENTOS, J.: The pharmacokinetics of halothane (Fluothane) anaesthesia. Brit. J. Anaesthesia **31**, 302—315 (1959).

EGER, E. I., II: On the variation of anesthetic potency with vapor pressure. Anesthesiology **29**, 1065—1066 (1968).

— BRANDSTATER, B., SAIDMAN, L. J., REGAN, M. J., SEVERINGHAUS, J. W., MUNSON, E. S.: Equipotent alveolar anesthetic concentrations of methoxyflurane, halothane, diethyl ether, fluroxene, cyclopropane, xenon and nitrous oxide in the dog. Anesthesiology **26**, 771—777 (1965).

ENGLIN, M. A., MAKAROV, S. T., KRUGLYAK, YU. L., MOISEEV, B. P., VIDEIKO, A. F., ANISIMOVA, A. N., YAKUBOVICH, A. YA.: Some reactions of alkyl difluoroamines. Zhur. Obshchei. Khim. **36**, (11) 1966—1968 (1966).

FORBES, A. M.: Halothane adrenaline and cardiac arrest. Anaesthesia **21**, 22—27 (1966).

FORRESTER, A. C.: Mishaps in anaesthesia. Anaesthesia **14**, 388—399 (1959).

GARMER, N. L., LEIGH, J. M.: Some effects of hexafluorobenzene in cats. Brit. J. Pharmacol. **31**, 345—350 (1967).

GLOVER, J. H., HODGSON, H. W.: An investigation of new fluorine compounds in anaesthesia (2). Analysis by gas chromatography. Anaesthesia **16**, 19—23 (1961).

HALL, L. W.: Private communication, 1968. School of Veterinary Medicine, Cambridge.

HASZLEDINE, R. N.: The fluorination of organic compounds containing nitrogen. J. Chem. Soc. **1950**, 1966—1968.

Imperial Smelting Co. Ltd. Unpublished work (1966).

KARIS, J. H., GISSEN, A. J., NASTUK, W. L.: The effect of volatile anesthetic agents on neuromuscular transmission. Anesthesiology **28**, 128—134 (1967).

KOBER, E., GRUNDMANN, C.: Triazines, XXII. Fluoro-s-triazines. J. Am. Chem. Soc. **81**, 3769—3770 (1959).

KRANTZ, J. C., JR.: CARR, C. J., LU, G., BELL, F. K.: Anesthesia XL. The anesthetic action of trifluoroethyl vinyl ether. J. Pharmacol. Exptl Therap. **108**, 488—495 (1953).

— RUDO, F. G.: The fluorinated anaesthetics. In: Handbook of Experimental Pharmacology, Vol. XX/I, p. 541. Berlin-Heidelberg-New York: Springer 1966.

LASSEN, H. C. A., KENRIKSEN, E., NEUKIRCH, F., KRISTENSEN, H. C.: Treatment of tetanus:
    severe bone marrow depression after prolonged nitrous oxide anaesthesia. Lancet **1956**
    I, 527—530.
LU, G. G., LING, J. S. L., KRANTZ, J. C., JR.: Anesthesia XLI. The anesthetic properties of
    certain fluorinated hydrocarbons and ethers. Anesthesiology **14**, 466—472 (1953).
MATHESON: Perfluoro-2-butene. Matheson Gas Data Book, p. 353. California: The Matheson
    Company Inc. 1961.
MCAULIFFE, C.: Solubility in water of paraffin, cycloparaffin, olefin, acetylene, cycloolefin,
    and aromatic hydrocarbons. J. Phys. Chem. **70**, 1267—1275 (1966).
MCDOWELL, S. A., HALL, K. D., STEPHEN, C. R.: Difluoromethyl-1,1,2-trifluoro-2-chloroethyl
    ether: Experiments on dogs with a new inhalational anaesthetic agent. Brit. J. Anaesthesia
    40, 511—516 (1968).
MERKEL, G., EGER, E. I., II: A comparative study of halothane and halopropropane an-
    esthesia, including method for determining equipotency. Anesthesiology **24**, 346—357
    (1963).
MEYER, H. H.: Zur Theorie der Alkoholnarkose. Naunyn-Schmiedebergs Arch. Exptl Pathol.
    u. Pharmakol. **42**, 109—118 (1899).
MILLER, K. W.: Brit. J. Anaesthesia **40**, 142 (1968).
— PATON, W. D. M., SMITH, B. E.: The anaesthetic pressure of certain fluorine-containing
    gases. Brit. J. Anaesthesia **39**, 910—918 (1967).
MILLER, S. L.: Theory of gaseous anesthetics. Proc. Natl. Acad. Sci. US **47**, 1515—1524
    (1961).
MULLINS, L. J.: Some physical mechanisms in narcosis. Chem. Revs **54**, 289—323 (1954).
NISBETT, H. B.: Anaesthetics: The Royal Institute of Chemistry Monograph (3) (1949).
OVERTON, E.: Studien über die Narkose. Jena 1901.
— STREET, W. B.: Animals at very high pressures of helium and neon. Science **157**, 97—98
    (1967).
PARBROOK, G. D.: The leucopenic effects of prolonged nitrous oxide treatment. Brit. J. An-
    esthesia **39**, 119—127 (1967).
PAULING, L.: The hydrate microcrystal theory of general anaesthesia. Anesthesia and An-
    algesia, Current Researches **43**, 1—10 (1961).
PITTINGER, C. B., FAULCONER, A., KNOTT, J. R., PENDER, J. W., LUCIEN MORRIS, E.,
    BICKFORD, R. G.: Electroencephalographic and other observations in monkeys during
    xenon anaesthesia at elevated pressures. Anesthesiology **16**, 551—563 (1955).
RAVENTOS, J.: The action of Fluothane — a new volatile anaesthetic. Brit. J. Pharmacol. **11**,
    394—410 (1956).
— LEMON, P. G.: The impurities in Fluothane. Their biological properties. Brit. J. An-
    aesthesia **37**, 716—737 (1965).
Report of a working party on anaesthetic explosions. H.M. Stationery Office, London 1956.
ROBBINS, B. H.: Preliminary studies of the anesthetic activity of fluorinated hydrocarbons.
    J. Pharmacol. Exptl Therap. **86**, 197—204 (1946).
SACHS, D. H.: On the variation of anesthetic potency with vapour pressure. Anesthesiology **29**,
    1064—1065 (1968).
SCHÖN, G., STEEN, H.: Explosion limits and ignition temperatures of some inhalational
    anaesthetics in mixtures with various oxygen carriers. Anaesthesist **17**, 6—10 (1968).
SCHREINER, H. R.: Technical Report: the physiological effects of argon, helium and the rare
    gases. Tonawanda Research Laboratory and Clearinghouse, 1965.
SEIFLOW, G. H.: The non-inflammability of Fluothane. Brit. J. Anaesthesia **29**, 438—439
    (1957).
SIMMONS, T. C., HOFFMANN, F. W. with BECK, R. B., HOLLER, H. V., KATZ, T., KOSHER, R. J.,
    LARSON, E. R., MULVANEY, J. E., PAULSON, K. E., ROGERS, F. E., SINGLETON, B.,
    SPARKS, R. E.: Fluorocarbon derivatives. II. Cyclic Nitrides. J. Am. Chem. Soc. **79**,
    3429—3432 (1957).
SMITH, B. E.: Discussion on "Prolonged inhalation of inert gases by rats". (Aldrete and
    Virtue). Anesthesia and Analgesia, Current Researches **46**, 564—565 (1967).
STIER, A.: Trifluoroacetic acid as metabolite of halothane. Biochem. Pharmacol. **13**, 1544
    (1964).
STRUCK, H. C., PLATTNER, E. B.: A study of the pharmacological properties of certain
    saturated fluorocarbons. J. Pharmacol. Exptl Therap. **68**, 217—219 (1940).
VAN POZNAK, A., ARTUSIO, J. F., JR.: Anesthetic properties of a series of fluorinated com-
    pounds. I. Fluorinated hydrocarbons. Toxicol. Appl. Pharmacol. **2**, 363—373 (1960).
VIRTUE, R. W., LUND, L. O., PHELPS, M., JR., VOGEL, J. H. K., BECKWITT, H., HERON, M.:
    Difluoromethyl-1,1,2-trifluoro-2-chloroethyl ether as an anaesthetic agent: results with
    dogs and a preliminary note on observations with man. Canad. Anaesth. Soc. J. **13**,
    233—241 (1966).

WINEK, C. L., COLLOM, W. C., WECHT, C. H.: Fatal benzene exposure by glue sniffing. Lancet 1967 I, 683.

YAKUBOVICH, A. YA., SERGEEV, A. P., FOGEL'ZANG, E. N.: Reaction of direct fluoroalkylenation. I. Synthesis of trifluorovinyl and chlorodifluorovinylamines. Zhur. Obshcheĭ. Khim. 36 (7), 1317—1325 (1966).

YOUNG, J. A., DRESDNER, R. D.: Fluorocarbon nitrogen compounds. II. Synthesis and properties of perfluorodimethylglycine, $(CF_3)_2NCF_2COOH$. J. Am. Chem. Soc. 80, 1889 to 1892 (1958).

— SIMMONS, T. C., HOFFMANN, F. W.: Fluorocarbon nitrogen compounds. I. Perfluorocarbamic acid derivatives, amides, and oxazolidones. J. Am. Chem. Soc. 78, 5637—5639 (1956).

Section 8.0

Comparative Aspects of Anesthesia in Animals

L. R. Soma and H. W. Calderwood

With 16 Figures

The interest in veterinary anesthesia has increased considerably, with greater focus on anesthesia as an important part of animal management and care. The approach and attitude has shifted from anesthesia as being only a necessary part of a surgical procedure to a greater overall awareness of its importance in the management of the animal from the preoperative through to the postoperative period. Along with the growing awareness of the practicing veterinarian in the greater use of newer anesthetic agents and techniques, has been an increased interest on the part of the experimental surgeon and research worker in better anesthetic methods. There has also been a greater concern for the impact of drugs and anesthetic agents on experimental results. Unfortunately, herein lies one of the greatest deficiencies of our knowledge of general anesthesia. The rapid development of the field of biomedical engineering has given the research scientist the means for the development of more sophisticated chronic models. This has placed a greater responsibility on the researcher for the use of better anesthetic techniques and a greater awareness on pre and postoperative care.

The following sections describe some of the techniques applicable to animals and point out some of the major anesthetic differences of depressants in some of the common species.

I. Inhalation Anesthetics

The inhalational anesthetics have within the last 5 years enjoyed a greater usage for both clinical and experimental surgery in the United States. The advantages of an anesthetic agent which is supplied and removed through the lungs are obvious. This coupled with the development of excellent equipment, more economically priced, has also spurred its use. The basic compromises which have been made to reduce the cost have been in cabinet design, not in vaporizer or circle construction (see following sections).

A detailed description of the action of the inhalational anesthetic agents in various species is beyond the intent of this chapter, but suffice it to say that of the broad scope of depressant drugs used in both man and animals, the inhalants have a greater uniformity of action. Because of this their actions, as measured from a clinical or applications point of view, are generally predictable when the clinician approaches an unfamiliar animal. Of course, some exceptions and variations in their actions among species are to be expected. For example, the ventilatory response of the canine species to diethyl ether is greater, with a marked increase in rate and decrease in tidal volume being a common observation. This greater response, as compared to man, may be related to a more predominant release of epinephrine, a tendency toward a metabolic acidosis, and a greater sensitivity of the Hering-Breuer reflex. The ventilatory response of the horse to ether anesthesia is the direct opposite to that of the dog, and very little reflex respiratory response occurs, from either the upper or lower airway. The ventilatory rates of ruminants during both ether and halothane anesthesia are high; the most probable reason being an increased sensitivity of the pulmonary reflex mechanisms.

The induction of anesthesia will vary somewhat with the species, the small mammals having a faster induction and recovery rates, related to greater ventilatory and circulatory capabilities when assessed on a body surface area basis. The induction of anesthesia in the cold blooded species, e.g. snakes, turtles, is prolonged because of very low rates of ventilation. The diving mammals are very sensitive to the respiratory depressant effects of barbiturates and require intubation and controlled ventilation shortly following the induction of anesthesia [SOMA, 1971 (2)]. The induction of anesthesia with a mask in the seal, for example, can be delayed because of the tendency of this aquatic mammal to hold its breath (diving reflex) with the detection of the anesthetic vapor. Under these circumstances the initial delivery concentration should be high, followed by intubation and controlled ventilation. With controlled ventilation the concentrations of anesthetic agents are comparable to those used in man and dogs.

The blood-gas solubility coefficients of the inhalants in the carnivorous dog are comparable to those of man (halothane = 2.40), whereas the herbivorous animals have considerably lower solubility coefficients. The blood-gas solubility coefficient of halothane in the sheep is 1.45. This varying solubility might also explain some of the differences noted in the induction and recovery from general anesthesia in some species.

The signs of anesthesia as described in man, generally can be applied, with some modification in the determination of the depth of anesthesia in animals. Slight variations can be noted among animals especially in ocular movements, abatement of oral tone, laryngeal reflexes and characteristics of ventilatory changes [SOMA, 1971 (2)].

The three most common inhalation agents used in veterinary anesthesia and anesthesia for experimental surgery are halothane, methoxyflurane, and nitrous oxide. The most important advantage of these agents is their non-explosive properties in the anesthetic ranges. Halothane is commonly used because of a more rapid induction and recovery from anesthesia. The need for an accurate vaporizer is just as important in veterinary anesthesia as it is in man. The development of accurate low flow vaporizers has also contributed to a greater use because of the capability of the use of lower flow techniques for the maintenance of anesthesia, especially in the smaller species. This has reduced considerably the expense of halothane anesthesia.

Methoxyflurane, a halogenated ether, is used a great deal for both clinical and experimental surgery. Because of its low vapor pressure, less elaborate equipment can be used for its vaporization. A common method of vaporization is the use of an in-the-circle glass vaporizer identical to the ones used for diethyl ether. As with the halothane vaporizers, there are out-of-the-circle vaporizers available which are capable of delivering a known vapor concentration over a wide range of fresh gas flows. Due to its high solubility coefficient, it is more convenient to use other agents for the induction of anesthesia.

Nitrous oxide is primarily used as a supplement to halothane and methoxyflurane, and in some circumstances in combination with narcotics and muscle relaxants. Diethyl ether is not generally used in clinical anesthesia because of the danger of explosions. It is still used in experimental work for small laboratory animals, usually using the more crude methods of vaporization, such as a bell jar and cotton pledget.

II. Tracheal Intubation

The ease of intubation varies from species to species and occasionally among breeds. With the exception of some rodents, the most difficult of species to intubate is man. The primary reasons are: (1) the angulation of the oral-tracheal axis, (2) the greater sensitivity of the larynx, (3) the greater tendency toward complete laryngospasms, and (4) the need for greater relaxation of the jaw and neck muscles for intubation. The angulation is diminished in the subhuman primates, and is markedly reduced in the prone species. The passage of an endotracheal tube in the canine is relatively easy except for the brachycephalic breeds such as the Boxer, Pug, and English Bulldog. In these particular breeds the pharyngeal soft tissue and tongue are enlarged relative to the size of the oral cavity. Even in the awake state these canines suffer from some degree of soft tissue obstruction which is increased under anesthesia. It is not uncommon to find the soft palate trailing into the larynx.

In animals, as in man, the proper angulation and positioning of the head facilitates intubation of the trachea [Soma, 1971 (2)]. The position for intubation in the dog can be either lateral or spinal recumbency. Large dogs with long and flexible necks can remain in lateral recumbency with the head twisted to a more supine position (Fig. 1). Cats and small dogs can be easily rolled into the supine position (Fig. 2). The dog and cat are intubated by direct vision using a straight or curved blade. In cats and smaller dogs the curved pediatric blades, placed at the base of the tongue facilitate exposure and better vision of the larynx. The soft palate of the dog is proportionally longer than in man and is lodged below the epiglottis and may interfere during tracheal intubation. This is a problem particularly in the brachycephalic breeds and the palate may have to be displaced with the endotracheal tube prior to insertion.

The feline species are more difficult to intubate than the canine because of the tendency to laryngospasm and persistent jaw tone during lighter planes of anesthesia. The dome shaped arytenoid cartilages will passively follow the respiratory exertion making intubation more difficult. Laryngospasms are more common in the feline species and the sensitivity of the larynx approaches that of man. Spraying the larynx with local anesthetics prior to intubation will prevent the spasms. The soft palate is shorter than in the canine so the larynx is easier to expose. As in the canine the brachycephalic breeds of cats such as the Persian and Himalayan also have a large tongue, but the degree of obstruction is usually not as severe as in the dog.

The intubation of the subhuman primate is similar to man. The tendency toward laryngospasm is not as marked but the spraying of the larynx with local anesthetic prior to intubation is advised.

The smaller ruminants and the pig can be intubated by direct vision with a laryngoscope blade of at least 250 mm in length. These can be made by adding an extension to a standard blade or by the use of the Rowan blade. Adding a curved stylet to the endotracheal tube will aid in its passage in the small ruminants. The pig should be placed in dorsal recumbancy and a straight endotracheal tube used. Intubation of the pig is difficult, due to the length of the oral cavity and minimal oral opening. In the sheep the use of 40 to 60 mg of succinylcholine chloride to produce muscle relaxation will aid in intubation. Preoxygenation via mask is necessary during spontaneous ventilation, because artificial ventilation with the mask is not possible in the paralyzed ruminant. Raising the head during intubation is recommended because of the possibility of regurgitation of ruminal fluids.

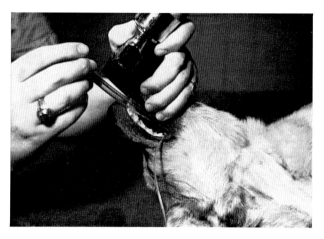

Fig. 1. Positioning of the dog for tracheal intubation. The dog can also be intubated in the lateral position. An assistant can aid intubation by opening the mouth. Courtesy of SOMA [1971 (2)]

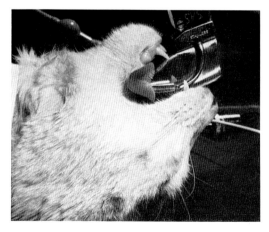

Fig. 2. Positioning of the cat for tracheal intubation. The tongue is pushed to one side with the blade. The tip of the blade is placed at the base of the tongue. Courtesy of SOMA [1971 (2)]

Blind intubation is necessary in the horse because of the long oral cavity, large tongue and minimal oral opening. By extending the head, a straight line is made of the oro-tracheal axis. A bite block is placed between the dental arcades, and the tongue is pulled forward slightly. Damage to the hyoid bones can occur if excessive traction is applied to the tongue. A slightly curved tube is passed on the midline toward the larynx. The tube should be passed during inspiration.

Tactile intubation is practiced in large ruminants. A bovine speculum or bite block is necessary because of stimulation of the chewing reflex under light planes of anesthesia. The arm should be kept on the midline to avoid being injured by the molars. The epiglottis is depressed by the index and middle finger and the endotracheal tube passed over them into the larynx. Another method is to place a small stomach tube into the larynx, as above, then thread the endotracheal tube over it. As with sheep the regurgitation of ruminal contents can occur. Tactile intubation of the dog and cat can be done but is not recommended.

Intubation of the mouse, rat and guinea pig is difficult. In these animals the use of a mask to administer the inhalation anesthetic can be used effectively, although a technic for the intubation of the rat has been reported (MEDD and HEYWOOD, 1970). A lighted speculum was made from a Gowlande auriscope. Endotracheal tubes were made from polyethylene tubing, 2 cm long and cemented into a larger tube which extends out of the mouth. Blind intubation of the rabbit is possible but consistency is dependent on experience and practice. Intubation under direct vision has been reported using a speculum or blade 6 to 7 cm long (WESTHUES and FRITSCH, 1965). The rabbit is placed on its back when under general anesthesia, and the tongue is pulled out to the side to avoid injury from the incisor teeth. The base of the tongue is depressed by the speculum. The cheek is pushed to the side by a endotracheal tube. A stiff tube or one with a stilette in it should be used. A lighting source such as that described for the intubation of the rat or a standard laryngoscope can be used to illuminate the epiglottis and larynx. It must be appreciated that the larynx is deep in the oral cavity with a minimal oral opening.

III. Complications and Species Differences of Tracheal Intubation

The complications of tracheal intubation are markedly reduced as skill in the method and the ability to recognize abnormal reactions to the tube increases. The advantages afforded by intubation in animals, as in man, far outweigh the potential complications [SOMA, 1971 (1)]. Mishaps can be categorized into: a) trauma, b) misplacement of tube, c) respiratory effects, d) and cardiovascular effects.

Trauma. Damage to the mucous membrane of the oral cavity, larynx and trachea can occur and is most likely to result from repeated attempts to intubate. Damage to teeth is uncommon in most animals because of the greater width of the oral cavity. Lips and tongue can be traumatized by pinching them between the laryngoscope and the teeth or by tying them between the tube and the teeth when securing the tube to the oral cavity. Marked edema of the tip of the tongue has occurred by pinching it between the incisor teeth and the tube, especially when the tube is secured by gauze to the mandible. Abrasions or lacerations of the mucous membrane of the upper respiratory tract can occur by the pushing of a dry tube into the larynx, especially if relaxation is incomplete.

Sore throats following tracheal intubation cannot be easily determined in veterinary patients. Laryngitis and tracheitis have been noted in some cases. Following endotracheal anesthesia excessive swallowing and a persistent dry cough are indicative of trauma and subsequent irritation.

Misplacement of the tube. Misplacement during intubation or displacement during anesthesia can result in a partial or complete respiratory obstruction. Endotracheal tubes are used to assure a patent airway; its insertion into the esophagus defeats this purpose. Lack of familiarity with the oro-tracheal structures, a hurried intubation, light anesthesia, or an oversized tube are the common causes of an esophageal placement. As the tip of the tube is placed into the glottis, vision of the inlet and surrounding structures are lost. If the tube is oversized or the laryngeal opening poorly relaxed, the tube can slip over the larynx into the esophagus.

An endotracheal tube can be inserted too far into the trachea and into the right bronchus, producing left lung collapse, especially in the smaller shorter necked animals. After intubation, the chest should be checked for equal expansion or auscultated for equal breath sounds on both sides. Displacement also can occur due to movement of the animal or weight of the anesthesia connections dislodging a poorly secured tube. Inflation of the cuff which is only partially inserted into the larynx, can push the tube out of the glottis.

Respiratory effects. The process of intubation in the lightly anesthetized dog or cat can produce transient increase in respiration or coughing (bucking) on the tube. Also under light planes of anesthesia apnea can occur shortly after intubation, due to reflex inhibition of respiration. Placement of the tip of the tube to the area of the carina, can stimulate respiration because of the persistance of this deep tracheal reflex. The respiratory pattern will be irregular.

Sensitivity of the larynx and its response to external stimuli varies from species to species (REX, 1966, 1967). Unfortunately, detailed information is not available. The larynx of the cat is very reactive and spastic closure is common. On the other hand, the horse can tolerate high concentrations of diethyl ether or other stimuli with no signs of laryngeal or tracheo-pulmonary sensitivity. Complete closure of the larynx, where no egress and ingress of air occurs, is impossible in most animals except some aboreal species and man (NEGUS, 1965). Man, the gibbon, the chimpanzee, and the gorilla are capable of preventing the escape of air by closure of the ventricular bands; a function dogs, cats, and most domestic species do not have. These arboreal species can fix the volume of the chest by preventing the escape of air, used as an aid in pulling themselves directly upward (NEGUS, 1965). Animals that climb, grasp, hug, or strike (e.g. cat, bear) do have more developed inlet valvular closure, either by a vaulted type of larynx, as seen in the cat, or a secondary inlet valve produced by a thyro-arytenoid fold (NEGUS, 1965). It has been noted clinically that some animals with a more highly developed inlet valve (man, cat, sub-human primates) are more prone to laryngospasms during tracheal intubation.

Respiratory obstruction, partial or complete, can occur during endotracheal anesthesia due to a mechanical obstruction, such as excessive flexion of the neck which can kink a rubber or plastic tube or the tube can kink in or out of the oral cavity due to the weight of the equipment connections, or because of extreme positions of the head. Veterinary patients have bitten down on tubes, creating an obstruction, or chewed a tube in half with the distal half sliding into the trachea.

Cardiovascular effects. The cardiovascular effects of manipulation of the larynx and intubation vary among species. There is minimal information in this area in all animals except man. The general effect in man is an increase in blood pressure and heart rate during manipulation of the epiglottis and intubation (BURSTEIN et al., 1950; ORR and JONES, 1968). Electrocardiographic changes in the form of bigeminal rhythms, ectopic ventricular contractions and sinus tachycardia have been reported in man (HUTCHINSON, 1964, 1967; LEWIS and SWERDLOW, 1964; ORR and JONES, 1968). These ECG changes have also been noted in the dog and cat, a response which may be caused by an increase in sympathetic activity or reflex excitation of the vagus nerve.

The cardiovascular changes in the dog are opposite to those of man; the common effect in the dog being bradycardia and hypotension (King et al., 1961). The vagotonic effects of narcotics, barbiturates, and halothane, for example, may exaggerate these effects (Burn et al., 1957; Johnstone, 1951; Redgate and Gellhorn, 1956). In the dog the vagolytic effects of atropine will minimize the effects of intubation and should be used. Atropine will not prevent laryngospasms, but its reduction of secretions may prevent inadvertant stimulation by these secretions. The cardiovascular effects in the cat are more similar to those in man, where an increase in blood pressure and heart rate can be expected. Cardiac arrest during intubation has been reported in man (Lewis and Swerdlow, 1964) and has occurred in dogs.

IV. Systems for Veterinary Anesthesia

Many circuits which have been developed for use in man can be easily adapted for use in animals except for the extremes in size, e.g. rodents, birds, and horses. At the small end of the scale a little ingenuity should suffice but for the larger animals special equipment such as larger endotracheal tubes and tubing as well as larger circle absorbers and valves are necessary.

Open drop technique. The "open-drop" or "cone method" of delivery is still applicable to the toy canine breeds, cats and small laboratory animals and can provide adequate planes of anesthesia with a minimal amount of equipment. The induction of anesthesia in the large dog is not recommended, because of the difficulty of restraint, amount of anesthetic agent needed and size of the mask. Major disadvantages even in the smaller species are: (1) it is wasteful and therefore can only be used economically with the older volatile agents, (2) there is considerable variation in anesthetic concentration and experience is required to provide a constant inspired vapor concentration, (3) there is no method of supporting ventilation if hypoventilation occurs, and (4) there is some rebreathing of exhaled carbon dioxide and a decrease of oxygen tension because of the increased dead space imposed by the mask (Dripps et al., 1961). The main advantages are that it can be readily applied to the smaller species with little equipment needs and there are no valves to impose resistance to respiration.

A common fault in this method is the use of a large cone packed at one end with cotton. Cotton or any other dense material will impede the exchange of respiratory gases with room air and the large cone will create a dead space further minimizing the ventilatory exchange. The resulting dead space can be a major hazard of the open-drop technique. The concentration (partial pressure) of oxygen below the mask when room air is being used will be lower than ambient pressure because of its dilution by accumulated water vapor, carbon dioxide and anesthetic vapor. The proper exchange of gas will depend upon the mask fit, the size of the mask, the thickness of the gauze and the patient's tidal volume in relationship to the dead space created by the mask. The concentration of carbon dioxide will be markedly increased as the patient's tidal exchange is decreased in the deeper planes of anesthesia. To insure an adequate concentration of oxygen and reduction of the accumulation of carbon dioxide a flow of oxygen of 200 to 300 ml/min should be maintained below the mask.

Other equipment that can be used consists of a wire mesh mask covered with eight layers of 16 ply surgical gauze (Fig. 3 and 4). The layers of gauze provide a good surface for vaporization of the volatile anesthetic agent, are a sufficient barrier to prevent facial contamination by the liquid anesthetic and are thin enough to insure adequate exchange of respiratory gases with room air.

The cat or small dog which has been premedicated is restrained gently by an assistant or the anesthetist and the face mask, after applying a few drops of liquid anesthetic, is held close to the face. Initial contact between the face mask and the animal should be avoided. The liquid agent should be dropped on the mask slowly at first in order to accustom the animal to the smell of the vapor. The rate of

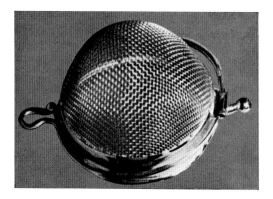

Fig. 3. Wire mesh mask used for open drop administration of volatile anesthetics. The mesh is covered by thin layers of gauze for vaporization. Courtesy of SOMA [1971 (2)]

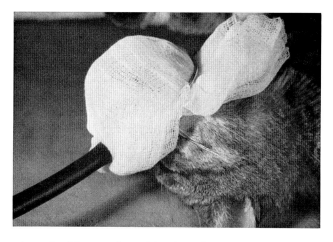

Fig. 4. Wire mesh mask with gauze in position for induction and maintenance of anesthesia in a cat. Tubing supplies supplemental oxygen and anesthetic vapors for maintenance. Courtesy of SOMA [1971 (2)]

dropping can be increased slowly as sedation occurs and the cat or dog becomes tolerant to the smell of the anesthetic vapor. Cats, especially, will resist vigorous restraint, and therefore the initial handling should be gentle. The cat should be approached from behind and allowed to back towards the body of the anesthetist as the mask is placed near the face. Struggling will occur when the excitement period (Stage II) is approached, and during this phase the cat or dog should be held on its side as anesthesia is deepened.

The open-drop method is relatively safe and can be used when it is difficult to induce anesthesia by intravenous barbiturates and other techniques are not available. It can be used effectively when a rapid recovery from a short period of anesthesia is desired. Important aspects of the method are as follows: (1) only 8 to 9 layers of 16 ply gauze should be used to cover the mask and tight wads of cotton should not be used, (2) the evaporization surface should be broad enough to insure sufficient area for the vaporization of the liquid agent, (3) the cone or mask should fit closely to the face of the animal, thereby minimizing dead space, (4) the eyes should be protected with a bland ophthalmic ointment, (5) shortly after the induction of anesthesia, supplemental oxygen should be administered below the mask, (6) the concentration of volatile anesthetic should be increased slowly, and discontinued if breath-holding occurs. This is to prevent the sudden build-up of high concentrations of anesthetic vapor, (7) the liquid anesthetic should be added evenly over the entire surface of the mask, developing a consistent pattern of application, (8) cooling of the mask surface will occur with the vaporization and at this point, the mask should be changed. A convenient method of maintaining general anesthesia after the induction of anesthesia is to administer the anesthetic-oxygen mixture below the mask through a catheter. An oxygen source and a vaporizer are necessary.

Diethyl ether is the most commonly used agent in the open-drop method and excessive loss of the anesthetic agent into the room cannot be avoided and large quantities are necessary to maintain general anesthesia even in smaller animals. A common method is to use more rapid acting agents such as divinyl ether for the induction of anesthesia and diethyl ether for the maintenance of general anesthesia. Hepatotoxicity can occur when ethyl chloride and divinyl ether are used for periods of anesthesia in excess of 20 to 30 min. Ideally, these agents should be used only for the induction of anesthesia and short periods of maintenance. Ethyl chloride and divinyl ether are extremely potent agents and can induce anesthesia very rapidly. Respiratory arrest and cardiac arrest can occur simultaneously, if care is not exercised.

A pledget of cotton placed in the apex of a small cone is a method commonly used for mice, rats and hamsters. For these small rodents halothane or methoxyflurane can be more economically used in this manner. This technique can be easily used for only short procedures.

In the past it has been common practice to use chambers or bell jars with ether soaked cotton balls placed in them to induce anesthesia. These chambers have been used for the small laboratory animals such as mice, rats and hamsters as well as larger animals such as rabbits and even cats. The disadvantages have been outlined above and hopefully emphasized sufficiently especially for the larger laboratory animals. Still, investigators find that the chambers are necessary when large numbers of animals must be anesthetized for short procedures. They often find inconsistent results and high mortality rates from the intraperitoneal injection of a barbiturate. Consequently these ether chambers have come into common usage. All in all it is still more desirable to utilize the non-explosive agents delivered from precision vaporizers capable of delivering anesthetic vapor at very low vehicular gas flows (Dräger, Vapor or Fluotec, Mark III). Other investigators have adapted these vaporizers into very satisfactory anesthetic chambers and report good results (BOUTELLE and RICH, 1969; SIMMONS and SMITH, 1968). Utilizing low flow capability vaporizers, adequate concentrations can be delivered at flows of between 200 to 250 ml/min.

Another equally satisfactory method of anesthesia which is superior to the use of a cone with a cotton ball is the designing of a mask fashioned from wire screening and liquid latex which fits a particular species (Fig. 5). Induction of anesthesia can be achieved and maintained with the same system.

Ayre's "T" piece system. The Ayres' technique is a semi-open method of delivering inhalation agents developed originally for pediatric anesthesia which is suitable for cats and the small breeds of dogs [Ayre, 1956; Clifford and Soma,

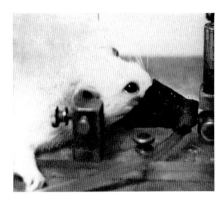

Fig. 5. Mask made from latex and wire screening to fit adult rats. Tubing delivers anesthetic gas mixtures directly from an out-of-the-circle halothane vaporizer (Vapor, Drazer) at a flow of 250 cc/min. The mask can be used for both induction and maintenance

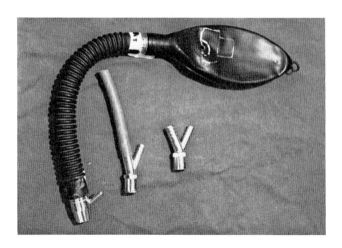

Fig. 6. The figure shows an Ayres "T" or "Y" piece and two modifications which permit their use with animals up to 4 to 5 kg

1964; Soma, 1971 (2)]. The equipment consists of a simple "Y" or "T" piece connected to an endotracheal tube or mask (Fig. 6). One arm of the "Y" piece is attached to a source of oxygen and is the inhalation limb. The second arm acts as an exhalation limb and is connected to a small reservoir. The unidirectional flow of gas is created by a constant flow of gas through one arm of the "Y" piece and the absence of valves assures a low resistance to respiration. The removal of carbon dioxide and flushing out of the system to prevent rebreathing of exhaled gases is accomplished by delivering a total flow higher than the patient's respiratory minute volume. The constant flow of oxygen anesthetic mixture assures the exhalation of respiratory gases through the expiratory limb.

The addition of the reservoir tube is employed in the system to eliminate the dilution of the oxygen-anesthetic mixture with room air during inspiration. The total capacity of the reservoir should be approximately one third of the animal's tidal volume. The internal diameter of the reservoir should be at least 1 cm; therefore, a piece of tubing 2.5 cm long will contain 2.5 ml of gas. The tidal volume of 2 to 4 kg cats under anesthesia varies between 12 to 25 ml; therefore, the expiratory arm should be between 4 to 8 cm long.

This reservoir can potentially increase the anatomical dead space by providing an area for the accumulation of exhaled carbon dioxide. To prevent rebreathing and assure the proper elimination of carbon dioxide, the size of the reservoir and flow of gas necessary to flush out the system should be considered. The flow of gas into the system should be approximately 2 times the respiratory minute volume (AYRE, 1956; BARATTA et al., 1969). This assures proper flushing of carbon dioxide from the expiratory limb. The respiratory minute volume of cats (2 to 4 kg) under anesthesia is 200 to 1000 ml/min; this dictates a flow of about 400 to 2000 ml/min. For most cats the flows are maintained at 1 to 1.5 l/min and these are increased or decreased slightly depending upon the size of the animal.

A modification involves the addition of a breathing bag which results in a greater capacity in the reservoir tube (Fig. 6) (HARRISON, 1964). This addition adds the capacity of administering positive pressure ventilation. The dilution of inspired gases cannot occur, because of the increased capacity of the reservoir, but rebreathing can. The fresh flow of gas should be maintained at two times the respiratory minute volume. The Kuhn's apparatus is an excellent adaptation of this modification, and can be used with both a mask or with an endotracheal tube (Fig. 7).

The Ayres' original method or its modifications are recommended only for animals under 4 to 6 kg. Larger dogs require higher gas flows through the system to provide adequate concentrations of anesthetic agent. The higher flows needed for the larger animals can create an increase in resistance to respiration because of the narrow diameter of the "Y" piece. In small patients the system is economical because relatively low flows can be used.

Modifications of the Magill Circuit. The Magill circuit, devised by Sir IVAN MAGILL, consists of a breathing bag, a length of corrugated tubing, a fresh gas inlet and a one-way valve adjacent to the patient (Fig. 8). It can be considered as a semi-open system (DRIPPS et al., 1961) and is similar in its application to the Ayres method. As in the Ayres method, fresh gas flows are used to eliminate carbon dioxide; the basic difference is the use of one valve and the direction of flow of the fresh gases.

In the Magill circuit the fresh gases enter into the distal segment of the system and leave through an exhalation valve at the face piece or endotracheal tube. With this arrangement the Magill circuit will prevent rebreathing, with a fresh gas flow less than the patient's respiratory minute volume (KAIN and NUNN, 1968). The efficiency of the system is based on the location of the exhalation valve which causes less mixing between the exhaled gas and fresh gas. The gas which is initially exhaled is anatomical dead space gas, and is identical in composition to the fresh gas. The remainder of the exhaled gas is alveolar gas, which has been in contact with the gas exchange portions of the lung. The rebreathing of this gas will raise alveolar and arterial carbon dioxide tensions (KAIN and NUNN, 1968). Purging of the system begins toward the end of exhalation. At this point in the respiratory cycle, the breathing bag is filling, and the pressure in the system is elevated sufficiently to open the exhalation valve. The fresh gas flow purges the system of alveolar gas. In theory, only the anatomical dead space gas has to be replaced with fresh gas flow to adequately remove exhaled carbon dioxide. The fresh gas flow necessary to remove the alveolar gas, therefore, must be correlated with the

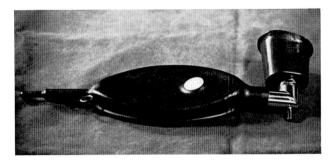

Fig. 7. The Kuhn's modified system with a mask suitable for cats, rabbits, and guinea pigs. Flows which are at least twice the respiratory minute volume are necessary to prevent rebreathing of alveolar gas

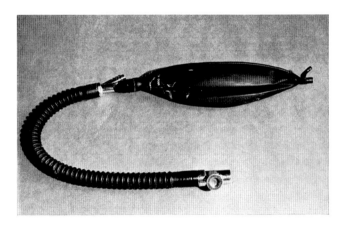

Fig. 8. A Magill type circuit in which fresh gas enters distal to the patient and exits just proximal to the face piece or endotracheal tube

patient's alveolar ventilation and not respiratory minute volume (MAPELSON, 1954). Because of this, the fresh gas flows necessary are smaller than measured respiratory minute volumes. There is inherent difficulty in attempting to equate fresh gas flows to body weight, because of the variation in ventilation of veterinary patients of similar weight when under anesthesia. Understandably, as respiratory rate increases, a rise in respiratory minute volume can be anticipated. A greater fresh gas flow may be needed because of the possible increase in alveolar ventilation, but more importantly, the exhalation pause is so short that high fresh gas flows are necessary to flush out the alveolar carbon dioxide prior to inhalation.

Using a 2 to 4 kg cat as a guide, fresh gas flows of between 500 to 600 ml/min are sufficient to prevent rebreathing. For larger cats or animals of other species slight increases may have to be made in flow to compensate for variations in rate and tidal volume.

The Magill system, like the Ayres system, is well suited for the small veterinary patient. As with the Ayres method, it is simple, cheap, and easy to clean. It is not well suited for controlled ventilation, as two hands are necessary, one for compression of the bag and the second for occluding the exhalation valve. If adequate spontaneous ventilation is anticipated, it is an excellent method for the delivery of anesthetic agents. As for other semi-open methods, halothane, methoxyflurane, and nitrous oxide are well suited and similar concentrations are employed.

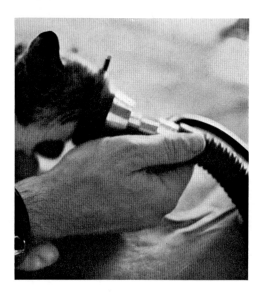

Fig. 9. Induction of anesthesia using a cat mask and Kuhn's system in a cat

Semi-Open System and Masks. Masks which conform to the facial structures of cats, small dogs and laboratory animals can be used with the Ayres and Magill systems (Fig. 9). For the induction of inhalation anesthesia in smaller animals, this is an excellent method. If the mask conforms somewhat to the facial contours and the gas flows are adequate, the additional respiratory dead space created by the mask can be minimized. In both the semi-open and the non-rebreathing systems the concentration of the anesthetic agent can be more easily controlled than the rebreathing systems. In these systems, the exhaled gases are expelled into the room and not rebreathed; therefore, the concentration delivered from the vaporizer and the inhaled concentration are the same.

Use of the Semi-Open Systems. The mask can be an effective and relatively safe method for the induction and also the maintenance of anesthesia in many small species and in young animals. Some of the basic principles of the open drop method also apply to the use of the mask. The patient should be restrained as gently as possible and the mask placed near the face. The initial concentration should be low, and then increased as the initial sedating effects are apparent.

A variety of anesthetic agents can be used, particularly halothane, methoxy-flurane and nitrous oxide. Halothane and methoxyflurane can be used alone or in combination with nitrous oxide. Nitrous oxide can provide a good base for volatile anesthetic agents, especially when a mask is being used for the induction of anesthesia. The anesthetic agent which induces sedation and anesthesia rapidly (nitrous oxide, halothane, and methoxyflurane in that order) will be the most effective and facilitate the easy induction of anesthesia. Nitrous oxide (75%) and oxygen (25%) is used as the base for the addition of halothane or methoxyflurane. Nitrous oxide-oxygen is started and 0.25% halothane is added and increased by 0.5% increments to 2 to 4%. The rapidity by which the inspired concentration is increased is determined by the animal's reactions to the induction of anesthesia. The maintenance concentration of halothane is approximately 1 to 2.5%, varying with the condition of the patient, preanesthetic medication and whether nitrous oxide is used. The induction concentrations of methoxyflurane are between 0.5 and 1.5% and the maintenance between 0.25 to 0.75%. Anesthesia can be maintained with the mask or the patient's trachea intubated and anesthesia continued with the

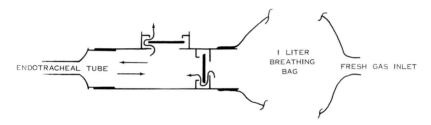

ENDOTRACHEAL TUBE

I LITER BREATHING BAG

FRESH GAS INLET

Fig. 10. Schematic representation of a non-rebreathing anesthetic system suitable for animals under 5 kg in weight. Courtesy of SOMA [1971 (2)]

endotracheal tube. Ultra-short acting barbiturates can be used to speed the induction of anesthesia even in cats and small dogs followed by the inhalation agents.

Non-Rebreathing Valves. The non-rebreathing method utilizes a set of valves which allows inspiration from a breathing bag (reservoir) and exhalation directly into the atmosphere (Fig. 10). If the valves are competent the only rebreathing which occurs is of the gas contained within the dead space of the valves. The basic design is an inhalation and an exhalation valve incorporated into a metal or plastic tube or mask (SYKES, 1959). These systems have been designed primarily for pediatric anesthesia, therefore, can be used for smaller patients in animal anesthesia; many types are available.

After the induction of anesthesia either with a mask or an ultra-short acting barbiturate and intubation of the trachea, the valve is attached to the endotracheal tube and flow of gas equal to or slightly higher than the animal's respiratory minute volume is added continuously to the breathing bag, as judged by watching the bag (Fig. 11). If it collapses, the respiratory minute volume of the patient is higher than the delivered gas and should be increased. The fresh gas flow requirements in a 2.5 kg cat or dog are approximately 700 ml. Compared to the semi-open system, the valves prevent the exhaled gases from entering the breathing bag and a flow of gas sufficient to flush out the exhaled gases is not necessary; low gas flows are used.

One of the disadvantages of the non-rebreathing method is the inability of the system to compensate for a sudden increase in ventilation. If this occurs the bag will be sucked empty by the increased ventilatory effort of the animal. Maintaining the flow of gas slightly above the actual needs of the patient will prevent this. The valve resistance is so low that gas from an overfilled bag will leak out through the valve system. A slight positive valve leak is an advantage and will flush out the small dead space between the valves.

Many of these valves are not spring loaded, and are dependent upon gravity for the closure of the exhalation valve. Periodic inspection of these valves is essential; since they are attached to an endotracheal tube, mucus can accumulate on the valves, preventing their free movement. Rubber valves will degenerate with time due to the accumulation of moisture and the action of inhalation agents on rubber. It is wise to maintain an extra set of valves for replacement.

The basic difference between the semi-open and the non-rebreathing system is the method of preventing the rebreathing of exhaled gases. Both systems are

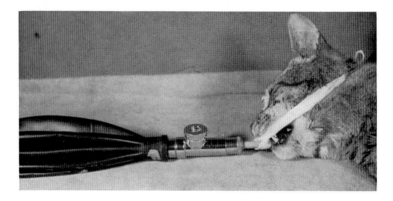

Fig. 11. Intubated cat maintained on a non-rebreathing system

applicable to smaller species of both laboratory and pet animals. When using the semi-open system, the size of the animal and not the specific species of animal determines the method which is most applicable. The end of the "Y" piece can also be used as a mask when the animal to be anesthetized is very small (Fig. 12). Most masks which have been developed for cats can be used for rabbits and large guinea pigs (Fig. 7). The anesthetic agents and the concentrations discussed in the previous section are applicable here.

Rebreathing Systems. In the rebreathing systems all or part of the animal's exhaled gases are passed back into the circuit. The differentiation between complete rebreathing (closed system) and partial rebreathing (semi-closed) is determined primarily by the inflow of fresh gases and also the size of the animal.

As compared to adolescents and adults where flows are somewhat standardized, the variation in veterinary anesthesia is great because of the patient size. The rebreathing system is used for pet animals (6 to 70 kg), the small farm animals and the horse and cow. For veterinary anesthesia, anesthetic machines with out-of-the-circle vaporizers are most commonly used (Figs. 12, 13). These machines conform to the standards designated for use in man, and are basically interchangeable.

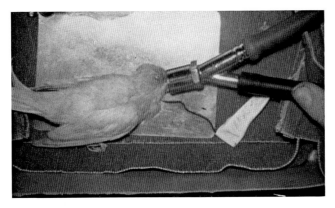

Fig. 12. Canary in which an inhalant is delivered using a Ayres "Y" piece as a mask. Flows of 100 are adequate to flush the mask and prevent rebreathing. Courtesy of SOMA [1971 (2)]

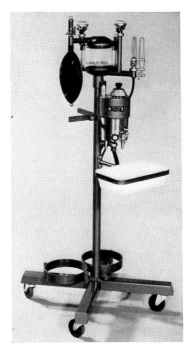

Fig. 13. Small animal anesthetic system (Narcovet) with an out-of-the-circuit vaporizer. Drawing shows ability to add extra flow meters for other gases such as nitrous oxide. Courtesy of North American Dräger, Telford, Pa.

Fresh Gas Flows in the Rebreathing System. The rebreathing system can be used as a closed (minimal oxygen flows) or semi-closed system (high oxygen flows). In the completely closed system, only the patient's minimum metabolic needs of oxygen and anesthetic are being delivered, and all exhaled gas minus the removed carbon dioxide are rebreathed. As the fresh gas flow of oxygen begins to exceed the needs of the animal, the system is no longer completely closed, but semi-closed.

The term semi-closed only indicates that the fresh gas flow is greater than the needs of the patient and when describing the system, the flows being used and the size of the patient should be indicated (Editorial, 1964). This becomes more important in veterinary anesthesia, due to the extremes of size encountered. For example the respiratory minute volume of a 5 kg dog under anesthesia would approximate 600 ml/min, and on the other hand the respiratory minute volume of a 50 kg dog would approach 5 l/min. The oxygen consumption of the smaller

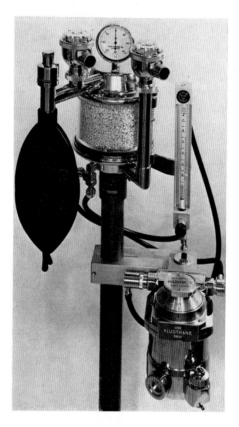

Fig. 14. VMS Small Animal Anesthesia Machine. The vaporizer is a Fluotec Mark III. Courtesy of Fraser Sweatman, Lancaster, N.Y.

dog approximates 50 ml/min, as compared to the larger dog which approximates 450 ml/min. With a fresh gas flow of 600 ml/min, for example, almost complete rebreathing of exhaled gases occurs in the larger dog, whereas in the smaller dog a non-rebreathing system is almost in effect. In both cases adequate amounts of oxygen are being delivered; in one case, in great excess of metabolic needs and in the other, minimal amounts. In the small dog the oxygen consumption is only 10% of the fresh gas flow. In the larger dog over 90% of the delivered oxygen is used for the metabolic needs and rebreathing is maximal.

The exact oxygen consumption of the patient is not known and cannot be easily calculated, and from a clinical use point of view exact numbers are not necessary.

But it does point out the fact that the flows of gas delivered to the rebreathing system should be chosen with some appreciation of the range of the oxygen requirements of the veterinary patients. The economic aspects of veterinary anesthesia would dictate that lower flows would be the most advantageous, but two other functions of the fresh gas flow, namely delivery of adequate volumes of anesthetic vapor and denitrogenation also must be considered, especially during the induction phases of anesthesia. These two aspects of fresh gas flow mandate

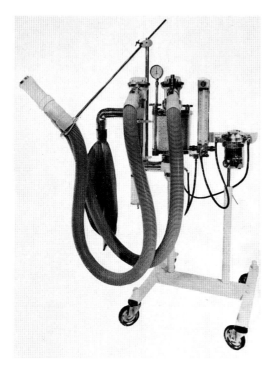

Fig. 15. VMS Large Animal Anesthesia Machine. Anesthetic equipment for animals the size of a horse or cow must be designed with larger tubing, valves, reservoir bag, canister. Courtesy of Fraser Sweatman, Lancaster, N.Y.

higher initial fresh gas flows for the induction of anesthesia which can be followed by lower flows for the maintenance of anesthesia. Denitrogenation is more of a problem in large animal anesthesia, where for greater economy, near metabolic flows are used for the maintenance of anesthesia. With fresh gas flows of 1.5 to 2.5 l/min, which equals the metabolic needs of a 500 kg horse, the nitrogen concentration will range between 23 to 57 % after 2 h of anesthesia (TEVIK et al., 1969). The concentration of oxygen can be appreciably increased by flushing the system 5 to 6 times during the first 15 min of anesthesia, and delivery of fresh gas flows of 6 to 10 l/min. It is important to denitrogenate the large animals early during the induction period prior to the reduction to maintenance flows of 1.5 to 2.5 l/min.

For all animals larger than 5 to 6 kg a circle system is the most efficient method of administering inhalational anesthetics. The unidirectional valves assure that the metabolic carbon dioxide passes through the CO_2 absorber. This eliminates the need for high flows of fresh gas which are necessary in the semi-open systems. These lower flows during maintenance have the advantage of reducing the loss of body heat and insensible body fluid, minimize cost and reduce room contamination. For animals larger than 6 kg and the smaller farm animals, equipment suitable for man is used. For animals under 50 pounds a 3 l bag is adequate, while for larger animals a 5 l bag is recommended. The diameters and lengths of corrugated tubing used in veterinary equipment are the same as for use in humans.

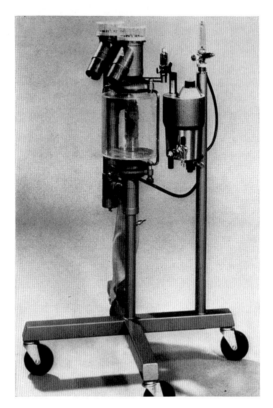

Fig. 16. Narcovet Large Animal Anesthesia Machine. Courtesy of North American Dräger, Telford, Pa.

The exception, of course, in the size of the circle system is in the design for the larger species. For the horse and cow (800 to 1500 lbs) a 30 l bag is used; the corrugated tubing is 5 cm in diameter and the valves are proportionally enlarged (Figs. 15 and 16). The cannister contains at least 4 kg of absorbant.

V. Intravenous Anesthetic Agents

The intravenous anesthetics in their broadest coverage would include a multitude of drugs, ranging from barbiturates which are the most commonly used, to many non-barbiturates. The non-barbiturates represent a wide number of non-related chemical compounds many of which are primarily used for basal narcosis and like the barbiturates, many are classified as hypnotic-sedative e.g., glutethimide, chloral hydrate, hydroxydione. On the other hand non-hypnotic drugs such as narcotics, tranquilizers, local anesthetics and alcohol, which generally are not considered intravenous agents, have been used in this manner in moderate amounts, many times in combination to produce a state of deep sedation almost bordering on general anesthesia. Unconsciousness is generally not produced with these latter compounds and arousal is possible. The unconscious state can be quickly created by the superimposition of small amounts of a barbiturate or an inhalation agent. The cyclohexamines, although discussed as preanesthetic agents, have been used both intramuscularly and intravenously to create levels of sedation bordering on general anesthesia.

Almost all clinicians generally associate barbiturates with intravenous anesthesia. From a pragmatic aspect this is true, but in the modern usage of drugs, many agents are used intravenously alone or in combination to establish varying degrees of central nervous system depression. Unfortunately many clinicians approach and compare many new compounds which can be injected intravenously as substitutes for the barbiturates, despite dissimilar actions, in the hopes that the disadvantages of intravenous barbiturates can be eliminated and the advantages preserved.

Barbiturates. The barbiturates are a widely used and very versatile group of agents. They are classified as hypnotic-sedatives based on their primary use for the production of sedation as preanesthetic drugs. In veterinary anesthesia they are used primarily for the induction or the maintenance of general anesthesia. The central nervous system actions of barbiturates are diverse and progressive; ranging from sedation, which implies mild depression, to hypnosis, which indicates a stronger degree of depression leading to sleep. The sedation and hypnosis produced by barbiturates can be considered gradations of the stage of general anesthesia, inasmuch as higher doses will produce excitement (Stage II) followed by general anesthesia (Stage III). An important distinction in comparing the actions of the sedative-hypnotic drugs with the actions or narcotics and tranquilizers is that increasing doses of barbiturates will produce anesthesia. Barbiturates are good enzyme inducers which must be taken into consideration with certain experimental designs (CONNEY, 1967).

Short Acting Barbiturates. The most commonly used short acting barbiturate is sodium pentobarbital and the safest method of administration is intravenously. Oral, intraperitoneal, intrapleural, intramuscular and even subcutaneous routes have been used, but are less reliable, more apt to produce tissue damage and are not recommended. The risk from the administration of a fixed dose which other routes necessitate should be obvious and is exceptionally dangerous when ill or aged animals are encountered. All animals to be subjected to venipuncture should be handled quietly and with a minimum of physical restraint, and in many instances preanesthetic drugs may be necessary to allow safe handling. Sodium pentobarbital for veterinary use is usually supplied as a 6 to 6.5% solution (60 to 65 mg/ml). When being administered to cats and other smaller animals it is advisable to dilute the solution with an equal amount of saline or water for injection.

The recommended method of anesthetizing a healthy dog or cat with pentobarbital is to inject rapidly, 1/3 to 1/2 of the calculated dose (25 to 30 mg/kg or approximately 60 mg/5 lbs). The rapid initial injection of a relatively large amount is important when using the short and intermediate acting drugs. This rapid injection of at least one third of the dose produces a high plasma level, and the excitement period (Stage II) of general anesthesia is rapidly passed, thereby avoiding massive excitement. If following this initial injection there are some indications that the animal is about to enter Stage II, a small additional amount should be given promptly before the needle is dislodged. When Stage III has been established the remaining amount of drug necessary to produce a surgical plane of anesthesia should be administered slowly to obtain the desired effect, while testing the animal's reflexes. The time period to produce general anesthesia is markedly slower than with the ultrashort-acting drugs and the injection time should be at least 5 min duration. This allows sufficient time for the anesthetic to cross the blood-brain barrier and for equilibrium of plasma-brain concentration. A too rapid injection of a large amount can cause apnea which will be prolonged in nature because of slow decline of the plasma level of pentobarbital. Alternately, too slow an administration of the initial dose will lead to excitement, which subsequently will necessitate an increased amount of barbiturate to produce adequate planes of anesthesia. This will increase the sleeping time and delay full recovery.

The total amount of pentobarbital required to produce surgical planes of anesthesia will vary according to the animal's age, nutritional state, weight, preanesthetic medication and many other factors. Because of this the recommended doses should only be used as a rough guideline for an approximation of the final total dose. There is marked variation in the dose range and preanesthetic medication will consistently reduce the amount but does not reduce the scatter (Table 1). The suggested dose range is from 30 to 40 mg/kg. This range should be scaled down by about 1/3 when preanesthetic medication has been administered; here again this is approximate depending on the preanesthetic drug, amount and sedative effect on the animal.

The recovery period from pentobarbital can be prolonged and stormy and because of this it is not used in the horse. Pentobarbital frequently causes post anesthetic delirium in dogs and occasionally in cats. They should be placed in a quiet, dark area, free of articles which could injure the animal. Whenever possible the animal should be given a tranquilizer or narcotic to sedate it during this recovery period. Occasionally cats may be somnolent for 24 to 48 h following surgical anesthesia with pentobarbital. It is not as common with the thiobarbiturates but may occur if repeated doses are given for one procedure. Pentobarbital causes splenic dilation in the dog and mouse and can cause significant changes in the hematocrit (Friedman, 1959).

Ultra Short Acting Barbiturates. The use of the thiobarbiturates, thiopental and thiamylal, in small animal practice has closely paralleled that of the oxybarbiturate, pentobarbital. The use of the ultrashort drugs is also common in large animal practice, especially in the equine for the induction of anesthesia. Methohexital, although not a thiobarbiturate, can be included in this group because of its ultrashort actions.

As with the oxybarbiturates, the preferred route of administration is intravenously. Although other routes have been used, these methods injure surrounding tissues. The perivascular injection of a 6% solution of pentobarbital or a 5% solution of a thiobarbiturate can cause necrosis and eventual sloughing of tissue, whereas a 2.5% solution of a thiobarbiturate is less likely to produce tissue damage unless large amounts are inadvertently injected subcutaneously. With the exception of the large domestic animals where a 10% solution is used primarily for the convenience of containment of the total dose in one syringe, the more dilute solutions are suggested for safety and to facilitate more accurate administration, especially in smaller animals.

In contrast to the pentobarbital, the thiobarbiturates can be given more slowly and "to effect". The transfer from plasma to brain is very rapid and the effect of an injection can be noted within one circulation time of 10 to 15 sec. Because there is no delay in the transfer of drug from perfusing blood into brain, the maximum effect from the intravenous injection of a quantity (bolus) of the drug is attained quickly and with no lag period. Subsequent doses can be given at short intervals to attain the desired depth of anesthesia, slowly and carefully. With careful observation this "foreleg to central nervous system time" can be used to assess somewhat the animal's circulation time and judge the subsequent effects of additional anesthesia. Again, using the skills of simple observation, differences can be noted in circulation time when comparing the healthy animal with those, for example, in shock or with cardiovascular disease.

The capability of injecting thiobarbiturates slowly with minimal expectation of excitement is an important asset, especially when anesthetizing ill and debilitated animals. In handling excitable or overly nervous animals, very low doses can be given initially in an attempt to quiet the animals; once a more serene state has been established, the induction of anesthesia can be continued. It must be pointed

Table 1. *Suggested dose ranges of barbiturates mg/kg*

Drug	Dog	Cat	Primate	Rabbit	Guinea pig	Rat	Mouse	Goat	Sheep	Swine
Thiopental Sodium	15—30	20—30	20—25	30[a]—50	—	—	25—50	22	25—37	10[b]
Pentobarbital Sodium	25—35	25—35	20—25	25—40	20 I.M. 15—30 I.P.	30—40	40—70 IV-I.P.	25	28—33	23—24

[a] Thiamylal Sodium.
[b] For intubation only. Dosage varies greatly with breed.
Compiled from VA Laboratory Guide (1969).

out that the induction of anesthesia in an extremely excitable animal is dangerous.

It should be remembered that thiobarbiturates are more potent than the oxybarbiturates; this combined with a more rapid effect can lead to respiratory arrest quickly and early in the induction period if given rapidly. As compared to the short acting drugs the respiratory arrest with the ultrashort-acting drugs is shorter in duration and can be easily managed by controlling ventilation for a period of time. The amount of thiopental and thiamylal necessary to produce surgical planes of anesthesia is approximately 18 to 26 mg/kg. As with the oxybarbiturates considerable variation can occur, which is not minimized by the addition of preanesthetic medication.

The thiobarbiturates are commonly used to induce anesthesia prior to the maintenance with the inhalation anesthetics. The amount necessary under these circumstances of use is considerably less than required for surgical planes of anesthesia, all that is necessary is adequate depth to produce sufficient muscle relaxation for tracheal intubation. A dose guide for this purpose is approximately 5 to 10 mg/kg.

Thiamylal is approximately 1.5 times the potency of thiopental; unfortunately the criteria for establishing a definite relationship are difficult to control, and opinions vary as to the actual figure (DUNDEE, 1956). If both drugs are administered slowly "to effect" it is difficult to distinguish between the two.

VI. Non-Barbiturate Injectable Drugs

Urethan

There are several drugs available which produce narcosis, and they are exalted for their ability to produce deep sleep for long periods of time without abolishing cardiopulmonary reflexes. These properties make them acceptable for experimental studies. Urethan does not markedly depress blood pressure or respiration and does not inhibit spinal reflexes. The onset of action is slow by any other route than intravenous and will last for many hours. The recovery is also prolonged and death can occur during this period. It may be given by the oral, rectal, intramuscular or subcutaneous route as well as intravenously (Table 2) at approximately 2 mg/kg in a 10 or 20% solution. The powder may be sprinkled on the moist frog's skin and then rinsed off when the desired depth of narcosis has been attained (Strobel and Wollman, 1969). Urethan is eliminated by the metabolic degradation to ethanol and carbonic acid. It is frequently used in mixtures of other injectable anesthetic agents because of its ability to increase the aqueous

Table 2. *Suggested doses of common non-barbiturate anesthetics (mg/kg or g/kg)*

Drug	Dog	Cat	Primate	Rabbit	Guinea pig
Urethan	1—2 g	1.5 g	—	1.6 g	1.5 g
Chlorolose	100 mg	50—70 mg	—	120 mg	—
Chloral hydrate	300 mg	250 mg	—	—	170—108 mg[a]
Phencyclidine	2.0 mg	1.1 mg	0.25—3 mg	10 mg	1.0 mg

[a] In combination with Pentobarbital.
Compiled from VA Laboratory Guide (1969).

solubility of organic compounds. This drug is not used for clinical anesthesia or survival experimental surgery.

Chloralose. Chloralose, like urethan, produces deep narcosis without serious depression of cardiopulmonary reflexes. It is said that chloralose will preserve or exaggerate baroreceptor and chemoreceptor reflexes (Killip, 1963). It resembles morphine in that it enhances spinal reflexes. The animals may be analgesic but show exaggerated responses to tactile or auditory stimuli. Chloralose may be given intravenously, intraperitoneally, or orally (Table 1). A 1% solution in water must be heated to dissolve and will precipitate on cooling. Frequently a 5% solution is made by adding a 25% urethan solution. Morphine is a common preanesthetic drug in the dog when chloralose is used for acute experiments, morphine is used to provide additional analgesia.

Chloral Hydrate. Chloral hydrate is a reaction product of ethanol and chlorine. It is commercially available in combination with pentobarbital and magnesium sulfate as an anesthetic product for horses. Its popularity has declined with the introduction of inhalational anesthetics. Singularly, when administered to the dog, it produces respiratory and cardiac depression as well as salivation, vomiting and micturation. The heart may be sensitized to sudden vagal arrest or arrhythmias. Concentrated solutions injected intravenously will produce hemolysis and hematuria. Hepatic and renal damage may follow large repeated doses. It is excreted as the glucuronide of trichloroethanal. Doses for several species are given in Table 2.

VIII. Preanesthetic Medication and Drugs for Restraint

Preanesthetic medication has been well established as an invaluable adjunct in anesthesia and in many instances it is more essential in animals than in man. Fractious or dangerous animals need preanesthetic sedation to enable their management and insure a smooth and safe induction of anesthesia. Some classical reasons for administering preanesthetic drugs are as follows: (1) To allay fear and apprehension and thus facilitate restraint, a condition which will vary greatly between species and is dependent on the previous experience of the animal; (2) to reduce pain or discomfort; (3) to facilitate induction of general anesthesia; (4) to serve as an adjunct to regional analgesia; (5) to minimize certain untoward effects (salivation) or reflex responses (vagal-vagal) in the patient, and (6) to act as pharmacologic adjuncts to the general anesthetic agents and thus reduce the amount of the general anesthetic (CLIFFORD and SOMA, 1964; DOBKIN, 1961).

Nearly every clinician favors a particular agent or combination of agents, and habits are established early, and in many instances there is little deviation in agents or dosages. Such stereotyped medication, especially in the amount administered, is potentially dangerous because it implies a lack of appreciation for individual variation and variation in response to drugs because of disease and altered physiological state.

The drugs which are used in veterinary anesthesia are similar to those used in man, and include narcotic-analgesics, tranquilizers, anticholinergic drugs, sedatives and cyclohexamines. It is not the purpose of this section to compare the pharmacological actions of the drugs in various species, but to point out the more obvious clinical differences in actions and usage. Admittedly the compilation of the former would be a worth-while contribution, but is beyond the current energies of the authors.

A. Narcotic-Analgesics

The narcotic-analgesics are an old and important class of drugs, and are used in dogs, subhuman primates and, depending upon the compound, in horses and cats. The analgesic and sedative properties of narcotics when needed are of great benefit to animals, as they are in man. Fortunately, in veterinary patients with no "subjective mind" the euphoric aspects which can lead to addiction are not important, but the respiratory and cardiovascular effects have to be considered. This is not to say that addiction and tolerance do not occur in animals, but they are man-made and not due to self-indulgence.

Morphine was recognized as an effective agent by CLAUDE BERNARD (ADRIANI and YARBERRY, 1959) and it continues to be commonly administered to dogs, primarily because it produces good sedation, has good analgesic properties, and is inexpensive. The sedation produced by morphine and other narcotics is of importance in veterinary anesthesia for restraint of fearful, anxious and sometimes vicious animals. Sedation is achieved at the expense of depression of the respiratory and cardiovascular system.

Respiration. The depressing effect of morphine and other narcotics on respiration is a disadvantage of the use of these drugs for preanesthetic medication. As in man, the respiratory effects of narcotics are difficult to assess with only the casual observation and measurement of tidal volume or rate of ventilation. More discriminating measurements such as arterial O_2 and CO_2 tension and CO_2 response curves are necessary to determine its actions on alveolar ventilation and the respiratory center. Numerous studies have been completed in man to determine the effects of various narcotics on the respiratory centers threshold to carbon dioxide stimulation (Smith et al., 1967). Similar studies starting with awake trained animals, e.g. dogs, have not been completed in an attempt to assess comparative sensitivities of the respiratory centers to narcotics and other depressants. This comparison would be interesting in view of the larger doses needed and tolerated in dogs to produce sedation and analgesia. Although comparative studies are not available, the effect on respiration is easily appreciated during the induction of anesthesia with either barbiturates or inhalation agents.

In the animals that pant to control body heat, the thermoregulating mechanisms can alter the respiratory effects of narcotics. After high doses of narcotics in the dog, thermoregulation is disrupted and the dog will begin panting at a lower body temperature. In the dog, the thermoregulating mechanism may predominate and the administration of a narcotic will not alter the established panting type of respiratory pattern and, occasionally, the rate may increase. This pattern can also persist under very light levels of thiobarbiturate anesthesia, which will eventually become depressed as anesthesia is deepened or ventilation controlled.

There are other factors which can influence the respiratory and also depressant effects of morphine and other narcotics. Pain and excitement will influence the ventilatory and sedative effects of narcotics. The administration of a drug on a mg/kg basis to animals without considering their temperament and excitability may account for part of the variability in response to many depressant drugs. In animals, as in man, age can alter the respiratory effects of morphine. This is due to a decrease in respiratory reserve, which includes an increased respiratory dead space, impaired elasticity of the chest wall, decreased vital capacity and a high incidence of pulmonary disease (Fowler, 1948).

Cardiovascular. The overall cardiovascular effects are less obvious than the respiratory changes, implying a lesser effect on the central vasomotor centers (Goodman and Gilman, 1965). The effects of morphine on the cardiovascular system become more evident upon challenging this system, and the veterinary patient is less able to compensate to stressful conditions. Changes in position, loss of blood, anesthetic agents and motion can disrupt cardiovascular stability and produce hypotension.

The cardiovascular effects of narcotics are primarily through a direct effect on the central vasomotor centers (Goodman and Gilman, 1965). Morphine and other narcotics also release histamine and how much this release contributes to the hypotensive effects is difficult to determine. This is especially true in the dog, cat, and rabbit where the release of histamine may be somewhat greater. The administration of morphine to the supine human has little effect on blood pressure, heart rate, and heart rhythm. Doses of 1 to 3 mg/kg have been administered to supine man (Lowenstein et al., 1969) producing respiratory depression and deep analgesia, with only minimal effects on the cardiovascular system. The therapeutic value of morphine in patients with left heart failure and especially pulmonary edema is well established in both human and veterinary patients. In the intact lightly anesthetized dog, an improvement of cardiovascular function was also noted after the injection of morphine (Vasko et al., 1966). Under these circumstances the cardiovascular system can still respond when the intact sympathetic system is stimulated. As with other drugs which depend on an intact sympathetic system for maintaining homeostasis, conditions or drugs which alter this system will compromise the final response. Unfortunately, much experimental data in animals has to be interpreted with a view of the effects of the previous administration of other drugs, anesthetics, and the experimental model itself, whether acute or chronic.

The effect of morphine on heart rate is more clear-cut, especially in the dog, and in comparison to man a bradycardia is more common. This is through a direct stimulation of the medullary vagal nuclei (KRUEGAR et al., 1943). A direct effect through the inhibition of acetylcholinesterase may also be a factor (GOODMAN and GILMAN, 1965). The bradycardia produced by morphine can be prevented or reversed with atropine. The intravenous injection of morphine in the standing awake animal produces a bradycardia and a drop in blood pressure; this reduction is transient, and pressures will return to control levels. The reduction in heart rate will persist.

The release of histamine by morphine and other narcotics, especially in the dog, adds a great deal of confusion to its effects on the heart rate and the cardiovascular system in general. The hypotension that can occur in the dog can be partially ascribed to the greater release of histamine in this species (FELDBERG and PATON, 1950). A similar pattern is noted with the administration of curare in both the dog and cat. The capacity to release histamine by various drugs varies considerably among species.

Gastrointestinal Tract. The effects of morphine on the gastrointestinal tract of the dog are salivation, nausea, vomiting, and defecation. These side effects are more likely to occur in upright ambulatory animals (WANG and BARISON, 1952), because of the vestibular stimulation which is enhanced by morphine. The initial effects of intramuscularly, asministered morphine in the dog is a slight ataxia and salivation which is followed by vomiting and defecation. This stimulatory phase of the gastrointestinal tract is followed by depression. Atropine reduces salivation, but not vomiting.

The final effects of morphine on the gastrointestinal tract are spasmogenic in nature. The initial increase in tone and motility is followed by a decrease in peristaltic activity with a continued maintenance of increased segmental tone, which delays the passage of its contents. The use of morphine should not be a substitution for an adequate withholding period prior to surgery. Vomiting does not occur under all circumstances of its administration and emptying of the stomach may not be complete. In many instances gastrointestinal stimulation is contraindicated and morphine should not be used. The administration of morphine postoperatively for its sedative and analgesic effects usually does not produce vomiting because of the depression of the patient and lack of movement. The rapid intravenous administration of morphine to an awake dog, with the rapid achievement of high blood levels prevents emesis by virtue of its antiemetic action.

Other Smooth Muscles. The overall effect of morphine and other narcotics on smooth muscle is an increase in tone. The bronchoconstrictor effect of morphine in the dog may be a direct action of morphine on bronchial smooth muscle or through the release of histamine. Morphine produces bronchoconstriction in doses of 0.5 to 2.5 mg/kg, the effect of which is reduced by bilateral vagotomy. This indicates a mechanism partially mediated through central vagal stimulation (SHEMANO and WENDEL, 1965).

Ocular Effects. In the species where the primary central nervous system effect is sedation (man, dog) narcotics produce miosis. In the animals where the primary effect is excitement (cat, horse, mice) mydriasis occurs. Intravenous injection in the awake dog will produce a mydriasis simultaneous with the occurrence of a brief excitement, followed by sedation and miosis.

Use of Morphine and Species Variation. Morphine is characterized by both excitement and sedation, depending on the species and the rate of administration. The excitement phase of morphine is characterized by mydriasis, nausea, panting, increased spinal reflex activity, and convulsions. The sedative aspects of morphine are miosis, respiratory depression, bradycardia, hypothermia, and the reduction in the response to external stimuli and reflex activity. The effects in the dog are biphasic and dose related; depression and analgesia at the lower therapeutic doses, and almost strychnine-like convulsions and death at the higher doses (Reynolds and Randall, 1957). The intravenous administration of morphine to the conscious dog produces a brief excitement with phonation, tremors, and mydriasis. This is shortly followed by a marked depression. The dose for minimal sedation in the dog is 0.1 mg/kg by parenteral administration; 0.5 to 0.75 mg/kg are adequate for premedication, and larger doses can be used if the animal is unmanageable or being premedicated for regional analgesia. It is important when using morphine that the dose be tailored to the patient's needs and general condition. Previous drugs, degree of excitement and amount of pain must be considered when selecting a dose.

The classic description of the effects of morphine in the cat is one of excitement commencing with restlessness and progressing to terminal convulsions. This is dose related, and a good sedative dose for the dog (0.5 mg/kg) will produce restlessness in the cat (Reynolds and Randall, 1957). Lower doses 0.1 mg/kg post anesthetically in the cat were found to be beneficial (Heavner, 1970). Other depressants will influence the excitatory effects of narcotics in the cat. Higher doses can be administered if tranquilizers are administered simultaneously, thereby depressing the excitatory effects. A dose of 0.5 mg/kg of morphine and 2 mg/kg of promazine will effectively sedate most cats. Barbiturates intramuscularly (pentobarbital 2 mg/kg) added to the above produces an extremely sedated cat. Under these conditions of sedation subsequent general anesthetic agents should be administered carefully and in reduced amounts. These concentrations of drugs are recommended for restraint of difficult to manage cats and are not suggested for routine premedication.

Morphine in the horse will produce some sedation and reduction of activity at intravenous dose levels of less than 200 mg for a 500 kg horse. The sedation is not outstanding. In doses exceeding 200 mg, motor excitement, stamping and neighing are seen (Westhues and Fritsch, 1961). A tranquilizer will suppress the excitatory activity of morphine in the horse.

Morphine in other farm animals (cow, sheep, goat, pig) is not recommended, again because of excitement. Subhuman primates respond in a dual manner to morphine as does the dog; lower doses producing sedation and the larger doses convulsions. In most subhuman primates the dose range suggested for the dog or slightly higher is necessary for adequate sedation to enable safe management of the primate.

Meperidine is used extensively in veterinary anesthesia. Unlike morphine it is devoid of gastrointestinal stimulatory effects. But, like morphine the rapid intravenous administration of meperidine in the unsedated animal is not recommended because of the excitatory effects on the central nervous system and its effects on the cardiovascular system (Robbins, 1945). This technique will produce hypotension in dogs. The cardiovascular effects of intravenous meperidine can be minimized by administering the drug slowly, preferably to a sedated animal. Pulse pressure, rate and rhythm should be monitored during intravenous administration to avoid any precipitious changes (Sugioka et al., 1957).

The dose for premedication in the dog varies from 2.5 mg/kg to 6.5 mg/kg. The amount used should be determined by the patient's physical status, clinical assessment of the degree of preanesthetic pain and excitability of the patient. Meperidine when given in the dose range suggested produces some sedation, which is one of its beneficial aspects. For postoperative analgesia in dogs the effective

dose is between 5 to 10 mg/kg. Here again, the amount selected should be dependent upon the condition of the patient, ventilatory stability and the overt
signs of pain. One of the main advantages of meperidine for premedication is the
lack of gastrointestinal stimulation.

Meperidine has been used in the feline species with some success, and is one
narcotic analgesic which when used in the correct dosage may not produce excitement (CARLSON, 1955). Compared to man, dog, and the subhuman primate sedation in the cat is poor and its analgesic properties are difficult to evaluate. The
dosage with or without a tranquilizer should not exceed 11 mg/kg by either the
subcutaneous or intramuscular route (BOOTH and RANKIN, 1954). Administration
of large amounts will produce signs which vary from incoordination and excitement to convulsions and death. These signs may be counteracted with a tranquilizer or barbiturate but not without added depression of the central nervous system
and hypoventilation. Occasionally lower doses will produce mild excitement in
cats or a very obvious lack of sedation. This obvious lack of sedation raises doubts
on the efficacy of narcotics when used alone in the feline species.

Table 3. *Suggested doses of other narcotic-analgesics in dogs*

	Dose	Reference
Anileridine (Leritine)	8 mg/kg	63, 71
Dihydromorphine (Dilaudid)	0.2 mg/kg	24
Thiambutine (Themalon)	4.5 mg/kg	1, 73, 83
Phenazocine (Prinadol)	0.5 mg/kg	—
Alphaprodine (Nisentil)	1 mg/kg	—
Methyldihydromorphine (Metapon)	4 mg/kg	33
Oxymorphone (Numorphan)	4 mg/kg	70

Courtesy of SOMA.

The value of meperidine in cats may be more from its potentiation of barbiturate anesthesia than predictable overt sedation in all animals. More effective
than meperidine alone is its combination with a tranquilizer. Meperidine alone,
or in combination with a tranquilizer potentiates general anesthesia, but unfortunately the marked overt signs of sedation, especially in very active cats, is
lacking. Irrespective of the overt signs in the cat the subsequent administration
of either intravenous or inhalational general anesthesia should be predicated on
the knowledge that the effects will be additive. The lack of marked sedation can
mislead the clinician into administration of general anesthesia with normal rates
and dosages. Meperidine has been used in the horse for pain especially in colic
cases and following orthopedic surgery. The suggested intramuscular dose is 500
to 1000 mg. Intravenous administration can produce hypotension. Doses of other
narcotics in the dog are given in Table 3.

B. Neuroleptanalgesia

Mixtures of fentanyl and droperidol (Innovar-Vet) are used for sedation and
analgesia in dog and subhuman primate. This neuroleptanalgesic mixture for
veterinary use contains 0.4 mg/ml of fentanyl and 20 mg/ml of droperidol. The
actions of the combined drugs are primarily those of the narcotic component. The
effect of the combination on respiration can vary and is primarily due to the

30*

narcotic. Panting can occur, but the overall effect is a depression of ventilation especially if the heat regulating mechanisms are not superimposed. Fortunately, compared to man the dog is more resistant to the respiratory depression produced by the narcotic component. But apnea can occur and all dogs should be watched carefully when high doses are administered.

Premedication with atropine is essential for the prevention of bradycardia, which is produced by the narcotic component. Sedation, ataxia and some analgesia occur in 3 to 4 min after I.M. injection. Other premonitory signs are flatulence, panting and ataxia. Complete sedation, immobility, and maximum analgesia will be noticed within 10 to 15 min (SOMA and SHIELDS, 1964). Innovar-Vet can be administered I.V., but at much lower doses.

A slow rhythmic oscillation of the eyeballs may be observed in some dogs; a more consistent finding is persistence of a vigorous eyelid reflex unrelated to the level of sedation. The pupillary constriction is not minimized by parenteral atropine. Muscular relaxation may be sufficient to enable oral examination and the reduction of many limb fractures. Oropharyngeal and laryngeal reflexes remain. Attempts at endotracheal intubation may evoke swallowing or laryngeal closure, but is possible in most cases. Some oral tone remains in the majority of dogs.

An interesting characteristic of neuroleptic-analgesia is the dog's ability to respond to auditory stimuli. A sharp noise, such as dropping an object or the crumpling of paper will evoke a response. The movement may be slight and consisting of lifting the head and some limb movement. This response persists despite the reduction or complete absence of a pedal reflex. It indicates the absence of complete unconsciousness despite deep sedation and analgesia. Unconsciousness is produced by administering nitrous oxide or small amounts of a barbiturate. Spontaneous movements of the head and limbs can occur, these are unrelated to auditory or painful stimulation.

Maximum analgesia is sustained for 30 to 40 min. Beyond this period the dog may react to cutaneous stimulation, although generalized sedation and some analgesia are still evident. Emergence delirium does not occur. Within 60 to 90 min after I.M. injection of the combined drugs, the majority of dogs are capable of maintaining sternal recumbency and responded to auditory stimuli by lifting their heads and "looking around". Some dogs attempt to stand. The majority will regain their righting and ambulatory capabilities within 2 h of injection.

Doses and use in Dogs. The fentanyl-droperidol mixture is administered I.M., I.V. or S.Q. at a dosage rate of 1 ml/10 kg to 1 ml/20 kg of body weight. The I.M. route produces an effect within 3 to 4 min, the subcutaneous route, a slower onset. Innovar-Vet is recommended for minor surgical procedures in combination with regional analgesia. It can substitute for a general anesthetic for many diagnostic procedures and for the restraint of difficult dogs. The dose should be reduced to $^1/_2$ to $^1/_4$ the suggested amount when used for preanesthetic medication. The smaller doses should also be used for dogs with a poor physical status and in older, obese and very large dogs.

C. Atropine Sulfate

Atropine is the anticholinergic (parasympatholytic) drug which is most frequently used to reduce secretions from the respiratory tract, salivary glands, and gastrointestinal tract and to inhibit the effects of vagal stimulation of the cardiovascular and respiratory systems. Its capability of suppressing secretory activity is effective in most species with the exception of the ruminants. The usual subcutaneous or intramuscular dose of atropine sulfate in dogs and cats is 0.02 mg/kg. Larger doses are required in many herbivorous animals because of higher levels of atropinesterase (GODEAUX and INNESEN, 1949). Suggested dose in the smaller farm animals is 3 to 5 mg, although in the smaller ruminants, as in the cow, salivation still continues but at a somewhat lessened degree. The actions persist for only $1^1/_2$ to 2 h. The dose in the horse is 40 to 60 mg. In the large ruminants atropine is of limited value, the flow of secretions is not appreciably reduced and the thickening of secretions make its removal more difficult.

In general the effectiveness of atropine in various species of animals is in the following ascending order: rodents, e.g. rabbit, rat; ruminants, e.g. cattle, sheep, goats; swine, horses, dogs and cats. The toxicity of atropine varies considerably with species, and most herbivores are like the rabbit in that they can feed on the belladonna plant without toxic effects.

D. Tranquilizers

The use of the term tranquilizer or ataractic in veterinary medicine is misleading and does not describe the use and function of these drugs. The term tranquilizer is a clinical term based on the drug's effect on psychomotor function, and the word ataractic is derived from the Greek word meaning without confusion, cool and collected (REMMEN et al., 1962). This descriptive terminology and others which related to psychic changes produced in man are not totally applicable in describing the effects in animals. The simple definition that a tranquilizer is a substance that reduces anxiety without clouding consciousness is certainly an oversimplified presentation of its effects (REMMEN et al., 1962). Its use in man is not only limited to the treatment of anxious states, which the definition implies, but the management of various degrees of psychological disorders. The psychomotor effects in man are varied and cannot be categorized by one definition. The end point and final effect depends on the mental state being treated.

Tranquilizers as opposed to other drugs used for premedication, are considered psychopharmacological agents, a class of compounds which depress many physiological functions, decrease motor activity, can produce mental calming, increase the threshold to environmental stimulation, but generally do not produce sleep, analgesia, or anesthesia. The sedation produced by tranquilizers differs from the state produced by barbiturates and narcotics in that sedation occurs without hypnosis The effect produced by the tranquilizers in animals can be reversed with an adequate stimulus. Tranquilizers are primarily used in man for their neuroleptic effects. Patients do not express anxiety, show little initiative, and exhibit a reduced response to external stimuli. The sedative effect may contribute to this reduced state of activity but it is not necessarily desirable or essential in man.

The desired effect in animals is sedation, without marked ataxia. This is especially important in large animals where maintaining the equilibrium may be essential. The basic difference in the administration of tranquilizers between man and animals, is that in man a mental disturbance is being treated, whereas in animals no such condition exists. Sedation in man is not the important aspect of the drug, and lower doses are generally used. In veterinary use, sedation and a tractable animal are the important aspects of the drug and higher amounts are needed [FLYGER, 1961; GRAHAM-JONES, 1964 (1); QUENTIN and SIRY, 1962].

In animals adequate doses produce quieting, sedation, ataxia, an increase in the threshold response to environmental stimuli, relaxation of the nictitating membrane and abolishment of conditioned reflexes. Phenothiazine compounds are drugs extensively used in veterinary medicine. Most congeners have been developed for their good antipsychotic effect and, unfortunately, higher doses are necessary to produce sedation in animals.

Tranquilizers when used in low doses impair the ability of animals to perform conditioned responses. Overt sedation may not be observed, but reaction time, avoidance response, and response to behavioral training are reduced. This typical inhibitor effect of low doses of neuroleptics has been observed in many species including the horse (Carey and Sanford, 1965). Promazine will reduce the horses' performance in a gallop and cavaletti tests. Tranquilizers also modify the increase in respiratory rate, pulse rate and body temperature produced by the exercising horse.

It must be emphasized that the sedation produced by tranquilizers is reversible and the animal can react in a coordinated manner. A horse can still react to painful stimuli and attempts at treatment, and a vicious dog can still bite. The degree of sedation and inactivity produced by the tranquilizers in many instances is dependent on the excitability of the animal being treated. This is especially true in wild animals, where the tranquilization of free living wild and captive undomesticated animals is not possible [Graham-Jones, 1960, 1964 (2); Harthoorn, 1971; Ratcliffe, 1962; Smits, 1964].

The phenothiazine derivatives have been used extensively for sedation and preanesthetic medication in a variety of animals. The agents commonly used in veterinary medicine are promazine, triflupromazine, and acetylpromazine. The original drug of this large series was the antihistamine promethazine. The classic tranquilizer chlorpromazine, has fallen into general disuse in veterinary medicine, because of its hypotensive action and in many species its inconsistent effect. Inconsistency and a prolonged sedation have been especially noted in the horse (Martin and Beck, 1958).

Chlorpromazine and the many analogous phenothiazine derivatives have similar basic structures and actions, but vary in potency and intensity of actions. The cardiovascular actions are through its multiple effects on the sympathetic nervous systems, the central nervous system, vascular and cardiovascular smooth muscle. These effects are both central and peripheral. The central manifestation is inhibition of centrally mediated pressor reflexes, which reduce both vascular tone and the animal's capabilities of responding reflexly to alterations in the cardiovascular system. The peripheral effects are alpha adrenergic receptor blockade, slight ganglionic blocking activity, and direct depression of the myocardium and vascular smooth muscle.

The effects on the cardiovascular system in the dog and horse are similar to the changes in man. In the awake dog, hypotension and a tachycardia occur after the administration of phenothiazine tranquilizers. In a comparative study of a group of tranquilizers, chlorpromazine and ethylisobutrazine produced the greatest fall, while promazine produced a moderate change. There was a rise toward control levels within 20 min (Hall and Stevenson, 1960). Chlorpromazine, flupherazine, trifluoperazine and promazine had similar effects in anesthetized dogs; hypotension followed by a gradual return toward normal (Bahga and Link, 1966; Bourgeois-Gavardin et al., 1955; Tavernor, 1962).

Studies in the standing horse were similar to the awake dog; a decrease in blood pressure and an increase in heart rate following I.V. promazine. The effect was maximal within 20 min. There was an increase in cardiac output when measured at the 15 min period (Gabel et al., 1964). The increase in cardiac output may reflect the peripheral vasodilatory effects with subsequent reduction in peripheral resistance. Tranquilizers are commonly administered to animals in the standing position, occasionally intravenously. This is especially true in horses. The cardiovascular actions have a more rapid onset than the sedative actions and orthostatic hypotension may be the explanation for the occasional collapse seen in the horse. A more frequent occurrence is indeed surprising. The hypotensive effects of a tranquilizer, as opposed to its sedative effect, are more variable, depending upon the state of the cardiovascular system and the relative degree of sympathetic tone when the drug is administered. Fatigue, hypovolemia, excitement and trauma are conditions which may increase sympathetic tone in attempts to maintain homeostasis. The administration of a sympatholytic drug under these circumstances can have a more profound effect. The cardiovascular systems under the influence of tranquilizers is less able to compensate for changes in vascular volume, position or stress. Chlorpromazine and other tranquilizers produce a hemodilution in the dog due to the sequestration of red blood cells by the spleen (COLLETTE and MERIWETHER, 1965; HOE and WILKINSON, 1957).

Table 4. *Suggested dose ranges of tranquilizers mg/kg (mg/lb)*[a]

Drug	Dog	Cat	Cow	Horse	Sheep goat	Swine
Chlorpromazine	1.0—2.0 (0.5—1.0)	1.0—2.0 (0.5—1.0)	0.3—0.6 (.15—0.3)	.2—1.6 (0.1—0.75)	1.0—2.2 (0.5—1.0)	— —
Promazine	2.2—4.4 (1—2)	2.2—4.4 (1—2)	0.4—1.1 (0.2—0.5)	0.4—1.1 (0.2—0.5)	0.4—1.0 (0.2—0.5)	— —
Acetylpromazine	.5—1.0 (0.25—0.5)	1.1—2.2 (0.5—1.0)	— —	0.04—0.09 (.02—.04)	— —	— —
Triflumeprazine	0.5—2.2 (0.25—1)	0.5—2.2 (0.25—1)	— —	— —	— —	— .9
Triflupromazine	1.0—4.4 (0.5—2)	2.2—4.4 (1—2)	0.11 (0.05)	.2—.3 (0.1—0.2)	1.1 (0.5)	.8—1.3 (0.4—0.6)
Ethylisobutrazine	2.2—11.0 (1—5)	2.2—11 (1—5)	0.5—2.2 (.25—1.0)	0.5 (.25)	—	4.4—11.0 (2—5)
Trimeprazine	— —	2.2 (1.0)	— —	— —	— —	— —

[a] Lower doses are the suggested intravenous doses.
Higher doses are the suggested intramuscular doses.
Courtesy of SOMA.

Preanesthetic Use. Animals sedated with tranquilizers can usually be handled and anesthetized more easily, however, loud noises or rough handling will arouse them. There are many exceptions, extremely high-strung nervous horses may still be difficult to manage and may not approach the surgical table. Under these circumstances barbiturates or other hypnotics may have to be administered. Vicious cats should also be placed in this category, tranquilizers may not produce sufficient sedation for safe management. Wild animals in general require higher doses than those suggested for their domestic counterparts. Dose ranges for various tranquilizers in some domestic species are suggested in Table 4.

Many phenothiazine derivatives have been used in veterinary medicine other than chlorpromazine (Thorazine) and promazine (Sparine). They include acetylpromazine (Acepromazine), trifluopromazine (Vetame), ethylisobutrazine (Diquel), promethazine (Phenergan), triflurpromazine (Nortran) and trimeprazine (Temaril).

Unusual Reactions to Tranquilizers. Most tranquilizers have a high therapeutic ratio. Unlike general anesthetics, tranquilizers produce an optimal effect within a dose range and increasing amounts do not produce a greater degree of sedation without marked undesirable side effects. Large doses in horses may produce muscle weakness and excessive sedation which can give rise to a state of panic. Under these circumstances the animal may be more difficult to control (Hall, 1966). Orthostatic hypotension can occur in the horse at therapeutic doses. Although rare, it is dramatic and distressing. This does not occur following the intramuscular route, which should be the preferred method. Accidental intracarotid arterial injections of tranquilizers and other drugs in the horse have produced disorders ranging from signs of mild disorientation to convulsive seizures and death. The microscopic changes have included endothelial swelling and necrosis (Gabel and Koestner, 1963). The initial cause of the violent response was probably vascular spasms and tissue ischemia. Drugs which deplete the stores of catecholamines (reserpine) and drugs which reduce the vasoreactivity of vessels (tranquilizers) will partially protect against intracarotid injections (Gabel and Koestner, 1963).

Common signs of exaggerated effects of tranquilizers usually following intravenous administration are: hypotension, hypothermia, recumbency and deep sedation. Acute administration of high doses can produce the extrapyramidal side effects. These include tremors, muscle spasticity, hyperirritability, spontaneous flexing and extension of forelegs and convulsions (Kaelber and Toynt, 1956). An interaction between parenteral chlorpromazine and piperazine has been reported in a child and duplicated in experimental dogs and goats (Boulos and Davis, 1969). The combination of these two drugs produced the extrapyramidal side effects whereas either drug alone produced no observable deleterious changes.

Unusual reactions to tranquilizers have occurred in dogs which include effects completely opposite to the anticipated one. Friendly dogs have become extremely savage (Collard, 1958) and actually attacked the owner. This may be similiar to the excitement and dissociation produced by chlorpromazine in young adults. Personality changes in dogs have also been reported by owners following the use of fentanyl and droperidol (Innovar-Vet). The animals were unfriendly, growled and were aggressive toward the owner. This effect is usually noted the day following its use and lasts for 24 h. This personality change has also been produced following the n-allyl nor-morphine of the narcotic component of Innovar-Vet. The unusual aspect of this reaction to a tranquilizer is that it can not be duplicated in the same dog.

E. Cyclohexamines (Dissociogenic Agents)

Cyclohexamines are a group of related compounds of which phencyclidine has had widespread usage in subhuman primates and wild cats. The state produced by the cyclohexamines has been termed "dissociative". These drugs are analgesic and in high doses produce a state which resembles anesthesia. The analgesia is not accompanied by central nervous system depression and hypnosis, but what appears to be a state of catalepsy. The specific effects will vary with species of animals but generally ocular, oral and swallowing reflexes are present, eyes remain open and muscle tone increases. Phencyclidine when used alone can have many undesirable side effects such as convulsions, vomiting and recovery periods which may run from 24 to 48 h (in Felidae) (Domino, 1964; Harthoorn, 1965; Kroll, 1962; Seal and Erickson, 1969). The characteristic pattern after administration in most animals is a progressive ataxia and loss of coordination, which culminates in loss of righting reflexes at higher doses. There is also head weaving, salivation, and occasional muscle twitching. There is usually an increase in muscle tone. The primates have a flaccid paralysis of the muscles of mastication whereas most other animals retain jaw tone. The eyes remain open with corneal and pupillary reflexes present. Nystagmus may occur. An increase in ventilation may be noted but death from over dosage is eventually due to respiratory depression. In some species of wild animals there is hypertension, convulsions and increased body temperature, especially in polar bears (SEAL and ERICKSON, 1969). These last effects are clinically lessened by the concurrent injection of atropine and a major tranquilizer, either a phenothiazine (SEAL and ERICKSON, 1969) or benzodiazepine derivatives which includes chlordiazepoxide (Librium) and diazepam (Valium). These tend to counter the effects of the phencyclidine drugs by depressing central nervous system excitation. The benzodiazepine compounds are important for their skeletal muscle relaxation. Because of the limited number of wild animals and wide varieties of species injected it is not possible to list doses for each. Interested readers are referred to the bibliography for more specific information [DOMINO, 1964; HARTHOORN, 1962 (1), 1965; KROLL, 1962; SEAL and ERICKSON, 1969].

Phencyclidine has had its greatest use in subhuman primates. Immobilizing or "sub-anesthetic" doses are particularly valuable in these and other animals which are difficult to handle [HARTHOORN, 1962 (1, 2)]. Its use as a total anesthetic should be questioned, because of the tremors and poor muscle relaxation. In many instances barbiturates are necessary to produce muscle relaxation even in the primates. Its adverse effects in species other than primates has reduced its value in most animals. The adverse effects could be minimized by the administration of tranquilizers. For the capture of the undomesticated feline and zoo animals the marked tremors and convulsive activity could be justified as the basis of complete restraint with relative safety to patient and clinician. The recovery period in both the primate and the feline species is prolonged with phencyclidine.

Two congeners of phencyclidine, tiletamine and ketamine, exhibit fewer of the undesirable properties. Tiletamine has shown taming and immobilizing effects in a number of species of animals (BENNETT, 1969; BREE et al., 1967; CALDERWOOD et al., 1971; CHEN et al., 1959; CHEN and ENSOR, 1968). Both drugs have an induction time of between 2 to 3 min following intramuscular injections. The duration of peak effect is approximately 60 min for tiletamine and 20 min for ketamine. This is followed by a variable but longer period of ataxia and sedation (CALDERWOOD et al., 1971).

Both drugs have been used in cats for restraint and minor surgical procedures. Cats lose their righting reflexes within 2 to 3 min after intramuscular injection. They lie quietly with their eyes open, maintaining palpebral, conjunctival, corneal, and swallowing reflexes. Lachrymal secretions persist and all cats salivate and atropine is recommended. Extensor rigidity of the forelegs with caudal deflection is observed with both drugs. The rigidity remains during the peak effect of the drug, with gradual subsidence during the recovery period. Hyperresponsiveness to tactile stimuli and ataxia has been noted during the recovery period.

The cardiovascular effects are a drop in heart rate and blood pressure which decreases to its nadir within 20 to 30 min, with a gradual return toward control (CALDERWOOD et al., 1971). As compared to intramuscular injections, intravenous administration produced a rise in blood pressure and heart rate. Arrhythmias were common with intravenous injections (CALDERWOOD et al., 1971). They included coupled premature ventricular beats which appeared as a bigeminal and trigeminal rhythm. There were fused ventricular beats and an increase in p wave amplitude. Tiletamine produces an irregular respiratory pattern which is apneustic in character; the animal "breath-holding" during the inspiratory period (CALDERWOOD et al., 1971). The consequence of this abnormal pattern is a respiratory acidosis. There was an increase in carbon dioxide tension and a decrease in pH. These alterations in arterial values occurred within the first 5 min and remained significantly different from the awake control during the first hour. Oxygen tensions were reduced and remained so for at least 30 min.

The persistence of this apneustic pattern with lower doses of tiletamine greatly reduced its usefulness as a preanesthetic agent. The subsequent induction of anesthesia with an inhalation agent was irregular and prolonged. Respiratory depression was more pronounced and general anesthesia could be adequately maintained only with controlled ventilation.

Ketamine is a recent derivative of phencyclidine, with further reduction in some of the undesirable effects of phencyclidine and tiletamine. It has been used in man and subhuman primates (BREE et al., 1967; CORSSEN and DOMINO, 1966; DOMINO et al., 1965; MATORRAS and FELIPE, 1970; TELIVUO and VAISANEN, 1970). The neuromuscular effects of ketamine in cats are similar to tiletamine but not as pronounced. This includes the apneustic respiratory pattern. The duration of the peak effect and recovery period are shorter.

The Use of Cyclohexamines. Phencyclidine has been used primarily in the subhuman primate and wild Felidae. The primary disadvantage is the long recovery period. This can be minimized by the reduction in the dose of phencyclidine and the simultaneous intramuscular injection of a tranquilizer. The dose in primates ranges from 0.5 to 2 mg/kg (STOLIKER, 1965), depending upon the state desired; reduced reactivity and catalepsis, to analgesia and "anesthesia". The dose in the undomesticated feline is 1 to 2 mg/kg. This should be administered with a tranquilizer to reduce the tremors and oculogyric movements. Atropine should be given to reduce salivation. The combination of phencyclidine, a tranquilizer and atropine has been effective orally in both domesticated and undomesticated cats.

Tiletamine has been used in a gorilla (1 mg/kg) and other primates for resttraint. The trachea can be intubated and anesthesia induced through the endoracheal tube. Tiletamine can be used in the cat for restraint and minor surgical procedures. The dose is 5 mg/kg. The extensor rigidity of the forelegs and tremors can be eliminated with intravenous diazepam (0.5 mg/kg), unfortunately the apneustic ventilatory pattern is not altered with diazepam.

The use of ketamine in humans for minor surgical procedures is still in the evaluation stages and its use in veterinary anesthesia has not been completely clarified. The muscle tremors and stiffness produced by these drugs certainly minimize their usefulness for abdominal and orthopedic surgery, both from a functional and esthetic point of view. The combination with a muscle relaxing tranquilizer (diazepam) minimizes some of the objectionable aspects of ketamine. Its combination with other anesthetics has not been evaluated and its potential use as a restraining prior to anesthesia needs further study. At the current stage of development ketamine has been used in man, subhuman primates and cats. The dose range for veterinary use is 10 to 20 mg/kg.

F. Rompun

Rompun (BAY-Va 1470) has recently been introduced in Western Germany as a sedative agent for cattle. With the knowledge available to date, it appears that it may be a useful drug for ruminants and horses. There is a wide variation in dosage between species of animals. The dosage for cattle ranges from 0.05 to 0.2 mg/kg I.M. or I.V. (CLARKE and HALL, 1969; SAGNER et al., 1968). The sedation produced is similar to that produced by chloral hydrate with analgesia present only at the higher doses. When administered I.M. cattle will usually "go down" within 15 to 10 min; the effects are noted within 1 min after I.V. administration.

The duration of sedation may last from 2 to 6 h. Sedation has been reported to last up to 24 to 48 h in isolated instances but without untoward effects or cause for alarm (CLARKE and HALL, 1969). A dosage of 2 mg/kg intramuscularly was sufficient to perform abdominal surgery in sheep, the effect lasting for 1 to 2 h.

Rompun has been given to horses intravenously (0.5 mg/kg) and intramuscularly (2 to 3 mg/kg) (CLARKE and HALL, 1969) producing a basal narcosis for 1 to 2 h. The horses are depressed but can be aroused by stimulation. There is one reported death from an overdose administered intravenously (CLARKE and HALL, 1969) and because of this the authors recommended that the drug be given only by the intramuscular route. Horses can develop second degree heart block and hypotension following intravenous administration. The bradycardia can be reversible with atropine. Although some horses were deeply sedated and ataxic, no horses were reported to have fallen down. An initial rise in blood pressure followed by a reduction to below the resting level has been demonstrated in horses. Sedation lasts about 30 min in horses without any clinical evidence of analgesia. Rompun has been given to horses as a premedicant prior to induction of general anesthesia with thiopental and maintenance with halothane/oxygen mixture. It was reported that the induction was smooth and clinically there appeared to be less respiratory depression then when acepromazine was used as a premedicant (CLARKE and HALL, 1969).

Rompun has been given to dogs and cats but insufficient data is available for any recommendations. Vomiting occurs initially in both dogs and cats. These is a decreased cardiac output, heart rate and blood pressure in the cats, with minimal changes in respiratory function (CALDERWOOD et al., 1970).

References

ADAMSON, D. W., GREEN, A. F.: New series of analgesics. Nature 165, 122 (1950).
ADRIANI, J., YARBERRY, O. H., JR.: Preanesthetic medication. Old and new concepts. Arch. Surg. 79, 976 (1959).
AYRE, P.: The T-piece technique. Brit. J. Anaesthesia 28, 520 (1956).
BAHGA, H. S., LINK, R. P.: Cardiovascular effects of two phenothiazines: fluphenazine and trifluoperazine. Am. J. Vet. Research 27, 81 (1966).
BARATTA, A., BRANDSLATER, B., MUALLEM, M., SERAPHIM, C.: Rebreathing in a double T-piece system. Brit. J. Anaesthesia 4, 47 (1969).
BENNETT, R. R.: The clinical use of 2-(ethylamino)-2-(2-thienyl) cyclohexanone HCl (CI 634) as an anesthetic for the cat. Am. J. Vet. Research 30, 1469 (1969).
BOOTH, N. H., RANKIN, A. D.: Evaluation of meperidine hydrochloride in the cat. Vet. Med. 49, 249 (1954).
BOULOS, B. M., DAVIS, L. E.: Hazard of simultaneous administration of phenothiazine and piperazine. New Engl. J. Med. 280, 1245 (1969).
BOURGEOIS-GAVARDIN, M., NOWILL, W. K., MARGOLIS, G., STEPHEN, C. R.: Chlorpromazine, a laboratory and clinical investigation. Anesthesiology 16, 829 (1955).
BOUTELLE, J. L., RICH, S. T.: An anesthetic chamber for prolonged immobilization of mice during tumor transplantation and radiation procedures. Lab. An. Care 19, 666 (1969).
BREE, M. M., FELLER, I., CORSSEN, G.: Safety and tolerance of repeated anesthesia with CI 581 (ketamine) in monkeys. Anesthesia Current Researches & Analgesia 46, 596 (1967).
BURN, J. H., EPSTEIN, H. G., FERGAN, G. A., PATON, W. D. M., BURNS, T. H. S., MUSHIN, W. W., ORGANE, G. S. W., ROBERTSON, J. D.: Fluothane: A report to the Medical Research Council by the Committee on Non-explosive Anesthetic Agents. Brit. Med. J. 2, 479 (1957).
BURSTEIN, C. L., LoPINTO, F. J., NEWMAN, W.: Electrocardiographic studies during endotracheal intubation; effects during usual routine technics. Anesthesiology 11, 224 (1950).
CALDERWOOD, H., KLIDE, A., COHN, B., SOMA, L.: The effects of tilitamine (CI 634) in the cat. Am. J. Vet. Research (in press).
— — SOMA, L.: Department of Clinical Studies, Section of Anesthesia, University of Pennsylvania Veterinary School, Philadelphia, Pennsylvania. Unpublished data, 1970.

Carey, F. M., Sanford, J.: A method of assessing the effect of drugs on the performance in the horse. Proc. Brit. Eq. Assoc. **52**, (1965).

Carlson, W. D.: A clinical evaluation of meperidine hydrochloride as a preanesthetic agent in the cat. Vet. Med. **50**, 229 (1955).

Chen, G., Ensor, C. R.: 2-(ethylamino)-2-(2-thienyl) cyclohexanone HCl (CI 634): A taming, incapacitating, and anesthetic agent for the cat. Am. J. Vet. Research **29**, 863 (1968).

— — Russell, D., Bohner, B.: The pharmacology of 1-(1-phencylcyclohexyl) piperidine HCl. J. Pharmacol. Exptl. Therap. **127**, 241 (1959).

Clarke, K. W., Hall, L. W.: Xylazine — a new sedative for horses and cattle. Vet. Record **85**, 512 (1969).

Clifford, D. H., Soma, L. R.: Chapter 22, Feline Medicine and Surgery, 1st Ed. Santa Barbara, Calif.: American Veterinary Publications, Inc. 1964.

Collard, J. A.: Unusual reaction to chlorpromazine hydrochloride in a bich. Australian Vet. J. **34**, 90 (1958).

Collette, W. L., Meriwether, W. F.: Some changes in the peripheral blood of dogs after administration of certain tranquillizers and narcotics. Vet. Med./Small Animal Clinician **60**, 1223 (1965).

Collins, R. J.: Potency of dihydromorphinone, methadone, and codeine compared to morphine in self-maintained addict rats. Federation Proc. **22**, 248 (1963).

Conney, A. H.: Pharmacological implications of microsomal enzyme induction. Pharmacol. Revs **19**, 317 (1967).

Corssen, G., Domino, E. F.: Dissociative anesthesia: further pharmacologic studies and first clinical experience with phencyclidine derivative CI-581. Current Researches Anesthesia & Analgesia **45**, 29 (1966).

Dobkin, A. B.: Potentiation of thiopental anaesthesia with Tigan, Panectyl, Benadryl, Gravol. Marzine, Histadyl, Librium, Haloperidol (R 1625). Canad. Anaesth. Soc. J. 8, 265 (1961).

Domino, E. F.: Neurobiology of phencyclidine (Sernyl), a drug with an unusual spectrum of pharmacological activity. Intern. Rev. Neurobiol. **6**, 303 (1964).

— Chodoff, P., Corssen, G.: Pharmacologic effects of CI-581, a new dissociative anesthetic in man. Clin. Pharmacol. Therap. **6**, 279 (1965).

Dripps, R. D., Eckenhoff, J. E., Vandam, L. D.: Introduction to anesthesia, 2nd ed. Philadelphia, Pa.: Saunders, W. B. 1961.

Dundee, J. W.: Thiopentone and other thiobarbiturates. London: E. and S. Livingstone, LTD 1956.

Editorial. Anesthesiology **25**, 3 (1964).

Epling, G. P., Rankin, A. D.: Metopon analgesia in the dog. Am. J. Vet. Research **15**, 338 (1954).

Feldberg, W., Paton, W. D. M.: Release of histamine by morphine alkaloids. J. Physiol. (London) **111**, 19 (1950).

Flyger, V.: Handling wild mammals with new tranquillizer. Trans. Twenty-Sixth North Am. Wildlife and Natural Resourses Conf., 230, 1961.

Fowler, W. S.: Lung function studies, respiratory dead space. Am. J. Physiol. **154**, 405 (1948).

Friedman, J. J.: Effect of Nembutal on circulating and tissue blood volumes and hematocrits of intact and splenectomezed mice. Am. J. Physiol. **197**, 399 (1959).

Gabel, A. A., Hamlin, R., Smith, C. R.: Effects of promazine and chloral hydrate on the cardiovascular system of the horse. Am. J. Vet. Research **25**, 1151 (1964).

— Koestner, A.: The effects of intracarotid artery injection of drugs in animals. J. Am. Vet. Med. Assoc. **142**, 1397 (1963).

Godeaux, J., Innesen, M.: Investigations into atropine metabolism in animal organism. Acta Pharmacol. Toxicol. **5**, 95 (1949).

Goodman, L. S., Gilman, A.: The pharmacological basis of therapeutics, 3rd ed. New York: Macmillan Co. 1965.

Graham-Jones, O.: (1) Restraint and anaesthesia of some captive wild mammals. Vet. Record **76**, 1216 (1964).

— (2) Discussion of Smits, G. M.: Some experiments and experiences with neuroleptic and hypnotic drugs on ungulates with special regard to Librium. Proceed. of Fifth Internat. Symp. on Disease of Zoo Animals. Royal Neth. Vet. Assoc. Tij. Dierg. **89**, 195 (1964).

— Tranquillizer and paralytic drugs. An international survey of animal restraint techniques. Intern. Zoo Yearbook **2**, 300 (1960).

Hall, L. W.: Wright's veterinary anesthesia and analgesia, 6th ed. Baltimore, Md.: William and Wilkings Co. 1966.

— Stevenson, D. F.: Effects of ataractic drugs on the blood pressure and heart rate of dogs. Nature **187**, 696 (1960).

Harrison, G. A.: Ayre's T-piece: A review of its modifications. Brit. J. Anaesthesia **36**, 118 (1964).

HARTHOORN, A. M.: Application of pharmacological and physiological principles in restraint of wild animals. Wildlife Monograph 14, 1 (1965).
— (1) On the use of phencyclidine for narcosis in the larger animals. Vet. Record 74, 410 (1962).
— (2) Producing "twilight sleep" in large wild mammals. J. Am. Vet. Med. Assoc. 141, 1473 (1962).
— Textbook of veterinary anesthesiology (SOMA, L. R., Ed.), Chapter 29. The capture and restraint of wild animals. Baltimore, Md.: Williams and Wilkins Co. 1971.
HEAVNER, J. E.: Morphine for postsurgical use in cats. J. Am. Vet. Med. Assoc. 156, 1018 (1970).
HOE, C. M., WILKINSON, J. S.: A diluting effect of chlorpromazine hydrochloride on the circulating blood of dogs. Vet. Record 69, 734 (1957).
HUTCHINSON, B. R.: Changes in pulse rate and blood pressure after extubation. Brit. J. Anaesthesia 36, 661 (1964).
— Electrocardiographic changes in children following extubation. Med. J. Australia 1, 151 (1967).
JOHNSTONE, M.: Pethidine and general anesthesia. Brit. Med. J. 2, 943 (1951).
KAELBER, W. W., TOYNT, R. J.: Tremor production in cats given chlorpromazine. Proc. Soc. Exptl. Biol. Med. 92, 399 (1956).
KAIN, L. M., NUNN, J. F.: Fresh gas economics of the Magill Circuit. Anesthesiology 29, 964 (1968).
KILLIP, T.: Sinus nerve stimulation in the chloralose anesthetized cat: Effect on blood pressure, heart rate, muscle blood flow and vascular resistance. Acta Physiol. Scand. 57, 437 (1963).
KING, B. D., HARRIS, L. C., JR., GREIFENSTEIN, F. E., ELDER, J. D., JR., DRIPPS, R. D.: Reflex circulatory responses to direct laryngoscopy and tracheal intubation performed during general anesthesia. Anesthesiology 12, 556 (1961).
KROLL, W. R.: Experience with Sernylan in zoo animals. Intern. Zoo Yearbook 4, 131 (1962).
KRUEGAR, H., EDDY, N. B., SUMWALT, M.: The pharmacology of the opium alkaloids. Supplement 165. Pub. Health Rep., U.S. Government Printing Office, Washington, D.C., Part I, 1941, Part II, 1943.
LEWIS, R. N., SWERDLOW, M.: Hazards of endotracheal anesthesia. Brit. J. Anaesthesia 36, 504 (1964).
LOWENSTEIN, E., MALLOWELL, P., LEVINE, H., DAGGETT, W. M., AUSTEN, W., LAVOR, M. B.: Cardiovascular response to large doses of intravenous morphine in man. New Engl. J. Med. 281, 1389 (1969).
MAPELSON, W. W.: The elimination of rebreathing in various semiclosed anesthetic systems. Brit. J. Anaesthesia 26, 323 (1954).
MARTIN, J. E., BECK, J. D.: Some effects of chlorpromazine in horses. Am. J. Vet. Research. 17, 678 (1958).
MATORRAS, A. A., FELIPE, M. A. N.: Selection of indications on the use of CI-581 and observations on 198 cases. Progress in Anaesthesiology, Proceedings of the Fourth World Congress of Anaesthesiologists, p. 1000, London 1968. Excerpta Med. Foundation, Amsterdam 1970.
MEDD, R. K., HEYWOOD, R.: A technic for intubation and repeated short-duration anesthesia in the rat. Lab. An. 4, 75 (1970).
NEGUS, V.: Biology of respiration. Edinburgh, London: E. and S. Livingstone, LTD 1965.
NYTCH, T. F.: Clinical observations on the preanesthetic use of oxymorphine and its antagonist N-allyl-noroxymorphane, in dogs. J. Am. Vet. Med. Assoc. 145, 127 (1964).
ORAHOVATS, P. D., LEHMAN, E. G., CHAPIN, E. W.: Pharmacology of Ethyl-1-(4-aminophenethyl)-4-phenylisonipecotate, anileridine, a new potent synthetic analgesic. J. Pharmacol. Exptl. Therap. 119, 26 (1957).
ORR, D., JONES, I.: Anesthesia for laryngoscopy. Current Researches Anesthesia & Analgesia 23, 194 (1968).
OWEN, L. N.: Thirambutene-thiopentone anesthesia for hysterectomy in pyometra of the bitch. Vet. Record 67, 580 (1955).
QUENTIN, J. R. L., SIRY, J. R.: Tranquillizers in veterinary medicine. Ag. Vet. Chem. 3, 136 (1962).
RATCLIFFE, H. L.: Diazepam (Tranimal) as a tranquillizer for zoo animals. Report Penrose Res. Lab. Zool. Soc. of Phila., 10, 1962.
REDGATE, J. D., GELLHORN, E.: The tonic effect of the posterior hypothalamus on blood pressure and pulse rate disclosed by the action of intra-hypothalamically injected drugs. Arch. intern. pharmacodynamic 105, 193 (1956).
REMMEN, E., COHEN, S., DITMAN, K. S., FRANTZ, J. R.: Psychochemotherapy, the physicians manual, Chap. 4. Los Angeles, Calif.: Western Medical Publications 1962.
REX, M. A. E.: Stimulation of larynospasms in the cat by volatile anesthetics. Brit. J. Anaesthesia 38, 569 (1966).
— The laryngeal reflex. New Zealand Vet. J. 15, 222 (1967).

Reynolds, A. K., Randall, L. O.: Morphine and allied drugs. Canada: University of Toronto Press 1957.
Robbins, B. H.: Studies on cyclopropane IX. The effect of premedication with demerol upon the heart rate, rhythm and blood pressure in dogs under cyclopropane anesthesia. J. Pharmacol. Exptl Therap. 85, 198 (1945).
Rubin, A. Winston, J.: The role of the vestibular apparatus in the production of nausea and vomiting following the administration of morphine to man. J. Clin. Invest. 29, 1261 (1950).
Sagner, G., Hoffmeister, F., Kroneberg, G.: Pharmacological basis of a new drug for analgesia, sedation and relaxation in veterinary medicine, Bayer Va 1470 or "Rompun". Deut. tierärztl. Wochschr. 75, 565 (1968).
Seal, U. S., Erickson, A. W.: Immobilization of carnivora and other mammals with phencyclidine and promazine. Federation Proc. 28 (1969).
Shemano, I., Wendel, H.: Effects of meperidine hydrochloride and morphine sulfate on the lung capacity of intact dogs. J. Pharmacol. Exptl Therap. 149, 379 (1965).
Simmons, M. L., Smith, L. H.: An anesthetic unit for small laboratory animals. J. Appl. Physiol. 25, 324 (1968).
Smith, T. C., Stephen, G. W., Zeiger, L., Wollman, H.: Effects of premedicant drugs on respiration and gas exchange in man. Anesthesiology 28, 883 (1967).
Smits, G. M.: Some experiments and experiences with neuroleptic and hypnotic drugs on ungulates with special regard to librium. Proc. of Fifth Internat. Symp. on Diseases of Zoo Animals. Royal Neth. Vet. Assoc., Ti; Dierg. 89, 195 (1964).
Soma, L. R.: (Ed.): (1) Textbook of veterinary anesthesia Baltimore, Md.: Williams and Wilkins Co. 1971.
— (Ed.): (2) Textbook of veterinary anesthesia, Chap. 21, Equipment and techniques for inhalation agents. Baltimore, Md.: Williams and Wilkins Co. 1971.
— Shields, D. R.: Neuroleptanalgesia produced by fentanyl and droperidol. J. Am. Vet. Med. Assoc. 145, 897 (1964).
Stoliker, H. E.: The physiological and pharmacological effects of Sernylan: a review. Experimental Animal Anesthesiology, pp. 148—184. U.S. School of Aerospace Medicine, Aerospace Medical Division (AFSC), Brooks Air Force Base, San Antionio, Texas, July, 1965.
Strobel, G. E., Wollman, H.: Pharmacology of anesthetic agents. Federation Proc. 28, 4 (1969).
Sugioka, K., Boniface, K. J., Davis, D. A.: The influence of meperidine on myocardial contractility in the intact dog. Anesthesiology 18, 623 (1957).
Sykes, M. K.: Non-rebreathing valves. Brit. J. Anaesthesia 31, 450 (1959).
Tavernor, W. D.: An assessment of promazine hydrochloride as a sedative in the dog. Vet. Record 74, 779 (1962).
Telivuo, L. J., Vaisanen, R.: Clinical experience with a phencyclidine derivative CI-581. Progress in Anaesthesiology Proceedings of the Fourth World Congress of Anesthesiologists. London, 1968. Excerpta Med. Foundation, Amsterdam 1970.
Tevik, A., Sharpe, J., Nelson, A. W., Berkely, W. E., Lumb, W. V.: Effect of nitrogen in a closed circle system with low oxygen flows for equine anesthesia. J. Am. Vet. Med. Assoc. 154, 166 (1969).
V.A. Laboratory Guide: Comparative anesthesia in laboratory animals. Federation Proc. 28. 4 (1969).
Vasko, J. S., Henney, R. P., Browley, R. K., Oldham, H. N., Morrow, A. G.: Effects of morphine on ventricular function and myocardial contractile force. J. Physiol. (London) 210, 329 (1966).
Wang, S. C., Barison, H. L.: A new concept of organization of the central emetic mechanism. Gastroenterology 22, 1 (1952).
Westhues, M., Fritsch, R.: Die Narkose der Tiere, Band I. Lokalanästhesie, Band II, Allgemeine Narkose. Berlin: Paul Parey 1961.
— — Animal anaesthesia: general, 1st ed. Philadelphia, Pennsylvania: J. B. Lippincott Co. 1965.

Toxicity of Impurities

ELLIS N. COHEN and H. WINSLOW BREWER

Present day manufacturers evidence considerable awareness in the problem of toxic impurities in anesthetic drugs. Rigid standards are set by the Food and Drug Administration and are carefully followed by the manufacturer. Fortunately, most impurities are harmless contaminants, or represent specific additives to the anesthetic, whose only disadvantage is to slightly dilute the agent. On the other hand, occasional toxic impurities are formed as by-products of the manufacturing process, and these may be difficult to remove. In addition, hazardous impurities may form during storage of the anesthetic, or appear after the container is opened and exposed to light, heat, moisture, or air. A recent report by CHENOWETH and BREWER (1968) calls attention to a number of important toxic impurities and breakdown products found in anesthetics.

The following pages present in some detail manufacturing processes and storage methods which on occasion lead to significant impurity formation in anesthetic agents. Table 1 indicates standards of purity which have been set by the F.D.A. or those accepted by the manufacturer. Finally, special attention is given to impurities in two anesthetic agents which are of current interest.

I. Hydrocarbons

Cyclopropane was first prepared for testing by LUCAS and HENDERSON (1929) because it was believed to be the impurity responsible for certain untoward cardiac effects observed when propylene was used as an anesthetic. Cyclopropane was not only exonerated by the tests, but proved to be superior to propylene as an anesthetic. Cyclopropane gas is stable for long periods of time in the steel cylinder in which it is stored and its purity exceeds 99.5%. Possible impurities present include propylene ($CH_3-CH=CH_2$), allene ($CH_2=C=CH_2$), cyclohexane, and bromochloropropanes. Propylene is the major impurity, with levels in the few hundred ppm range. Occasionally, levels as high as 1% have been encountered, and these are permissible.

Since cyclopropane is prepared by treating 1,3-dibromopropane with zinc dust, the olefinic impurities are formed when reductive debromination or hydrogen bromide elimination takes place, rather than the desired ring closure.

$$BrCH_2CH_2CH_2Br \xrightarrow{Zn} \underset{CH_2-CH_2}{\overset{CH_2}{\triangle}} + ZnBr_2$$

Purification is usually achieved by washing and liquification of the crude **gas**.

Ethylene occurs in varying amounts in natural gas. It can also be prepared by "cracking" other components of natural gas. Isolation and purification from natural sources, however, is so laborious that the dehydration of ethyl alcohol with sulphuric or phosphoric acid is preferable.

$$CH_3CH_2OH \xrightarrow[150\,°C]{H_2SO_4} H_2C = CH_2 + H_2O \,.$$

The latter procedure leads to a relatively pure product, while ethylene from natural or "cracking" sources may be contaminated with oxides of sulfur and phosphorous, nitrogen, acetylene, low molecular weight hydrocarbons, acetaldehyde, and carbon monoxide. The latter impurity is especially hazardous with its strong affinity for hemoglobin. It is customarily removed by compression and liquification processes.

II. Ethers

Of the various gaseous anesthetic agents the ethers are probably the most labile. If impurities are found in other inhalation anesthetics. they are most likely present because the manufacturer was unable to remove them. On the other hand, very pure preparations of the anesthetic ethers may decompose on standing in the presence of light, heat, or moisture. Peroxides, acids, and aldehydes all form on standing. The unsaturated ethers are especially labile. The simple aldehydes which arise by decomposition often polymerize to form precipitates. All ethers are stable for considerable periods of time when stored under cool, dry, dark conditions, and it is only after they are opened that the user must be concerned with maintaining their purity.

Divinyl ether is prepared by the chlorination of diethyl ether. Fusion with molten potassium hydroxide removes two molecules of hydrogen chloride.

$$ClCH_2CH_2\text{–O–}CH_2CH_2Cl \xrightarrow{KOH} H_2C=CH\text{–O–}CH=CH_2 + 2KCl + H_2O \,.$$

A variety of side products, including hydrogen, acetylene, ethylene and partially dechlorinated ethers are also formed, but all of these can be successfully removed. Of primary concern to the anesthetist is the stability of divinyl ether after the container has been opened and is in use. Most manufacturers recommend using the drug within 2 years after preparation, and discarding of any unused portion 24 h after opening.

0.01% N-phenyl-α-naphthylamine is added as a stabilizer to prevent polymerization and precipitation of aldehydic polymers formed by ether decomposition. Interestingly, a 3—4% "impurity" in the form of ethyl alcohol is added to elevate the boiling point and alleviate the problem of ice formation during vaporization.

Diethyl ether for anesthesia is prepared by treating ethyl alcohol with sulphuric acid below 130 °C:

$$C_2H_5OH + H_2SO_4 \longrightarrow C_2H_5OSO_3H + H_2O \,,$$
$$C_2H_5OSO_3H + C_2H_5OH \longrightarrow C_2H_5\text{–O–}C_2H_5 + H_2SO_4 \,.$$

Some ethyl alcohol passes over during the preparation. It is difficult to exclude traces of water, oxygen, and alcohol from the ether. All of these agents promote the formation of peroxides, aldehydes, and acids. Decomposition takes place slowly during storage in the sealed container, but increases considerably once the sample is exposed to air and light. The presence of alcohol in impure ether serves to compound the difficulties since it is easily oxidized to acetaldehyde by any peroxides present. Diethyl ether should be stored in glass under dark, cool conditions and not allowed to stand open. For anesthetic use, copper plated metal containers are frequently utilized. The copper lining inhibits oxidation and the formation of impurities during storage. In this container, the ether will actually remain stable for days even after opening.

III. Halogenated Compounds

Trichloroethylene is prepared by boiling tetrachlorethylene with lime.

$$2\ Cl_2CHCHCl_2 + CaO \longrightarrow 2\ \underset{\underset{Cl}{|}}{\overset{\overset{Cl}{|}}{C}}=\underset{\underset{Cl}{|}}{\overset{\overset{H}{|}}{C}} + CaCl_2 + H_2O\,.$$

It contains 100 ppm thymol as a stabilizer, and Waxoline Blue (5 ppm), is added as a colorizing agent to distinguish it from chloroform.

A significant danger in the administration of anesthetic trichloroethylene exists in its reaction with soda lime to form highly toxic dichloroacetylene [FABIAN et al. (1956)]. In turn, dichloroacetylene reacts with oxygen and moisture to form phosgene ($COCl_2$) and methylene chloride (CH_2Cl_2), which are also toxic.

$$1)\ \underset{\underset{Cl}{|}}{\overset{\overset{H}{|}}{C}}=\underset{\underset{Cl}{|}}{\overset{\overset{Cl}{|}}{C}} \xrightarrow{\ NaOH\ } \overset{\overset{Cl}{|}}{C}\equiv\overset{\overset{Cl}{|}}{C} + HCl$$

$$2)\ \overset{\overset{Cl}{|}}{C}\equiv\overset{\overset{Cl}{|}}{C} \xrightarrow{\ O_2\ } \underset{\underset{Cl}{|}}{\overset{\overset{O}{\|}}{C}}-Cl + C=O$$

Rebreathing systems utilizing soda lime are hazardous when employed with trichloroethylene and should not be used. Flame pyrolysis, as with the electrocautery, may promote the conversion of trichloroethylene to dichloroacetylene, and phosgene.

Chloroform is supplied essentially free of impurities except for 1% ethyl alcohol which is added as a stabilizer. It is prepared by the reduction of carbon tetrachloride in the presence of iron.

$$CCl_4 + H_2 \xrightarrow{\ Fe\ } CHCl_3 + HCl\,.$$

When allowed to stand in the presence of light and air, phosgene may form. Phosgene reacts with water to form HCl, producing respiratory tract irritation and pulmonary edema.

Ethyl chloride is prepared from ethyl alcohol and hydrochloric acid,

$$HCl + C_2H_5OH \xrightarrow{\ ZnCl_2\ } C_2H_5Cl + H_2O\,.$$

It is supplied essentially pure but may contain traces of alcohol. Aldehydes, chlorides, and halogenated ethanes may form on standing or exposure to heat and moisture.

Trifluoroethyl vinyl ether is prepared from trifluoroethanol and acetylene. It is stabilized by the addition of 0.01% N-phenyl-α-naphthylamine and protected from light by storage in brown bottles, since light promotes the decomposition of trifluoroethyl vinyl ether to acetaldehyde and trifluoroethanol. It is stable in aqueous solution through the pH range 2—11.

Methoxyflurane 2,2-dichloro-1, 1-difluoroethyl methyl ether, (II) can be prepared from methyl alcohol and 1,1-dichloro-2, 2-difluoroethylene (I).

$$
\begin{array}{ccc}
\underset{\underset{Cl}{|}}{\overset{\overset{Cl}{|}}{C}} = \underset{\underset{F}{|}}{\overset{\overset{F}{|}}{C}} + CH_3OH \xrightarrow{\text{alkali}} & H - \underset{\underset{Cl}{|}}{\overset{\overset{Cl}{|}}{C}} - \underset{\underset{F}{|}}{\overset{\overset{F}{|}}{C}} - OCH_3 + & \underset{\underset{Cl}{|}}{\overset{\overset{Cl}{|}}{C}} = \overset{\overset{F}{|}}{C} - OCH_3 \, . \\
I & II & III
\end{array}
$$

The reaction temperature is maintained in the range 10—20° in order to minimize side reactions and the loss by evaporation of dichlorodifluoroethylene (b.p. 17 °C). Although the preparation of 2,2-dichloro-1,1-difluoroethyl methyl ether (II) had been described earlier by Tarrant and Brown (1951), it showed little promise as an anesthetic agent because of a tendency to decompose at room temperature with the formation of various acidic substances and the liberation of hydrogen fluoride. Subsequently, it was shown that even pure preparations of (II) were contaminated by small amounts of (III), which is exceedingly unstable at room temperature. The extensive and rapid decomposition of this impurity causes trouble far beyond that which its concentration level (ca. 3500 ppm) might suggest, since the acidic products which accumulate during its breakdown proceed to promote the rapid destruction of the 2,2-dichloro-1,1-difluoroethyl methyl ether, (II) and the final mixture is complex and exceedingly toxic.

The key to the successful production of pure 2,2-dichloro-1,1-difluoroethyl methyl ether was the finding of Larsen (1966) that the contaminant (III) could be removed by treatment of the reaction product mixture with various oxidizing agents, such as ozone, permaganate and oxygen. Since the oxidization products are more easily removed, subsequent washing, drying and careful distillation affords a highly purified stable product. Total impurities do not exceed 1000 ppm. Only rarely are all of the impurities present in the same sample.

Halothane is prepared by the high temperature (above 400 °C) bromination of 2-chloro-1,1,1-trifluoroethane.

$$ CF_3CH_2Cl + Br_2 \longrightarrow CF_3CHBrCl \, . $$

Under these conditions a number of impurities may be expected to be formed. In addition, the starting material also contains three trace impurities, (2,2-dibromo-1,1,1-trifluoroethane, 1,2-dichloro-1,2,2-trifluoroethane, and 1,2-dichloro-1,1-difluoroethane) which perist in the final product. In a recent discussion of halothane impurities, Chapman et al., (1967) outlined the sources of these impurities, and the extent to which they are removed. Five of the possible impurities are substituted butenes which are probably formed by dimerization of various free radicals such as $CF_3\text{-}\overset{\cdot}{C}\text{-}Cl$ and $CF_3\text{-}\overset{\cdot}{C}\text{-}Br$ which are also intermediates in the formation of the halothane itself. 2-bromo-2-chloro-1,1-difluoroethylene may arise by the elimination of hydrogen fluoride from halothane.

Halothane may be also prepared in a similar manner by chlorination of 1,1,1,-trifluoro-2-bromoethane, hydrogenation of 1,1,1-trifluoro-2-chloro-2,2-dibromoethane, or by chlorination of 1,1,2-trifluoro-1,2-dibromoethane.

An alternative preparation for halothane is a two step synthesis under milder conditions (90 °C)

$$ CF_2 = CFCl \xrightarrow{\text{HBr}} BrCF_2\text{-}CHFCl \xrightarrow[\substack{(X=Br, Cl)}]{\text{AlX}_3} CF_3CHBrCl \, . $$

Halothane prepared by this method contains small amounts (up to 20 ppm) of hexafluoro-1,2-dichlorocyclobutane, presumably formed by dimerization of the starting material.

IV. Nitrous Oxide

Anesthetic grade nitrous oxide is prepared by heating ammonium nitrate (NH_4NO_3) in the range 245—270 °C,

$$NH_4NO_3 \longrightarrow N_2O + 2\ H_2O\ .$$

This equation is somewhat oversimplified. The real mechanism(s) of the decomposition are complex and the source of considerable disagreement. AUSTIN (1967) has suggested that a proton transfer in the melt leads to the formation of ammonia and nitric acid,

$$NH_4NO_3 \rightleftarrows NH^+ + NO^-{}_3 \rightleftarrows NH_3 + HNO_3\ .$$

Pyrolysis of HNO_3 would produce nitronium ion (NO_2^+) which would combine with ammonia to form nitramide (NO_2NH_2), whose decomposition would lead to nitrous oxide,

$$HO\,.\,NO_2 \xrightarrow{\ H^+\ } H_2O\,.\,\overset{+}{N}O_2 \longrightarrow NO_2{}^+$$

$$\xrightarrow{\ NH_3\ } O_2N\,.\,NH_2 \longrightarrow N_2O + H_2O$$

Dinitrogen trioxide (N_2O_3) and hydroxylamine (NH_2OH) have also been suggested as intermediates.

Nitrous oxide production in this manner is accompanied by the formation of various amounts of nitric oxide (NO) and nitrogen dioxide ($NO_2 \leftrightharpoons N_2O_4$). The reaction is exothermic and when properly controlled provides its own heat energy. Overheating produces a vigorous reaction with formation of large amounts of nitrogen, nitric oxide, and nitrogen dioxide. Elaborate precautions are taken to scrub, wash, dry and purify anesthetic grade nitrous oxide since the presence of the so-called "higher" oxides (NO and NO_2) constitute an extreme hazard.

The following table lists a number of impurities of manufacture which may be present in commonly used anesthetic agents. Where indicated by asterisk, acceptable safe limits for these impurities have been specified by the U.S. Pharmacopeia (Editions 15 and 17). Where otherwise noted, limits are those established by the manufacturer.

*Diethyl ether**

ethylene glycol	10	ppm
ethyl peroxide	0.5	ppm
acetaldehyde	1	ppm
acetone	5	ppm
alcohol	23,000	ppm
water	7,000	ppm
chloride	0.3	ppm
unsaturated compounds	3.5	ppm
non-volatile glycol	10	ppm
acetic acid	10	ppm

Trifluoroethyl vinyl ether*

aldehydes	100	ppm
fluoride ion	5	ppm
phenyl α-naphthylamine	100	ppm
trifluoroethanol	100	ppm
water	100	ppm
1,1,1-trifluoroethyl acetal of trifluoroacetaldehyde		

Ethylene*

carbon dioxide	300	ppm
carbon monoxide	15	ppm
acetylene, aldehydes, hydrogen sulfide,		
phosphine	1	ppm

Cyclopropane*

carbon dioxide	300	ppm
halogens	225	ppm
propylene, other unsaturated hydrocarbons	740	ppm

Nitrous oxide*

nitrogen	30,000	ppm
carbon dioxide	300	ppm
halogens	1	ppm
nitric oxide, nitrogen dioxide	1	ppm

Halothane*

2,3-dichloro-1,1,1,4,4,4-hexafluorobutene-2	15	ppm
2-chloro-1,1,1,4,4,4-hexafluorobutene-2	300	ppm
2-bromo-1.1,1,4,4,4-hexafluorobutene-2	2,500	ppm
1,1-difluoro-2-bromo-2-chloroethylene	50	ppm
1,1,2-trifluoro-1,2,2-trichloroethane	5	ppm
1,1,1-trifluoro-2,2-dichloroethane	15	ppm
1,1,1-trifluoro-2-chloroethane	10	ppm
1,1,1-trifluoro-2,2-dibromoethane	10	ppm
1-fluoro-2-bromo-2,2-dichloroethane	10	ppm
1,1,1-trifluoro-2-bromo-2,2-dichloroethane	20	ppm
1,1,1-trifluoro-2-bromoethane	5	ppm
1,1—difluoro-1,2-dichloroethane	5	ppm
trichloromethane	10	ppm
1,1,1-trifluoro-2,2-dibromo-2-chloroethane	10	ppm

Methoxyflurane*

Methyl chloride	70	ppm
1,1-difluoro-2-chloroethylene	10	ppm
1,1-dichloro-2,2-difluoroethylene	10	ppm
1,2,2-trichloro-1,1-difluoroethane	70	ppm
2-chloro-1,1-difluoroethyl methyl ether	70	ppm
dimethyl carbonate	300	ppm
1,1,1,2-tetrachloro-2,2-difluoroethane	300	ppm
Methyl chloroacetate	600	ppm
Methyl dichloroacetate	50	ppm

Chloroform

ethyl alcohol   10,000   ppm

phosgene
acetone
halogens
hydrochloric acid   traces may form on
ethyl carbonate   standing or exposure
aldehydes   to light or air
peroxides
halides

Trichlorethylene

phosgene
hydrochloric acid   traces may from on
chlorides   standing or exposure
acetylene   to air and moisture
acetylene dichloride

Ethyl chloride

alcohol
aldehydes   traces may form on
chlorides   standing or exposure
halogenated ethanes   to light or moisture

Divinyl ether

ethyl alcohol   35,000   ppm
dioxane
aldehydes   traces may form on
acetylenes   exposure to air
ethylene   or moisture
chloro-ethyl-vinyl ethers

Although certain impurities listed in the above table are exceedingly toxic, their concentration is carefully maintained several magnitudes below dangerous levels. Nonetheless, situations occasionally have arisen in which impurities have accumulated to toxic or potentially harzardous levels. In recent years, considerable attention has centered on certain impurities present in nitrous oxide and in halothane.

Higher Oxides of Nitrogen. The first suggestion that dangerous impurities might be present in anesthetic nitrous oxide was made by BUXTON (1907). WARNER (1915) recorded a death from nitrous oxide poisoning in which he implicated impurities present in the nitrous oxide. In 1966, CLUTTON-BROCK reported two patients given nitrous oxide anesthesia which was later found to be severely contaminated with nitrogen dioxide and nitric oxide. Although the second patient was saved by prompt treatment, the outcome in the first patient was fatal.

As indicated earlier, nitrogen dioxide and nitric oxide are by-product impurities of manufacture against which the precautions of scrubbing, gas washing, and fractionation of liquid gas are usually effective. Although the thermal decomposition of ammonium nitrate occurs in a controlled fashion at temperatures up to 260—270 °C, the reaction proceedes more vigorously above 290 °C with a considerable increase in formation of NO and NO_2. For this reason, strict precautions against overheating are observed.

The wide variation in boiling points of NO (-151 °C), N_2O (-85 °C), and NO_2 ($21°$) presents a special danger in the use of contaminated cylinders for the administration of anesthesia. Due to its greater volatility, NO is present in highest concentration in the first flow of gas leaving the cylinder. Conversely, the relative involatility of NO_2 causes this compound to concentrate in that portion of gas present in the nearly empty cylinder. The mathematics and physical chemistry of this problem have been presented in detail by AUSTIN (1967).

Severe hypoxia quickly follows the inhalation of the higher oxides of nitrogen through a combination of two mechanisms. Cyanosis develops from the formation of methemoglobin, and as a result of arterial desaturation due to changes in pulmonary gas exchange. The latter results from intense irritation of the lower respiratory tract by the higher oxides. Diffuse inflammation of the lungs leads to fulminating pulmonary edema. Treatment consists of oxygen therapy and in the use of intermittent positive pressure ventilation, the intravenous injections of methylene blue to reconvert the methemoglobin, and the administration of steroids and antibiotics to treat the resultant chemical pneumonitis.

A study by GREENBAUM et al. (1967) in dogs indicates that inhaled concentrations of 2% NO or 2% NO_2 for periods of 15—50 min are fatal. Concentrations as low as 0.5% are also fatal when continuation of exposure exceed 24 min. At postmortem, the lesions included pulmonary edema, hyperinflation, hemorrhage, desquamation of mucosa, and bronchopneumonia (SHIEL, 1967).

Unsaturated Hydrocarbons in Halothane. Recent reports of possible hepatotoxicity following the anesthetic administration of halothane (LINDENBAUM and LEIFER, 1963; BUNKER and BLUMENFELD, 1963) have generated interest in a possible causal relationship of the contaminants present in this anesthetic and the question of hepatotoxicity. Reports by COHEN et al. (1963, 1965) of the isolation of a toxic impurity, dichlorohexafluorobutene, in halothane were later followed by reports of at least three other unsaturated hydrocarbons of high toxicity present as impurities in this agent (RAVENTOS and LEMON, 1965). The major impurity, dichlorohexafluorobutene, was present in concentrations of 0.018% in stock halothane and tended to increase in concentration under conditions of clinical use. Although the importance of the impurity as a hepatoxin in man, its precise cause of increase, and the degree to which this increase occurs remain controversial, several reports validate the facts of its presence and its increase in concentration (CHAPMAN et al., 1967; SEXTON, 1963).

Studies in a number of experimental species (rats, mice, rabbits, dogs, and monkeys) demonstrated wide species difference in the determined L.D. 50's (COHEN et al., 1965; RAVENTOS and LEMON, 1965). The primary lesion appeared to be in the lung, but certain species, including the monkey, evidenced hepatic lesions at concentrations uncomfortably close to those present during clinical anesthesia. Additionally, evidence for the metabolic degradation of dichlorohexafluorobutene was obtained in the monkey and in man (COHEN et al., 1965). In light of this evidence, the manufacturer has developed new methods of purification for halothane, and present concentrations of this and other impurities (see table) are many-fold removed from a hazardous level.

Acknowledgement

Appreciation is expressed to the Dow Chemical Company, Squibb Professional Services Department, and the Ohio Chemical and Surgical Equipment Company for data provided in the table of impurities.

References

AUSTIN, A. T.: The chemistry of the higher oxides of nitrogen as related to the manufacture, storage and administration of nitrous oxide. Brit. J. Anaesthesia **39**, 345 (1967).

BUNKER, J. P., BLUMENFELD, C. M.: Liver necrosis after halothane anesthesia: Cause or coincidence. New Engl. J. Med. **268**, 531 (1963).

BUXTON, D. W.: Anaesthetics: Their uses and administration. London: Lewis 1907.

CHAPMAN, J., HILL, R., MUIR, J., SUCKLING, C. W., VINEY, D. J.: Impurities in halothane: Their identities, concentrations and determination. J. Pharm. Pharmacol. **19**, 231 (1967).

CHENOWETH, M. B., BREWER, H. W.: Toxic impurities and breakdown products of anesthesia, toxicity of anesthetics, p. 65, (FINK, B. R., Edit.). Baltimore: Williams and Wilkins Co. 1968.

CLUTTON-BROCK, J.: Two cases of poisoning by contamination of nitrous oxide with higher oxides of nitrogen during anaesthesia. Brit. J. Anaesthesia **39**, 388 (1967).

COHEN, E. N., BELLVILLE, J. W., BUDZIKIEWICZ, H., WILLIAMS, D. H.: Impurity in halothane anesthesia. Science **141**, 879 (1963).

— BREWER, H. W., BELLVILLE, J. W., SHER, R.: The chemistry and toxicology of dichlorohexa-flurobutene Anesthesiology **26**, 140 (1965).

FABIAN, L. W., STEPHEN, C. R., BOURGEOIS-GAVARDIN, M.: Place of trichlorethylene in obstetrical and anesthetic practice. South. Med. J. **49**, 808 (1956).

GREENBAUM, R., BAY, J., HARGREAVES, M. D., KAIN, M. L., KELMAN, G. R., NUNN, J. F., PRYS-ROBERTS, C., SIEBOLD, K.: Effects of higher oxides of nitrogen on the anaestetized dog. Brit. J. Anaesthesia **39**, 393 (1967).

LARSEN, E. R.: U.S. Patent 3,264,356 (1966), Dow Chemical, Midland, Mich.

LINDENBAUM, J., LEIFER, E.: Hepatic necrosis associated with halothane anesthesia. New Engl. J. Med. **268**, 525 (1963).

LUCAS, G. H. W., HENDERSON, K. E.: New anesthetic gas: Cyclopropane, preliminary report. Can. Med. Assoc. J. **21**, 173 (1929).

RAVENTOS, J., LEMON, P. G.: The impurities in fluothane: Their biological properties. Brit. J. Anaesthesia **37**, 716 (1965).

SEXTON, W. A., Hendrickson, W. G.: Purity of halothane ("Fluothane"). Science **142**, 621 (1963).

SHIEL, F. O. M.: Morbid anatomical changes in the lungs of dogs after inhalation of higher oxides of nitrogen during anaesthesia. Brit. J. Anaesthesia **39**, 413 (1967).

TARRANT, P., BROWN, H. J.: The addition of alcohols to some 1,1-difluoroethylenes. J. Am. Chem. Soc. **73**, 1781 (1951).

WARNER, A. R.: Manufacture and administration of nitrous oxide for anesthesia: The experience of Lakeside Hospital. J. Am. Med. Assoc. **65**, 1973 (1915).

Section 10.0

Interaction of Drugs*

J. Weldon Bellville

With 7 Figures

Drug interactions are important causes of unexpected pharmacologic effects — toxic or therapeutic. The clinicians' interest has been focused on drug interaction recently, since in an affluent society a large number of patients entering the hospital are receiving medication. Certainly the average patient in the hospital today receives at least six drugs daily (Smith, J. W. et al., 1966) — some drugs that were not even known to medical practice two decades ago. Furthermore, since the end of World War II, the practice of anesthesia has changed drastically in that instead of relying upon one drug to provide anesthesia, analgesia, amnesia and muscular relaxation, a combination of specific drugs is often employed to provide each of these effects in an attempt to assure ideal surgical conditions with minimal physiologic disturbance. The larger the number of drugs a patient receives, the greater the probability for a drug interaction to occur. This increase is not linear but is almost exponentially related to the number of different drugs given (Smith, J. W. et al., 1966).

In this chapter some of the complexity of understanding drug interaction will be discussed. References to complete works on the subject are given since it is impossible to present a complete theoretical discussion of drug interaction in the limited space provided here. Some possible errors in interpreting experimental results are illustrated with examples of interest to the anesthetist. However, I do not attempt to provide the practicing anesthetist with a guidebook that considers all the potential drug interactions of clinical importance. Rather various *types* of drug interaction are considered and often studies from the anesthesia literature are used to illustrate that particular type.

From reading the medical literature it is apparent that the terms *synergism* and *antagonism* are poorly understood by the clinician. Whether a combination of drugs produces antagonism, simple addition, or synergism is pertinent. Carefully controlled studies need to be carried out to define which of these three conditions exist.

Drug interaction has been discussed in detail by Clark (1926); Loewe (1928, 1955, 1957); Gaddum (1926, 1957); Schild (1947, 1957); Ariens (1954); Ariens et al. (1957), and many others. For the student reading these theoretical discussions of drug interaction it is apparent that one must start from the simplest model of the drug interacting with a receptor to produce some effect. From this one can progress to two drugs interacting with a receptor to produce an effect; two drugs interacting with different receptors that each produce the same effect — and so forth.

* Supported in part by NIH Grant GM 12527 and FO3 GM 16, 732-02.

The simplest interaction to consider is that of an active compound whose activity is enhanced in the presence of an ordinarily ineffective compound. A factorially designed study (FINNEY, 1964) might be considered to study such a proposed model. The simplest factorial design would evaluate the effects of the active compound, the inert compound, their combination *and a placebo*. It is then possible to analyze the contribution of each drug alone as well as the combination. It had been taught that atropine, when given in conjunction with morphine, decreases the respiratory depressant effects of morphine, the atropine itself not being a respiratory stimulant. This hypothesis was tested by STEINBERG et al. (1957) in a factorially designed study in which morphine 10 mg, atropine 0.6 mg, morphine 10 mg plus atropine 0.6 mg and placebo were each administered to volunteers on successive weeks and their respiratory response curves (BELLVILLE and SEED, 1959) determined. These data were analyzed statistically and no significant interaction of atropine and morphine was demonstrated.

If one is studying two compounds both of which produce pharmacologic effects (a change in the respsonse variable) then the problem is complex. It is necessary to compare the drugs and their combination at equal effect levels or define dose-effect curves for the drugs individually and in combination if meaningful statements are to be made.

One approach to studying drug interaction is to employ the concept of the isobologram as developed by LOEWE (1955, 1957). This is, perhaps, the simplest approach to use and one that may be most readily understood. In essence it involves developing a three dimensional dose-effect curve plot and determining if the plane so defined is flat (simple addition) or curved (indicating an interaction). A review of the use of isobolograms in anesthesia has been written by SMITH, N. T. (1966). While the isobologram may be a useful concept for analyzing data from clinical studies, the mathematical modeling approach of SCHILD (1947) is a more fundamental contribution.

An example of how an investigator might go awry by not comparing drugs at equal effect levels can be appreciated from analysis of a study carried out by GREENE and WHITTAKER (1957). They did a study in which the anesthetic effects of pentobarbital were compared with ether in a group of mice. They found that when pentobarbital was given, in dose of 20 mg/kg, the sleeping time was 56.8 min $\pm$ 20.6 min, and when 3.6 vol-% of diethyl ether was administered, the sleeping time was 50.0 min $\pm$ 8 min, and when the same dose of pentobarbital plus 3.6 vol-% of ether was given, the sleeping time was 164 $\pm$ 72.8 min. Since the combination produced an anesthetic effect in terms of sleeping time that was more than the arithmetic sum of the individual effects, BAEKELAND and GREENE (1958) infered that the effect resembled potentiation. Whether this represents synergism, additivism, or indeed, antagonism cannot be determined from these data without knowing the slope of the dose-effect curve. That this actually represents antagonism can be understood from the following analysis, using the author's values as stated above. Assume a slope of the dose effect curve of 400 (Fig. 1). From the equation for the dose-effect curve, $y = a + b \log x$ where y is the sleeping time in minutes, a the intercept, b the slope and x the dose of the drugs, one obtains the plot shown in Fig. 1. We know the effect of the combination of 3.6 vol-% ether and 20 mg/kg of pentobarbital. If we cut across these dose effect curves at this level (pass a plane perpendicular to Fig. 1), we construct an isobologram plot (LOEWE, 1957; SMITH, N. T., 1966). We find that at this exact level it would require 6.95 vol-% of ether alone to produce this effect, or 36.5 mg/kg of pentobarbital. A straight line connecting these last two points (an isobologram plot) describes additivism (Fig. 2). Points falling inside the line would represent syn-

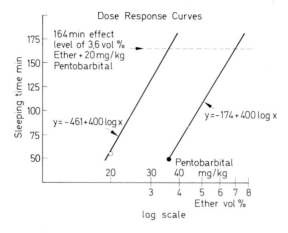

Fig. 1. The sleeping time in minutes is plotted against the dose of ether and pentobarbital. The three experimental results are shown: the response to 20 mg/kg pentobarbital (open circle), the response to 3.6 vol-% ether (solid circle) and the response to 3.6 vol-% ether plus 20 mg/kg pentobarbital (dashed line). Hypothetical parallel dose-effect curves are drawn through both circles [By permission Anesthesiology **20**, 724 (1959)]

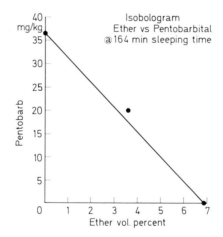

Fig. 2. Isobologram obtained by passing a plane perpendicular to Fig. 1 through the dashed line. The concentrations of ether (6.95 vol-% and pentobarbital [36.5 mg/kg]) were obtained by dropping perpendiculars from the intersection of their dose-effect curve and the dashed line in Fig. 1 to the x axis. The point falling to the right of the line in Fig. 2 represents the concentration of a combination of ether (3.6 vol-%) and pentobarbital (20 mg/kg) which produces a sleeping time of 164 min. Since this point falls to the right of the line, the effect of this mixture represents a type of antagonsim (see text). [By permission Anesthesiology **20**, 724 (1959)]

ergism. Points falling outside the line, such as that represented by 20 mg/kg pentobarbital plus 3.6 vol-% of ether, would represent antagonism. Thus, whether antagonism, additivism, or synergism occurs is a function of the slope of these two dose-effect curves. If the slope is 372, additivism is present. If it is greater than

372, antagonism is present, and if it is less, synergism is present. Thus, in this case it is clear that drugs must be compared at equal effect levels, or the slope of the dose response curve must be known to make a meaningful conclusion.

In the foregoing discussion it is assumed that the dose effect curves for ether and pentobarbital are parallel. This may not be true. If the slopes are not parallel, the problem is even more complicated.

Another common error is for the investigator to make statements in reference to drug interaction without evaluating the sensitivity of the method. If two drugs are compared, and no difference is detected, this may not mean that no difference exists but merely this method is not sensitive enough to detect the pharmacologic differences that do exist. An example of this type error is the study of BENTLEY and SAVIDGE (1958). They stated that when β, β-ethylmethylglutarimide (Megi-

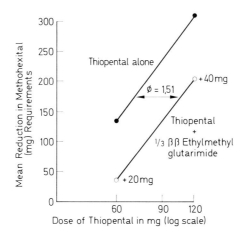

Fig. 3. The reduction in methohexital required to maintain the dog in a steady state of anesthesia is plotted versus the disturbance dose of thiopental administered. When β, β-ethylmethylglutarimide was added, the potency of thiopental was decreased. Thiopental alone was 1.5 times as potent as the 1:3 mixture. [By permission of J. Pharmacol. Exptl Therap. **130**, 364—366 (1960)]

mide) and thiopental are administered simultaneously in a 1:3 ratio, hypnotic potency is not decreased but that there is less respiratory depression. They studied the dose of thiopental and the dose of the 1:3 mixture required to abolish the paw withdrawal reflex in the dog. These authors did not demonstrate the sensitivity of their method, which could have been done by defining, say, the threshold level for abolishing the paw withdrawal reflex. It is probable that a 50% decrease in potency of the anesthetic would not have been appreciated. (This is another argument for defining dose-effect curves in pharmacologic research. The ability to discriminate between the effects of graded doses of a drug is a measure of the sensitivity of the method.) To investigate this problem in dogs, we developed a method wherein a dose effect curve could be determined for thiopental alone and for the mixture of thiopental plus β,β-ethylmethylglutarimide in a 1:3 mixture (BELLVILLE et al., 1960). When this was done, it was found that the hypnotic potency was decreased by the addition of β,β-ethylmethylglutarimide (Fig. 3).

The effect of a drug may be modified in many ways, such as: direct chemical inactivation, absorption prior to reaching the receptor site, interaction at several sites, alteration in metabolism or drug inactivation, temperature effects, and factors related to the patient.

I. Chemical Reactions

When we administer an anesthetic to a patient, we must be aware that factors in the system can influence the response of the patient. Certainly anesthesiologists are aware of mechanical factors especially in children and debilitated patients that can be critical. Also the drugs employed themselves may produce depression of circulation and respiration and if not controlled may affect the distribution of the anesthetic and the course of anesthesia. But even beyond this, direct chemical reactions have been reported that are not commonly regarded as a drug interaction.

Direct chemical reactions that may influence the anesthetics effect on a patient may occur outside the patient. The reaction of trichloroethylene with soda lime to produce dichloracetylene is taught to every beginning anesthetist (ADRIANI, 1962). Recently the reaction of halothane in the presence of copper and oxygen to yield highly toxic dichlorohexafluorobutene has been described (COHEN et al., 1965) (see Section 9.0).

The latter reaction raises the question of drug purity. Is the effect seen due to the primary agent or a contaminant? Unsaturated fluorinated hydrocarbons have been described whose LD_{50} is as low as 0.5 ppm (CLAYTON, 1962) (several hundred times as toxic as hydrogen cyanide) so that the presence of unsaturated fluorinated hydrocarbons in anesthetics is not solely academic. Fortunately dichlorohexafluorobutene, which at one time was found in halothane synthesized by the high thermal reaction, is no longer present in that sold in the United States (COHEN et al., 1965). Nitrous oxide also has been reported to contain the toxic contaminant nitric oxide (CLINTTON-BROCK, 1967) which produced death in at least one patient, and both these illustrations emphasize the need for stringent quality control in the manufacture of pharmaceuticals.

ADAMS et al. (1944) called attention to the fact that citrate intoxication can and does occur during massive blood transfusion. This represents chelating of plasma calcium by the citrate ion present in banked blood. This has been studied in detail by many investigators (BUNKER et al. 1955; HOWLAND et al., 1957).

A direct chemical combination that *is* used therapeutically is the reaction of protamine with heparin. It is accepted practice in some institutions to administer protamine upon termination of a cardiovascular pump bypass procedure to reverse the effect of heparin used to anticoagulate the blood. This represents a direct chemical reaction in which protamine combines with heparin and it is no longer effective.

II. Transport Phenomena

While transport of drugs across membranes is often governed by their oil-water solubility (for weak acids and bases this may be dependent on the pKa of the compound) there are often other factors that directly affect the absorption of the drug, and interfere with its transport to the receptor site. For instance, aspirin is very weakly soluble, and if compressed too tightly, it may fail to decompose in the stomach, and pass through the entire gastrointestinal tract unchanged.

Instances have been reported wherein the preservative in the vehicle has influenced the toxicity of the compound. The best known of these to anesthesiologists is probably the "bisulfite phenomenon". RICHARDS and KUETER (1943) determined that the toxicity of procaine was influenced by the reducing agent sodium bisulfite added as a preservative.

The drug itself may also modify uptake and distribution by altering body physiology locally. For example, morphine when given intramuscularly has a time effect curve that has a longer duration of action and less marked peak effect than is seen following some of the synthetic analgesics (FORREST and BELLVILLE, 1968). This may be due to the local release of histamine from the tissues following the injection of morphine. The histamine alters circulation to that particular area of muscle and thus delays the morphine absorption. No such effect is seen after many of the synthetic narcotics — thus they have a faster absorption (higher peak effect) and shorter duration of action.

While ultimately it is the drug interacting with a receptor that produces a pharmacologic effect, drugs are bound by many non-specific proteins (GOLDSTEIN, 1949). Instances occur wherein drugs may be displaced from the non-specific sites by competing compounds. This means that a much higher concentration of unbound drug is available for diffusion into tissues and sites of alteration and excretion. Thus the pharmacologic action of the drug is altered. Bilirubin bound to albumin in newborns can be displaced by sulfonamides (ODELL, 1959). The unbound bilirubin is then free to diffuse into the brain and produce harmful effects.

d-tubocurarine is bound to plasma protein (COHEN, 1963). BARAKA and GABALI (1968) have shown a correlation between the gamma globulin concentration and the d-tubocurarine dose requirements of an individual during surgery. It may be that the binding of d-tubocurarine to plasma protein is pH dependent. COHEN et al. (1965) studied this in dogs and found that during alkalosis the amount bound was higher, with an inflection peak occurring at pH 8.2. In an early study, COHEN et al. (1957) observed a fall in plasma d-tubocurarine concentration in human beings given meostigmine to reverse curare. BARAKA (1964) studied this phenomen on humans and found that plasma binding was pH dependent. Some of the difference between these several studies may be related to species differences. It may also be due to alterations in drug distribution, since in the study of BARAKA (1964) blood pressure was not controlled while in the study of COHEN et al. (1965) it was. It does appear that there is some pH dependence of curare binding to protein in man.

III. Interaction at Receptor Site

The affinity as well as intrinsic activity of a drug must be considered when defining the action of a drug at a receptor site. Affinity describes the force with which a drug is bound to a receptor, whereas intrinsic activity describes the change in some physiologic process the drug-receptor complex produces (ARIENS et al., 1957). It is possible for compounds to have affinity for a receptor but to have no intrinsic activity. This is well known to anesthesiologists in that atropine bound to receptors has, in itself, no effect, but prevents subsequent acetylcholine having an effect on the receptors.

A drug bound to a receptor may be displaced if a second drug with a higher affinity for the receptor is available to compete with it. This is thought to be the most likely mechanism to explain the antagonism of morphine poisoning by nalorphine (BELLVILLE and FLEISCHLI, 1968). Nalorphine has a higher affinity than morphine but a lower intrinsic activity than morphine. Thus, after nalorphine is administered the morphine and nalorphine compete for the receptor; the morphine is displaced and since nalorphine has a lower intrinsic activity the severe respiratory depression due to morphine is replaced by the mild respiratory depression due to nalorphine. From this example it can be appreciated that the best antagonist would be one that has a high affinity for the receptor but a low, or ideally, zero intrinsic activity. Narcotic antagonists with lower intrinsic activity than nalorphine such as naloxone (LASAGNA, 1965) are currently under study. They are of particular interest now since nalorphine is not effective in treating overdosage of pentazocine (an analgesic that also has some narcotic antagonist properties) but naloxone appears to be effective (KALLOS and SMITH, 1968).

IV. Interaction at Several Sites

There have been a number of studies of the interaction of halothane and curare on skeletal muscle (SMITH, N. T. et al., 1963; KATZ and GISSEN, 1967; BARAKA, 1968 (2)]. In the cat, SMITH et al. showed that when the intact sciatic nerve was stimulated and the response of the tibialis anticus muscle recorded, halothane alone would cause depression of the twitch response (Fig. 4). They carried out a series of experiments in which in one group of cats anesthesia was induced with nitrous oxide and the twitch response to d-tubocurarine studied. Arterial blood samples were drawn to relate concentration of d-tubocurarine (COHEN, 1963) to twitch height. After recovery of the twitch height to control levels, halothane was added and arterial blood samples drawn for determination of halothane and d-tubocurarine concentrations. Supplemental doses of curare were also given to study the twitch heights with combinations of the two drugs. A similar study was carried out wherein the procedure was reversed. Anesthesia was induced with nitrous oxide-halothane and the twitch height response to various concentrations studied. Then curare was introduced. From these studies dose-effect curves were constructed for halothane and d-tubocurarine (Fig. 5). By cutting across these curves at effect levels corresponding to that observed with measured combinations of d-tubocurarine and halothane it was possible to construct an isobologram plot (Fig. 6). In every instance the point fell within the straight line joining the halothane and d-tubocurarine concentrations predicted from Fig. 5 necessary to produce the same (75%, 93.3%, 99.3%) depression in twitch height. This clearly shows synergism.

KATZ and GISSEN (1967) studied this phenomena in human beings by stimulating the intact radial nerve and recording the twitch response of the thumb. With halothane alone there was no effect on the twitch response. In the presence of halothane the effect of d-tubocurarine on the twitch response was augmented although concentrations of d-tubocurarine were not measured.

BARAKA [1968 (2)] also studied this interaction in man by stimulating the ulnar nerve supramaximally and recording the twitch response of the ring finger. Halothane (2%) caused an increase in response. Curare when administered during nitrous oxide anesthesia caused a decrease in twitch height. After recovery of the twitch was complete, adding 2% halothane caused the block to be reestablished.

Although synergism occurs between halothane and curare, the mechanism is still undefined. None of these experiments rule out retrograde stimulation of the nerve and might be affected by halothane acting on the central nervous system. However, SABAWALA and DILLON (1958) observed that 4% halothane produced a rise in the twitch response to direct human muscle stimulation *in vitro*. Thus halothane might have a positive inotropic effect *in vivo*. Depression by halothane of the post-junctional depolarization evoked by iontophoretically applied acetyl-

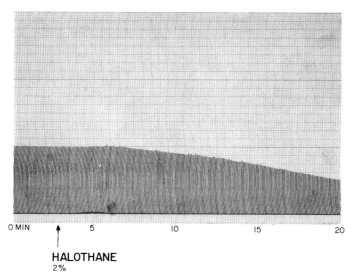

O MIN   5   10   15   20

HALOTHANE
2%

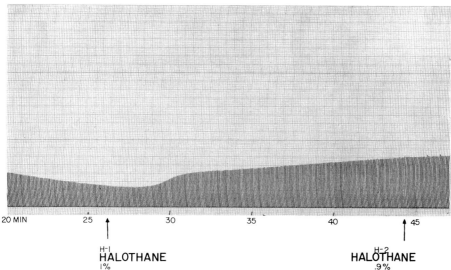

20 MIN   25   30   35   40   45

H-I
HALOTHANE
1%

H-2
HALOTHANE
.9%

Fig. 4. The twitch response of the tibialis anticus recorded continuously for 47 min is shown. The intact sciatic nerve was stimulated supramaximally every 5 sec. Anesthesia consisted of 80% nitrous oxide-20% oxygen. The arrows indicate when 2% halothane commenced and when the inhaled concentration was changed. Note the depression following introduction of 2% halothane

choline has been demonstrated by GISSEN et al. (1966) using *in-vitro* preparations of frog muscle. The positive inotropic effect of 2% halothane probably predominates in man except in the instance where d-tubocurarine occupies the endplate receptors. Then the depressant effect of halothane becomes manifest. Thus it appears that halothane and curare probably have different sites of action but act synergistically.

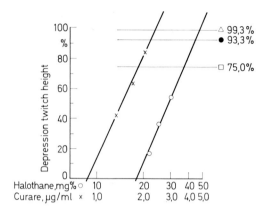

Fig. 5. Dose effect curves obtained in an experiment from one cat for halothane and d-tubo-curarine are plotted versus percent of twitch height. Planes are passed at 75, 93.3 and 99.3% depression corresponding to twitch height depression obtained for combinations of halothane and curare. By dropping perpendicular lines from the intersections of the dose-effect curves and these planes the arterial blood concentration of d-tubocurarine or halothane (above) required to produce this amount of depression can be calculated

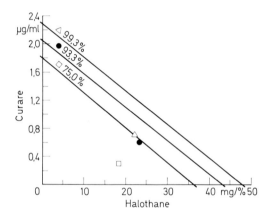

Fig. 6. The isobologram (LOEWE, 1957) showing the interaction of d-tubocurarine and halo-thane. On the ordinate and abscissa are plotted the points computed from Fig. 5 to give that particular level of depression. The straight lines (75, 93.3 and 99.3%) connecting these points indicate concentrations of halothane plus d-tubocurarine that would be required to produce that degree of depression if the interaction were additive. The points indicating arterial blood concentration of d-tubocurarine plus halothane which produced these three degrees of depression all fall inside the respective straight line. This indicates a synergism between these two drugs

Recently KRANTZ and LOECHER (1967) published an interesting study of the effect of the inert fluorinated gas, fluoroform (CHF_3), on the anesthetic effects of fluroxene. They observed that although fluoroform appeared to have no effect itself, it increased the anesthetic potency of fluroxene. Another inert gas, Freon[R] E-1 ($CF_3CF_2CF_2OCFHCF_3$), had little effect on fluroxene anesthesia other than increasing movement and excitation of the mice. The convulsant gas, flurothyl [bis-(2,2,2-trichloroethyl) ether], did not produce seizures when administered with fluroform. Both these observations raise the question as to whether fluroform is truly inert (is one on a low portion of the dose-effect curve?) or would it show anesthetic effects at higher partial pressures.

From the same laboratory (CASCORBI and LOECHER, 1967) has come an interesting study of the interaction of volatile anesthetics and the convulsant, flurothyl. All anesthetics in suitable dose would protect against the lethal effect of flurothyl. They observed that with methoxyflurane, fluroxene, and ether in suitable mixtures the gases were inert. This was not true with halothane or chloroform. In fact when combined with a subanesthetic dose of chloroform, flurothyl produced anesthesia in 30% of mice and when given with an anesthetic dose of chloroform induction time was shortened and recovery time prolonged.

In both these studies one is dealing with a very complex system. The oil-water solubilities of the various compounds studied vary so that observations during induction and recovery are almost impossible to interpret. But most important, what do these studies mean in terms of the theories of PAULING (1961) and MILLER (1961)? First, it will be necessary to define in detail the interaction of flurothyl and an anesthetic in much the same way LOEWE (1955) studied the barbiturates and analeptics. The question then will be to relate such an interaction to a receptor model. Only then will it be possible to know if one is dealing with an interaction involving one or several receptors.

The interaction of nitrous oxide and halothane has been of particular interest to anesthesiologists. SAIDMAN and EGER (1964) showed that 70% nitrous oxide decreased the minimum alveolar concentration required to prevent response to pain from .74%—.29% halothane. Although from their experiment it is not possible to determine what type interaction one is dealing with in terms of the primary anesthetic effect, investigators have studied this interaction in terms of many responses with the hope that, if the effects were not strictly additive, the combination of these two drugs might permit the maintenance of adequate anesthesia with less physiologic derangement. PRICE and PRICE (1967) studied this interaction in terms of its ganglionic blocking properties and thought the interaction was additive (although there was no rigorous statistical analysis of the type interaction). SMITH, N. T. et al. (1968) found that addition of nitrous oxide to halothane-oxygen anesthesia produced stimulation of the peripheral vascular system. This response was not seen during light (1%) halothane anesthesia but during deeper anesthesia (1.6—2%) with holathane. They thought the effect of nitrous oxide in stimulating the peripheral vascular system was mediated through norepinephrine release since norepinephrine levels increased from 0.97—1.33 μg/ml. Thus some of the cardiovascular depressant effects of halothane are counteracted by nitrous oxide which stimulates the release of norepinephrine.

V. Altered Drug Metabolism

The action of a drug may be modified if its metabolism is altered. Perhaps one of the best known examples is the enhanced oxidation of ethyl alcohol to acetaldehyde which occurs when alcohol is taken after disulfiram, an inhibitor of aldehyde dehydrogenase.

Presently the most widely used enzyme inhibitors are the monamine oxidase inhibitors (isocarboxazide, nialamide, phenelzine and tranylcypromine). These compounds, used in the treatment of mental depression, inhibit monoamine oxidase, an enzyme that plays a major role in the degradation of intracellular

biogenic amines [epinephrine, norepinephrine, dopamine and 5-hydroxy trypt-
amine (serotonin)]. Recently many articles have been published to emphasize
that the change induced by these drugs on normal metabolic pathways may profoundly affect the reaction of the individual to drugs (Sjöqvist, 1965). The
hypertensive crises in patients receiving monamine oxidase inhibitors (MAOI)
who eat cheese containing tryamine has been well publicized (Asatoor et al.,
1963). The effects of ganglion-blocking agents may be enhanced by MAOI.
Anesthesiologist have been cautioned that patients receiving these anti-depressant
drugs may show prolonged effects following the administration of meperidine,
pentobarbital and the phenothiazines, possibly due to deceleration of the metabolism of these compounds by a non-specific inhibition of liver microsomal enzymes.

Conversly, attention has also been called to the phenomenon of a decreased
effect of a therapeutic agent due to enhancement of metabolism by means of
enzyme induction. Conney et al. (1960) showed that animals exposed to insecticides such as chlordane stimulated drug-metabolizing enzyme activity and shortened the duration of action of hexobarbital. This phenomenon is known as enzyme
induction. Phenobarbital causes enzyme induction. After chronic administration
of phenobarbital there is a marked increase in the activity of the liver microsomal
enzyme which metabolizes bishydroxycoumarin (Dicumarol) so that patients
receiving bishydroxycoumarin have a decrease in drug level and prothrombin
time while they are receiving phenobarbital.

Drug metabolism can be stimulated by many different types of drugs such as
barbiturates, other hypnotics, analgesics, tranquilizers and antihistamines.
Recently it has been shown that inhalation anesthetics such as ether, chloroform
methoxyflurane and halothane are metabolized mainly in the liver (van Dyke
and Chenoweth, 1965; Cohen et al., 1965; Cohen and Hood, 1969). The clinical
import of enzyme induction in relation to inhalation agents is not known. It is
possible, however, that the untoward reaction to a halogenated general anesthetic
might be related to unusual metabolic pathways, induced or inborn.

VI. Effects of Temperature

Eger et al. (1965) published a provocative study of the effects of temperature
on the minimal alveolar concentration of halothane or cyclopropane necessary to
abolish the reaction to pain in the dog. They observed that for both halothane and
cyclopropane the alveolar concentration of drug necessary to abolish reaction to
pain was lowered with decreasing temperature. Although, whether this is simple
additivism or synergism has not been determined, it remains of fundamental
importance due to its implications in terms of the theories of Miller (1961) and
Pauling (1961) on action of gaseous anesthetics.

VII. Patient Factors Affecting Drug Action

There are inumerable patient factors that affect drug action. Certainly, physical status is the most important for it is clearly related to operative mortality.
The role of the anesthetic in contributing to operative mortality is difficult to
establish and a complete discussion of this may be found in the report of the
National Halothane Study (1969).

While we know about many factors that influence drug action some have only
recently been called to anesthetists' attention. Gunther and Bauman (1969)
recently showed that parity of the mother is important in determining the dura-

tion of effect of a caudal anesthetic. In multipara the duration of action of the anesthetic is shorter. We have also recently found that in a population of patients the pain relief afforded by 10 mg morphine increases with increasing age (Fig. 7).

These and other physical factors, while important in themselves, are most important in relationship to the design of clinical studies. Randomization of treatment is one method of balancing out bias that might otherwise be introduced by some patient variable. Or, patients might be stratified according to known

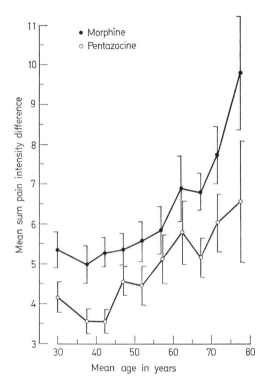

Fig. 7. The mean pain relief (Sum Pain Intensity Difference) is plotted versus the age in a population of patients (673) receiving 10 mg morphine sulfate intramuscularly. The vertical lines about each point represent one standard deviation. By Permission of J. Amer. Med. Ass. 1971

important patient variables and treatments randomized within these subgroups. Consultation with a biostatician is essential before embarking on any clinical pharmacologic study. Few clinical pharmacologic studies supposed to evaluate drug interaction permit any meaningful statement. Therefore, I maintain that for the investigator interested in studying a drug interaction, consultation with a competent biostatician is *mandatory*.

References

ADAMS, W. F., THORNTON, T. F., ALLEN, J. G., GONZALES, D. E.: The danger and prevention of citrate intoxication in massive transfusion of whole blood. Ann. Surg. **120**, 656—669 (1944).

Adriani, J.: The chemistry and physics of anesthetic, 2nd ed. Springfield, Ill.: Charles C. Thomas 1962.

Ariens, E. J.: Affinity and intrinsic activity in the theory of competitive inhibition. Part I. Problems and theory. Arch. intern. pharmacodynamie **99**, 32—50 (1954).

— van Rossum, J. M., Simonis, A. M.: Affinity, intrinsic activity and drug interactions. Pharmacol. Revs **9**, 218—236 (1957).

Asatoor, A. M., Levi, A. J., Milne, M. D.: Tranylcypromine and cheese. Lancet **1963 II**, 733—734.

Baekeland, F., Greene, N. M.: Effect of diethyl ether on tissue distribution and metabolism of pentobarbital in rats. Anesthesiology **19**, 724—732 (1958).

Baraka, A.: The influence of carbon dioxide on the neuromuscular block of tubocurarine chloride in the human subject. Brit. J. Anaesthesia **36**, 272—278 (1964).

— (2) Effect of halothane on tubocurarine and suxamethionium block in man. Brit. J. Anaesthesia **40**, 602—606 (1968).

— Gabali, F.: (1) Correlation between tubocurarine requirements and plasma protein pattern. Brit. J. Anaesthesia **40**, 89—93 (1968).

Bellville, J. W., Fleischli, G.: The interaction of morphine and nalorphine on respiration. Clin. Pharmacol. Therap. **9**, 152—161 (1968).

— Murphy, T., Howland, W. S.: Potency of thiopental plus β, β-ethylmethylglutarimide. J. Pharmacol. Exptl Therap. **130**, 364—366 (1960).

— Seed, J. C.: A respiratory carbon dioxide response curve computer. Science **130**, 1079 to 1083 (1959).

Bentley, G. A., Savidge, S.: The simultaneous administration of thiopental plus bemegride or other derivatives of glutaric acid to dogs. Brit. J. Anaesthesia **30**, 506—514 (1968).

Bunker, J. P., Stetson, J. B., Coe, R. C., Grillo, H. C., Murphy, A. J.: Citric acid intoxication. J. Am. Med. Assoc. **157**, 1361—1367 (1955).

Cascorbi, H. F., Loecher, C. K.: Antagonism and synergism of six volatile anesthetic agents and flurothyl, a convulsant ether. Anesthesia & Analgesia **46**, 546—550 (1967).

Clark, A. J.: The antagonism of acetylcholine by atropine. J. Physiol. (London) **61**, 547—556 (1926).

Clayton, J. W.: The toxicity of flurocarbons with special reference to chemical constitution. J. Occup. Med. **4**, 262—273 (1962).

Clintton-Brock, J.: Two cases of poisoning by contamination of nitrous oxide with higher oxides of nitrogen during anaesthesia. Brit. J. Anaesthesia **39**, 388—392 (1967).

Cohen, E. N.: Fluorescent analysis of d-tubocurarine hydrochloride. J. Lab. Clin. Med. **61**, 338—345 (1963).

— Brewer, H. W., Bellville, J. W., Sher, R.: The chemistry and toxicology of dichlorohexafluorobutene. Anesthesiology **26**, 140—153 (1965).

— Hood, N.: Application of low-temperature autoradiography to studies of the uptake and metabolism of volatile anesthetics in the mouse: II. Diethyl Ether. Anesthesiology **31**, 61—68 (1969).

— Paulson, W. J., Bernice, E.: Studies of d-tubocurarine with measurements of concentration in human blood. Anesthesiology **18**, 300—309 (1957).

Conney, A. H., Davison, C., Gastel, R., Burns, J. J.: Adaptive increases in drug-metabolizing enzymes induced by phenobarbital and other drugs. J. Pharmacol. Exptl Therap. **130**, 1—8 (1960).

Eger II, E. I., Saidman, L. J., Brandstater, B.: Temperature dependence of halothane and cyclopropane anesthesia in dogs: Correlation with some theories of anesthetic action. Anesthesiology **26**, 764—770 (1965).

Finney, D. J.: Statistical method in biological assay. London: Charles Griffin Company, Ltd. 1964.

Forrest, W. H., Jr., Bellville, J. W.: Respiratory effects of alphaprodine in man. Obstet. Gynecol. **31**, 61—68 (1968).

Gaddum, J. H.: The action of adrenaline and ergotamine on the uterus of the rabbit. J. Physiol. (London) **61**, 141—150 (1926).

— Theories of drug antagonism. Pharmacol. Revs **9**, 211—218 (1957).

Gissen, A. J., Karis, J. H., Nastuk, W. L.: Effect of halothane on neuromuscular transmission. J. Am. Med. Assoc. **197**, 770—774 (1966).

Goldstein, A.: The interaction of drugs and plasma proteins. Pharmacol. Revs **1**, 102—165 (1949).

Green, N. M., Whittaker, D. J.: Duration of action of pentobarbital as influenced by ether anesthesia in rats. Anesthesiology **18**, 165 (1957).

Gunther, R. E., Bauman, J.: Obstetrical caudal anesthesia I: a randomized study comparing 1 % mepivacaine with 1 % lidocaine plus epinephrine. Anesthesiology **31**, 5—19 (1969).

HOWLAND, W. S., BELLVILLE, J. W., ZUCKER, M. B., BOYAN, C. P., CLIFTON, E. E.: Massive blood replacement V. Failure to observe citrate intoxication. Surg. Gynecol. Obstet. **105**, 529—540 (1957).

KALLOS, T., SMITH, T. C.: Naloxone reversal of pentazocine-induced respiratory depression. J. Am. Med. Assoc. **204**, 932 (1968).

KATZ, R. L., GISSEN, A. J.: Neuromuscular and electromyographic effects of halothane and its interaction with d-tubocurarine in man. Anesthesiology **28**, 564—567 (1967).

KRANTZ, J. C., LOECHER, C. K.: Anesthesia LXX: effect of inert fluorinated agents on fluoroxene and flurothyl. Anesthesia & Analgesia **46**, 271—274 (1967).

LASAGNA, L.: Drug interaction in the field of analgesic drugs. Proc. Roy. Soc. Med. **58**, 978 to 983 (1965).

LOEWE, S.: Die quantitativen Probleme der Pharmakologie. Ergeb. Physiol. **27**, 47—187 (1928).

— Isobols of dose-effect relations in the combination of pentamethylenetetrazole and phenobarbital. J. Pharmacol. Exptl Therap. **115**, 6—15 (1955).

— Antagonisms and antagonists. Pharmacol. Revs **9**, 237—242 (1957).

MILLER, S.: A theory of gaseous anesthetics. Proc. Natl. Acad. Sci. US **47**, 1515—1524 (1961).

ODELL, G. B.: Studies in kernicterus I. The protein binding of bilirubin. J. Clin. Invest. **38**, 823—833 (1959).

PAULING, L.: A molecular theory of general anethesia. Science **134**, 15—24 (1961).

PRICE, H. L., PRICE, M. L.: Relative ganglion blocking potencies of cyclopropane, halothane and nitrous oxide, and the interaction of nitrous oxide with halothane. Anesthesiology **28**, 349—353 (1967).

RICHARDS, R. K., KUETER, K.: Studies on procaine toxicity: Effects of calcium levulinate and of sodium bisulfite. Anesthesia & Analgesia **22**, 283—289 (1943).

SABAWALA, P. B., DILLON, J. P.: Action of volatile anesthetics on human muscle preparation. Anesthesiology **19**, 587—594 (1958).

SAIDMAN, L. J., EGER II, E. I.: Effect of nitrous oxide and of narcotic premedication on the alveolar concentration of halothane required for anesthesia. Anesthesiology **25**, 302—306 (1964).

SCHILD, H. O.: pA, a new scale for the measurement of drug antagonism. Brit. J. Pharmacol. **2**, 189—206 (1947).

— Drug antagonism and pAx. Pharmacol. Revs. **9**, 242—246 (1957).

SJÖQVIST, F.: Psychotropic drugs, interaction between monoamine oxidase (MAO) inhibitors and other substances. Proc. Roy. Soc. Med. **58**, 967—978 (1965).

SMITH, J. W., SEIDL, L. G., CLUFF, L. E.: Studies on the epidemiology of adverse drug reaction. Ann. Internal Med. **65**, 629—640 (1966).

SMITH, N. T.: Use of isobolograms in anesthesia. Anesthesia & Analgesia **45**, 467—473 (1966).

— BELLVILLE, J. W., COHEN, E. N.: Interaction of halothane and d-tubocurarine on skeletal muscle in the cat. Pharmacologist **5**, 276 (1963).

— EGER II, E. I., STOELTING, R. K., WHITCHER, C. E., WAYNE, T. F.: The circulatory effects of the addition of nitrous oxide to halothane anesthesia in man. Anesthesiology **29**, 212 to 213 (1968).

STEINBERG, S. S., BELLVILLE, J. W., SEED, J. C.: The effect of atropine and morphine on respiration. J. Pharmacol. Exptl Therap. **121**, 71—77 (1957).

4.4. The Liver

CHARLES TREY

With 1 Figure

I. Clinical and Biochemical Assessment of Liver Function

This chapter is concerned with the clinical approach to the pre- und post-operative assessment of the patient who may have liver disease and the effect of anesthesiology and surgery on such a patient. The anesthesiologist needs to be able to recognize signs of mild and sub-clinical liver disease, as these may be aggravated by surgery. Common examples of these liver diseases in America are alcoholic hepatitis, viral hepatitis, the effects of shock on the liver, and sub-clinical cirrhosis. We will discuss the systemic effects of liver disease and the role of the anesthesiologist in the management of these during surgery and the post-operative period. The physician is assumed to have basic knowledge of the structure and function of the liver, as these will only be briefly mentioned in this review [1—7].

The liver is the largest gland in the body and weighs some 1500 grams in man. It is both an exocrine and endocrine organ, and is situated in the right upper quadrant. The liver is divided into four partially-separated lobes and covered by a capsule, and its parenchyma is divided into numerous small lobes. These lobes are formed by plates of cells separated by sinusoids. At the middle of the lobule is a central vein which drains blood from the sinusoids. At the periphery of the lobule are portal canals containing a branch of the hepatic artery, portal vein and bile duct.

The hepatic circulation is a double efferent blood supply which consists of the hepatic artery and portal vein. The portal vein drains the viscera of the mesenteric circulation, spleen, stomach, intestines and pancreas, and supplies 60%—80% of the blood flow to the liver. The hepatic artery, a branch of the celiac artery, supplies the remaining 20%—40% of the blood flow. Of practical clinical importance is the fact that there is about a 30% chance of anomalous arterial or venous supply; for example, the right hepatic artery can arise from the celiac or the superior mesenteric artery. Thus the importance to any surgical approach to the liver of performing angiography to delineate the vascular supply to the liver. The vascular intra-hepatic pressure of the liver varies, whether it is the hepatic arterial pressure of about 98 mm of mercury or the portal venous perfusion pressure of about 8 mm of mercury. The hepatic blood flow can be influenced by various anesthetic agents. Both halothane and spinal analgesia decrease the hepatic blood flow by reducing perfusion pressure. Nitrous oxide-diethyl ether anesthesia can also reduce hepatic blood flow. The blood from the portal vein and hepatic artery flow through the sinusoids and into the central vein. Bile flows in the opposite direction from the blood to the bile duct and into the portal canals. The hepatic parenchymal cells are situated as cell plates, and the sinusoids are vascular canals between the liver plates. In the sinusoids are also the acidic cells of Kupffer. The hepatic parenchymal cell may or may not have stored glycogen or fat. There is a correlation of the cytology in altered structure of the hepatic cell with its numerous functions. These have been well described [9—11].

The liver function embraces the vast majority of metabolic functions and is responsible for homeostasis of carbohydrates, protein and fat. In liver disease, there is impairment or decrease of function. Approximately two-thirds of an oral glucose load is taken by the liver, and much of it is stored by the liver as glycogen. The liver releases glucose at about the rate of 8—16 g/h in the adult, and the glucose is derived from glycogenolysis and gluconeogenesis. Thus, the clinical consequence of severe hepatic failure is hypoglycemia due to glycogen depletion and impaired gluconeogenesis. The liver plays a major role in protein metabolism. In lipid metabolism, it facilitates lipid absorption through bile salt synthesis and plays a role in fatty acid formation and fatty acid utilization. Derangement of lipid hepatic metabolism can lead to the fatty liver. It synthesizes non-essential amino acids and excretes nitrogen by the formation of urea. It also detoxifies ammonia. These functions are used as a measurement of the liver function and failure. The liver synthesizes plasma clotting factors, 1, 2, 5, 7, 9, and 10, all of which, except for 1 and 5, are vitamin K dependent. Because of the short half-life of the clotting factors, prothrombin time is a very sensitive test of early signs of severe liver failure. The liver synthesizes albumin at the rate of about 15 g/day so that hypoalbuminemia can be associated with liver failure, but is slower in onset then the clotting factors.

The liver is important in drug detoxification, most probably at the smooth endoplastic reticulum. The smooth endoplastic reticulum is induced by pheno-barbital, alcohol, etc.; thus, these metabolites increase enzymatic drug metaboliz-ing activity. The liver also metabolizes hormones, especially cortisone and estrogens. It conjugates and excretes bilirubin, stores vitamins, for example B-12 and folic acid, as well as minerals, such as iron and copper. In severe liver failure, the blood reflects the derangement in the hepatocyte. Thus, vitamin B-12 is grossly elevated in massive liver disease and can be used as a measurement of this. The enzymes usually stored in the mitochondrial endoplastic reticulum, as well as lysosomes, are also elevated in mild liver damage, for example serum glutamic oxaloacetic transaminase (SGOT) is raised in many forms of liver damage. SGOT is measured in tissues of other organs, but the enzyme is most prevalent in hepatocytes. For example, the rise in myocardial damage is twice or three times normal, whereas in liver disease, the SGOT elevation is much more than that, between four times to usually 10 times normal value.

II. The Diagnostic Approach to Liver Disease

In the pre- and post-operative assessment of the suspected of liver disease, the presence and severity, pathology and specific etiology of hepatic disorders are mainly determined by clinical and biochemical evaluations. Ancillary tests such as radiology or liver biopsy may be necessary. A careful history needs to be taken, especially as regards possible exposure to toxins; whether there was recent exposure to patients with hepatitis or blood or blood products, or whether he had recent injections or parental drug abuse. There should be a listing of the various drugs the patient is at present taking or had recently received. Allergies, especially to drugs, are to be noted. Previous effects of anesthesia on the patient need to be carefully and comprehensively considered. This is especially important if the patient gives a previous history of post-operative jaundice, post-operative fevers or post-operative nausea or vomiting. The dietary habits and alcoholic intake have to be evaluated and many patients are modest and underestimate ethanol intake. In these latter, patients are asked about morning nausea, delirium tremens and other withdrawal symptoms.

Specific points to note in the physical examination are the presence of jaundice and signs of chronic liver disease. The commonest skin manifestation is spider angioma, which consists of a central arteriole from which radiate small vessels; pressure on the arteriole causes blanching of the area. Spider angioma should be looked for in the face and trunk and upper arms. These spider angioma are present during pregnancy and occasionally in normal individuals, but their presence should alert the examiner to the possibility of liver damage. The skin should be examined for purpura. Palmar erythema, gynecomastia, and Dupuytrens' contractions are frequently present in patients with chronic liver disease. Parotid gland enlargement is fairly common to these patients, especially with alcohol-associated liver disease, and testicular atrophy may be present. Clinically, the liver itself is best measured by percussion. The surface markings are: the upper border of the liver is at the level of the fifth rib at a point one-inch medial to the right mid-clavicular line, and the upper border of the left lobe corresponds to the upper border of the sixth rib. The lower border of the liver extends to the costal margin, and this lower border passes obliquely upwards from the right ninth rib to the eighth ridge costal margin crossing the midline somewhat above the mid-point between the base of the sternum and umbilicus to the ninth left costal margin. The gall bladder is situated just internally to the ninth right costal cartilage. The edge of the liver may thus be felt in health as it moves downwards with inspiration. Riedel lobe is a fairly common normal finding, especially in women. This is noted as a projection from the inferior surface of the right lobe. If the liver is enlarged, the size, texture and tenderness should be assessed. In examining the abdomen, other organomegaly should be noted, especially whether the patient has an enlarged spleen. Ascites can be noted by bulging of the flanks and by the presence of shifting dullness. The central nervous system needs to be examined for evidence of localizing neurological signs or central nervous depression.

The biochemical tests in liver disease need to be interpreted in relation to the clinical setting. Many of these abnormalities in the tests are non-specific, and some may be due diseases other than those of the liver. (Table 1 gives an analysis and interpretation of the various common liver function tests and their relation to liver diseases.) Serum transaminases, glutamic oxaloacetic, as well as glutamic pyruvic, usually measure hepatic cellular injury, but can be modestly elevated in myocardial necrosis or hemolysis. If the elevation, however, is above 200 to 300 units, this is usually associated with liver disease. The serum alkaline phosphatase may be derived from liver, bone, intestines or placental origin, and is excreted in the bile. It is elevated commonly in obstructive or cholestatic liver disease and rarely in hepatocellular disease. Bilirubinemia can be elevated and may be due to hemolysis, cholestasis or hepatocellular disease. The prothrombin time is a measure of the liver's ability to synthesize and retain coagulation factors. A prolonged prothrombin time is usually an index of liver disease, but may be due to anti-coagulant therapy or malabsorption. In these instances, the prothrombin time could be corrected by the parenteral administration of aqueous vitamin K. A depressed prothrombin time is one of the earlier signs of severe liver disease. Depressed serum albumin not due to albumin loss may be a sign of liver disease. Serum ammonia levels can also be increased in hepatic disease, as the liver is the site for ammonia metabolism. The level of blood ammonia in liver disease is influenced by both the severity of the hepatic dysfunction and by factors which could elevate ammonia. In this regard, the protein intake, presence of gastrointestinal bleeding or hypokalemia need to be considered. Patients with renal tubular acidosis are more sensitive to diuretics and the potassium is easily lost. The ammonia is elevated in the renal veins and can aggravate the hepatic encephalopathy. The bromsulphalein excretion is a sensitive measurement of hepatic uptake and storage.

The liver functtion tests need to be re-assessed on a daily or frequent basis in patients with severe liver disease; otherwise, at less frequent intervals. Fluctuations or progression of liver function tests are useful in the diagnosis and assessment of these patients. We have mentioned in Table 1 the importance of urinalysis and biochemical tests. Evaluation of the hematocrit, hemoglobin, and white cell count are important in the detection of infections. Red cell morphology as regards the target cell, and the presence of burr cells, is well correlated with liver damage. Burr cells in liver disease may be due to the excessive bile salt content of the serum, causing increase in storage of cholesterol and triglycerides in the cell membrane, and the enlargement of the cell walls. In patients with cirrhosis or chronic liver disease, the burr cells reflect a poor prognosis [12]. The presence or absence of platelets on the smear and platelet count is important in liver disease. Thrombocytopenia could be due to hypersplenism but, on occassions, especially in alcoholic patients, is a reflection of the effects of alcohol on the bone marrow.

More specific immunological tests for detection of various forms of liver disease have been described. The presence of hepatitis-associated antigen can now be tested by radio immunoassays, which is more sensitive than the double immunodiffusion technique. The presence of the antigen is invariably associated with serum hepatitis or a carrier state, and the antibody to hepatitis-associated antigen, when present, can now also be detected. The detection, and now the elaboration, of the constituents of the hepatitis-associated antigen is a major scientific achievement [13—15]. α-Fetal globulin in man is usually an indication that the patient has a hepatoma [16]. Antimito chondrial antibodies in patients with liver disease are usually seen in primary biliary cirrhosis, but now titres of these antibodies have been reported in post-operative hepatic disease due to halothane anesthesia [17]. Anti-nuclear factors or smooth-muscle antibodies have been reported in chronic active hepatitis and primary biliary cirrhosis. Ascitic fluid examination by diagnostic paracentesis and evaluation of fluid and cellular constituents are most important. Radiology of the gastrointestinal tract, gall bladder and biliary tract and angiography have also been most useful in diagnosing liver diseases. Liver biopsies are valuable clinical tools in diagnosing various patterns of liver disease. These will be discussed later. The pre-operative hepatic tests in patients with liver disease are important for anethesiologists in evaluating the type of anesthetic and the possible risks of morbidity and mortality to patients [18].

III. Systemic Effects of Liver Failure

The physician and anesthesiologist caring for the patient with liver disease need to be aware of early signs of liver failure. The initial changes of liver failure may be subtle. The correlation between liver disease and its systemic effects on the body must be carefully examined. The observation and treatment of patients in severe liver failure illustrates the clinical application of our present physiological knowledge. To understand the effects of liver dysfunction on the body, we have studies the effects of severe liver failure on animals. In the Rhesus monkey, we have observed these sequence of events after a large dose of intra-

Table 1. *Comments on Frequently Used Liver Function Tests*

Tests	Normal value	Changes in		Comments
		Hepato-cellular	or　Cholestatic and Obstructive liver disease	
Urine Bilirubin	—	+ +	+ +	Present in liver disease-sensitive test.
Urobilinogen	0.2—0.8 mg (in 2 h)	+ + +		Test for entero-hepatic circulation of bilirubin and renal excretion. Increased in hemolytic anemia. Increased in hepatocellular disease. Absent in complete obstruction of biliary tract. May be absent if patient on antibiotics.
Urinary electrolytes				Low urinary sodium and increased potassium excretion in hepato-renal syndrome associated with rising serum creatine.
Serum Bilirubin				
Direct or conjugated	< 0.2 mg-%	↑	↑	Clinical jaundice recognized if bilirubin above 2 to 3 mg-%.
Total	< 1.2 mg-%	↑	↑	
I. V. Bromsulphalein (5 mg/kg)	< 6% Serum retention in 45 min	↑ ↑	↑	Also elevated in shock. A sensitive test for liver function in absence of jaundice. Danger of reactions.
Alkaline Phosphatase	0.5—4.0 Bodansky Units 10—70 International Units	N or ↑	↑ ↑	Greatest elevation in obstructive jaundice Also in conditions of osteoblastic activity; e.g., fractures, Paget's Disease: congestive cardiac failure

Test	Normal values	Change	Comments
Serum Glutamic Oxaloacetic Transaminase (GOT)	5—40 Karmen Units; 5—20 International Units	↑↑ 100's—1,000's; ↑ Usually less than 300	Liver injury leads to increase in serum. Useful in non-icteric patients. Serial estimations more useful. Screening for drug liver injury. Moderately elevated in obstructive jaundice.
Serum Glutamic Pyruvic Transaminase (GPT)	5—40 Karmen Units; 4—13 International Units	↑ ↑	GPT more abnormal than GOT in hepatitis. Mildly elevated in myocardial infarction. Usually less than 400 in alcoholic hepatitis.
Serum Cholesterol	180—250 mg. %	↓; ↑	Usually elevated in obstructive jaundice.
Serum Albumin Globulin	4.0—5.5 mg-%; 1.3—3.0 mg-%	↓ ↑; ↑	Albumin usually low in long-standing hepatocellular disease. Exclude albumin loss from urine or stool and also low intake. With fever, may be indication of liver abscess. Serum electrophoresis may be useful.
Prothrombin Time	50—100% of normal	↓ ↓; No ↓	If suspect impaired absorption, repeat after administration of aqueous vitamin K. Low values in viral hepatitis can be poor prognostic sign.
Blood Ammonia (NH_3)	40—70 mg-%	± on ↑; N	Elevated in hepatic failure or portal-systemic shunting of blood and excessive protein in gastro-intestinal tract;
Cephalin Flocculation Thymol Turbidity Thymol Flocculation	0 to 2+; < 5 Units; 0 to 2+	↑ ↑ ↑; ± N	Usually abnormal in hepatocellular disease, now rarely measured.

portal carbon tetrachloride, which causes massive destruction of the liver cells [20]. In order to develop fatal liver failure, 80% of the liver needs to be destroyed [21—23]. Within 1—3 h of the injury, the animal develops profound hypoglycemia and dies, unless the hypoglycemia is corrected by adequate amounts of glucose. When glucose is given, the animal remains conscious and alert for about 8—10 h, and then slowly develops increased muscle tone, rapid respiration, lethargy and later manifests decortical and decerebrate neurological states. These observations correspond closely to the various planes of anesthesia noted in animal and man. Finally, during the deep state of anesthesia, the monkey dies in coma with either respiratory failure or if the animal's ventilation is assisted, in cardiovascular failure.

The early stages of hepatic coma are best assessed clinically, as there are no good biochemical tests which correlate well to the patients state. The anesthesio-

Table 2. *Table of Clinical Stages and Correlation with Electroencephalography in the Onset and Development of Hepatic Coma*

Stage	Mental Stage	Tremor-"Flap"	E.E.G.
I	Euphoria, occasionally depression. Fluctuant, mild confusion. Slowness of mentation and effect. Untidy. Slurred speech. *Disorder in sleep rhythm.*	Slight	Usually normal
II	Accentuation of Stage I. Drowsiness. *Inappropriate behavior.* Able to maintain sphincter control.	Present (Easily elicited)	Generalized Abnormal — Slowing
III	Sleeps most of the time, but is rousable. Speech is incoherent. Confusion is marked.	Usually present if patient can cooperate	Always abnormal
IV	Not rousable. May or may not respond to noxious stimuli. Decorticate or decerebrate posturing.	Usually absent	Always abnormal

logist, in examining and assessing a patient for operation, must recognize early stages and onset of hepatic coma (Table 2). The pre-coma stage is usually diagnosed in retrospect. The most important feature is the disorder in sleep rhythm; the patient complains that he is sleepy in the daytime but has difficulty in sleeping at night. The patient has also been noted to be slow in speech and effect, untidy, and mildly confused. He may show slight hepatic "flap", which is the sudden dropping of the wrist when the joint is held against gravity, and then the rightening of this effect. The flap seems to be due to a sudden asyncope in neural conduction. The patient, during this stage, may become obstreperous and, if the hepatic encephalopathy is not recognized, may injudiciously receive sedation. Fetor hepaticus, a musty odor in the breath, charitably described as similar to the smell of new-mown hay, but which is more pungently sweet, is an ominous sign. It may be a reflection of decreased metabolism of methyl mercaptan. The second stage of hepatic coma is more easily recognizable, as it is an accentuation of the pre-coma state. The patient is now more drowsy; his behavior is even more inappropriate, but he is still able to maintain sphincter control. An electroencephalogram taken in this stage would show generalized slowing. As the patient progresses into stages of deeper hepatic encephalopathy, the hepatic flap is now easily elicited. The patient is difficult to arouse, loses sphincter control, and eventually becomes unresponsive to noxious stimuli. It is in stage four that the patient exhibits decorticate or decerebrate posturing. These stages of coma may fluctuate, and the neurological examination of the patient may vary from the detection of mild increase of reflexes to decorticate posturing. The swallowing reflex is depressed at an earlier stage than the breathing reflex, so that the

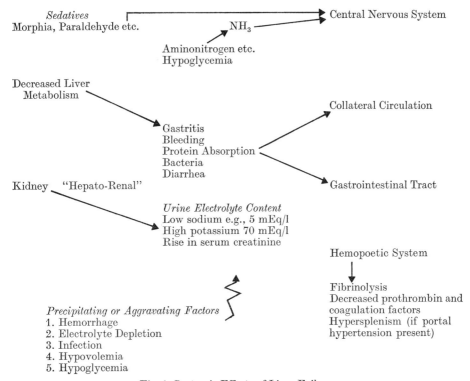

Fig. 1. Systemic Effects of Liver Failure

physician must test for swallowing. Early intubation or tracheostomy is indicated in a patient with liver failure where the swallowing reflex is depressed. The precise mechanism or pathogenesis of hepatic encephalopathy remains to be elucidated. However, clinical and experimental studies have shown factors which aggravate or precipitate these cerebral disorders (Fig. 1). Sedatives, such as morphine or paraldehyde, which are chiefly metabolized in the liver, and are sometimes given to these patients in an agitated state, can aggravate the coma. Ammonia or nitrogenous products given intravenously or absorbed through the gastrointestinal tract will increase the levels of ammonia in the blood and aggravate hepatic encephalopathy. It has been noticed that the level of consciousness in chronic encephalopathy can be improved by decreasing the protein intake, decreasing the intestinal flora with antibiotics or changing the flora by the introduction of lactic bacillus or by colonic exclusion. Experimentally, the brain actively takes up ammonia via α-ketoglutarate to form glutamine which can react with more ammonia to form glutamine, so that cerebrospinal fluid glutamine is markedly elevated in hepatic encephalopathy. This increase in ammonia is facilitated by hypokalemia, hyponatremia or anoxia.

Severe renal failure can accompany hepatic failure. The pathogenesis of this effect on the kidney is not clear. Serum aldosterone levels are high. Decreased cortical perfusion and intermittent arterial spasm in the kidneys have been reported in the presence of severe liver disease. In the patients who succumb to the so-called hepato-renal syndrome, there is no demonstrable organic renal disease, and kidneys from these patients used in transplantation recipients have found to function similarly to other kidneys. The syndrome of the hepato-renal disease is characterized by urine of normal to high specific gravity and osmolality. The urinary electrolytes show a low sodium concentration and a high potassium concentration. This is compatible with good renal tubular function, as the urine is concentrated normally. These urinary findings distinguish this syndrome from renal tubular failure. The serum creatinine rises in the blood, but the blood urea concentration is not as sensitive an index of renal failure, as the urea is synthesized by the liver.

There is a marked effect of liver failure on the cardiovascular system. In patients with severe liver failure, the cardiac output is high, and the patient is sensitive to volume depletion. With anesthesia there may be a further drop in peripheral resistence, and on occasions, correction of the blood pressure would require added colloid volume supplement.

The patient with severe liver disease also has difficulty in hemostasis. The prothrombin time and other clotting factors are depleted. Generalized bleeding is a frequent terminal event in hepatic failure. Where the liver is sufficiently damaged, there is fibrinolysis, but this may not be gross enough to cause the syndrome of disseminated intravascular coagulopathy. Severe systemic effects of liver failure should be recognized by the physician as these can be life-threatening. We have described the extreme events occurring in a patient of severe liver failure to illustrate these points more readily. The effects in the less severely affected patient are more subtle. Also, patients with mild or quiescent liver disease such as cirrhosis or chronic hepatitis may be more easily precipitated into hepatic failure. The effects, for example, of shock; bleeding from the gastrointestinal tract; stress of extensive operation or sepsis on patients with cirrhosis can cause severe encephalopathy.

IV. The Treatment of Patients with Fulminant Hepatic Failure before and during Anesthesia

The anesthesiologist may be called on to administer anesthesia and to maintain the patient during surgery while the patient is in mild or severe liver failure. The usual surgical procedures would be tracheostomy, laparotomy and operations for severe gastrointestinal bleeding which may be due to ulcers, gastritis or esophageal varices, and may be considered life-saving by the physicians and surgeons. In some patients, there may be a need for surgery because of obstructive biliary tract disease and cholangitis. The patient may come in with a surgical condition and at the same time, have alcoholic hepatitis and cirrhosis. Patients with hepatocellular disease can simulate acute surgical emergencies. An example of this is the post-operative fever and jaundice which can occur after halothane anesthesia exposure. Intra-operative treatment of patients with chronic or acute liver disease follows the principles discussed in countering the systemic effects of liver failure. Pre-operative assessment and biochemical tests are essential in detecting the degree of hepatic damage, and its effect on the patient. Aggravating and precipitating factors which could cause the patient to go into hepatic encephalopathy or shock should be investigated. The blood glucose should be tested, monitored and, when needed, glucose should be supplemented intravenously. Electrolytes, especially potassium, need to be monitored and supplemented. A urinary electrolyte estimation can be of help in calculating the minimum amount of potassium supplement required. In certain operative conditions, the serum potassium can drop precipitously. This is especially true in liver transplant operations where there is initial hypokalemia. Then, as the liver is removed, there may be a state of hyperkalemia and with the re-introduction and functioning of the new transplanted liver, potassium may again drop precipitously. Apnea can occur in these patients, and they need to be constantly monitored and ventilated. Sudden gastrointestinal bleeding can occur during operation. This could raise the blood ammonia and further depress the patient.

Shock is poorly tolerated. The patient in hepatic disease, and especially in cirrhosis, can have a high cardiac output. Volume depletion can easily cause shock. This can occur during the administration of anesthesia or during the operation when even minimal volume loss can cause shock. These patients need to be treated by additional blood or colloid to maintain their blood volumes. Vasopressor agents in these patients can be harmful as they can further aggravate a decreased perfusion in the liver and will not compensate for the volume loss. Ascites is frequently present in the patients. The incision may cause a sudden release of this ascitic fluid and thus the decrease of the extravascular pressure, causing hypotension. As a dynamic exchange exists between the ascitic fluid in the peritoneum and the patient's intravascular volume, the anesthesiologist needs to measure the fluid loss, but may only need to replace the colloid loss in the form of plasma or low-salt albumin. Colloid replacement of the ascitic fluid could be calculated by the estimation of the protein content of the ascitic fluid. The administration of protein in the form of amino acids could lead to an aggravation of hepatic encephalopathy. The coagulation factors need to be measured before, during, if the operation is prolonged, and after the operation. As mentioned previously, patients with liver disease can have sub-clinical fibrinolytic activity. This could be aggravated in the presence of infection and may need to be treated. These patients should be treated by the administration of heparin. The judgment for this form of treatment may be more difficult in patients with an already low fibrinogen and platelet level in the blood. In these patients, it is useful to have serial estimation of their fibrinogen and coagulation factors, as the decrease of clotting factors in liver disease is slow and not as acute as the sudden onset of disseminated intravascular coagulation. In the postoperative period, the patient may need to be managed with respiratory assistance with ventilation; the parameters of electrolytes, level of consciousness, clotting factors, and blood pressure again need to be estimated frequently. The hallmark of treatment, again, is attention to details. The liver in most diseased states usually has the capacity for regeneration and improvement, and the aim of the physician is to maintain the patient until such an event occurs. This may take from hours to days to weeks. In patients with fulminant hepatic failure, and in severe Stage IV coma, more heroic measures to maintain the patients are indicated. Exchange blood transfusions in the hope of decreasing the noxious effects of metabolites on the central nervous system have been frequently used. Ex vivo liver perfusions, cross circulation with human or primate livers and transplantations of the liver have been reported, but these measures have only been used in selected special cases.

V. Post-Operative Acute Hepatic Failure

Post-operative hepatic failure is a rare but serious event. The occurrence of unexpected jaundice, liver failure and, on occasion, death, can be of great concern to physicians. The National Halothane Study examined the clinical cause of 856,500 general anesthesia administrations in 34 participating institutions over a four-year study period [24]. There were 16,840 deaths, with an autopsy rate of 60.4%. The incidence of massive hepatic necrosis which was found in 82 of the patients, was 0.96 per 10,000. The commonest type of severe hepatic failure was shown to be that of vascular or shock category, and was recognized in 73 of the 82 patients with acute post-operative liver failure. The histology of the liver in all the patients in the vascular category were similar and showed acute coagulation necrosis, and congestion, but the lobular architecture was well-preserved. There was little or no polymorphonuclear or other cellular response [25, 26]. The cause of these patients' deaths was readily attributed to recognizable factors such as shock, infection, especially gram-negative organisms, pre-existing disease, and/or extensive surgical manipulation. The pre- and post-operative clinical course reflected these causes. Only 9 cases of the 82 with massive hepatic necrosis were considered to be of unexplained origin as to the etiology of the hepatitis. In these patients, there was no obvious shock, sepsis, or extensive surgical manipulation, which could explain massive hepatic necrosis which occurred and was attributed to their death. These patients showed the syndrome of fulminant hepatic failure characterized by the acute onset of progressive jaundice, hepatic coma, and shrinkage of the liver. Liver histology in these nine patients showed histologic changes similar to viral hepatitis. Loss of lobular architecture, periportal inflammation with eosinophils and polymorphic leukocytes, and inflammation of the hepatocyte were noted. The liver cells in some areas were showing inflammation, undergoing ballooning of the cell and, at times, shrinkage of the cell with acidophilic bodies interspersed in the lobule. The histological changes could easily be distinguished from the previously described vascular category. Death of these patients is of serious concern as the cause of the failure is not easily explained. In the Fulminant Hepatic Failure Surveillance Study, there were reported patients in fulminant hepatic failure who had previously been presumed to have normal liver function [27, 28]. About 20% of them were found to be post-operative liver failures. The cause of the hepatic failure in these patients was not always established. There are many presumed causes of fulminant hepatic failure, viral hepatitis and drug hepatitis being the most frequently cited [26, 27]. In many of the viral hepatitis patients, the hepatitis-associated antigen is usually positive. There is no good diagnostic test for other viral causes or to distinguish viral from drug hepatitis. The diagnosis is thus based in many on clinical judgment.

The establishment of the drug cause in many of the affected individuals is through circumstantial evidence by excluding other causes of hepatitis and, when possible, by direct challenge to patients under controlled circumstances [37, 38]. Table 3 showed the syndromes of drugs associated with liver disease. The sensitizing drug syndrome is the one which leads to the most difficult decision in a differential diagnosis as in these, there is no dose-related effect of the drug on the liver, nor can this syndrome of hepatic failure be demonstrated in animals. This is the syndrome that has been frequently reported in patients presumed to have hepatitis as the result of single or repeated exposure to halothane anesthesia. In these reports, other obvious causes of hepatitis have been excluded and the clinical course of the patients helps in the detection of this cause. In order to fall into this syndrome, it has been decided that jaundice should occur within 21 days of exposure to the anesthetic agent [33]. Eighty percent of the patients we studied with presumed halothane hepatitis had multiple exposures to halothane within a

Table 3. *Syndromes of Drugs Associated with Liver Disease*

I. *Direct Hepatotoxins*

a) Dose-related liver damage.
b) Reproducable in animal.
E. G. Carbon Tetrachloride, Chloroform, Tannic Acid, Tetracycline, 6-Murcaptopurine, Ethyl Chloride, Phosphorus, Aflatoxins, Plant Poisons of mushrooms.

II. *Sensitizing Drugs*

a) In susceptible individual, can produce syndromes of hepatitis and sensitivity reactions; e.g., fever, eosinophilia.
b) Syndrome can be reproduced by re-challenging patient with agent. Can be hazardous.
c) Not dose-related.
d) Cannot be reproduced in animal.
E. G. Halothane, Iproniazide, Pheniprazine, Phenelzine, Sulphonamides, Isoniazid, Para-Aminosalicylic Acid, Pyrazinamide, Ethionamide, Indomethicin, Gold, Chlorpropamide, Methaheximide, Methotrexate, Oxyphenacin Acetate, Phenurone, Aldomet, Phenindione, ? Methoxyflurane.

III. *Interference with Bilirubin Metabolism*

a) Can cause jaundice, but no fatalities reported.
E. G. Gall Bladder Dyes, i.e., Iopanoic Acid Sulfonamides, 17-α-Alkylated Steroids, i.e., Methyltestosterone.

IV. *Syndrome of Cholestasis*

a) Presents as obstructive jaundice and hepatitis.
E. G. Phenothiazine and derivatives, Chlorpropamide, Erythromycin Estolate, Estrogenic components.

V. *Syndrome of Hepatocellular Disease Associated with Vascular Effects on Liver*

a) Direct venous inflammation.
b) Congestive cardiac failure.
c) Shock.
E. G. Senecio Alkaloids, Vasopressors and Ergot Alkaloids.

period of 60 days. The incidence of multiple exposure in a similar time period in the 856,000 patients studied in the National Halothane Study was 9%. Frequency of multiple exposures in patients who subsequently developed fulminant hepatic failure after halothane anesthesia was noted in many of the early and subsequent reports. The duration of anesthesia or extent of surgery was unrelated to the development of halothane hepatitis. The majority of patients developed un-expected hepatitis after low death rate operations, such as gynecological, ortho-pedic or eye surgery, and in these forms of treatment, multiple operations are common practice. Unexplained fever was noted in 80% of the patients-in most of them, after minor surgery. On occasions. patients may have elevated SGOT's and other enzymes found in liver disease, and eosinophilia after an initial exposure to halothane. Jaundice usually occurs after multiple exposure and is commonly noted after the third post-operative day. Hepatitis, after exposure to halothane when this occurs, may vary from an anicteric through icteric to fulminant hepatic failure, and the biochemical tests show abnormalities similar to that described with other causes of hepatitis. The clinical syndrome of halothane hepatitis (see Table 4) occurs usually in adults, predominantly in females, usually after multiple exposures. Severity of the liver failure is not related to the length of exposure to halothane or extent of the operation. Jaundice usually occurs on the third or later post-operative day, and the hepatitis is similar to that seen with other infectious

Table. 4. *Clinical Syndrome of Halothane-Associated Hepatitis Noted in 74 Patients*

Age and Sex: Usually adult, female more than male.

Associated Factors:

1. Multiple exposures to halothane. Commonly within 60 day period (about 80% of patients reported had multiple exposures).

2. Not influenced by length of exposure or extent of surgery.

3. Syndrome noted in surgery where multiple exposure is common — gynecological, orthopedic, plastic or eye surgery.

4. May be cross-sensitivity between halogenated anesthetic agents.

Clinical Presentation:

1. Post-operative unexplained fever and elevated S.G.O.T., S.G.P.T. and/or bilirubin.

2. *Post-operative jaundice* of hepatocellular or cholestatic presentation in 70% of patients between 3d—9th post-operative day and rest up to 21st post-operative day.

3. *Presentation* varies from anicteric hepatitis to acute hepatitis or cholestatic phase of hepatitis to fulminant hepatic failure.

4. *Prognosis* — Overall prognosis not known, as there may be many mild cases. Prognosis if patient lapses into severe hepatic coma — 5% recovery.

5. *Incidence* — Not known. Presumed 1:10,000 or 1:1,000 multiple exposures.

6. *Pathophysiology:*
a) Presumed sensitivity type of hepatitis. Rare instances of individual case reports of positive challenge.
b) Occasionally eosinophilia, lymphocyte transformation or low antimitochondrial antibody titre.

hepatitis causes. Hepatitis may present as cholestasis and can be difficult to distinguish from organic obstruction of the biliary tract and in some instances, exploratory operations frequently using halothane anesthesia have been performed and have aggravated the previous hepatitis. The patients may present with high fever, mild elevation of liver function tests and the differential diagnosis may include intra-abdominal sepsis which again could lead to surgery. It is thus most important to be aware of the syndrome of halothane-associated hepatitis.

There has been considerable debate [39 to 42], about whether such a syndrome occurs and whether there is such an association. There needs to be evidence of the existence of halothane hepatitis, and also that certain individuals are at risk of developing hepatitis on repeated exposure to halothane. This latter criteria has been confirmed by case reports of halothane rechallenge under controlled circumstances. In these instances, a small dosage of halothane reproduced the clinical syndrome of hepatitis, and when the agent was removed in these patients, the clinical conditions of the liver lesions improved. Halothane hepatitis has been reported as a rare occupational hazard among anesthesiologists and other workers with halothane. By radio isotope labelling the halothane molecule, halothane is shown to be metabolized in man as trifluoroacetic acid and halogens. These metabolize and can persist in the serum and urine for as long as 21 days after exposure [43]. Individuals vary in the biotransformation of the halothane [44]. In patients with halothane-associated hepatitis and occasional patients in a study, eosinophilia and the presence of antimitochondrial bodies in titres much lower than that rated in primary biliary cirrhosis have been reported. The lymphocytes from affected patients were found to undergo transformation in vitro when treated with halothane. Some investigators report characteristic liver histology and electromicroscopic changes, but in most reports, the histology of massive hepatic necrosis is similar to that of the hepatitis type.

The incidence of halothane hepatitis and death from massive hepatic necrosis is not known. The National Halothane Study calculates a mortality rate from multiple halothane exposures developing massive hepatic necrosis to be about 7.1 in 10,000 anesthesias. Reviews of the incidents in anesthesiology practice vary from no deaths seen to the majority of one in 1,000 multiple exposures. Retrospective reports also vary. A report from Brisbane, Australia, reported 6 patients with hepatitis, and 2 deaths from massive hepatic necrosis after the multiple use of halothane in 360 patients, in the management of carcinoma of the cervix. There were no outbreaks of hepatitis in the community at the time, and this form of postoperative hepatitis was not seen in the hospital prior to the use of halothane. In the subsequent 300 patients who had multiple exposures to other anesthetic agents for management of carcinoma of the cervix, the incidence was 2 cholestatic hepatitis, both of which recovered and which were attributable to phenothiazine [36].

In the assessment of patients with post-operative fever and jaundice for further surgery, the clinical syndrome of halothane hepatitis must be considered. Consideration should be given to variety of presentation, and the syndrome may be considered in the differential diagnosis of post-operative obstructive jaundice or in patients with post-operative fever and suspected intra-abdominal sepsis. If there is a doubt of the diagnosis, repeat SGOT and prothrombin time should be performed and if they are still deranged, surgery can be delayed. In doubtful anicteric patients, the BSP estimation can be helpful if elevated and cardiac failure is absent. Anesthesia other than halogen agents should be used. During surgery, a liver biopsy should be obtained to determine whether hepatitis is present. Hepatitis-associated antigen should be estimated at intervals, or hepatitis-associated antibody may appear transiently.

Other causes of post-operative hepatic dysfunctions should be investigated. Transient elevations of the alkaline phosphatase, serum transaminases and bromsulphalein have been reported sometimes within 72 hours of uneventful surgery under general anesthesia.

Post-operative hepatic dysfunction associated with jaundice occurs less frequently than transient elevation of the biochemical tests associated with liver functions. The investigation of the causes of the jaundice is usually considered in three broad groups as regards the pathophysiology of bilirubinemia. Over-production of bilirubin can occur from hemolysis, either because of the susceptibility of the patient, for example if he also has chronic hemolytic states, such as sickle cell anemia or glucose-6-phosphate deficiency, or the patient's liver may not be able to cope with excessive bilirubin load. Circumstances in which the latter cause apply are when large amounts of stored blood may be needed for open heart

surgery or in patients with excessive bleeding, during or after surgery, and large
hematomas are formed [46]. Pulmonary embolism can also cause hyperbilirubinemia. In these instances, jaundice occurs early in the post-operative period, and
is usually cleared within the first few days. Clearance of the bilirubin will depend
on liver and, to a lesser extent, renal function. Patients with Gilbert's syndrome
will have a high ratio of unconjugated bilirubin similar to that of patients with
hemolytic anemia.

The second type of post-operative jaundice is that associated with extra-
hepatic biliary tract obstruction. This can occur post-operatively in patients who
have undergone biliary tract surgery or pancreatic surgery, or who have developed
pancreatitis or edema around the porta hepaticus in the post-operative period.
These patients need to be distinguished from those with intra-hepatic cholestasis
due to drugs or shock.

Hepato-cellular disease following surgery forms the third category of post-
operative jaundice. Hepatitis in these patients must be distinguished from drug
hepatitis, and these patients jaundice needs to be investigated after any anesthetic
exposure and before further anesthesia is considered. Diagnosis and clinical
symptoms of these conditions will be discussed later in the chapter. Perhaps the
commonest event in the post-operative period causing hepatic dysfunction is that
associated with a shocked liver. This can occur in patients who have had under-
perfusion of the liver, either from the trauma prior to surgery, or from the events
during or in the immediate post-operative period. In these patients, the liver
function tests are similar to that of acute hepatitis, and the clinical course will
vary according to the reason for the shock and sepsis. A similar event can occur
in patients with post-operative congestive cardiac failure. Severe hepatic congestion can lead to hepatic dysfunction and hepatic encephalopathy, and the
syndrome of fulminant hepatic failure. Therapy for these patients is similar to
that discussed in patients with severe hepatic dysfunction. A post-pump syndrome
of jaundice and fever has been reported three to eight weeks after extra-corporeal
circulation. This syndrome is characterized by fever, splenomegaly, atypical
lymphocytosis and in some, focal hepatic necrosis. Cytomegalovirus has been
isolated in the peripheral blood in some patients [47]. Hepatic abscess is an
uncommon lesion that can occur, more frequently in elderly patients. The principal
route of infection is through the portal vein or from intraabdominal sepsis, such as
cholecystitis, appendicitis, or diverticulitis. This is more likely to develop in
patients who already are prone to infections. These patients could either be
diabetic, have leukemia, Hodgkins disease or some immunological abnormality.
Leukocytosis is commonly seen, but in most of these with severe sepsis, the
characteristic liver dysfunction is that of persistently low albumin in the blood.
The transaminase and alkaline phosphatase elevation occurs much later. The
mortality rate in these is high unless the abscess is suspected and drained.

VI. Toxic and Drug Injuries to the Liver

The liver is the principle organ for drug metabolism and as such, can be
expected to manifest signs which may mimic other types of hepatic disease. The
effect of drugs on the liver can usually be classified in five categories according to
the manifestation of effects on the liver. These have been classified in Table 4.
In one, the syndrome of hepato-cellular disease which can mimic other types of
hepatitis, can initially present in a cholestatic phase where the biochemical tests
may be indistinguishable from organic obstruction of the biliary tract. The types

of hepatitis associated with drugs are those which have a direct hepatotoxic effect syndrome. The syndrome is characterized by non-specific symptoms such as nausea, vomiting and fever, and later jaundice, changes in liver size, elevation of liver enzymes and bilirubin and prolonged prothrombin time unaltered by parenteral administration of vitamin K may be noticed. Patients in the first two groups with the direct hepatotoxins or the sensitizing drugs can develop acute liver failure, and the syndrome of fulminant hepatic failure previously described, and in these patients, death can rarely occur. Drugs causing direct hepatotoxic effects are those in which doses are related to liver damage, and these drugs can cause similar effects in experimental animals. Extensively studied examples of this are carbon tetrachloride, chloroform and tannic acid, as well as mushroom and organic toxins, which are other examples. Tetracycline can also cause a dose-related hepatotoxicity and since tetracycline is excreted in the kidneys, impaired renal function will aggravate the hepato-cellular damage. Although the original case reports have been in woman, and the most quoted ones have been in pregnant women, hepatitis can develop in the other sex and at any age [48, 49, 50]. The dose reported to cause hepatitis in adults is usually about 2 grams administered intravenously per day for 5 to 10 days. This dose-related syndrome has been reproduced in animals. The anesthesiologist, in pre-operative or post-operative assessments of patients with jaundice should consider this in a differential diagnosis. A liver biopsy in patients with tetracycline-associated hepatitis is distinguishable from that of viral hepatitis or toxic hepatitis, in that the liver cells have intracellular vacuoles of fat, and hepatic necrosis is not evident. The disease is that which in other hepato-toxic situations can be reversible on discontinuing the drug and initiating appropriate measures for maintaining the patient similar to that discussed in fulminant hepatic failure patients.

There is another group of drugs which causes hepatitis indistinguishable from viral hepatitis, and this group is not dose related to the severity of the infection, nor can this syndrome be reproduced by the administration of the drugs in animals. These drugs include tranquilizers and anti-depressants such as pheniprazine, anti-tubercular drugs such as iproniazide, as well as anesthetics such as halothane and methoxyflurane. We have discussed the syndrome of halothane-associated hepatitis previously. The method of action of the drugs in causing the hepatitis is not clear, but it is presumed that many are sensitizing drugs and, in certain instances, early drug-associated phase can be diagnosed prior to the patient's becoming seriously ill. For example, in halothane hepatitis, unexplained fever and mild elevation of liver function tests have been reported after first or subsequent exposures before the development of jaundice and severe liver disease. In para-aminosalicylic acid, the rash and fever and eosinophilia precedes the advent of severe liver failure [51]. Hepatomegaly can also be noticed. It is important for the clinician to heed these warning signs. Interference with bilirubin metabolism can occur after the administration of gall bladder dye, such as iopanoic acid, sulfonamides, 17-alpha alkyl steroids [52]. These patients can become jaundiced or have alteration of the bilirubin and alkaline phosphate. There have been no fatalities reported in this group. Patients with this syndrome can be confused with acquired or hereditary bilirubinemia such as Gilbert's disease or Devlin Johnson's disease. The condition improves on stopping administration of the drug. A syndrome of cholestasis which presents with elevation of the alkaline phosphatase and liver function tests which is indistinguishable from obstructive jaundice or hepatitis has been reported, after phenothiazine or its derivatives, estrogenic compounds, or chlorpropamide. Few fatalities have been reported, and these patients can improve on the withdrawal of the drugs. The syndrome of surgical import is that associated with the erythromycin estolate which can mimic acute cholecystitis. In these patients, occasionally eosinophilia is seen, and an oral cholecystogram can visualize the biliary ducts and gall bladder. These tests are helpful in the pre-operative assessment of the patient. Withdrawal of the drugs will reverse this condition [53].

Syndromes of hepato-cellular disease have been associated with the vascular effect on the liver, especially congestive cardiac failure and pre- or post-operative shock with under-perfusion of the liver. The administration of vasopressors can cause further under-perfusion of the liver. A direct vascular inflammation of the hepatic veins has been reported in patients who have been exposed to senecio alkaloids, found in Jamaica or South Africa. The patients can present as a Budd-Chiari syndrome with portal hypertension, splenomegaly, ascites and esophageal varices.

On detecting a patient with a suspected drug-associated hepatitis, investigation and proving of this association may be difficult [54—56]. Rarely, such as in tetracycline-associated hepatitis, there may be a relatively characteristic liver biopsy [56], but in most instances, it may be more prudent to consider the probability of an association and warn the patient against repeated exposures than to attempt rechallenge. This is especially true of the direct hepatotoxins or sensitizing drugs which can cause fulminant hepatic failure. Rechallenging in these patients must be done with a full understanding of the untoward consequences. Most of the case reports have usually been those in which rechallenging has been inadvertently performed. In these patients, epidemiological studies and evolution of a clinical syndrome or prospective studies may be more appropriate. Criteria for a clinical syndrome of sensitizing drug hepatitis have been discussed. Drugs which cause cholestasis or interfere with bilirubin metabolism are easily amenable to rechallenging, as fatalities have not been well documented. Challenges should be performed with the full knowledge and consent of the patient, and appropriate studies should be undertaken. Registry of patients with untoward drug-associated or suspected hepatitis should be instituted as many new drugs coming on the market may present with some of the syndromes of drug-associated liver disease.

VII. Viral Hepatitis

Viral hepatitis is a common infectious disease with a world-wide distribution. There is usually little difficulty in arriving at a diagnosis of viral hepatitis. The patient may present with anorexia, nausea, and symptoms of ill health associated with prodromal stage of infectious illness and later jaundice. A history of either contact with jaundiced patients, blood transfusion or blood products administration can establish the etiology better. The patient may admit to parenteral drug abuse. The clinical syndrome, however, from the epidemiological point of view is produced by two separate agents: type A virus, or infectious hepatitis, and type B, or serum hepatitis [57]. There may be many other epidemiological entities awaiting elaboration. Type A or infectious hepatitis, has an incubation period of two to six weeks. There may be a history of contact with patients with hepatitis. The young adult or child between 5 to 40 years are commonly affected, and the route of infection is usually fecal-oral and, rarely, parenteral. Studies have been performed for the infectivity. The infectious period seems to be a week prior to the onset of jaundice in the prodromal stage and a week after the onset of jaundice. Viral hepatitis affects many organ systems. In 20% of patients, there may be an arthralgia or, rarely, other systemic manifestations, such as rash or red cell cast in urine, have been described. It has been estimated that up to 90% of the patients with infectious or serum hepatitis may not develop an icteric phase. The course of infectious hepatitis varies, but usually lasts four to six weeks and, in about 95% of patients, recovery is complete, even after severe attacks. Death from infectious hepatitis is rare, and chronic hepatitis is a rare complication. The administration of γ-globulin has been shown to protect susceptible patients and, at times, to attenuate the disease [58].

Serum hepatitis is transmitted parenterally through blood or blood products, but can on occasions be transmitted in the oral route through the ingestion of blood or blood products. Chance of an infection from blood transfusions in America range from 1 in 100, and an average of two units of blood is given to 1 in 10 when more than 10 units are used. The incidence varies according to the source of blood. Commercial sources have a higher incidence than voluntary blood donor services. There is a suggestion that it could also be transmitted through sexual intercourse [57]. The onset is more insidious and the incubation period varies between two to six months. In many patients, the hepatitis-associated antigen (H.A.A.) is positive and, on occasion, the hepatitis-associated antibody may be detected. These tests are useful markers for diagnosing this condition. The hepatitis-associated antigen is thought to be a virus particle and the ultra-structure has been visualized by electron microscopy. Use of fluorescent antibody techniques has found hepatitis-associated antigen to be in hepatocytes, arterioles and glomerular membrane of the kidney [58]. The hepatitis-associated antigen may precede the advent of elevation of the SGOT or bilirubin in patients who develop hepatitis and, as such, is a more useful screening measure. Period of infectivity with patients with serum hepatitis varies, but the usual in patients who develop hepatitis is two to six months. Morphological features in viral hepatitis are similar to that of severe injury to the liver from either infectious agents or certain drugs as discussed previously. Features include hepato-cellular alteration of both nucleus and cytoplasm, involves neighbor cells and is not restricted to any zone. Changes are seen of ballooning of cells and occasional cell degeneration leading to dehydration of the cytoplasm (acidophilic bodies) with or without nuclei in the cell. There is cellular exudation with portal inflammatory reaction and accumulation of lymphocytes and eosinophils. An intra-lobular inflammatory reaction and a proliferation of sinusoidal microphages is seen. Biliary ductules are surrounded by inflammatory exudates and, on occasion, there is stagnation of bile similar to extra hepatic obstruction. In the severe illness, there may be spotty necrosis or even sub-massive hepatic necrosis with central lobular necrosis and loss of liver cells with collapse of the interstitial parenchyma. This bridging is considered an ominous sign and there is an increased fatality in patients who show this manifestation. Hepatic necrosis is a rare condition, and usually shows wipeout of cells with collapsed architecture. Physicians and staff of dialysis units, operating theatre units, and technicians handling blood are at greater risk of developing hepatitis. Immunological incompetence may facilitate a carrier state in patients, and this has been frequently reported in patients with chronic renal failure undergoing dialysis, patients with Hodgkins disease and mongol children who have been exposed to the virus, thus the suggestion that the infectivity is related to the dosage and to the host response. Infectious hepatitis is a more benign diseases than serum hepatitis. In serum hepatitis, the fatality rate is much higher, and it has been estimated that patients admitted to hospitals in the Boston area who have been admitted because of jaundice and hepatitis have a fatality rate of about 6% to 8%. The clinical features in both hepatitis can be divided in similar stages, although the prodromal stage is much less evident in patients with serum hepatitis. Rarely, these patients can develop peripheral neuropathy and even periarteritis nodosa. The stage of obstructive jaundice is seen in about 10% to 20% of patients and rarely lasts longer than 2 to 3 weeks. In this period, it may be difficult to differentiate these patients from patients with organic obstruction of the biliary tree. Efforts should be made to confirm the diagnosis of organic obstruction prior to laparotomy, as there may be an increase in morbidity and mortality in surgery and anesthesia during the acute phase of hepatitis. After recovery from the jaundice phase, the convalescence may be prolonged — it may take as long as 6 months before restoration to full health. During this period, the patient is easily fatigued. There may be occasions of transient jaundice and bilirubinemia or elevation of liver enzymes. If this phase lasts longer than 6 months, it is usually termed remitting hepatitis. Rarely, a phase of persistent hepatitis which can last a few years is seen. In rare patients, there may be continual destruction of liver cells with destruction of the area between the portal and liver lobules called aggressive hepatitis.

Chronic hepatitis may develop after an acute attack and is usually manifest in three pathological entities. In one which is similar to acute hepatitis but in a more persistent form, the inflammatory cells do not spill over into renal parenchyma, and there is still balloning in a few acidophilic bodies in the parenchyma. Chronic aggressive hepatitis is characterized by conspicuous inflammation in the portal tract which extends into the surrounding parenchyma and the hepatocytes between the lobule and the portal tract show inflammatory cell infiltration and necrosis of the liver cell, with some fibroplasia. This type of hepatitis potentially progresses to cirrhosis. These conditions need to be differentiated from drug-induced hepatitis, alcoholic hepatitis, and mechanical obstruction.

Immunity to type A virus does not confer immunity to type B, and the serum, or type B, hepatitis can usually not be attenuated by the γ-globulin commercially available. Care needs to be taken by the surgeon and anesthesiologist in these patients not to infect themselves or the theatre personnel. Anesthesiologists should be aware of these certain patients who are at more risk of being carriers of the hepatitis-associated antigen and these patients should be screened prior to the administrations of anesthesia. If the patient needs surgery despite having his liver disease, the usual care in the administration of anesthesia is indicated. There is no evidence that the sensitizing type of anesthetic agents, such as halothane or methoxyflurane are more prone to give untoward hepatic effects than that of any other anesthetic agent. If the anesthesiologist or other member of the surgical team is inadvertently exposed to patients with serum hepatitis, and is inoculated with the blood of these patients, a preventive treatment is not yet clearly defined. Unlike infectious hepatitis, γ-globulin has not been found to be effective, although it would be prudent to have an administration of γ-globulin in the exposed patient. The usual dose is 0.04 ml/p (0.10 per kg). Trials on the effect of γ-globulin derived from patients with antibodies to hepatitis-associated antigen are in progress, but the results are not yet available. There may be a theoretical reason for not using this, as it has not been ascertained whether the serum hepatitis is an antigen-associated disease or an immune complex associated disease. Patients who have been exposed to serum hepatitis or viral hepatitis should be followed at frequent intervals.

There have been conflicting experiences of the effects of surgery on patients with viral hepatitis. In some the mortality was as high as 9.5%, while in others there was no mortality associated with the hepatitis per se [59, 60]. The morbidity of surgery would vary and could be difficult to distinguish from the continual course of the viral disease. The effects of surgery would also depend on the severity of the hepatitis and the indications and extent of the surgical procedure. In patients with fulminant hepatic failure, surgery can be hazardous, but this may be due to the severity of the hepatitis. We have at times followed patients with hepatitis and concommitant illness requiring surgery, as in patients who were operated on for suspected obstructive jaundice, and the patients have not had any untoward effect post-operatively. However, in patients with sub-massive or massive hepatitis, it can be difficult to decide whether the patient's conditions is aggravated by the surgery. We have followed patients with fulminant hepatic failure and active bleeding from duodenal ulcer, where the surgery was life-saving, and patients subsequently recovered from the hepatitis. The principles of management are similar to those described for fulminant hepatic failure. The indications for surgery thus need to be defined and pre-operative measures to correct electrolyte abnormality, hapoglycemia and coagulation defects should be instituted.

VIII. Chronic Hepatitis

Chronic hepatitis may follow acute infectious hepatitis but in the majority, it is an insidious disease which may usually be detected after a period of ill health and investigation finding abnormal liver functions. A liver biopsy will usually establish the diagnosis. There are many forms of chronic hepatitis, the commonest being chronic active hepatitis. This is more frequently seen in young women or menopausal women, but can occur in either sex and at all ages. There is usually no history of an acute hepatitis. The patients have a slow onset of ill health and usually evidence of chronic liver disease as evident by spider angioma, palmar erythema, and some have developed the syndrome of portal hypertension. There have been many sub-groups of this illness described; in young girls, syndrome of amenorrhea, polyarthritis and high γ-globulins may present. Primary biliary cirrhosis is another variety. Here an obstructive-like picture predominates, and these patients present with itch, hyperpigmentation and later jaundice. A liver biopsy usually shows excessive involvement of the biliary and portal areas and the serum in these patients may show antimitochondrial antibodies. The clinical course can resemble extra-hepatic biliary obstruction and many of the patients operated to exclude this diagnosis. The operative risk in patients with chronic active hepatitis depends on the extent of liver involvement [60]. Patients with persistent or relapsing hepatitis usually are good surgical risks, whereas patients with cirrhosis, portal hypertension and aggressive hepatitis can be poor surgical risks. If surgery is indicated, similar precautions to that used in patients with possible liver failure should be exercised. Hepatitis-associated antigen may be present in about 10%, and the surgeon and anesthetist should be alerted for the possibility of transmission.

IX. Alcoholic-Associated Liver Disease

The association of alcohol and hepatitis has been recognized for many years. Although cirrhosis with portal hypertension is common, alcohol can cause, in certain individuals, a picture of acute hepatitis [61]. This form of hepatitis is important to recognize as the evolution of the syndrome can occur after the patient withdraws from alcohol ingestion. Up to 95% of ingested alcohol is oxidized in the liver. First is the conversion to acet aldehyde. The latter is further oxidized to acetate. This is oxidized to carbon dioxide by the Krebs citric acid cycle, and part is utilized for fatty acid synthesis. Alcohol dehydrogenase is the important enzyme. Alcohol causes an accumulation of fat in the liver and also triglycerides in the serum. A bout of drinking may be followed by acute alcoholic hepatitis. Usually the patients are known alcoholics with cirrhosis, but occasionally there may be denial on the part of the patient as to the extent of his alcoholic consumption. These patients may be admitted for a concommitant illness, usually gastrointestinal bleeding from gastritis, ulcers, or varices, for investigation of fever of unknown origin. Systemic response to alcoholic ingestion may be prolonged, and the patient may enter hospital with a relatively low bilirubin and low enzymes, and over the course of 4 to 6 weeks, may develop the clinical picture of high fever, elevation of SGOT, usually in the level of 300 to 400 range, elevation of the bilirubin and, on ocassion, prolonged prothrombin time, which does not respond to the administration of aqueous vitamin K. The patient may develop leukocytosis and fever, and in about one-third of the patients, may develop the stage of cholestatic jaundice, which may be difficult to distinguish from organic biliary tract obstruction [62]. The patient may also manifest delirium tremens, myopathy, or peripheral neuropathy. In these patients, the diagnosis may be more easily made. In some patients, the differential diagnosis may be difficult. If the patient is suspected of having the syndrome of alcoholic hepatitis, operations should be deferred, as there is an increase in morbidity and mortality during this phase of acute alcoholic hepatitis. As the diagnosis can mimic such diseases as obstructive jaundice, intra-abdominal sepsis or head injuries, there must be adequate indication for surgery under these conditions. Alcoholic hepatitis per se can be a fatal disease with progressive loss of liver function and terminal hepatic encephalopathy, hepato-renal syndrome, or gastrointestinal bleeding. Diagnosis, where possible, is best established by percutaneous liver biopsy. The microscopic findings may be an abundance of acute inflammatory response in the periportal area, and large amounts of intra-cellular fat, which displaces the nucleus and, in the cytoplasm of hepatocytes, one can see hyaline bodies first described by Mallory. These are fairly characteristic of alcoholic liver disease.

Cirrhosis can be observed concomitantly with acute alcoholic-associated hepatitis. The cirrhosis was occasionally thought to be due to nutritional effects, but it has now been observed that alcohol per se may play an etiological role through direct toxic effects on the liver. The diagnosis is best made by liver biopsy, which shows disarray of lobules with fibroseptum replacing necrotic liver cells, and the surviving liver cells regenerate to produce these nodules of an irregular nature. The cirrhotic liver is thus rough and composed of many small and large nodules. Examination of the patient may show stigmata of both alcoholic and liver disease, spider angioma, parotid swelling and gynecomastia. The liver may be enlarged on palpation and is usually hard and occasionally nodules can be felt. There may be associated splenomegaly and ascites, and the syndrome of portal hypertension will be noticed. These patients usually have a high-output cardiac state and if operations are necessary, can manifest with shock due to hypovolemia. In assessing the patient pre-operatively, bleeding and evidence of pupura must be looked for, as well as evidence of portal hypertension. Gastro-intestinal bleeding is a common hospital admission diagnosis. The commonest cause of gastrointestinal bleeding in an alcoholic is acute gastritis. This can occur even in the presence of varices or ulcers, and as such, appropriate pre-operative assessment with esophagoscopy, gastroscopy, and radiology are indicated. In considering operation on a patient with alcoholic-associated liver disease, the systemic effects of alcohol per se need to be considered. The bone marrow is suppressed by alcohol, thus thrombocytopenia is common and can last for many weeks. Alcohol causes a direct effect on macrophage function and decreases phago-cytosis so that patients with alcoholic-associated liver disease are prone to in-fection, especially from pneumococcal organisms. During the stage of acute alcoholic hepatitis, the patient may also bleed more easily. Because of the poor socio-economic environment and poor nutrition, these patients are liably to have associated diseases such as tuberculosis. If the patient needs general anesthesia, enzyme induction by alcohol must be considered. Severe hypoglycemia can occur in these patients and blood sugar should be monitored [63]. The requirements for pentobarbital and other anesthetic agents may be greater than calculated during the acute alcoholic phase, but may be less if the patient has been in hospital for a few days. The planning of the anesthesia and prevention of untoward effects of alcohol on the patients undergoing operation will depend on the state of the patient and the time from alcohol withdrawal when the operation is being performed [64]. The patient may be admitted after motor accident or other trauma and immediate operation may be indicated. At this stage, the patient may require a higher dose of anesthetic. He may be agitated and pre-operative sedation will be necessary, i.e. chlordiazepoxide or phenothiazine derivatives rather than paraldehyde or chloral hydrate. Chloral hydrate may give depression as it inhibits oxydation of alcohol [65]. Paraldehyde can have a depressant effect if the patient is in shock and liver failure.

In the event of the patient's requiring anesthesia after withdrawal from alcohol for a day or two, the syndrome of alcoholic withdrawal should be in-vestigated. The syndrome is characterized by nervousness, tremor and, in severe instances, tachycardia, fever, hallucinations and convulsions. Delirium tremens is an acute syndrom which can last for several days. Because of excessive sweating and high output states, there is loss of fluid and electrolytes. Respiratory alkalosis is common. Serum magnesium has been noted to fall to low levels and is considered a cause of the withdrawal convulsions seen in some patients. Surgery during this period carries high mortality and morbidity and, if needed, the patient should be managed with adequate fluid and colloid replacement, as they do not tolerate volume loss. There is usually concommitant liver disease and, as such, requires similar treatments previously described.

X. Anesthesia for Patients with Liver Disease

The selection for appropriate drugs for use in patients with hepatic disease is a difficult one, and an understanding of the metabolism of the drugs is necessary. Although they metabolize in the liver, many drugs may be excreted by the kidneys and on occasions, can be excreted pre-dominantly by kidney. The choice of drugs in liver disease should be those which are excreted by kidney, lung, or other organs. Consideration of the extent of liver disease, the requirements of the surgeon, and the nature of the operation are necessary in assessing which drugs are to be used. Most narcotics are metabolized in the liver. This is especially true of morphine and its derivatives and, if necessary, these drugs should be given in smaller amounts because of the cumulative effect. Barbiturates may be necessary for the induction of anesthesia, and the barbiturate which is mainly excreted in the kidney should be used. Phenobarbital and barbital are excreted unchanged in the kidneys and thus these drugs are recommended in patients with liver disease. Some fraction is metabolized in the liver and can thus have a cumulative effect because of its slow metabolim and excretion under ordinary conditions. About 28% of paraldehyde is normally excreted unchanged in the lungs, but the

Table 5. *Pre-Operative Assessment of Patients with Suspected Liver Disease*

A. *History*

1. Liver disease, alcoholic intake, exposure to jaundiced patient, blood or blood products or parenteral drug abuse. Exposure to hepatotoxic drugs or chemicals. Alcoholic withdrawal or gastrointestinal bleeding.
2. Previous post-operative course, especially unexplained post-operative fever, elevated S.G.O.T., S.G.P.T., alkaline phosphatase or bilirubin.
3. History of allergies.

B. *Physical Examination*

1. Skin stigmata of chronic liver disease: jaundice, palmar erythema, spider angioma, gynecomastia in the male, purpura.
2. *Abdomen* — Liver by percussion and palpation. Presence of splenomegaly or ascites.
3. *Other signs* — Fetor hepaticus, flap, encephalopathy.

C. *Biochemical tests*

1. Blood count, platelet count and red cell morphology (presence of target, or burr-cells).
2. Prothrombin time. If prolonged, effect of aqueous vitamin K and other clotting parameters.
3. S.G.O.T., S.G.P.T., alkaline phosphatase and bilirubin. Serum electrolytes, glucose, serum protein and albumin, creatinine, Hepatitis-Associated Antigen.
4. Urinalysis and, if indicated, urine electrolytes.
5. If hepatic coma suspected, blood ammonia and electroencephalogram.

D. *Check special investigations: Liver biopsy, liver scan, radiological test.*

Table 6. *Intra-Operative and Post-Operative Management of Patient with Liver Disease*

1. Monitor vital signs. Electrocardiographic changes for potassium derangement. Blood sugar and serum electrolytes.

2. If drop in blood pressure, consider hypovolemia as likely course and replace blood or colloid volume.

3. In presence of cirrhosis or hepatitis, consider patient to have high output state and replace volume.

4. Consider probability of peripheral neuropathy in patient with alcoholism.

5. Follow and replace volume loss, especially if patient has ascites.

6. Consider possibility of cumulative dosage of anesthetic agent, especially d-tubocurarine, phenobarbital, phenothiazines.

7. Consider vasopressor effects on liver blood flow.
a) *Post-operative monitoring*, correct hypovolemia.
b) *Serum* glucose and electrolytes, especially potassium; creatine.
c) *Urine* electrolyte measurement useful in estimating potassium loss and distinguishing effect of liver disease on kidney from tubular damage.
d) *Prothrombin time* and clotting factors.
e) Patient's level of consciousness and whether swallowing reflex present.
f) Chart of measurements should be at bedside.

major part of it is metabolized in the liver and caution should be exercised in using it. Phenothiazines can cause cholestasis, but rarely, if ever, cause severe hepatitis but they have a cumulative effect in patients with liver disease. In the choice of inhalation anesthesia, most studies have shown that liver disease per se is not necessarily associated with sensitizing-drug hepatitis and, as such, there seems to be no contraindication for the use of halothane or others, except those previously discussed under drug-sensitizing hepatitis. Muscle relaxants such as d-tubocurarine have been used in patients with liver disease, but there have been reports that patients with hepatic disease may require greater amounts of the drug than in normal patients [66]. The muscle relaxants may be more prolonged in their action in patients with liver disease, as hepatic disease could result in impairment of plasma cholinesterase synthesis, but actual incidents of prolonged apnea in patients with hepatic disease are rare. Anesthesia and surgery may affect specific hepatic diseases, and these have been discussed previously. Tables 5 and 6 give a brief outline of the pre- and intra-operative protocol of the investigation and management of patients with suspected liver disease.

References

1. SCHIFF, L.: Diseases of the liver, 3rd Ed. Philadelphia: Lippincott 1968.
2. SHERLOCK, S.: Diseases of the liver and biliary system, 4th Ed. Philadelphia: F. A. Davis 1968.
3. POPPER, H., SCHAFFNER, F.: Progress in liver disease. New York: Grune and Stratton, Vol. 1, 1963; Vol. 2, 1965; Vol. 3, 1970.
4. ROUILLER, CH.: The liver — morphology, biochemistry, physiology. New York: Academic Press, Vol. 1, 1963; Vol. 2, 1964.
5. SCHEUR, P. J.: Liver biopsy interpretation. Williams and Wilkins Co. 1968.
6. Symposium on liver disease. Amer. J. Med., Nov. 1970.
7. DAVIDSON, C. S.: Liver pathophysiology. Its relevance to human disease. Boston: Little Brown and Comp. 1970.
8. BRUNI, C., PORTER, K. R.: The fine structure of the parenchymal cell of the normal rat liver. I. General observations. Amer. J. Path. **46**, 691 (1965).
9. ELIAS, H.: A re-examination of the structure of the mammalian liver. Amer. J. Anat. **84**, 311, **85**, 379 (1949).
10. — SHERRICK, J. C.: Morphology of the liver. New York: Academic Press 1969.
11. RAPPAPORT, A. M., BOROWY, Z. J., LOUGHEED, W. M., LOTTO, W. N.: Subdivision of hexagonal liver lobules into a structural and functional unit; role in hepatic physiology and pathology. Anat. Rec. **119**, 11 (1954).
12. COOPER, R. A., GARCIA, F. A., TREY, C.: The effect of lithocholic acid on red cell membranes in vivo. J. Lab. clin. Med. **79**, 7—18 (1972).
13. BLUMBERG, B. S.: Australia antigen and hepatitis. New Engl. J. Med. **283**, 349 (1970).
14. PRINCE, A. M.: Immunologic distinction between infectious and serum hepatitis. New Engl. J. Med. **282**, 987 (1970).
15. SHULMAN, N. R.: Viral hepatitis. Ann. intern. Med. **72**, 257 (1970).
16. PURVES, L. R.: Serum alpha-fetal protein and primary carcinoma of the liver in man. Cancer **25**, 1261 (1970).
17. DONIACH, D., WALKER, G. G.: A unified concept of auto viral hepatitis. Lancet **1969**, I, 813.
18. WHITCOMB, F. F., TREY, C., BRAASCH, J. W.: Preoperative preparation of the jaundiced patient. A review of current practice. Surg. Clin. N. Amer. **50**, 663—682 (1970).
19. TREY, C., DAVIDSON, C. S.: The management of fulminant hepatic failure. Rep. from Progress in Liver Disease, Vol. III. Grune and Stratton 1970.
20. — GARCIA, F. G., KING, N. W., LOWENSTEIN, L. M., DAVIDSON, C. S.: Massive liver necrosis in the monkey. The effects of exchange blood transfusions on fulminant liver failure. J. Lab. clin. Med. **73**, 784—794 (1969).
21. MANN, F. C.: The effects of complete and partial removal of the liver. Medicine (Baltimore) **6**, 419 (1927).
22. MADDOCK, S., SVEDBERG, A.: The effect of total removal of the liver in the monkey. Amer. J. Physiol. **121**, 203 (1938).
23. LAMSON, P. D., GARDNER, G. H., GUSTAFSON, R. K., MAIRE, E. D., MCLEAN, A. J., WELLS, H. S.: The pharmacology and toxicity of carbon tetrachloride. J. Pharmacol. exp. Ther. **22**, 215 (1924).
24. Subcommittee on National Halothane Study of Committee on Anesthesia, National Academy of Sciences-National Research Council. Summary of national halothane study: possible association between halothane anesthesia and postoperative hepatic necrosis. J. Amer. med. Ass. **197**, 775—788 (1966).

25. GALL, E. A.: Report of the pathology panel, National Halothane Study. Anesthesiology 29, 233—248 (1968).
26. BABIOR, B. M., DAVIDSON, C. S.: Post-operative massive liver necrosis, clinical and pathological study. New Engl. J. Med. 276, 645—652 (1967).
27. TREY, C.: Fulminant hepatic failure surveillance study: effect of age, etiology and treatment on survival. Preliminary analysis of 488 patients. Canad. med. Ass. J. 1971.
28. — LIPWORTH, L., CHALMERS, T. C.: Fulminant hepatic failure: presumable contribution of halothane. New Engl. J. Med. 297 798—801 (1968).
29. COMBES, B.: Halothane-induced liver damage — an entity. New Engl. J. Med. 280, 558—559 (1969).
30. SHARPSTONE, P., MEDLEY, D. R. K., WILLIAMS, R.: Halothane hepatitis — a preventable disease ? Brit. med. J. 1971, I, 488—550.
31. LINDENBAUM, J., LEIRFER, E.: Hepatic necrosis associated with halothane. New Engl. J. Med. 268, 525—530 (1963).
32. HERBER, R., SPECHT, M. W.: Liver necrosis following anesthesia. Arch. intern. Med. 115, 266—272 (1965).
33. TREY, C., LIPWORTH, L., DAVIDSON, C. S.: The clinical syndrome of halothane hepatitis. Anesth. Analg. Curr. Res. 48, 1033—1042 (1969).
34. PETERS, R. L., EDMONDSON, H. A., REYNOLDS, T. B.: Hepatic necrosis associated with halothane. Anesthesia 47, 748—764 (1969).
35. KLION, F. M., SCHAFNER, F., POPPER, H.: Hepatitis after exposure to halothane. Ann. intern. Med. 71, 467—477 (1969).
36. HUGHES, M., POWELL, L. W.: Recurrent hepatitis in patients receiving multiple halothane anesthesias for radium treatment to the cervix uteri. Gastroenterology 58, 790—797 (1970).
37. BELFRAGE, S., AHLGREN, L., AXELSON, S.: Halothane hepatitis in anesthetist. Lancet 1966 II, 1466—1467.
38. KLATSKIN, G., KIMBERG, D. V.: Recurrent hepatitis attributable to halothane sentitization in an anesthetist. New Engl. J. Med. 280, 515—522 (1969).
39. SLATER, E. M., GIBSON, J. M., DYKES, M. H. M.: Postoperative hepatic necrosis: its incidence and diagnostic value in association with administration of halothane. New Engl. J. Med. 270, 983—987 (1964).
40. MUSHIN, W. W., ROSEN, M., BOWEN, D. J.: Halothane and liver dysfunction: retrospective study. Brit. med. J. 1964 II, 329—341.
41. STEPHEN, C. R.: Halothane and liver damage. New Engl. J. Med. 280, 561—562 (1969).
42. Anesthesia and the liver. (DYKES, M. H. M., Ed.) Intern. Anesth. Clin. 8, 175—492 (1970).
43. REHOER, K., FORBES, G., ALTER, H.: Halothane biotransfusion in man: a quantitative study. Anesthesiology 28, 711—715 (1967).
44. CASCORBI, H. F., BLAKE, D. A., HELRICH, M.: Differences in the biotransformation of halothane in man. Anesthesiology 32, 119—123 (1970).
45. DAWSON, B., ADSON, M. A., DOCKERTY, M. B., FLEISHER, G. A., JONES, R. R., HARTRIDGE, V. B., SCHNELLE, N., McGUCKIN, W. P., SUMMERSKILL, W. H.: Hepatic function tests; postoperative changes with halothane or diethyl ether anesthesia. Proc. Mayo Clin. 41, 599 (1966).
46. KANTROWITZ, P. A., JONES, W. A., GREENBERGER, N. G., ISSELBACHER, K. G.: Postoperative hyperbilirubinemia simulating obstructive jaundice. New Engl. J. Med. 276, 591 (1967).
47. FOSTER, J. M., JACK, I.: A prospective study of the role cytomegalovirus in post-transfusion mononucleosis. New Engl. J. Med. 280, 1311 (1969).
48. SCHULTZ, J. C., ADAMSON, J. S., Jr., WORKMAN, W. W.: Fatal liver disease after intravenous administration of tetracycline in high dosage. New Engl. J. Med. 269, 999—1004 (1963).
49. POPPER, H., SCHAFFNER, F.: Drug-induced hepatic injury. Ann. intern. Med. 51, 1230 to 1252 (1959).
50. EDMONDSON, H. A., MIKKELSEN, W. P., PETERS, R. L., TATTER, D.: Tetracycline-induced fatty liver in nonpregnant patients. A report of six cases. Amer. J. Surg. 113, 622 (1967).
51. SIMPSON, D. G., WALKER, J.: Hypersensitivity to para-aminosalicyclic acid. Amer. J. Med. 29, 297 (1960).
52. CHESROW, E., POPPER, H., SCHAFFNER, F.: Cholestasis produced by the administration of norethandrolone. Amer. J. Med. 26, 249 (1959).
53. HAVENS, W. P.: Cholestatic jaundice in patients treated with erythromycin estolate. J. Amer. med. Ass. 180, 30 (1962).
54. BABIOR, B. M., TREY, C.: Drug hepatitis. Intern. Anesth. Clin. 8, 329 (1970).
55. GRINER, P. F.: Epidemiology of drug-induced liver disease. Intern. Anesth. Clin. 8, 343 (1970).

56. WRUBLE, L. D., LADMAN, A. J., BRITT, L. G., CUMMINS, A. J.: Hepatotoxicity produced by tetracycline overdosage. J. Amer. med. Ass. **192**, 92—94 (1965).
57. MOSELEY, J. W.: Viral hepatitis: a group of epidemiologic entities. Canad. Med. Ass. J. **106**, 427 (1971).
58. KRUGMAN, S., GILES, J. P.: The natural history of viral hepatitis. Canad. Med. Ass. J. **106**, 442 (1971).
59. HARVILLE, D. D., SUMMERSKILL, W. H. G.: Surgery in acute hepatitis. Causes and effects. J. Amer. med. Ass. **184**, 257 (1963)
60. HARDY, K. J., HUGHES, E. S. R.: Laparotomy in viral hepatitis. Med. J. Aust. **1**, 710 (1968).
61. HARDISON, W. G., LEE, F. L.: Prognosis in acute liver disease of the alcoholic patient. New Engl. J. Med. **275**, 61 (1966).
62. DAVIDSON, C. S., PHILLIPS, G. B.: Liver disease of the chronic alcoholic simulating extrahepatic biliary obstruction. Gastroenterology **33**, 236 (1957).
63. ARKY, R. A., VERVERBRANTE, E., ABRAHAMSON, E. A.: Irreversible hypoglycemia: a complication of alcohol and insulin. J. Amer. med. Ass. **206**, 575 (1968).
64. SHIBUTAWI, K.: Anesthetic management of alcoholic patients, chapter 5. The alcoholic patient in surgery. (LOWENFEL, A. B., Ed.) Baltimore: Wilkins and Wilkins 1971.
65. GESSNER, P. K., CABANA, B. E.: A study of the interaction of hypnotic effects and of the toxic effects of chloral hydrate and ethanol. J. Pharmacol. exp. Ther. **174**, 247 (1970).
66. DUNDEE, J. W., GREY, T. C.: Resistance to d-tubocurarine chloride in presence of liver damage. Lancet **1953** II, 16.

Author Index

The numbers shown in square brackets are the numbers of the references in the bibliography.
Page numbers in *italics* refer to the bibliography

Rankin, A. D., see Booth, N. H. 467, *475*
— see Epling, G. P. *476*
Rapaport, E., see Hamilton, W. K. 165, 170, 174, 177, *233*
Rapicavoli, E., see Wyant, G. M. 92, 202, 204, 206, 207, 211, *240*
Rappaport, A. M., Borowy, Z. J., Lougheed, W. M., Lotto, W. N. [11] 503, *525*
Ratcliffe, H. L. 470, *477*
Rausch, D. A., Davis, R. A., Osborne, D. W. 21, *31*
Raventós, J. 33, 34, 35, 36, 38, 52, 56, *74*, 125, 133, *147*, 165, 170, 174, 175, *237*, 311, 312, 315, 316, *324*, 365, *386*, 409, *432*, *438*
— Dee, J. 173, 176, *237*
— Lemon, P. G. 34, 35, *74*, 418, 429, *433*, *438*, 486, *487*
— Spinks, A. *432*
— see Duncan, W. A. M. 411, 428, *437*
— see Suckling, C. W. 4, 6, 7, 21, *32*
Rawlinson, K., see Wells, C. 318, *325*
Ray, B. S., see Poznak, A. van *92*
Rea, J. L., see Black, G. W. 192, 203, 205, *230*
Read, D. J. C. 263, *270*
Redfield, A. C., see McIver, M. A. 318, *323*
Redgate, J. D., Gellhorn, E. 446, *477*
Reeves, J. T., Grover, R. F., Filley, G. F., Blount, S. G., Jr. 202, *237*
Regan, M. J., Eger, E. I., II., 41, *74*, 265, *270*
— — Munson, E. S. 267, *270*
— see Eger, E. I. II 41, *68*, 95, *101*, 412, 413, *437*
— see Munson, E. S. 45, *73*, 98, *102*, 257 *269*
Rehder K., Forbes, G., Alter, H. [43] 515, *526*
— Forbes, J., Alter, H., Hessler, O., Stier, A. 41, *74*, 348, *355*
— see Stier, A. 348, *355*
Reichenberg, S., see Gold, M. I. 266, *269*
Reichlin, S., see Schalch, D. S. 296, *298*
Reid, C., see Banerji, H. 276, *284*

Reier, C. E., see Gardier, R. W. 130, 137, 140, *144*
Rein, J., Austen, W. G., Morrow, D. H. *74*, 138, *147*, 170, 174, 176, 200, *237*
Reinke, D. A., Rosenbaum, A. H., Bennett, D. R. 314, 315, *324*
Reivich, M., see Alexander, S. C. 279, *284*
Rember, R. R., see Virtue, R. W. 277, 281, *287*
Remmen, E., Cohen, S., Ditman, K. S., Frantz, J. R. 469, *477*
Remmer, H. 353, *355*
Renn, C. 364, *386*
— Lanoir, J., Bimar, J., Naquet, R. 364, *386*
— Vuillon-Cacciuttolo, G., Jutier, M., Bimar, J., Naquet, R. 380, 385, *386*
— see Bimar. J. 364 380, 384, 385, *385*
Rennick, B. R., see Moe, G. K. 197, *236*
Renoll, M. W., see Henne, A. L. *432*
Renwick, W., see Hogg, S. 112, *120*
Restall, C. J., Milde, J. H., Theye, R. A. 202, 206, *237*
Rex, M. A. E. 445, *477*
Reynell, P. C., Spray, G. H. 307, 312, *324*
Reynolds, A. K., Randall, L. O. 466, *478*
Reynolds, A. L., see Macleod, D. P. 197, *235*
Reynolds, R. C., see Chenoweth, M. B. 131, *142*
Reynolds, T. B., see Peters, R. L. [34] *526*
Rhamy, R. K., see Miller, J. R. 180, 226, *236*
Riccio, J. S., see Keet, J. E. 38, *71*
Rich, S. T., see Boutelle, J. L. 448, *475*
Richards, A. B., see Gardier, R. W. 126, 131, 134, 138, *143*, *144*
Richards, C. C., Bachman, L. 211, *237*
Richards, R. K., Kueter, K. 493, *501*
Richardson, J. A., see Hamelberg, W. 54, *70*, 140, *144*, 198, 226, *233*
Richter, D., see Dawson, R. M. C. 400, *404*

Richter, D., see Gaitonde, M. K. 399, *405*
Riding, J. E. 305, 306, *324*
Rigler, R., see Kobacker, J. L. 132, *145*
Rikans, L. A., see van Dyke, R. A. 353, *355*
Riker, W. F., Werner, G., Roberts, J., Kuperman, A. *92*
Riker, W. K., Komalahiranya, A. 133, *147*
Riley, P. A., Jr., see Segar, W. E. 179, *238*
Rinaldo, J. A., Jr. 300, *324*
— Levey, J. F. 302, *324*
Ringsted, A., see Andersen, K. 318, *320*
Risinger, K. B. H., see Bagwell, E. E. 97, *101*, 215, 216, *229*
Robbins, B. H. 306, 311, 312, *324*, 418, *432*, *438*, 466, *478*
— Thomas, J. D. 133, *147*
Robért, A., Nezamis, J. E., Phillips, J. P. 312, *324*
Roberts, H. L., see Crowther, A. F. 9, 10, *30*
Roberts, J., see Riker, W. F. *92*
Roberts, R. B., Cam, J. F. 203, 213, *237*
Robertson, D. N., see Chenoweth, M. B. *91*
Robertson, J. D., Swan, A. A. B., Whitteridge, D. 111, *122*, 123, *147*, 246, *253*
— see Burn, J. H. 446, *475*
— see Burns, T. H. S. 174, *230*
Robidoux, H. J., Jr., see Israel, J. S. *91*, 193, 212, 217, *234*
Robinson, A., Denson, J. S. 35, *74*
Robles, R., see Jong, R. H. de 41, 43, *70*, 107, *119*
Robson, J. G., Davenport, H. T., Sugiyama, R. 43, *74*
Robson, J. M., see Neal, M. J. *433*
Rocco, A. G., see Galla, S. J. 108, *120*
Roe, F. C., see Goldberg, M. J. 112, *120*
Roe, R. B. 319, *324*
— see Rosen, M. 194, *238*
Roger, A., Rossi, G. F., Zirondoli, A. 108, *122*

Subject Index

Cyclic AMP 288, 291
Cyclobutanes; Perfluoro, Anesthetic
    Action 415
Cyclohexamines, Animal Effects 472
    et seq.
Cyclohexane, Toxicity of 479
Cyclohexyl Vinyl Ether 420
Cyclo-octatetraene 419, 420
Cyclopropane, Analgesia 117
    Autonomic Effects 129
    Autonomic Nervous System Effects
        133
    Baroreceptors and 128
    Baroreceptor Effect 123, 124
    Cardiac Output and 139
    Cardiovascular Effects 117
    Chemoreceptor Effect 125
    Electroencephalographic Effects 117
    Evoked Potentials 117
    Ganglionic Depression 133
    Henry's Law and 341
    Impurities in 484
    Local Adrenergic Function and 139
    MAC 117
    Medullary Effects 129
    Metabolism of 351
    Myoglobin Complex 361
    Preganglionic Effects 132
    Propylene in 479
    Protein Interaction 360
    Renal Function and 295
    Spinal Cord, Effect on 129
    Sympathetic Activity, Action on 131
Cyprane Inhaler 84
Cytoplasmic Structure, Halothane on 63

Dead Space, Physiologic 254
Decafluorocyclohexene, Toxicity of 416
Decerebration, Arrythmias and 128, 130
    Cardiac Arrhythmias and 128
Decomposition, Halothane 11
Definition, MAC 256
Deglutition, Details of 300
Dehalogenation, Rules for in Metabolism
    352
Dehydration, Methoxyflurane and 251
Delirium, Anesthetics Produce 107
Delirium, Tremens 522
Delivery, See Labor
Delta Rhythms, Normal 109
Denitrogenation 457
Depression; Organ, Nonspecific 139
    Tissue Response by Ether of 133
Diabetes Insipidus, Anesthetics and 245
Diazepam, Electroencephalographic Effects
    385
2,2-Dibromo-1,1,1-Trifluoroethane 482
Dichloroacetylene, Trichloroethylene
    Produces 481
Dichlorohexafluorobutene 35
    Toxicity of 486
1,2-Dichloro-1,2,2-Trifluoroethane 482
Diethyl Ether, Impurities in 483
Diffusion, Anesthetics 342
    Anoxia 268

Diffusion, Facilitated 275
    Tissues, Between 343
    Tissues, Within 342
Digitalis, Anesthetics and 188
    Arrhythmias and 197
    Halothane and 56
Digoxin, Versus Halothane 188
Dilution Effect 268
Dimethyl Carbonate, in Methoxyflurane
    484
Diphosphoinositide 400
Disease States, Gut Motility and 307
Dissociogenic Drugs 472 et seq.
Distribution; Anesthetics, Water Analogue
    326 et seq.
    Halothane 38, 40
    Modelling of 330 et seq.
    Tissue Groups Related to 328
Diving Mammals, Anesthesia of 441
Divinyl Ether, Analgesia and 113
    Hepatotoxicity 448
    Impurities in 485
    Stability of 480
Dog, Bradycardia from Morphine 465
    Morphine on Gut of 465
Dopamine, Cardiac Effect 196
Dosage, Barbiturates 461
Dosage, Non-Barbiturate Injectable Drugs
    462
Dose Effect Curve, Drug Interaction 491
Dose, Narcotics in Dog 467
Doses, Tranquilizers in Animals 471
Doxapram, Respiratory Effect 262
Drug Interaction, Anesthetics with
    488 et seq.
    Chemical Basis 492
    Nonspecific protein Binding 493
    Pentobarbital-Ether 489
    Receptor Sites 493
    Thiopental Megimide 491
Drugs, MAC of Halothane on 42
    Liver and 517
    Liver Disease and, Tabulated 513
Drug Metabolism, Multiple Drug Effects
    497
Duke Inhaler 84

ECG (Electrocardiogram), Anesthetics on
    190
Effect, Second Gas 40
Ejection, Aortic 159
Electrocorticogram, Halothane and 364
Electroencephalogram, Anesthetics and
    108
    Anesthetics on Power Spectrum
        380 et seq.
    Autocorrelation Functions 380
    Benzodiazepines on 385
    Cyclopropane on 117
    Differences Between Halothane and
        Methoxyflurane 384
    Ether on 112
    Fluroxene on 98
    Halothane and 43, 114
    Hepatic Coma and 508